THE PSYCHOLOGY OF HEALTH AND HEALTH CARE: A CANADIAN PERSPECTIVE

Gary Poole
Simon Fraser University

Deborah Hunt Matheson
University of Victoria

David N. Cox
Simon Fraser University

Prentice Hall
Toronto

For our families
Marsha, Colleen and Graeme Poole
Owen and Wyatt Matheson
Susan, Kelsi, Kieran, and Dylan Cox

Canadian Cataloguing in Publication Data

Poole, Gary Douglas, 1950–
The psychology of health and health care : a Canadian perspective

Includes bibliographical references and index.
ISBN 0-13-022529-0

1. Clinical health psychology. 2. Medicine and psychology. I. Matheson, Deborah Hunt, 1966– . II. Cox, David Neil, 1947– . III. Title.

R726.7.P66 2001 610'.1'9 C00-930921-7

ISBN 0-13-022529-0

Vice President, Editorial Director: Michael Young
Acquisitions Editor: Jessica Mosher
Marketing Manager: Kathleen McGill
Signing Representative: Katherine McWhirter
Developmental Editor: Lise Creurer
Production Editor: Matthew Christian
Copy Editor: Craig Wilson
Production Coordinator: Wendy Moran
Page Layout: Kelly Gervais
Art Director: Mary Opper
Cover Image: PhotoDisc, Inc.

1 2 3 4 5 05 04 03 02 01

Printed and bound in the United States.

Prentice Hall

Contents

Preface

Why did we write this book? More relevant to you, why should you read it? Or, if you are an instructor, why should you require your students to read it? If you are a student who is new to health psychology, you will learn that the field is growing in leaps and bounds (the reasons for this growth are discussed in Chapter 1). If you have been teaching health psychology for any length of time, you will know that, until now, no textbook has presented a Canadian perspective to the field. These two factors—the rapid growth of the field and the need for a book that captures the Canadian context—motivated us to write *The Psychology of Health and Health Care: A Canadian Perspective*.

What exactly do we mean by a "Canadian perspective?" It does not mean simply changing behavi*or* to behavi*our*. There is much more to it than that. While it is true that many psychological theories developed in the United States "cross the border" quite well, when it comes to health and health care, our geography, demography, history, and health care system make Canadians unique. While writing this book, we found it surprisingly easy to capture this uniqueness. As a country, Canada does a very good job of documenting the health of its citizens. Statistics relevant to that documentation are found throughout the book. Some good examples can be found in Chapter 1 in our introduction to the field and in Chapter 4 when we talk about health promotion.

While writing this book, it was also gratifying to confirm that Canadians are very active in research that goes beyond descriptions of our health to explore factors affecting it. Again, this research is discussed throughout the book. To get a sense of this, turn to Chapter 14, where we discuss in detail examples of health psychology research programs found at Canadian universities and in health care settings. Equally exciting is the changing landscape of health research funding in Canada. In Chapter 14, we also discuss the introduction of the Canadian Institutes for Health Research (CIHR) and explain how this new system will bring more research dollars to a wider range of health-related researchers, including psychologists, in Canada.

It is not just its Canadian focus that makes this book unique among health psychology textbooks. Another distinguishing feature stems from our attempts to provide in-depth coverage of important psychological issues in health and health care. To this end, you will find an entire chapter dedicated to psychoneuroimmunology (PNI) (Chapter 3) and another to research methods as they apply to health psychology (Chapter 2). Chapter 4 focuses on health promotion and Chapter 12 on the role of exercise and sport in well-being. We have tried to make these chapters comprehensive and at the same time engaging and readable.

HOW BEST TO USE THIS BOOK

Health psychology is relevant to many other fields of study. For this reason, a textbook in the field may be read not only by students of psychology but also of nursing, medicine, public health, and epidemiology, to name a few. For a textbook in health psychology to be useful, then, it must be flexible. To achieve this objective, *The Psychology of Health and Health Care:*

A Canadian Perspective has been written in a modular fashion. Each chapter can be assigned independent of the others. At the same time, at appropriate places in each chapter, we have directed the student to related material in other chapters to show connections among topics.

The first four chapters of this book provide an introduction to the field of health psychology. Subsequent chapters provide detailed discussions of specific topics. Therefore, if you are an instructor teaching the course over a short timeframe (e.g., 20 hours or less) you may want to assign the first four chapters then select other chapters that are most relevant to your students' needs. Nursing and medical students may want to focus on Chapter 6 (Communication in Medical Settings), Chapter 7 (Hospital Stays and Medical Procedures), Chapter 8 (The Health Care Provider), Chapter 10 (Pain), and Chapter 11 (Chronic and Life-Threatening Illness).

If your course is intended for students who must be able to read research papers or at some point conduct research, then you may want to assign all of Chapter 2, which provides a detailed introduction to a wide variety of research methods, statistics, and terminology relevant to health psychology. If your students do not need to learn how to read journal articles or conduct their own research, you can assign selected sections of that chapter.

It has become increasingly evident that an understanding of the key issues related to health and health care demands a multidisciplinary approach. This approach is clearly evident in *The Psychology of Health and Health Care: A Canadian Perspective* in at least two important ways. First, we have adopted a biopsychosocial approach to virtually every major topic. In so doing, we have attempted to explain the ways biological, psychological, and sociological factors interact to affect health and health care. Second, we have dedicated Chapter 13 to an explanation of the ways health-related topics are studied in other disciplines. Health psychologists must have an appreciation for cultural factors (medical anthropology), societal factors (medical sociology), and environmental factors (medical geography). Now and in the future, answering vital questions regarding why some people suffer from a given illness while others do not will require teams of researchers from these and other fields.

Health psychology is primarily an applied discipline and so any textbook in the field should feature an ample number of applications. Each chapter of *The Psychology of Health and Health Care: A Canadian Perspective* opens with a vignette intended to provide students with a realistic context for what they are about to read. In this way, we begin each chapter with an applied focus. Students will also find case studies throughout the book. In addition to the analysis we provide, students can discuss these case studies in lectures or seminars.

We have also included "Focus on Research" features throughout the book. In these, we have taken one or two studies and described them in more detail than we would if they were in the main body of the text. We have included descriptions of procedures to give students a sense of the ways in which research is conducted in the field. They may be used in lectures and seminars as examples of research for students to critique.

In writing this book, we have learned an enormous amount. We have tried to adopt a student's perspective as we have read the relevant literature, and we have written about it in ways students will understand. In so doing, we feel that we have become better teachers as well. It is our hope that you, too, will learn from *The Psychology of Health and Health Care: A Canadian Perspective*, and enjoy the same enthusiasm we do for the potential of health psychology to improve people's lives.

Acknowledgments

The Psychology of Health and Health Care: A Canadian Perspective benefited greatly from the thoughtful feedback we received from Lois Hunt, Dennis Krebs, and Tina Niwinska. Helpful research was provided by Jody Bain, and we are very grateful to Peter Gibson for sharing his remarkable story with us in Chapter 12.

The editors would like to thank Larry M. Leith of the University of Toronto, Wolfgang Linden of the University of British Columbia, and Gerry Goldberg for their helpful comments in preparing this manuscript.

Gary Poole

Deborah Hunt Matheson

David N. Cox

Part 1

AN INTRODUCTION TO HEALTH PSYCHOLOGY

Chapter 1

THE DEVELOPMENT OF THE FIELD

Chapter Outline

Key Questions

1. What is health psychology, and what other terms are used to describe the work conducted in this area?
2. How did health psychology get started and how has it changed over the years?
3. Why has health psychology grown rapidly in recent years?
4. What is meant by a biopsychosocial approach to health?
5. What are some of the prominent theories used in health psychology?
6. What sorts of career opportunities are available in the field, and what training is required for them?

In a small lecture theatre, buried somewhere in the basement of a large urban hospital, a psychologist stands before a group of physicians. They are radiologists who have just spent a rather long and demanding working day examining pictures from x-ray, computed tomography (CT), magnetic resonance imaging (MRI), ultrasound, and nuclear medicine scans. The machines used represent the cutting edge of diagnostic technology. The physicians are here to listen to the psychologist introduce them to health psychology.

The psychologist displays a slide showing a CT head and neck scan. He asks his audience if they can detect anything remarkable about the scan. They take to the challenge en masse, leaning forward, examining the slide closely. It seems normal, though. No one provides an answer.

The psychologist continues. "Nothing evident? Well, I'll tell you what is remarkable about this scan. That happens to be *my* head you're looking at. Well, that might not be all that remarkable to you, but I can assure you, it is to me."

He then asks another question. "When you were examining this scan, whose heart was beating the fastest in this room?" The answer, of course, is the psychologist's heart. "Every time I use this example, I'm afraid one of the specialists is going to find something!"

On another day, in the same hospital, there are a series of research seminars being presented. A nuclear physicist and a psychologist are on the same program. Both of them do research in nuclear medicine. While the physicist studies radioactive isotopes, the psychologist looks for ways to make these procedures less anxiety-arousing for patients.

Both these examples illustrate some of the fundamental work of health psychologists. For every CT procedure or injection of radioactive isotopes, there is a *person* to consider. Indeed, there are many people to consider when the medical staff involved is included. In its simplest terms, health psychology is the consideration of these people.

In this chapter, we will develop our definition of health psychology to include its many facets. We will document the development of the field and provide a rationale for why health psychology has risen to prominence. We will then look at health psychology as it exists today, explaining some of its theoretical foundations and exploring some of the ways psychologists work in health-related settings.

CASE 1-1 When the Heart Stops

Alan was admitted to hospital with classic symptoms of a heart attack, though that wasn't how he was explaining his chest pain, difficulty breathing, and profuse sweating. He had been suffering from a cold for the past week and he thought the virus had flared rather badly. However, Alan was wrong. Tests revealed an *infarct*, or tissue that has died because of a lack of oxygen. Other tests showed the reason for the infarct. A coronary artery was completely blocked. In fact, so were two others—not the stuff of viruses. Alan was advised that he needed emergency bypass surgery.

WHAT IS HEALTH PSYCHOLOGY?

After reading Case Study 1.1, ask yourself what might have caused Alan's heart attack. From the case study, we might conclude that the cause was the arterial blockage, and this would certainly be correct. But is that *all* that caused it? Why did bypass surgery like Alan's become so common in the latter half of the twentieth century? Did millions of people in North America develop blocked coronary arteries because of some colossal biological coincidence? No. To understand Alan's heart attack and the growth industry that bypass surgery has become, we must look beyond biology. We must consider psychological causes, such as Alan's outlook on life, his lifestyle, and his stress level. We must consider sociological causes, such as the nature of his employment as well as his social network. Finally, we must consider environmental causes, such as the air he breathes.

Not only is this collection of causes relevant to Alan's heart, it is, indeed, at the heart of this book. In this first chapter, we want you to develop an appreciation for the fact that an understanding of health is best achieved by a partnership between medical and social science. We will explore, in detail, the contributions of the social science of psychology to this understanding.

Clinical psychologists have long recognized that there are psychological consequences associated with ill health. Conversely, there are physical consequences associated with many psychological disorders. It wasn't until the 1970s, however, that psychologists from other non-clinical subdisciplines began to recognize that there were many ways psychological principles could be applied to health and health care in contexts that were psychologically *normal*.

It was out of this recognition that the fields of behavioural medicine and ultimately health psychology emerged. There were a range of terms introduced as names for the new discipline linking psychology and health. All these terms can be somewhat confusing, because some psychologists use them interchangeably while others believe they refer to distinctly different subcategories. We will begin our investigation of the field's development by trying to sort out the different names that have been used as labels.

One of the first terms commonly used when people talked about psychology and health was **biofeedback** (Birk, 1973), which involves the use of techniques designed to provide individuals with visual or auditory feedback on particular physiological responses they want to modify. For example, a person might hear a tone that drops in pitch as her blood pressure drops. Thus the tone provides audible *feedback* for a *biological* process.

However, the first formal definition of the field used the term **behavioural medicine**.The term was defined at the Yale Conference on Behavioral Medicine in 1977 and improved upon the following year by the Academy of Behavioral Medicine Research. Here is their definition:

> Behavioral medicine is the interdisciplinary field concerned with the development and integration of behavioral and biomedical science knowledge and techniques relevant to the understanding of health and illness, the application of this knowledge and these techniques to prevention, diagnosis, treatment and rehabilitation (Academy of Behavioral Medicine Research, 1978).

This definition stressed the importance of a model integrating biomedical and behavioural approaches. It should also be noted that it was in 1978 that the first issue of the *Journal of Behavioral Medicine* was published and the Society of Behavioral Medicine was formed.

Within the field of behavioural medicine, four subdomains were described (Blanchard, 1977). The first of these involves psychological interventions in areas that had traditionally been considered medical problems, such as obesity or headaches. The behavioural approach emphasizes *adjunctive methods* or alternatives to traditional pharmacological or surgical interventions through the development of effective strategies for behavioural change. The focus of the second subdomain is the use of psychological interventions to improve compliance or adherence to medical care. The third involves the use of the previously described biofeedback techniques to detect and ultimately modify physiological response patterns. The fourth focuses on the area of *primary prevention*, which emphasizes establishing and maintaining appropriate health behaviours.

Other terms have been proposed to deal with various components of the relationship between psychology and health. For example, Matarazzo (1980) discussed three terms that he did not feel should be used synonymously. The first, described above, is *behavioural medicine*, emphasizing a broad interdisciplinary approach to health and illness. The second is **behavioural health**, which Matarazzo defined as an interdisciplinary subspecialty within the framework of behavioural medicine, concerned with the maintenance of health and the prevention of illness and dysfunction in currently healthy individuals. In a behavioural health approach, people are helped to take personal responsibility for such maintenance and prevention. The third and more all-encompassing term is **health psychology**, for which Matarazzo proposed the following definition:

> Health psychology is the aggregate of the specific educational, scientific and professional contributions of the discipline of psychology to the promotion and maintenance of health,

> the prevention or treatment of illness, and the identification of etiologic and diagnostic correlates of health, illness, and related dysfunction (Matarazzo, 1980).

Notice that this definition includes not just maintenance of health but also treatment of illness. Health psychology, then, is the compilation of all that psychology has to offer to the diagnosis and treatment of illness as well as people's attempts to maintain health and well-being. In this context, the word "health" means more than just the absence of illness. As far back as the 1940s, the World Health Organization promoted the notion that being "healthy" also means being able to enjoy a desired quality of life in terms of physical, mental, and social functioning.

Let's apply this notion of health to Alan, who has just had a heart attack. We can, with some accuracy, assess the extent of his tissue damage. However, what will it take to help Alan be *healthy* again, and what does this mean? If we adopt the World Health Organization's definition of health, our role as health psychologists becomes clearer. We must help Alan return to a level of functioning that restores his sense of quality of life. This may include addressing his fears of having another heart attack, helping him change his approach to life so that it is less hostile, and helping him develop the conviction that these changes are possible.

In this example, and in Matarazzo's definition of health psychology, we form an image of psychologists working at the interface of medicine and psychology. This work has been recognized by the Canadian Psychological Association in its creation of a section on Health Psychology, and by the American Psychological Association through its creation of Division 38, the Division of Health Psychology. To put these definitions in context, we might describe ourselves as psychologists working in the field of health psychology within the interdisciplinary fields of behavioural health (when our focus is on prevention) or behavioural medicine (when our focus is on remediation).

Another term common to the field is **psychosomatic medicine**, in which a particular medical complaint is viewed as being the result of an underlying chronic emotional conflict that ultimately surfaces in the form of physiological symptoms. Specific symptoms are linked to particular kinds of conflicts. Probably the most well-known example of this relationship between psychological conflict and physical symptoms is the understanding that essential hypertension (high blood pressure) is connected to an inability to express feelings of anger in an appropriate manner.

As you might expect, psychotherapy is the treatment of choice in such cases because it intends to provide insight into the impact that unresolved conflicts are having on a particular individual's life. It is hoped that insight will be accompanied by symptom reduction. However, treatment of medical disorders based on this approach has not been successful. In comparison, treatment in behavioural medicine is focused on the individual's current *behaviour* that is viewed as being strongly influenced by learning. Symptoms are considered to be important in their own right and the emphasis is on defining them in observable and measurable terms.

In summary, there are many terms that are used to describe the work done by psychologists working in health-related areas. Some focus on behavioural interventions, some on enhancing people's abilities to maintain their own health. All these terms relate to the same process—the application of psychological principles to the understanding of and improvement of our health.

THE DEVELOPMENT OF HEALTH PSYCHOLOGY AS A DISCIPLINE

When health psychology began to emerge as a field, the *Annual Review of Psychology* began publishing articles summarizing the "state of the art", as it were. First there was Neal Miller's 1983 article on behavioural medicine (Miller, 1983). This article was followed by a number of reviews over the years. Some of the more comprehensive include Krantz, Grunberg, and Baum, who reviewed the field in 1985, Rodin and Salovey in 1989, and Cohen and Herbert in 1996. Taken collectively, these articles provide a good overview of how the field has developed, especially in terms of the topics given attention over the years. By looking at the highlights of each article, we will get a sense of the field's development.

The Early Stages of Health Psychology's Development: Applying the Principles of Behaviourism to Health

In 1983, Neal Miller reviewed the state of the field in an article entitled "Behavioral Medicine: Symbiosis between Laboratory and Clinic." In this article, Miller traced the development of the biomedical perspective on illness, starting with the invention of the microscope and moving to the development of **germ theory**, the discovery that many illnesses were caused by the activity of microorganisms such as bacteria. From germ theory came the refinement of antibiotics to fight these germs; the biomedical perspective was in full flight, realizing considerable success by reducing illnesses to a cellular level and treating them with medicines.

At least two important developments resulted from this history. First, the success of antibiotics brought about a change in the profile of life-threatening illnesses, as we will see later in the chapter. Germs were replaced by lifestyle as the number one killer. Second, an emphasis on technical aspects of medicine came to replace a consideration for emotional factors in health.

When behavioural medicine emerged, it did so in response to these two factors. It was called **behavioural medicine** because of the emphasis placed on the link between *behaviour* and health. This emphasis was consistent with the theoretical stance adopted by some of the field's pioneers, such as Neal Miller. Miller was a **behaviourist**, which means that he believed that most behaviour was learned, rather than innate.

As the term implies, behaviourists focus on overt or observable behaviour. They are less concerned with internal processes such as cognition. Instead, behaviourists study the ways in which reinforcers in the environment shape our behaviour. Behaviours that pay off are repeated, those that don't are extinguished.

People adopting a behavioural perspective believe that our health is affected primarily by what we *do* rather than what we *think*. You will see later in this chapter how this perspective contrasts with modern theories in health, like the health belief model, which is primarily about the way our thinking can affect what we do.

In Miller's article, then, the key issues of the day were explained using the language of behaviourism. For example, Miller identified non-compliance with medical regimens as an important problem. He explained it in terms of what he called a **gradient of reinforcement**. By this, he meant that the greater the lag time between behaviour and reinforcer, the weaker the behaviour would be. Non-compliance could be explained in these terms because the reinforcement for following a medical regimen was often delayed. When we exercise, we don't suddenly get fit. High blood pressure doesn't drop to a normal range after one low-sodium meal. These benefits take time to realize. Behaviourists call this time lag between behaviour and reinforcer **delayed gratification**. From our case study, Alan would have to contend with problems of delayed gratification as he recovered from his heart attack and tried to change his behaviour and thinking.

There is research support for the delayed gratification explanation of what Miller termed "non-compliance." Specifically, we know that compliance rates are higher for regimens bringing about a rapid reduction in symptoms than they are for those in which improvement takes longer. Lowest of all are compliance rates for conditions that are **asymptomatic**—conditions not accompanied by palpable symptoms or sensations (Buckalew, 1991).

For example, the delayed gratification approach helps explain why significantly more people will follow instructions to take an antibiotic to relieve them of a painful ear infection than will change their lifestyle to reduce hypertension. According to the behavioural explanation, this is because taking the antibiotic is reinforced by pain relief; lifestyle changes for the usually asymptomatic condition of high blood pressure, however, are reinforced by longer life expectancy, which is far less immediate. This problem is further compounded by the fact that behaviours worsening hypertension, like eating a high-fat diet, are immediately reinforced—these foods taste good. Miller provided a similar analysis to explain why it is hard to quit smoking cigarettes.

Other issues introduced by Miller included alcohol abuse, obesity, and the Type A behaviour pattern. At the time of Miller's article (1983), it was believed that the entire constellation of attributes identified by the Type A pattern were linked to heart disease. These included time urgency, achievement orientation, and hostility. Large-scale studies, such as the Framingham study, published around the time of Miller's article, showed that people exhibiting the Type A pattern were generally at greater risk for coronary heart disease (CHD) (Haynes, Feinleib, & Kannel, 1980). More recent work, however, has shown that hostility is the trait most reliably linked to CHD (Dembroski & Costa, 1988).

Finally, Miller devoted considerable space to a discussion of stress. True to his behaviourist leanings, he examined animal studies, in which researchers measured the effects that variables such as control over aversive stimuli had on stress responses and mortality. For example, in one series of studies, mice placed in environments that brought on confrontations and prevented the formation of social networks developed high blood pressure (Henry & Stephens, 1979; cited in Miller, 1983). In addition, Miller introduced stress-related topics that are still pursued today. For example, he talked about social support as a way of reducing stress and the possibility that stress levels were related to immune system functioning. We will see below that these topics received considerable attention in later review articles.

Health Psychology Expands to Include Cognition and Personality Factors

Shortly after Miller's review, Krantz and colleagues (1985) published another major review that identified a number of key areas health psychology had made contributions to and in which more research was needed. They continued Miller's discussion of stress. By the mid-1980s, psychologists were working with physiologists and others to identify the mechanisms whereby stressful environments put people at risk for health problems. Further, Miller's behavioural perspective had been expanded to include the study of cognitive and personality factors predisposing some people to view a situation as being stressful that others may not.

At the same time, psychologists were studying ways that stress could be reduced. For example, social support had grown as a significant area of study, as had therapeutic interventions such as *cognitive restructuring*, aimed at changing people's stress-prone interpretations of events (for a review, see Matarazzo et al., 1984).

Closely related to these investigations was the study of the relationship between behaviour and cardiovascular health. The link between cigarette smoking and disease had been sufficiently established, so the next logical step was to study the psychology of smoking. To this end, studies looked at when people (usually young people) started smoking (Kozlowski, 1979; Pomerleau, 1979), how their habit was maintained (Kozlowski & Herman, 1984), and why smoking cessation programs were less successful than they might be (Schachter, 1981).

Krantz and colleagues took a more detailed look at the Type A construct introduced in the late 1950s when two cardiologists identified behaviour patterns that they claimed were more common among their cardiac patients than in the general population (Friedman & Rosenman, 1959). They called this the Type A Coronary Prone Behaviour Pattern. The Type A construct generated a considerable number of studies in the 1970s and early 1980s. Some of these studies supported the assertions of Friedman and Rosenman, others did not. We will review the balance of these findings in Chapter 5 in our discussion of stress and coping. For now, it is important to understand that the Type A construct proved to be an important catalyst for general research attempting to link psychology with health.

Eating disorders was another topic that rose to prominence in the 1980s, specifically obesity, anorexia, and cachexia (malnourishment). Obesity was discussed from biological, behavioural, and social perspectives; today we call this a *biopsychosocial approach*, discussed later in the chapter. In their discussion, Krantz and colleagues addressed the problem of maintaining a healthy weight. Anorexia was also discussed from a biopsychosocial perspective.

Finally, Krantz and colleagues continued the study of compliance by introducing perspectives other than behaviourism. The study of compliance was very important historically for a number of reasons. First, the work of Howard Waitzkin in the United States (Waitzkin, 1985), Philip Ley in Great Britain (Ley, 1977), and others showed that communication between physicians and their patients often lacked clarity and relevance. Through this work, physicians discovered that their impression of an interview with a patient could be quite different from that of the patient. Specifically, less information was being conveyed and patients' understanding of that information was poorer than physicians realized. Communication in medical settings continues to be an important topic in health psychology (see Chapter 6).

The study of compliance was also important because it led to a more in-depth study of the patient-physician relationship. Indeed, the term "compliance" has come under fire because of its implication that the physician-patient relationship is unidirectional (DiMatteo, 1991). Some analysts criticized the value of the expectation that the physician should give the orders and patients must passively follow them.

More Attention is Paid to the Ways People Cope

Four years after the review paper by Krantz and colleagues, Rodin and Salovey (1989) published another review of health psychology. At that time, further work was being done to investigate dispositional, or personality, variables as well as the relationship between thinking and health. Social support and health promotion continued to be topics of importance.

Some new topics had emerged by 1989. For example, research attention was being paid to the ways in which people *coped* with illness and all that came with it, such as hospital stays and relationships with others. Consistent with the investigation of dispositional variables, health psychologists were attempting to identify **coping styles**—patterns in the ways people deal with difficult situations.

One good example is Suzanne Miller's notion of monitors and blunters (Miller, 1980). **Monitors** are information seekers. **Blunters** are information avoiders. The coping style of each type is consistent with their desire for receiving or avoiding information. This is just one example of how people differ in the ways they cope with illness and the challenges it brings. We will look more closely at these and other coping styles in Chapter 7 when we talk about hospital stays and medical procedures, and again in Chapter 11 in our discussion of chronic and terminal illness.

Another topic that continued to be prominent from the time of Miller's review was substance use and abuse. The analysis moved away from the addictive properties of the substance to the cognitions and behaviours of the addicted. Combined with this was a study of the possibility of a genetic predisposition to substance abuse.

The Introduction of Psychoneuroimmunology: Finding Links between Psychological and Biological Processes

In 1996, Cohen and Herbert summarized the state of health psychology by focusing exclusively on **psychoneuroimmunology (PNI)**. This is the study of the relationship between our psychological state and the functioning of our immune system, a relationship alluded to by Miller in 1983 and studied in more detail in more recent years. The breakthrough in this area came with the development of techniques to quantify the status of our immune systems (called **immunocompetence**) through blood tests and saliva samples. This made PNI extremely important because it provided an opportunity for health psychology to produce empirical proof of hypothesized relationships between mind and body.

In truth, PNI was introduced well before the mid-1990s. In fact, a prominent book on the subject was published in 1981 (Ader, 1981). Our knowledge of PNI has been significantly advanced by a number of researchers since then. One of the more prolific is Janice Kiecolt-Glaser, who has been publishing extensively in the area of PNI since the mid-1980s. She has looked at such diverse psychological states and situations as marital conflict (Kiecolt-Glaser et al., 1987a) and caregiving for patients with Alzheimer's disease (Kiecolt-Glaser et al., 1987b) in terms of their effects on the immune system. We present a detailed examination of PNI in Chapter 3.

The most recent *Annual Review of Psychology* article to summarize the field is that of Andrew Baum and Donna Posluszny (1999). Their paper provides an excellent overview of the ways in which all the major relevant topics since Miller's 1983 article have coalesced and evolved into what health psychology is today.

Summary

By comparing these major reviews of health psychology, we can see that the actual topics being studied have changed much less than the ways in which these topics are viewed. From the strong behavioural roots of Miller and others, we have expanded to include theories featuring a more cognitive approach. Today, health psychologists employ interventions that combine behavioural and cognitive theories, evidence of which we will see in this book.

The research in health psychology continues to proliferate, though questions have been raised as to whether the work is building upon itself to create a body of knowledge or just going off madly in all directions with few interconnections being made among studies (Belar, 1997). We have reached the point in health psychology where we have established that tangible links exist between numerous psychological phenomena and physical health. The next step is to hone and test interventions to affect these phenomena in ways that increase well-being and save time, money, and lives. If health psychology is to thrive, or indeed survive, as a field, it must reach this level of accountability.

WHY HAS HEALTH PSYCHOLOGY COME INTO PROMINENCE?

Health psychology is a growing field. The Health Psychology section of the Canadian Psychological Association (CPA) is one of the larger CPA sections, with approximately 200 members (CPA web site, 1999,/www.cpa.ca). There are many reasons for this growth, not the least of which are the changes in health and illness patterns in this country and elsewhere in the latter half of the twentieth century. Let's begin with a close look at some of those changes.

Changing Profiles of Illness and Health In Canada

One important reason for the emergence of health psychology as a discipline can be demonstrated by comparing mortality statistics over the course of the twentieth century. This reveals that the causes of death today are different from those of just 50 or 100 years ago.

At the turn of the century, the most common cause of death in North America was acute, infectious disease, namely, respiratory diseases (influenza and pneumonia) (Sexton, 1979) (see Figure 1.1). By 1950, the leading cause of death in Canada had become circulatory diseases (heart and cerebrovascular disease). Cancer had become the second leading cause, ahead of respiratory diseases (Wilkins, 1995) (see Figure 1.2).

When psychologists look at this change, they focus on the *preventability* of these diseases. Some time around the middle of the twentieth century, lifestyle replaced microbiology as our major source of life-threatening toxins. Hence the rationale for **behavioural medicine**, which, as we have seen, is concerned with the relationship between health and behaviour. Indeed, a comparison of 1950 and 1993 death rates in Canada reveals a dramatic 57 percent drop in deaths from circulatory disease (Figure 1.2). Much of this decline can be attributed to lifestyle change, which is, in many ways, a psychological phenomenon. It is very possible that lifestyle change will be the most pressing challenge Alan from our case study will face as he approaches life after his heart attack.

FIGURE 1-1 Death Rates per 100 000, 1900

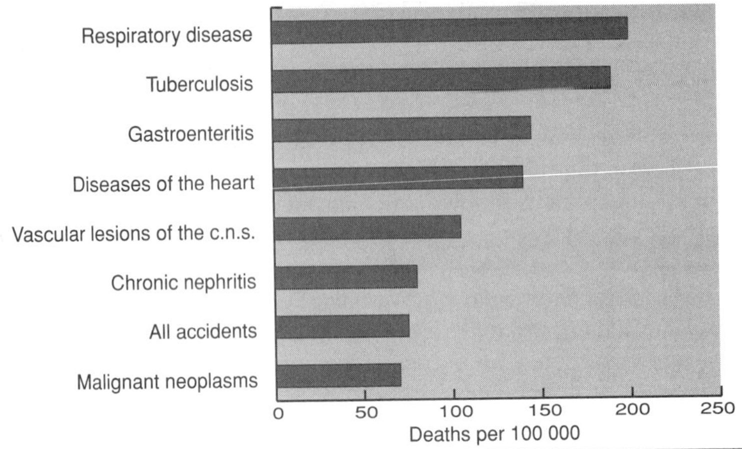

Source: Sexton (1979). Adapted by permission.

FIGURE 1-2 Major Causes of Death in Canada, 1950 and 1993, per 100 000

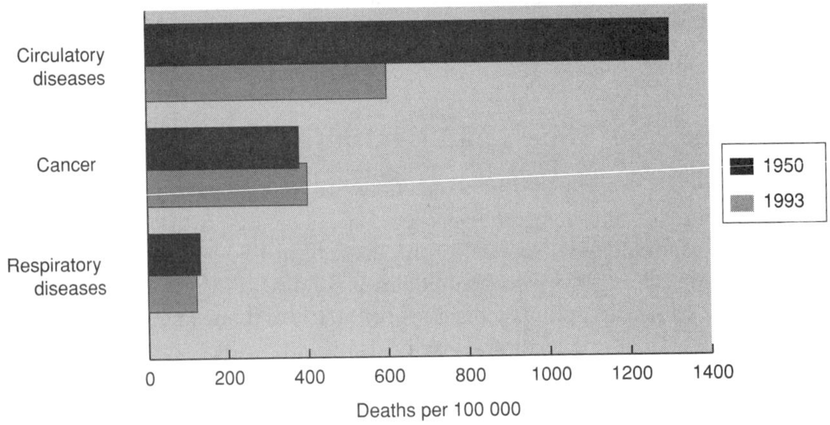

Source: Wilkins, K. (1995). Adapted by permission.

According to Statistics Canada, 56 percent of men and 58 percent of women report that they exercise regularly. This means that they engage in vigorous activities such as calisthenics, jogging or racquet sports, team sports, dance classes, or brisk walking for a period of at least 15 minutes at least three times per week. Only 21 percent of men and 22 percent of women say they rarely exercise. Figure 1.3 shows the percentage of men and women reporting regular exercise across various age groups. While this graph indicates a slight decline in exercise rates as people age, it is perhaps more noteworthy that Canadian seniors are maintaining exercise rates that are not remarkably below those of people in early adulthood. The result is improved cardiovascular health for all ages.

Activity level is one aspect of lifestyle relevant to health. Cigarette smoking is another. In 1990, over 840 000 people in Canada tried to either quit smoking or reduce the amount they smoked (Statistics Canada). If you have ever tried to do this or make some other

FIGURE 1-3 Exercise Frequency for Men and Women in Canada 1996–97

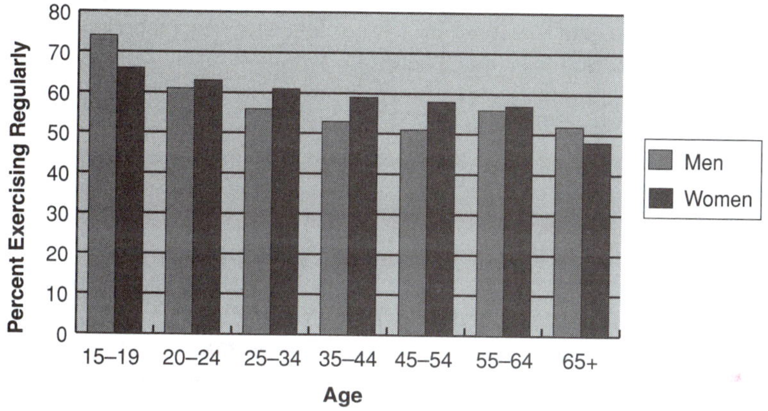

Source: Health Indicators, Catalogue No. 82-221. Adapted by permission.

significant and lasting change to your lifestyle, it is likely that you encountered some psychological barriers along the way. You had to *learn* new behaviours and *unlearn* old ones. You had to *believe* that you were capable of making the change, and other people may have been involved who made the change easier or harder. Even from this brief analysis, we can see that learning theory, cognitive psychology, and social psychology are very relevant to lifestyle change, which has become an integral part of our health and wellness in the new millennium.

Alan will be encouraged to learn new ways of thinking and behaving that will result in reduced stress, greater relaxation, and improved fitness. These changes will also have a social component, as family and friends will be called upon for support.

Multiple Perspectives are Needed to Understand Health and Health Statistics

Another reason for the growth of health psychology is that it provides helpful ways to understand the statistics describing our health. For example, between 1950 and 1993 male deaths from cancer in Canada rose 35 percent (Wilkins, 1995). Which perspective provides us with the best way to respond to this in ways that will affect that statistic? Biomedical research may focus on the biology of **malignant neoplasms**, which are cancerous growths that may be treated by radiation and chemical therapy. This is a valuable perspective but is there more to the story? Just as we discovered when talking about Alan's heart attack, there are additional perspectives that will help us better understand cancer statistics.

Perhaps we can learn something further by looking at the *types* of cancer that account most for this 35 percent increase. When we do, we find that lung cancer showed the greatest increase, accounting for nearly one-third of all male cancer deaths in 1993 in Canada. The next sharpest increase was in prostate cancer, which accounted for about one-eighth of male cancer deaths in the same year (Wilkins, 1995).

These data indicate that there is more at work than a random and unfortunate growth of neoplasms. Lung cancer is linked to a behaviour—smoking. Psychologists can make valuable contributions to the modification of this behaviour from what they know about attitude change, persuasion, and addiction. They can help reduce the number of smokers and thus reduce death rates resulting from lung cancer.

There is even more to this picture, however, than can be captured within biomedical and psychological perspectives. Environmentalists may argue that increases in lung and prostate cancer rates have resulted from breathing toxic air and eating foods containing chemicals that are potentially **carcinogenic**, or cancer causing. From this perspective, the field of **medical geography** has developed. Clearly, some environments are healthier than others; medical geographers study these differences (see Chapter 13).

Thus far, we have identified biomedical, psychological, and geographical perspectives used to understand cancer deaths, and we still haven't exhausted our list of useful perspectives. For example, we also know that there are **demographic differences** in the health of Canadians—differences that depend on culture, affluence, employment status, gender, and so on.

When asked, the majority of Canadians report that they are in good health. In the provinces, 63 percent of residents gave this rating to their health. In a study of residents in the Yukon and Northwest Territories, 69 percent of non-aboriginal residents rated their health as very good or excellent; however, only 47 percent of the aboriginal residents of the Northwest Territories called their health very good or excellent (Diverty & Pérez, 1998). We must be cautious when comparing health statistics across cultures. Nevertheless, data such as these invite further study of cultural and demographic differences in diet, social support, the use of medical services, and many other factors. If Alan is a member of a culture in which high-fat foods are common, he will find it harder to adopt a heart-healthy lifestyle. Cultural factors are studied by **medical anthropologists** and demographic factors are studied by **medical sociologists** and **epidemiologists**.

The patterns of illness and health are changing in Canada. Also, there has been a change in emphasis from cure to prevention. To understand these changes and to improve health and health care, we need to acquire the knowledge of many disciplines. This is the essence of the **biopsychosocial approach** (Engel, 1977). As the term implies, this model considers biological, psychological, and social factors affecting health. We will take a close look at this approach in the next section. At this point, it is important to understand that psychology has much to offer in our attempt to best understand health and illness.

HEALTH PSYCHOLOGY TODAY

Now that you have some idea of what health psychology is about, let's look at the key issues for people working in health psychology today. We'll begin by introducing the most fundamental assumption of the field, as captured by the biopsychosocial approach. We'll then look at what this approach means for psychologists working in health care settings. From there, we'll move to an overview of prominent theories in the field today and conclude with a look at what people with training in health psychology actually do.

A Biopsychosocial Approach to Health

It is essential to understand that good and poor health can be attributed to a multitude of causes. Further, these causes are varied enough that they cannot be understood from any one perspective, whether in medicine or the social sciences. The **biopsychosocial approach** to health takes these various perspectives into account, acknowledging that biological, psychological, and social factors combine to influence our health.

The term "biopsychosocial", then, refers to three major perspectives or causes of health and illness. As we move from the biological to the psychological and finally to the social, we move from a *microscopic* perspective to a *macroscopic* one. For example, we can study cancer at a *biological*, cellular level by analyzing neoplasms (new growths), at a *psychological* level by assessing patients' coping abilities and correlations between stress and immune function, and at a *sociological* level by identifying government policies that affect environmental toxins or hospital regulations that affect the nature of treatment.

Why is a Biopsychosocial Approach so Important?

Health psychologists believe that no medical condition exists that can be fully understood from one perspective alone. Mortality statistics make it clear that many life-threatening conditions are preventable, in some cases by inoculation, in others by lifestyle changes, and in others by government policies such as seatbelt legislation. Only the biopsychosocial approach encompasses all these levels.

Even the common cold has psychological and sociological causes. Our immune systems are affected by our psychological state (for a review, see Cohen and Herbert, 1996), so we are more likely to catch a cold when we have endured something stressful, and we often catch colds from other people with whom we interact at work and in other social settings.

What are the Implications of the Biopsychosocial Approach for Health Psychologists?

Today, the adoption of the biopsychosocial approach demands clear communication among health care practitioners and social scientists as well as a mutual respect for the potential contributions each can make to health and health care. It makes no more sense for a physician to downplay psychological factors affecting patients than it does for psychologists to say that viruses, tissue damage, and neoplasms are of little consequence.

Clear communication between practitioners and social scientists requires mutual understanding. This doesn't mean that social scientists must have all the knowledge of a physician or that physicians must be trained psychologists, but it does require a mutual appreciation for each other's potential contributions to the understanding of health and illness. For a number of reasons, however, achieving this mutual appreciation can be difficult. One important reason for this stems from the different ways in which people are trained.

Medical practitioners are trained in the **biomedical model**. According to this model, as the name implies, health is best understood in terms of our biology. Students of this model are taught that it is precise and concrete. The concreteness of the model might make it easier to understand; however, it is a daunting task to learn enough human biology to be able to practise medicine. The time required often results in the exclusion of other models of health and well-being. It stands to reason that the dedication required to cope with the reams of material presented in medical school demands a strong belief in the efficacy of the biomedical model.

The end result, understandably, is a medical school graduate who is firmly entrenched in that model. Other approaches, for example those from the social sciences, seem much less precise and far too abstract by comparison. Psychosocial causes can't be viewed under a microscope or measured directly via blood tests or a CT scan. This abstractness can affect a physician's view of the credibility of disciplines like health psychology.

Writing in the *Journal of the American Medical Association*, Norman Cousins quotes a physician who captures the feelings of a number of others in the profession:

> I am not interested in charming or entertaining my patients or winning popularity contests. I want to give them the benefit of my special knowledge and ability. If I myself were seriously ill, I would have no difficulty in expressing my preference for a physician who is capable of making an absolutely correct diagnosis and who would know exactly what has to be done—rather than choose a physician who is adept at sweet talk, or in making friends and influencing people, or in gaining recognition as one hell of a fine fellow (Cousins, 1988, p. 1610).

The problem with this position is that it assumes biomedical and psychosocial competencies to be mutually exclusive—if you have one you can't have the other. Norman Cousins became well known for his book *Anatomy of an Illness*, in which he documents his personal experience with the therapeutic effects of humour on cancer (Cousins, 1979). In his *JAMA* commentary containing the above passage, Cousins calls for a balance between biomedical and psychosocial perspectives. This balance is what the biopsychosocial approach is all about.

For their part, psychologists have their own set of beliefs specific to their discipline that are not always considered reasonable by people outside the field. For example, psychologists are trained to believe that behavioural phenomena can be reliably measured, that correlations as small as .3 can be meaningful, and that there are attributes shared by large groups of people that go beyond how many kidneys or lungs they have. As part of their training, psychologists are sensitized to the *psychological impact* of events on our lives.

The different levels of emphasis in training produce graduates with different perspectives. This is well illustrated by health psychologist Robin DiMatteo, who describes a tour a physician gave her through their intensive care unit (ICU). The physician was justifiably excited by the recent acquisition of new equipment for ICU. Dr. DiMatteo, on the other hand, had her attention drawn in different directions:

> I remember feigning interest in the newly acquired machinery, little of which I understood, and I congratulated everyone on this up-to-date facility. But as I looked around to where the loved ones of the intubated people were waiting, I tried to catch a glimpse of their faces. My concern was not with the tremendous technical advances in the intensive care unit (ICU). As a psychologist, my focus was on the loved ones of those in the ICU, people who were suddenly forced to have their lives revolve around the ICU, where they waited day after day for some

news that their child, spouse, relative, or friend might survive and someday be normal again (DiMatteo, 1995, p. 217).

The point of this example isn't that the physician was misguided in his focus on the new equipment in ICU. Rather, it is that there are many phenomena needing attention in a place like ICU. Robin DiMatteo and other health psychologists provide expertise that fills in other pieces of the puzzle implied by the biopsychosocial approach.

As we mentioned earlier, this realization grew, in part, from a change in the causes of life-threatening illnesses. Psychological and behavioural factors became more significant. From this, it became clear that there were psychological causes and consequences associated with *many* aspects of our health, not just those that resulted in mortality statistics.

Prominent Theories in Health Psychology

In this chapter, we are attempting to tell the story of health psychology. We began by defining what health psychology is. We then looked at how it developed from its early years and why it has grown so rapidly. We then looked at the overarching model in modern health psychology—the psychosocial approach. Now it is time to look into the "tool kit" of today's health psychologists. In it, we will find a number of very useful theories they use to help them understand health issues and help people recover from illness or injury and stay healthy. Our list of theories will not be exhaustive at this point. Rather, we will talk about some of the more prominent theories in the field to give you a sense of the work health psychologists do in research and intervention. Let's start by returning to Alan who, as you will see in Case Study 1.2, is home from the hospital and has been put on a rehabilitative plan for his recovery.

CASE 1-2 Alan Revisited: The Road Back

Alan spent 5 days in the cardiac care unit of the hospital. His moods swung between fear and frustration. He certainly didn't want another heart attack, but he had a business to run and countless other responsibilities. The people in cardiac care didn't seem to appreciate this. They kept telling him to try and relax—easy for them to say.

Now that he was home convalescing, it was even harder to "relax." He had so much to do and think about. On top it all, the cardiologist had given him a bunch of pills to take and a strict diet to follow. And then there was the Healthy Heart program at the hospital that he was expected to start attending on a weekly basis. He had been asked to rethink his life's priorities, change the way he ate, and start the Healthy Heart program. Would Alan do all these things? It is an important question, since Alan's life might depend on it. The theories we look at in this section will help us predict the answer.

The Health Belief Model

One of the most well-developed and useful contributions psychology has made to the understanding of health is the **health belief model** (Becker, 1974; Rosenstock, 1974). As such, it represents a good entry point for our exploration of the psychological component of the biopsychosocial approach. A "health belief", as the term implies, is something we think to be true concerning our health. For example, we might believe that a low-fat diet will improve cardiovascular health or that modern medicine can cure most ailments. There are many different health beliefs.

The health belief model starts with the reasonable assumption that health behaviours are explained by our health beliefs. This is a good start, but we really need to know *which* specific health beliefs are most closely linked to behaviour, if the model is to be of value.

The health belief model is valuable because it identifies a manageable number of relevant, measurable types of health beliefs that often do a reasonable job of predicting health behaviour. In its most basic form, the model focuses on two beliefs: the belief that a health threat exists and the belief that a given course of action will affect the threat.

Social psychologists have learned that beliefs don't exist in isolation (e.g., Schroder, 1971). Rather, they co-exist interdependently in *belief systems*. Consistent with this, the health belief model expands to include several other beliefs that influence these two basic ones concerning health threat. Specifically, our belief about the existence of a health threat is influenced by the extent to which we believe we are personally vulnerable to that threat as well as by our beliefs about the severity of the consequences.

Let's illustrate these beliefs with an everyday example. When the weather channel reports a 100 percent chance of rain on a day when you must go outdoors, you know you are personally vulnerable to the threat of rain, but the *consequence* isn't particularly severe, so you don't believe a threat exists. On the other hand, if you read that one in three people will get cancer, you develop a belief regarding the likelihood that you could be that one (personal vulnerability), as well as a belief regarding how bad it would be to get cancer (severity of consequences). These beliefs affect your perception of threat and, in turn, affect your cancer preventing behaviours, such as using sunscreen.

Similarly, there are two beliefs that influence the fundamental belief that a course of action will *reduce* a threat. First, there is something called an **efficacy belief**. This refers to the extent to which you think a course of action (e.g., a preventive behaviour or treatment) will actually work. Second, there is a **cost-gain belief**. This refers to your assessment of the costs (such as effort, discomfort, embarrassment, or inconvenience) associated with this action compared to the benefit of the behaviour to your health. For example, if someone believes that the gains of exercise seem distant and minor compared to the costs such as effort and short-term fatigue, then exercise behaviour is unlikely. This belief is reminiscent of Miller's behaviourist approach we discussed earlier in the chapter.

Table 1.1 diagrams the health belief model and contrasts the beliefs of two people (Person A and Person B). In this case, the model is being used to predict condom usage. At the top of the table, we begin with the two general beliefs regarding the existence of a threat and the possibility that a behaviour can affect the threat. Beneath that, specific beliefs related to these general beliefs are listed. The next two rows provide examples of those related beliefs for each of these fictitious people.

Person A believes himself to be somewhat vulnerable and also that the consequences of contracting acquired immunodeficiency syndrome (AIDS) are severe (i.e., fatal). He also

TABLE 1-1 The Health Belief Model Applied to Condom Usage

General Belief	A Health Threat Exists		A Behaviour Will Affect the Threat		Result
Related Beliefs	Beliefs regarding personal vulnerability to the threat	Beliefs about the severity of the consequences	The belief that a course of action will actually work or not	The assessment of the costs and benefits associated with this action	
Person A	*"I could get AIDS."*	*"AIDS is a fatal disease."*	*"Using condoms will greatly reduce my chances of getting AIDS."*	*"I get embarrassed when I buy condoms, but they will reduce the risk of getting AIDS."*	Condoms are used
Person B	*"Other people might get AIDS but I won't."*	*"With new drugs, AIDS isn't as life-threatening as it once was."*	*"Condoms don't always work."*	*"I feel very embarrassed when I buy condoms and using them ruins sex."*	Condoms are *not* used

believes that condoms work and that the costs of using them are outweighed by the benefits. As a result, Person A uses condoms. In contrast, Person B feels little vulnerability, doesn't think AIDS is necessarily fatal, does not believe in the effectiveness of condoms, and thinks the personal costs of using them are high. Not surprisingly, this person doesn't use condoms.

The beliefs in this example have been intentionally polarized to make the contrast clear. In reality, a person may hold a range of beliefs adding up in such a way that prediction of behaviour is more difficult. For example, a woman might believe that she could get breast cancer and that it could be fatal. She might think the costs of breast self-examination (BSE) are low but lacks confidence in her ability to do BSE correctly, so she doesn't think the behaviour will work. What could we predict here? Perhaps sporadic attempts at BSE? It is difficult to be certain.

And what about Alan? The health belief model can help us predict the likelihood that he will attend the Healthy Heart program. To start, we would need to know if Alan believes he is vulnerable to a second heart attack and, if so, whether he thinks its consequences would be severe. In fact, he does believe that people who have had a heart attack are at increased risk for a second one and that people are much less likely to survive a second one than they were their first. Now we move to his beliefs regarding the behaviour that is supposed to affect that threat—the Healthy Heart program. We already know that he has considered the costs of attending. He is busy and thinks it will be inconvenient. There is his efficacy belief as well. Does he think the program will reduce the threat of a second heart attack? If he does, then he might attend. The problem is that he must *keep attending*, therefore his beliefs must be quite strong to keep him going.

Health Beliefs and Health Values. The health belief model attempts to predict behaviour using a person's specific beliefs regarding two main topics—the existence of a threat and the effectiveness of that behaviour to reduce the threat. There is one more important factor to consider, however. This is the extent to which the person values good health. Even if a person's beliefs would appear to predict a certain behaviour, such as condom use or breast self-examination, the behaviour will not follow unless the person values his or her health.

At first, it may be difficult to imagine that there are people who don't place a high value on their health. However, research indicates that people do vary in terms of their health values. To understand this, we must view values as being *relative* to each other. For example, an adolescent might value health to a certain extent, but he or she might value group acceptance more. This person might take up smoking, in spite of the fact that it compromises health, to achieve the more valued outcome of group acceptance.

It is also possible that some people can *afford* to place health values high on their list while other people must be more concerned with basic survival (Larson & Sutker, 1966). *Gender differences* also exist regarding health values. Women tend to value their health more than men do (Felton, Parsons, & Bartoces, 1997). Clear reasons exist, then, for individual differences in health values. These differences are important to consider because research has shown that the health belief model is most predictive for people who place a high value on their health (Lau, Hartman, & Ware, 1986).

How Well Does the Health Belief Model Predict Behaviour? If the health belief model is to be useful and thereby provide a good starting point for our study of health psychology, it must do a better-than-chance job of explaining and predicting health-related behaviour for those individuals who place a relatively high value on their health. For health psychologists, it is important to investigate the model's utility because, as we mentioned earlier, the model has the potential to make significant contributions to the **biopsychosocial** understanding of health and illness.

Given this importance, it is not surprising that a great deal of research has been conducted over the years testing the ability of the health belief model to explain and predict behaviour in a wide variety of health-related contexts, from exercise behaviour (Taggart & Connor, 1995) to motorcycle safety (Rutter, Quine, & Chesham, 1995).

One area in which the health belief model has been used extensively is AIDS-risk-related behaviours. DiFranceisco and colleagues (1998) used the health belief model to predict whether gay/bisexual men would complete a small-group program in HIV-risk reduction. The health belief model has also been used to explain some of the variance in sexual risk behaviours among college students, such as having multiple partners and being intoxicated or high during sexual encounters. It did not help, however, when it came to predicting condom usage for this group (Lollis, Johnson, & Antoni, 1997).

Some studies have produced more encouraging results than others when it comes to the ability of the health belief model to predict HIV-risk behaviour. Differences of opinion regarding the usefulness of the health belief model could be attributed to differences in the way the beliefs are measured and just what is being predicted. Specifically, some researchers use the model to predict *behaviour*, such as dropping out of a prevention program, while others use it to predict *intention* to engage in or avoid a particular behaviour. For example, some researchers (e.g., Bakker et al., 1997) argue that the health belief model can be used to explain differences in people's *intention* to practise safe sex. Taken in sum, the research using the health belief model in AIDS-related contexts appears promising, but it cannot be used exclusively to explain differences in sexual behaviour putting people at risk for HIV infection.

The health belief model has also been used to predict breast self-examination. It stands to reason that self-examination behaviours would be well suited to analysis by the health belief model. These behaviours are likely to be motivated, in part, by beliefs about vulnerability and the importance of early detection. Consistent with this, the health belief model has been proven useful in predicting BSE (Barron, Houfek, & Foxall, 1997; Champion, 1990, 1993; Ellingson & Yarber, 1997; Savage & Clarke, 1996).

In general, behaviours associated with screening for cancer can be analyzed reasonably well using the health belief model, given that important issues of perceived vulnerability and belief in the value of early detection fit well within the model. The model is far less than perfect in this context, though, because of other psychological factors. Perhaps the most notable is the role that *emotion* plays in cancer screening.

FOCUS ON RESEARCH 1-1

Checking Yourself Out

Roger Katz, Kelly Meyers, and Jennifer Walls (1995) have conducted research on cancer awareness and self-examination practices in young men and women. Their purpose was to test the usefulness of the health belief model in predicting whether college students practise self-examination (SE) for breast or testicular cancer.

To test this, 178 college men and women completed a series of questionnaires, including the Testicular Cancer Awareness Survey (completed by the men) and the Breast Cancer Awareness Survey (completed by the women). Personality scales were also completed, including measures of health locus of control, perceived social support, and hypochondriasis.

They found that women were more fearful of developing breast cancer than men were of developing testicular cancer. Consistent with this perception of vulnerability, women were significantly more likely to practise SE. Thirty percent of women practised SE compared to 19 percent of the men. Fear of cancer and confidence in doing the SE correctly were significantly correlated with actually practising SE. Women were better informed about breast cancer than men were about testicular cancer, however those practising SE were not necessarily those with the most knowledge.

The authors concluded that the health belief model is supported by their data to the extent that fear of cancer (vulnerability beliefs) and confidence in ability (efficacy beliefs) help predict SE. Getting more people to practice SE involves more than making them knowledgeable. We must also send messages regarding vulnerability and efficacy.

Consider the example of a woman who feels vulnerable to breast cancer, believes the disease to be serious, and believes that BSE can work as an easy early detection strategy, but *does not want to know* if she has breast cancer because of fears associated with the disease. With this in mind, Millar (1997) has argued that a woman's emotional state associated with BSE must be considered. In support of this argument, it has been found that women whose coping style could be called anxious and defensive are less likely to practise BSE (Barron et al., 1997).

Of course, this consideration of emotion is not restricted to women's health behaviours. Indeed, among college students, men are significantly less likely to practise self-examination for, in their case, testicular cancer (Katz, Meyers, & Walls, 1995).

CASE 1-3 Surgery or Bed Rest for Back Pain? An application of the Health Belief Model

Stan is a 45-year-old construction worker with persistent low back pain. The first indication that something was wrong came when he tried to get out of bed one morning. An intense shot of pain in his back and down his left leg sent him back onto the bed. He got to his feet carefully and managed to get to work, where the pain came and went during the day. This persisted for 2 weeks, with Stan missing 3 days of work during that period.

Stan's family physician referred him to a neurologist. The neurologist told Stan that he had a herniated disk between his third and fourth lumbar vertebrae.

The condition persisted. Finally, on a return visit to the neurologist, Stan was told that he had two options: surgery or prolonged bed rest. The neurologist recommended surgery, explaining that the success rates for the procedure were high and the risks relatively low. He emphasized, though, that the final decision would be Stan's.

The health belief model can be used in this case study to understand the decision faced by Stan. If we can get an accurate measure of Stan's beliefs relevant to this decision, we can do a better-than-chance job of predicting what his decision will be. Let's refer to Table 1.2 and fill in Stan's beliefs.

In this case, Stan's beliefs are such that he chooses surgery. Given the existence of the debilitating pain, it would be difficult, if not impossible, for him to ignore the existence of the threat. This means that we can focus on his beliefs regarding the behaviour or action—in this case, the surgery.

If he doubts the effectiveness of the surgery, or if he believes there would be serious costs, Stan would probably try bed rest first, which could last from 3 to 6 weeks. Of course, we could chart his beliefs regarding bed rest too. These could then be weighed against his beliefs regarding surgery. The advantage of bed rest, according to the health belief model, is that Stan may perceive it to have fewer potential costs than surgery. Others, though, might consider the prospect of up to 6 weeks in bed to be a high cost and thus opt for the surgery if they believed it would be effective.

TABLE 1-2 The Health Belief Model Applied to the Decision to Have Back Surgery

General Belief	A Health Threat Exists		A Behaviour Will Affect the Threat		Result
Related Beliefs	Beliefs regarding personal vulnerability to the threat	Beliefs about the severity of the consequences	The belief that a course of action will actually work or not	The assessment of the costs and benefits associated with this action	
Stan	*"I definitely have a back problem."*	*"I am in pain. I can't work and I can't enjoy my life."*	*"Surgery will correct this problem."*	*"I'm nervous about the possibility of being paralyzed but the risk is low."*	Stan chooses surgery

We have introduced the health belief model in this first chapter because it is a good example of the way in which psychological constructs can be applied to our understanding of health and health behaviour. It is a model that continues to be widely used and refined, with research going into the improvement of measurement tools and appropriate applications (for a review, see Strecher, Champion, & Rosenstock, 1997). We will return to the health belief model in Chapter 4 when we discuss health promotion.

The health belief model was derived from other theories in social and cognitive psychology designed to predict behaviour from beliefs. Two of these related theories, the *Theory of Reasoned Action* and its relative, the *Theory of Planned Behaviour*, have been applied directly to health-related thinking and behaviour. Let's take a look at each.

The Theory of Reasoned Action

The **Theory of Reasoned Action** (Ajzen & Fishbein, 1980; Fishbein & Ajzen, 1975) shares a number of things in common with the health belief model, while adding some other considerations. As we explain the theory, it will be helpful if you can appreciate these similarities and differences. One important assumption of the Theory of Reasoned Action is that behaviour is preceded by *intention*. Alan will not attend the Healthy Heart program until he *intends* to do so. Thus, understanding the link between thinking and intention is an important step to understanding how beliefs lead to behaviour.

The two main elements of the Theory of Reasoned Action are a person's attitudes toward a behaviour and the person's beliefs regarding other people's thoughts about the behaviour. It is this introduction of other people's beliefs that most strongly differentiates the Theory of Reasoned Action from the health belief model. In the language of the theory, other people's beliefs help us to develop **subjective norms**—what we think other people want us to do.

To illustrate the potentially powerful role that other people can play in our health-related decisions, let's revisit Case Study 1.3. Stan has to decide whether to treat his back pain with surgery or bed rest. In that case study, we did not include a discussion of what other people think. We could have included discussions Stan may have had with friends and coworkers who faced a similar decision, or we could have taken a broader perspective and included information regarding the prevailing beliefs within the health care system regarding surgery. According to the Theory of Reasoned Action, this would have increased our understanding of the nature of Stan's decision and increased the accuracy of our prediction regarding what that decision would be.

For example, if Stan lived in Ontario, he would be one-third as likely to receive surgical treatment for his back problem than if he lived in Washington State (Taylor et al., 1998). To be sure, there are many possible reasons for this regional difference beyond the Theory of Reasoned Action, such as who controls hospital budgets and what technology is available across each province or state. Still, it is interesting to speculate on the potential influence of different subjective norms in these settings. For one thing, people in Washington State are three times more likely to know people who have had surgery, which will affect their norms.

According to the Theory of Reasoned Action, we consider our attitudes toward a behaviour and our subjective norms to determine our *intention* regarding the behaviour. As in the health belief model, we have related beliefs to consider for each of these two main elements of the Theory of Reasoned Action. Specifically, our attitudes toward a behaviour are influenced by our beliefs regarding the *outcomes* it will bring about and the extent to which we *value* that outcome.

Subjective norms are composed of beliefs regarding what others think we should do and the extent to which we are motivated to go along with these people. To put all this together and apply the theory to health, let's look at Table 1.3.

Table 1.3 charts two people facing a decision similar to the one faced by Stan in Case Study 1.3. Person A believes that the surgery will work, so he sees a connection between the behaviour (surgery) and the outcome (pain relief). He values a pain-free existence. His friends and family are in favour of surgery and he wants them to have a favourable impression of him. These beliefs lead to a decision to choose surgery.

In contrast, Person B is not convinced of the efficacy of the surgery, nor does he place as high a value on being pain free. His subjective norms oppose surgery; namely, his wife favours bed rest and he values his wife's opinion. Consistent with these beliefs, surgery is not chosen.

As we did with Table 1.1 in relation to the health belief model, in Table 1.3 we have created two people with diametrically opposed views. In reality, our beliefs are more mixed than this. We may really want to engage in a health-related behaviour (be it surgery, a low-sodium diet, etc.) but find that our friends are opposed to it. It should also be noted that the process by which we *choose* people when creating subjective norms can be quite complicated (Kahneman & Miller, 1986). For example, we take into account such things as friendship and how similar they are to us. This is part of what we mean by the *social* component of the biopsychosocial approach.

How Well Does the Theory of Reasoned Action Predict Health Behaviour? It isn't surprising that modern research using the Theory of Reasoned Action has addressed many of the same phenomena as that using the health belief model. Thus, we find studies testing the power of the Theory of Reasoned Action for predicting HIV risk and prevention behaviours (e.g., Baker et al., 1996) and cancer screening behaviours (e.g., Barling & Moore, 1996). The Theory of Reasoned Action has also been applied to an understanding of exercise behaviour (e.g., Olson & Zanna, 1987).

TABLE 1-3 The Theory of Reasoned Action

General Belief	Attitudes Toward the Behaviour		Subjective Norms		Result
Related Beliefs	Belief that the behaviour will produce a given outcome	The value placed on the outcome	Beliefs regarding what other people think regarding the behaviour	Motivation to do what other people think should be done	
Person A	*"Surgery will relieve the pain in my back."*	*"I would love to be pain free again."*	*"My friends and family think I should have the back operation."*	*"I want my friends and family to know I have the courage to have the operation."*	Surgery chosen
Person B	*"Surgery might not work. There's no guarantee."*	*"Being pain free isn't really possible. Everyone lives with some degree of pain."*	*"My wife thinks I should try bed rest before risking surgery."*	*"My wife is usually right."*	Surgery not chosen

In a scan of the literature, we see that the Theory of Reasoned Action does a good job of predicting behaviours related to HIV and AIDS prevention. The addition of social norms tends to increase its predictive power over that of the health belief model. For example, Baker and colleagues (1996) surveyed over 700 heterosexual clients at a sexually transmitted disease (STD) clinic. They discovered that social norms and attitudes toward condom use were significant predictors of respondents' intentions to use condoms. For men in that study, social norms worked better as a predictor of intended condom use if the men had a steady partner than if they were with casual partners. This is consistent with the Theory of Reasoned Action, in that men with steady partners are probably more motivated to follow their partners' beliefs, a factor related to the social norms component of the theory. Similarly, Morrison, Gillmore, and Baker (1995) found that the Theory of Reasoned Action worked well to predict both intention and actual condom use among high-risk heterosexual adults, again attending an STD clinic.

In terms of cancer screening behaviour, the Theory of Reasoned Action predicts the intention to do self-examination (breast and testicular) very well (Moore, Barling, & Hood, 1998). The theory has also been used to explain differences in women's intentions to be screened for cervical cancer via a Pap smear test (Barling & Moore, 1996).

Interestingly, the Theory of Reasoned Action has also been used to predict *physician* behaviour. Susan Millstein (1996) used the theory to explain differences in physicians' delivery of preventive services (in this case, the education of adolescents about STD transmission). Millstein found that the predictive power of the theory increased significantly if she included a measure of **perceived behavioural control**. By this, she was referring to the physicians' beliefs that they were, in fact, in control of the delivery of those preventive services.

The Theory of Planned Behaviour

Millstein's finding that the predictive power of the Theory of Reasoned Action is generally improved with the addition of the notion of perceived behavioural control is consistent with the thinking of Fishbein and Ajzen, the psychologists who proposed the theory in 1975. In fact, Fishbein and Ajzen developed a hybrid theory, by including perceived behavioural control, and named it the **Theory of Planned Behaviour** (Fishbein & Ajzen, 1975).

The only difference between the two theories is the addition of the belief that the person is actually capable of performing the behaviour. "Can I really quit smoking?" "Can I go through with the operation?" These are questions about perceived behavioural control. The answer must be "Yes" for the Theory of Planned Behaviour to predict that intention will follow belief.

The Theory of Planned Behaviour can be a powerful tool to help explain variation in health-related intention and behaviour. For example, Marcoux and Shope (1997) found that the theory explained 76 percent of the variance in adolescents' intention to use alcohol. In other words, the elements of the theory combine to correlate highly with adolescents' reports of intention to drink. As one might expect, the Theory of Planned Behaviour has been used as widely as the Theory of Reasoned Action to analyze a wide range of behaviours, such as when students begin to smoke cigarettes (Hill et al., 1997), whether college students will use sunscreen (Hillhouse, Adler, Drinnon, & Turrisi, 1997), and whether people will practise safe sex (Helweg-Larsen & Collins, 1997).

How can the Theory of Planned Behaviour help us predict whether Alan will attend the Healthy Heart program? To answer this question, let's consider each of the elements of the theory. First, like the health belief model, there are Alan's beliefs regarding the efficacy of the program and the value he places on not having another heart attack. Then there are the subjective norms. Would other people want him to go to the program? For example, his wife might really encourage him to attend, or she might see it as an unnecessary inconvenience, as Alan does. Also, we must know whether Alan is motivated to do what his wife thinks he should do, or whether he would rather assert his independence and either not go or go in opposition to her wishes. Finally, there is perceived behavioural control. Does Alan really believe that he can do the things the Health Heart program will expect of him in terms of exercise, diet, tests, and so on? According to the Theory of Planned Behaviour, the answers to these questions will determine whether Alan intends to go to the program.

Beliefs about Personal Control: Locus of Control and Self-Efficacy

Social psychologists would not be surprised to find that we learn more about health behaviour by taking control beliefs into account. It was, after all, back in the late 1950s that Phares (1957) introduced the notion of **locus of control**, the extent to which we believe the events in our lives are controlled internally by us or externally by outside forces. This construct was refined by Rotter (1996) and a scale was devised to measure it.

Our beliefs regarding control can affect our behaviour. We choose different courses of action depending upon whether we believe we have the power to affect outcomes or that we are helpless. As demonstrated by the Theory of Planned Behaviour, control beliefs specific to health behaviours play a role in determining that behaviour. Given this relationship, it would make sense to develop a scale that measured health-specific control beliefs. This is what

Wallston and colleagues did when they created the **Multidimensional Health Locus of Control Scale (MHLC)** (Wallston, Wallston, & DeVellis (1978).

This 18-item scale presents a series of straightforward statements intended to assess the extent to which people think their health is under their control, under the control of such factors as luck or fate, or under the control of "powerful others" such as physicians and other health care staff. People's scores on these three dimensions (internal, external, and powerful-other) are correlated with health-related behaviour. The MHLC has been widely used in studies that have attempted to find correlations between thinking and health behaviour. There have been over 900 studies published in the past 10 years using health locus of control as a variable.

Some of the best applications of the MHLC have been in settings in which people must be motivated to comply with a program or to overcome adversity. For example, locus of control is related to diabetics' ability to control their diabetes (Stenstroem, Wikby, Andersson, & Ryden, 1998); people with an internal orientation control their diabetes better. It is also related to physical functioning among people who are in rehabilitation for returning to work (Wiegmann & Berven, 1998). In their study, Wiegmann and Berven found that people with higher scores on the internal and powerful-other dimensions showed the most improvement. Similarly, people with spinal cord injuries have been shown to make better life adjustments if they have an internal orientation (Krause, Stanwyck, & Maides, 1998).

Because of studies like these, health psychologists generally view an internal orientation to be a good thing. Yet, there are other important issues to consider before we try to convince everyone to adopt this orientation. These issues relate primarily to the realities of being sick.

For many people, being sick means giving up a certain amount of control over their lives. This is especially true for hospitalized patients who find themselves in what sociologists call a **total institution**—a place in which almost all of a patient's behaviours are controlled by hospital staff. This is compounded, of course, by the fact that most illnesses wrestle some control away from us by confining us to bed or otherwise restricting our activities.

Given these realities, how reasonable is it for health psychologists to encourage an internal orientation in their clients? This is an important question, because an overemphasis on internal control in the face of strong external factors can be stressful. It can also be upsetting if the patient takes personal responsibility for disease progression or recovery rates that might, in truth, be beyond his or her control.

With this in mind, Newsom and colleages looked at the relationship between perceptions of control and symptoms of depression among people with recurring cancer (Newsom, Knapp, & Schulz, 1996). One important assumption of this study was that we don't simply have a set of general control beliefs; they also come in a number of specific forms. For example, we have beliefs about what should be blamed for cancer, the extent to which onset can be prevented or controlled, or to what degree symptoms and side effects can be controlled. The researchers found that, over an 8-month period, depression among patients with recurrent cancer was significantly related to what they called **onset control**—the greater the patient's belief that the onset of the illness could have been controlled or avoided, the greater the depression when it recurred.

This depression could develop from a number of different thoughts. It may stem from a sense of **learned helplessness**, in which the patient despairs that his or her situation cannot be remedied no matter what he or she does. It may also be related to **self-blame**, the patient's belief that somehow he or she is personally responsible for the illness. Though little current research has been conducted on the nature of self-blame in cancer patients, one study (Malcarne, Compas, Epping-Jordan, & Howell, 1995) did find that self-blame was *not* related to control beliefs, though it was related to psychological distress. Presumably, then, while self-blame is a problem for those coping with cancer, it is not necessarily the result of an internal orientation. We'll have more to say about control beliefs in Chapter 5 when we look at stress and coping.

The Stages of Change Model

When we look at the topic of health promotion in Chapter 4, we will see that an important challenge for health psychologists involves helping people make changes to their lives. In many cases, these changes involve aspects of lifestyle, as we have seen with Alan in Case Studies 1.1 and 1.2. In others, changes are forced upon us by illness, accident, or aging. Because change is such a major topic, a model that describes the ways people go about effecting change (or not) would be most helpful.

The *Stages of Change Model* provides just such a description (Prochaska & DiClemente, 1983; 1986). In this model, change is broken down into five stages: precontemplation, contemplation, action, maintenance, and relapse. Though these stages are simple enough to comprehend, they can be very valuable as a way to understand health behaviour and, in particular, behaviour involving a lifestyle change. One of the most common applications of the Stages of Change Model is to smoking cessation. The people in the precontemplation stage have not thought about quitting and see no need to do so. People in the contemplation stage may have some symptom or nagging thought that has them considering quitting. In the next stage, they take action. Perhaps they see their physician, or use patches, or make a pact with a friend. If the action works, then they must maintain their non-smoking behaviour.

One of the most valuable contributions of the model is the acknowledgment of relapse as a stage rather than as failure. This allows the person to deal with a bout of cigarette smoking as something that is part of the process, rather than as a sign that the entire lifestyle change has failed. They can then get back into the maintenance stage, rather than starting over.

Summary of the Models

You may have wondered, as you read through these theories, just how well they apply across different cultures. For example, the notion of internal locus of control tends to make more sense to people who have been raised in **individualist** rather than **collectivist** cultures (Hart & Poole, 1995; Triandis et al., 1988). Individualists focus on independence and self-reliance, whereas collectivists see themselves as part of a greater whole in which one's individualism is less important than allegiance to the group.

The Theory of Reasoned Action and the Theory of Planned Behaviour have been tested with Latin American, English-speaking Caribbean, and South Asian participants (Godin et al., 1996). The conclusion was that the Theory of Planned Behaviour was more useful in these three cultures than the Theory of Reasoned Action, even though these cultures would be considered more collectivist than most Western cultures. This would suggest that the Theory of Planned Behaviour's inclusion of a measure of perceived control was still useful for cultures in which the orientation was more collectivist.

This brief introduction to some of the major theories and models common to health psychology was presented to give you an idea of some of the ways psychological theory has been applied to health and health care. The theories and models presented in this chapter grow, for the most part, from a cognitive perspective, with their focus on people's thought processes, attitudes, and beliefs. Of course, there are many other theories, some with a stronger behavioural emphasis, others more humanistic or psychodynamic. We will be referring to such models and theories throughout the remaining chapters of this book. We invite you to think critically about their utility and about ways in which they could be further developed to be even more useful.

WORKING IN HEALTH PSYCHOLOGY

Health psychology is a field that offers a number of interesting career opportunities. The vast majority of these require a graduate degree, usually a PhD. There are two main paths you can take when preparing for a career in health psychology. One is to be trained as a clinical or counselling psychologist. The other is to be trained as a researcher. Let's take a look at what these paths entail and what opportunities they provide.

Clinical and Counselling Psychologists Working in Health Psychology

Clinical and counselling psychologists require training that it distinct from one another. As a result, the roles each play in health psychology differ. Clinical psychologists must have either a master's or doctorate degree, depending upon the province or territory in which one is practising. The Canadian Psychological Association has recommended that all clinical psychologists hold a PhD. Clinical training usually involves a year of internship and, in some jurisdictions, students must pass a certification exam to be considered clinical psychologists.

Counselling psychologists do not require a PhD, though some will have one. The certification process for counselling psychologists tends to be less rigourous than for clinical psychologists. In fact, in some jurisdictions, no formal training is required to call oneself a counsellor. It is usually the case, though, that counsellors working in health settings have formal training at least at the master's level.

Clinical health psychologists work with people who are experiencing psychological problems that are either the result of illness or a cause of it. They may work with cancer patients who are suffering from depression, or breast reconstruction patients who are grappling with issues related to self-image. They may also work with people who suffer from anxiety and, as a result, are dealing with psychosomatic disorders. These are just a few of the types of people who benefit from a clinical health psychologist's intervention.

Clinical health psychologists might be employed by hospitals or they might work in private practice. Their salaries tend to be quite good, in keeping with what one might expect for a person with an advanced degree and considerable training who is dealing with challenging psychological issues related to health.

Counselling psychologists work with people in similar circumstances. For example, a counselling psychologist might work with a family in which a member is seriously ill. Another might work with someone who is recovering from an injury or illness and is trying to integrate back into work and society. As is the case with clinical health psychologists, there is plenty of work for a skilled counselling psychologist working in health-related settings. Their salaries tend to be somewhat lower than those of clinical psychologists, though they can still do very well financially. Similar work might also be conducted by people in other helping professions, such as social work.

Research Careers in Health Psychology

Not all people working in health psychology have clinical training. Some are trained in other fields, such as social or developmental psychology, and they apply the theories of those disciplines to health and health care. Indeed, some of the major theories we introduced earlier in the chapter were forwarded by social psychologists. A good example is the Theory of Reasoned Action developed by Fishbein and Ajzen. Instead of providing clinical services, psychologists from these other areas conduct research and consult with health professionals regarding aspects of health care delivery.

Most people conducting research in health psychology hold academic appointments at universities, though some are employed by other institutions such as hospitals and cancer agencies. Most hold doctorate degrees. Those working in universities combine their research duties with teaching and other responsibilities common to an academic position. Of course, it is important to point out that clinical work and research are not mutually exclusive. Many people do both, either from private practice, institutional appointments, or university positions.

KEY TERMS

biofeedback
behavioural medicine
behavioural health
health psychology
psychosomatic medicine
germ theory
behaviourist
gradient of reinforcement
delayed gratification
asymptomatic
coping styles
monitors
blunters
psychoneuroimmunology (PNI)
immunocompetence
malignant neoplasms
carcinogenic
medical geography
demographic differences
medical anthropologists
medical sociologists
epidemiologists
biopsychosocial approach
biomedical model
health belief model
efficacy belief
cost-gain belief
theory of reasoned action
subjective norms
perceived behavioural control
theory of planned behaviour
locus of control
multidimensional health locus of control scale (MHLC)
total institution
onset control
learned helplessness
self-blame
stages of change model
individualist cultures
collectivist cultures

Chapter 2

CONDUCTING RESEARCH IN HEALTH PSYCHOLOGY

Chapter Outline

Key Questions

1. What are the different ways researchers learn about health psychology?
2. How much control can researchers actually exert over situations when conducting studies in health psychology?
3. What terminology must I learn to be able to understand health psychology research?
4. What challenges do health psychology researchers face, and what would it be like to conduct this research?
5. When I read studies in health psychology, what do I need to know to evaluate them intelligently?

A group of psychologists and students is sitting around a table. The group has been asked to submit a research proposal to investigate some important psychosocial aspect of cancer. The group is considering a set of research questions. The possibilities are both exciting and daunting. With so much to study in this area, where should they begin? Should they look at personality variables? Communication issues? Social variables? Fortunately, they have a fairly good knowledge of the literature in these areas, so they know what has already been done.

After discussing this literature, the group decides that, though social support has been studied quite extensively in women with cancer, more study is needed in this area for men who have cancer. Now they must decide *how* they will study social support in male cancer patients. Do they want to do a descriptive study that finds out how much support there is and what forms it takes? Do they want to know if social support is related to coping or disease progression? Do they want to know if social support is *causally* linked to experiences with cancer?

The answer to all these questions is probably, "Yes." However, no single study can address them all. The research group has to decide whether their study will be descriptive, correlational, experimental, or some combination of the three. Do they want to do longitudinal work in which they follow patients through the entire progression of their disease, or do they want to do cross-sectional work using a number of groups from different age categories? How will they measure social support and the other variables of interest? These are just a few of the decisions the group will have to make.

In this chapter, you will develop an understanding of the way research is conducted in health psychology. In so doing, you will take a step toward being able to make the sorts of decisions facing the research group investigating social support in male cancer patients, as well as those faced by others doing research in health psychology.

Health psychology is an *applied* discipline. This means that psychologists working in this field spend more time *using* theories to explain real-world phenomena than they do *developing* the theories. This doesn't mean that health psychologists don't ever develop theories. You learned in Chapter 1 that there are a number of key theories in the field. You might have noticed, though, that these theories grew from pre-existing theories taken from other domains in psychology, such as social psychology.

THE GENERAL CHALLENGES OF APPLIED RESEARCH

This applied focus in health psychology means that much of the research conducted in the field is **applied research**, which is designed to solve real-world problems. This type of research is usually contrasted with **basic research**, where the primary goal is to learn about fundamental psychological processes like memory or sleep patterns. Applied research comes with its own unique set of challenges. Primary among these is that applied research must be *relevant.* While basic researchers can study a phenomenon for its own sake, applied researchers usually need some *practical outcome* for their work. For example, program improvement, improved coping, and wellness are goals of applied research.

This is not to imply that one kind of research is better or more virtuous than the other. Obviously, some vital discoveries have been made by those doing basic research in psychology. In fact, without basic research applied research would have little to apply! It is often the job of those doing applied research to take those discoveries and put them to work solving problems in a field like health psychology. For example, many years ago psychologists doing basic research in memory function found that when items were presented in a series or list, the items at the beginning and end of that list were more likely to be remembered. This is called the *serial-position effect*. Health psychologists have conducted applied research by taking that finding and determining if it is applicable to the way physicians give instructions to patients. Can communication be improved if physicians state the most important point of their instructions at the beginning and then again at the end? You won't be surprised to learn that the answer is "Yes." This takes advantage of the serial-position effect and of repetition.

In addition to requiring practical outcomes, applied research is challenging because it often takes place in the actual settings in which the application is to be made. In health psychology, this means doing a great deal of research in hospitals and clinics. These field experiments, which are conducted in real-life settings, can be difficult to carry out. Hospitals are very busy places with mandates that do not always include cooperation with research projects. The primary focus of the professionals working in hospitals is the care of the patient, not the completion of someone's research.

Psychosocial research in hospitals can be very intrusive. Imagine conducting a study in which nurses were asked to follow a script that differed from what they were used to. Now, in addition to concentrating on the patient, the nurses must also pay attention to this new protocol. Through all of this, patient care cannot be compromised. This means that close consultation must take place between practitioners and researchers before conducting hospital research in which routine is altered. To complicate matters, this consultation is time consuming, and practitioners usually don't have the luxury of spare time.

The intrusions of this research are not restricted to the practitioners. There are the patients to consider as well. For example, just trying to enlist the participation of patients in hospital settings can be problematic. Patients might not be at their most receptive immmediately before undergoing a nuclear medicine test in which they may find that they have cancer, or before cardiac catheterization, in which a probe is going to be inserted into one of their coronary arteries. All the same, it is vital that we learn about the psychology involved in patients undergoing such tests and procedures to help patients cope and to guide practitioners (see Chapter 7, Hospital Stays and Medical Procedures).

Psychologists deal with these methodological challenges by devising careful ways of enlisting patient participation. We will look at one of these methods in this chapter. These procedures are more labour intensive than putting up a sheet for university students to sign so they can get course credit, which is a common way of soliciting participants in many laboratory studies.

Perhaps the greatest challenge is that field research is never "tidy", in that there are always going to be numerous variables that a researcher cannot control. Imagine being the researcher in the following example:

> A patient arrives 30 minutes early for her computed tomography (CT) scan so that she can fill out your questionnaires. However, the clinic is running a bit ahead of schedule on this day and the patient is asked to come in for her scan before she has finished completing the questionnaires. She offers to finish them after the scan. Other patients in the study completed all the questionnaires before the scan, but you don't want to lose valuable data, since so few patients fit the inclusion criteria for the study. So you take her up on her offer to complete them afterwards. The patient returns from her scan 45 minutes later, willing to complete the questionnaires. Unfortunately, she was feeling a bit anxious just before her scan and so she was given a mild tranquillizer. Will her data still be of value?

Unlike laboratories, hospitals are not controlled environments. Each patient brings a host of unique variables into the equation. As you will see later in this chapter, researchers try to control for these differences by matching the characteristics of patients in various treatment groups. But the match is never perfect.

This does not mean that good psychological research cannot be conducted in hospitals or other field settings. Indeed, we believe that a person trained in psychological principles can hardly walk through a hospital without generating important hypotheses about its workings. It must be kept in mind, however, that such research is very challenging and, by its very nature, less precise than laboratory experimentation. In response to this, researchers in health psychology *do* conduct laboratory work when feasible. When they conduct field work, they are careful to control as many extraneous variables as possible. Even so, researchers draw conclusions that take unavoidable limitations of such work into account.

DESCRIPTIVE VERSUS EXPLANATORY RESEARCH

In our opening example, we met a group of researchers who were in the early stages of designing a research program. It was at this time that they had to make decisions regarding the fundamental goals of the research. If their primary purpose was to measure the extent to which certain phenomena existed, they would be conducting descriptive research. As the term clearly implies, the goal of this research is to take "snapshots" of the way things are. What forms does social support take for men with cancer? Are they satisfied with their support? Does it differ from one type of cancer to another? These are some of the questions that could be answered with descriptive research.

If you are reading a journal article and the authors state that their work was descriptive in nature, don't expect to find hypotheses tested. Descriptive studies don't make predictions about results. Instead, their contribution is derived from careful methods that shed light on phenomena we knew little about before the research. Data from descriptive studies tend to be in the form of frequency distributions, group means, correlations, and qualitative anecdotal summaries. You might already know that these are often called descriptive statistics. Descriptive studies often represent important starting points for research programs.

In contrast, explanatory research is designed to discover relationships between phenomena, often in the form of cause and effect (Jackson, 1999). Hypotheses, which are predictions about expected results, are formulated and tested in explanatory research. As such, explanatory studies are much more likely to have a theoretical basis, which is to say the hypotheses and methods are justified by referring to established theory. For example, the researchers in our example may formulate the hypothesis that men who attend support groups cope with cancer better than men who do not attend such groups. This hypothesis is consistent with social comparison theory, which states that, in times of uncertainty, we turn to others for important information or to gauge our well-being. If the researchers adopt this theoretical stance, then they will want to include questions about this comparison process when they collect data from cancer patients who either attend or don't attend support groups.

There are those who believe that adopting a given theoretical stance prior to collecting data might result in biased research. As an alternative, they propose that the theory should be developed *as data are collected*. In other words, the theory should be grounded in the data. Hence, this research method is called grounded theory (Glaser & Strauss, 1967). Grounded theory provides a particularly useful approach for observational research, because it reduces the likelihood that observers will enter into the research with preconceived notions that will blind them to certain observations or cause them to see things that actually aren't there. We will discuss observational research in more detail shortly.

Data from explanatory studies tend to be more complex in nature. Such studies will report inferential statistics. These are statistics that allow us to draw *inferences* regarding real differences between groups in the population and about cause-effect relationships. For example, in their study of cancer patients, the researchers will want to know more than mean coping scores. They will also want to know if these differences are significant, and thus attributable to support group attendance, or if they could have occurred by chance.

Now that we know something about the general purposes of research in health psychology, let's look at the different types of research that are conducted. As we do so, you will notice that other purposes become evident. For example, some research is intended to *evaluate* programs while other research attempts to improve our ability to *predict* certain outcomes. Of course, it is also common for one research project to have more than one of these purposes.

OBSERVATIONAL METHODS: LEARNING BY LOOKING

One of the most fundamental ways to learn about phenomena in health psychology is to observe them. The research group in our opening example could choose to attend support group meetings and take notes on what goes on there. They could try to learn something about group dynamics, leadership, and the content of the sessions. This is observational research, and it is almost always descriptive in its purpose. This method might seem straightforward on the surface, but there are many challenges inherent in this form of research. We'll explore some of these challenges in the following example.

Imagine that you wanted to study communication between physicians and their patients. You might decide that the best place to start would be with an observational design. To be of value, your observations would have to be made in real-life settings—actual consultations between physicians and their patients. Your first challenge presents itself: how do you make your observations without getting in the way? In the language of observational methodology, how can you be **unobtrusive**? Just by being there, you would change the nature of the interaction you were hoping to observe. Will you hide behind a screen? A one-way mirror? Not likely. These solutions are both awkward and unethical. The patients and physicians must consent to being observed, and so they will know their behaviour is being monitored.

Maybe technology can help. There is audio tape. This method is much less obtrusive but you would lose valuable visual information that might help you understand non-verbal behaviour. There is videotape. The camera is more obtrusive, but perhaps if you set it up inconspicuously enough people will forget it is there and you will get to observe some fairly natural behaviour.

Let's say that you did manage to get these videotapes and participants report afterwards that they did forget the camera was in the room. This is a good start. But what are you going to do with these tapes? When you begin to view them, you realize that there is a great deal going on in them. Body positions are shifting, words are zipping back and forth between patient and practitioner, other non-linguistic sounds like "uh" and "mmm" are coming out, and it's all happening so fast. You have just encountered another challenge of observational research: knowing *what* to observe. You're lucky. You have videotape that you can replay and even slow down if necessary. Those making real-time observations with the naked eye don't have these luxuries.

To help meet the challenge of having so much to observe, researchers adopting this method often pick one of two kinds of observation: **natural** or **systematic** (Cozby, 1993). Natural observation is more global in nature. It looks at larger pictures, attempting to determine, generally, what is going on in a give situation or context. Systematic research takes a more focused approach. It is intended to discover things like how often a specific phenomenon happens, or what specific forms a phenomenon takes. In our example, people using natural observation would try to get an overall impression of the nature of a medical encounter of this type. This might then provide direction for systematic observation, in which trained observers kept track of such things as the physical distance between participants, the number of questions a patient asks, or the body posture of the physician.

In observational research, nothing is manipulated. Observers try to become "part of the furniture", beginning with global, natural observation then moving to more systematic observation in subsequent stages of the program. From this, researchers might then try to identify variables that appear important enough to manipulate in research that takes on experimental, rather than observational, forms.

CASE STUDIES: CLOSE LOOKS AT ONE PERSON AT A TIME

In each chapter of this textbook, you will find a case study. These are usually narrative in nature, providing details about one person's life (or in some cases, comparing two or more individuals) that help us learn about some aspect of health psychology. In this book, some of these case studies are hypothetical. In research, real stories are used. **Case studies**, then, present such things as individual histories, symptoms, specific reactions, or treatment outcomes (Cozby, 1993). They can also be used at a more sociological level. As such, they would present descriptions of programs or institutions.

Our research group may want to trace the life of a prostate cancer patient to discover what role, if any, social support plays in his story. How does he describe his relationship with his wife? Did attending a support group represent some sort of turning point for him in his ability to cope with his prostate cancer? These case studies, and the testimonials they feature, can provide valuable insights into men's experiences with the disease.

The basic assumption behind case studies is that much can be learned by looking at individual cases on an in-depth basis, as opposed to analyzing large groups through statistics such as averages or correlations. This latter method employs what is called a **nomothetic approach**. Behaviour is studied by looking at group trends. Case studies use an **idiographic approach**, in which the richness of individual stories is considered valuable.

If you examine major medical journals like the *Canadian Medical Association Journal*, the *New England Journal of Medicine*, or the *Journal of the American Medical Association*, you will find numerous case studies. Some are very biomedical in nature, but some are more psychosocial. Try looking for cases in which psychological issues or ethical dilemmas are presented by contributing physicians. For example, a case study about whether to put an 80-year-old man through difficult cancer treatment can provide real insights into the kinds of decisions practitioners face on a daily basis.

If you were to work with case studies, you would find that, as useful as they can be, there are also some problems with them as sources of data. Most obvious is the fact that

CASE 2-1 Taking Medicine by Mouth or through the Skin?

If we were to use a case study method to investigate communication in medical settings, we might discover that a particular patient had considerable difficulty controlling his high blood pressure using medication. A closer look at his story reveals that, at one point in his treatment, he was given *transdermal patches*. He had dutifully taken this medicine, but it had made him sick. The reason was that he was taking the patches orally rather than sticking them on his skin as directed. No one had told him what "transdermal"meant (literally, "through the skin"). And so, he had taken the medicine the way he had taken all other medicine in his life—he swallowed it. This one story speaks volumes for the problems that can arise when communication in medical settings is poor. Further complications arose when the man was given oral medication to take for his hypertension. He had become sensitized to it and was sick again. Now his physician had to deal with the problem of having a hypertensive patient who, for a time at least, could not take medication for his condition.

you are working with a very small sample size so you cannot be sure that it is representative of a larger population. Perhaps, when you were reading about the man with high blood pressure in Case Study 2.1, you commented, "How many people would swallow a transdermal patch?" It is a good question. We can't answer it through individual case studies, unless of course we did a large number of them, which would make our work nomothetic. Clearly, the tradeoff with case studies is that you get a great deal of detail at the expense of sample size. Case studies are often described as "*n* of 1, repeated measures." This means that the sample size is one, but you have many pieces of data. Perhaps you have been able to chart this person over the entire course of his or her life.

To do this type of charting, you probably will be working with case studies that are in the past tense. You are looking up files that fortunately contain quite a bit of detail. The problem is that you have no control over the collection of that data because the collection is over. It is not uncommon to be reading a case study and wish that the person who documented the story had paid attention to a detail that is central to your work. For example, in the case study of the man who swallowed the transdermal patch, we are not told what languages he speaks. This would be very helpful information when trying to learn about the problem he encountered.

In summary, case studies can be very valuable because they provide rich sources of data that are rarely obtainable using other methods featuring large groups. Also, the data become "personalized" rather than "dehumanized", which is important in a discipline like health psychology that prides itself on its human focus. The problems with case studies involve difficulties generalizing them to other people and in working with stories that, though detailed, are sometimes unavoidably incomplete.

SURVEY METHODS: TAKING SNAPSHOTS OF LARGE SAMPLES

Much of the data collected by social scientists working in health-related applications comes in the form of surveys. A well-designed survey can produce a wealth of information about a large group of people. It is particularly good for assessing trends in health behaviours and in the use of a health care system. For these reasons, you will find that much of the data available from sources like Statistics Canada have been collected through surveys. Statistics Canada publishes its findings in a number of forms. One of the most informative is a publication entitled *Health Reports*. Reviewing some of the titles featured in this quarterly publication will give you a sense of the kinds of things that can be learned through surveys. Table 2.1 provides some of the more recent titles.

TABLE 2-1 Sample Titles of Survey Research from Recent Issues of *Health Reports*

Issue	Title	Author(s)
Spring, 1999	Living with Heart Disease—The Working-Age Population	Helen Johansen
Spring, 1998	Multiple Medication Use among Seniors	Wayne J. Miller
Spring, 1998	Smoking Prevalence, Quit Attempts, and Successes	Megan Stephens and Jason Siroonian
Spring, 1998	Work Stress and Health	Kathryn Wilkins and Marie P. Beaudet

The Health Statistics Division of Statistics Canada provides extensive survey data on the health of Canadians. In fact, many of the articles featured in *Health Reports* derive their data from one large Canadian survey—the National Population Health Survey (NPHS). There are a number of obvious advantages of the NPHS to health researchers. First of all, the numbers are large and so the trends indicated by the survey are reliable. Second, the NPHS is administered regularly, which allows for comparisons across time periods. In recent years, it has been administered in 1994/95 and then again in 1996/97. Interestingly, a number of differences appeared in just 2 years. For example, it was discovered that smokers who reported having no activity limitations on the 1994/95 survey started to show such limitations by the 1996/97 survey, due to respiratory, heart, and other circulatory problems (Swain, Catlin, & Beaudet, 1999).

In British Columbia, the Adolescent Health Survey (McCreary Centre, 1993) collected data on adolescent health and risk behaviours from 15 549 youth in high schools throughout the province. Like the NPHS, the survey was administered again to allow for comparisons over time to be made. This was done in 1998, with approximately 25 500 high school students completing the survey. For more information on the Adolescent Health Surveys I and II, see Box 2.1.

BOX 2-1 The Adolescent Health Survey

In 1992, the McCreary Centre Society, with the support of British Columbia Health Units, carried out a survey of health status and risk behaviours in high school students in the Province of British Columbia. In 1990, the McCreary Centre Society began the development of the Adolescent Health Survey under the guidance of its Executive Director, Dr. Roger Tonkin. It was Dr. Tonkin's concern that there was relatively little information available on the health status of adolescents in British Columbia and that existing programs were based more on the attributions of adults than on the demonstrated needs of the population.

In 1992, the survey was administered to 15 549 students between grades 7 through 12 in approximately 840 classrooms across 174 schools in British Columbia. As the questionnaire was given in schools, 87 percent of all youth in the province were included in the sampling frame by virtue of their school attendance. This means that while the findings do not represent all youth in the province, they are very representative of those who attend school. The questionnaire is a self-administered paper and pencil format and contains 123 questions that were derived from sources such as the U.S. Centers for Disease Control and the World Health Organization. Extensive field testing in 1991 confirmed that the questionnaire could be comfortably administered within one school period.

The domains covered in the questionnaire include: physical health, chronic illness/disability, and mental health; behaviours resulting in intentional and unintentional injuries; sexuality, STDs, and pregnancy; tobacco, drug, and alcohol abuse; physical activities, school achievement, and self-esteem; nutrition, eating behaviours, and dietary disorders; and individual and family demographics.

Once school boards, superintendents, and/or principals gave their permission, a trained representative from the health unit went to the school to administer the questionnaire. The parents of students were contacted about the survey through a letter and informed that participation was anonymous and voluntary. This process highlights the distinction between *active* and *passive* consent. Clearly, research of this nature requires the consent of the parents, but the school districts varied in the manner in which parental consent was obtained. In 16 districts, students required the approval of their parents to participate in the study. This is *active* consent. By contrast, parents in the other 32 districts were only required to indicate if they did not want the child to participate. This is *passive* consent. Passive consent produced a response rate of 86 percent while active consent resulted in a response rate of 65 percent. The overall response rate was 74 percent. If one is planning to do survey research of this type, the form of consent required will clearly be important in determining the response rate.

Response rate was calculated by comparing the number of students in the selected schools who provided useable data with the number of students available. Non-responses occur for different reasons. In this survey, the largest source of non-responses was the failure to return active consent forms. The next two were absenteeism and parental refusal.

In the "data cleaning" process, approximately 1 percent of the questionnaires were deleted according to the following criteria: fewer than 50 percent of the questions were answered by an individual; inconsistent answers (for example, an individual who is not old enough to have a driver's licence indicating that they drink and drive; a *response set bias*—endorsing all items in the same manner even when they contradict one another.

Subsequent research using the survey has looked at such issues as street youth in Vancouver, chronic illness and disability among youth, and youth and AIDS. A research group of Simon Fraser University students has used the data to do research is such areas as eating disorders, resilience, sexual orientation, high-risk sexual behaviours, suicidality, quality of life, and participation in physical activity. In a general sense, the data have been used extensively by planners in health and education to develop programs, services, and prevention and health promotion initiatives for youth at the local, provincial, and national levels.

Following on the success of the initial survey, the project team decided to administer the survey again in 1998 to examine trends and emerging health issues in students in British Columbia since 1992. The 1998 survey included most of the questions from the 1992 survey, although a few items were deleted and some new questions added to increase the length to 127 items. The new questions were designed to cover such issues as: safety at school and at home; vegetarian diets; leisure activities (e.g., television, videos, Internet, and computer games) sunburn and skin cancer risk; sexually transmitted diseases; gambling; volunteering; and injury-prevention behaviour.

While it was considered important to add new items, it was also important to maintain the integrity of the questionnaire to allow for comparisons from 1992 to 1998. The selection process was a difficult one and involved an interesting tradeoff between change and stability in the questionnaire. Given the success of the 1992 survey, the Adolescent Health Survey II received increased participation from school districts around the province. Once again, the survey was based on a representative sample of students in grades 7 to 12 in 20 provincial regions. In the second administration, over 25 000 students completed the questionnaire.

Sample Items from the 1992 Survey

How often do you wear a seat belt when riding in a car driven by someone else?

- ❑ Never
- ❑ Rarely
- ❑ Sometimes
- ❑ Most of the time
- ❑ Always

How old were you when you smoked a whole cigarette for the first time?

- ❑ I have never smoked a whole cigarette
- ❑ Less than 9 years old
- ❑ 9 or 10 years old
- ❑ 11 or 12 years old
- ❑ 13 or 14 years old
- ❑ 15 or 16 years old
- ❑ 17 or more years old

At this time, how satisfied are you with your weight? (Mark the number which seems the closest to how you feel)

- ❑ 1 Not at all satisfied
- ❑ 2
- ❑ 3
- ❑ 4
- ❑ 5
- ❑ 6
- ❑ 7 Very satisfied

Conducting Survey Research Well

There are two fundamental questions that have to be answered at the outset of planning for conducting survey research. What do you want to know and who do you want to ask? These are straightforward enough questions, but researchers interested in survey methods soon discover that much planning must go into answering them. Let's look at them one at a time.

Designing a Survey: What Do You Want to Know?

It's amazing how often a research group goes over survey results only to have one of the group say, "If only we had asked ___!" This happens, in part, because it can be difficult to anticipate what all the important questions are the first time you administer a survey. For example, the second administration of the Adolescent Health Survey in 1998 included most of the questions from the initial survey in 1992, although a few items were deleted and some new questions were added. This was done to reflect current issues among youth. New items were concerned with topic areas such as: safety at school and in the home; vegetarian diets; gambling activities; sunburn (skin cancer risks); leisure activities (TV, videos, Internet, and computer games); and participation in sports and athletic activities.

Of concern here is striking a balance between keeping the survey relevant, allowing for comparisons across different administrations of the survey, and keeping the administration within acceptable time limits—one high-school period in this case. Items that are deleted from one administration of the survey are lost for purposes of comparison, yet it is not possible to continuously add new items without deleting others. It can be a difficult tradeoff.

Survey Wording

There are instances when the survey items should be worded directly. By "directly", we mean wording items in ways that make it perfectly clear what you are looking for. For example, imagine being given the task of designing a survey to measure anxiety in people undergoing a magnetic resonance imaging (MRI) examination. Many MRI scanners feature a rather narrow space, called a "bore", that the patient is placed in so pictures that look like sophisticated x-ray images can be taken. When designing your questionnaire, you might want to take this into account by exploring the extent to which *claustrophobia* (fear of enclosed spaces) is part of the patient's anxiety. You could design an item that asks directly, "Do you suffer from claustrophobia?" As relevant as this item appears, there may be problems with it. First, it requires a simple yes/no answer, so the patients don't get a chance to indicate the *degree* of claustrophobia they might have experienced or how many times they experienced it. Second, mentioning claustrophobia before the MRI examination might *sensitize* patients to its possibility and thereby increase their anxiety.

For these reasons, you might want to adopt a more indirect approach by including items in which patients are given hypothetical situations and asked how often they have felt uncomfortable in them. Among these you could include elevator rides, for example. Another indirect approach would be to focus on physical sensations such as heart rate that are associated with anxiety, rather than directly referring to anxiety or tension.

Obviously, the more indirect your items, the greater risk you run of measuring something other than what you intended. In many surveys designed by health psychologists, a direct approach works best. Still, when asking direct questions about a person's health or health-related behaviour, there are privacy issues and potential embarrassment to consider. Both of these concerns might affect the extent to which respondents reply honestly to the survey.

In the 1940s and 1950s, Alfred Kinsey and his associates conducted extensive interviews to learn about the range and frequency of people's sexual behaviours (Kinsey, Pomeroy & Martin, 1948; Kinsey et al., 1953). Of all survey research, Kinsey's must rank among the most problematic in terms of getting honest responses. Not only were respondents being asked questions about the most intimate aspects of their lives at a time when discussion of sexual topics was somewhat less liberated than it is today, they were being asked in face-to-face interviews. One of the researchers doing some of these interviews became as interested in the process as in the data (Pomeroy, 1972).

One of the valuable things that was learned from the Kinsey work was that the honesty of a response is affected by the way the item is worded. In particular, Kinsey and colleagues found that they got a wider range of responses if the options that respondents had to choose from implied a wide range of what was normal or acceptable. Compare these two items, for example:

How many times per week do you masturbate? ___

How many times per week do you masturbate? (Circle the correct number)

0   1–3   4–6   7–9   10–12   More than 12

In the second example, the respondent is given a scale that implies a broad range of normality. In Kinsey's face-to-face interviews, this technique was employed, along with a non-judgmental manner on the part of the interviewer.

There are other things to consider when deciding upon the wording of survey items. For example, researchers must decide if they want people to respond to statements or to questions. Statements allow for an assessment of how much the respondent agrees or disagrees with the statement, believes it to be true, believes it to be an accurate description of themselves, and so on. Questions can be closed- or open-ended (see Cozby, 1993). Closed-ended questions yield yes/no type answers. They are easy to code and quantify but provide limited insight into the thinking of the respondent. Open-ended questions yield prose. The data are richer but harder to code and summarize.

Another consideration is whether one item actually makes two statements or asks two questions. These are sometimes called **double-barrelled items**. Here is an example:

I overeat during exam time because of the stress of exams.

Never Rarely Sometimes Often Always

Let's say our respondent circles "never." Does this mean that the person never overeats at exam time, or that he or she overeats, but doesn't attribute it to exam stress? Maybe he or she thinks eating more aids concentration or increases energy levels.

Finally, it is important to keep one's biases out of the wording. For example, when constructing a survey about people's experiences in hospitals, the researcher's own beliefs would enter into an item that reads:

The quality of my hospital stay is diminished when hospital staff ask me needless questions.

Strongly Disagree Disagree Undecided Agree Strongly Agree

Let's say that 90 percent of survey respondents agreed or strongly agreed with this item and the researchers conclude that "Ninety percent of hospital patients have the quality of their stay diminished by needless questions asked by hospital staff." Perhaps this is an extreme example. Nevertheless, it illustrates the point that the wording of an item can "push" respondents in certain directions that are consistent with the researcher's bias, especially when the researchers draw conclusions that go beyond the meaning of the item, as is the case with our example.

Closely related to wording is question *order*. There are two important things to consider here. First, if a number of questionnaires are being administered together, is it possible that responses to one survey could be influenced by an earlier survey? For example, might people complete a patient satisfaction survey differently if they had just completed a survey on anxiety? To answer this question, half of the respondents should complete the anxiety survey first and the other half should complete the satisfaction survey first. This method, called **counterbalancing**, allows the researchers to assess possible order effects. Finally, it is generally accepted practice today to put questions about demographics (age, sex, income, and so on) at the end of the questionnaire rather than at the beginning. This decreases the likelihood that people will feel their responses are valued more or less because of the demographic group they fall into.

CORRELATIONAL METHODS: LOOKING FOR THINGS THAT CHANGE TOGETHER

For men with prostate cancer, it is possible that their ability to cope with the disease is related to their satisfaction with their social support. We might hypothesize that coping is *positively correlated* with social support. This means simply that as social support satisfaction increases, so does coping ability. These two variables change together—they *covary*. To test this hypothesis, we would conduct **correlational research**. This means that we would use statistical analyses to determine if these variables did, in fact, covary. Of course, the main statistic we would rely on would be correlation. Not surprisingly, correlational research is very common in health psychology.

Conceptually, correlations are not particularly complicated. For example, you need three things to do correlational analysis in our prostate cancer study. First, you need pairs of scores for a given individual. In this case, each man has a social support satisfaction score and a coping score. It would make no sense to correlate one man's satisfaction score with another man's coping score. Second, you should have a large sample of these men and it would be best if they varied on these scores. Third, you need variables with multiple levels, preferably measured on a continuum. Correlation would not be an appropriate statistic if you wanted to compare support group attendance (attenders and non-attenders) with surgical status (had surgery or have not had surgery). In fact, there are other variables that are more ideally suited to correlational analysis than satisfaction and coping scores. For example, age works well in correlational analysis because you can measure it right down to the day if necessary, whereas satisfaction scores are usually measured on a five- or seven-point scale, in which you cannot guarantee that the intervals between the points are arithmetically equal (e.g., is the distance between "somewhat satisfied" and "satisfied" the same as the distance between "satisfied" and "very satisfied"?)

Once you have your pairs of scores on appropriate variables, you can calculate your correlation. Basically, you have only three possibilities:

1. As one variable increases (or decreases), so does another. This would result in a **positive correlation**. For example, we would hypothesize a positive correlation between social support satisfaction and coping. Look at Figure 2.1A. This is a **scatterplot**. It is simply a plotting of the pairs of values for social support and coping. You will notice that the plot forms a pattern that slopes upward. The line drawn through the scatterplot is the one that comes closest to as many data points as possible. It is called the **line of best fit**. Notice that it has a positive slope. The slope of the line is positive and so is the correlation—this isn't just a coincidence.
2. As one variable increases, the other might decrease. This would result in a **negative correlation**. For example, we might hypothesize a negative correlation between social support satisfaction and illness progression. The better the support, the slower the illness progression (as measured by some biomedical indicator in which higher scores meant more progression of illness). Figure 2.1B illustrates a negative correlation. You can see that, as support satisfaction goes up (moving to the right on the x-axis), illness progression goes down. Remember that each data point represents a pair of scores for one individual. This means that many men would have to take part in this study to provide all the data points. Figure 2.1B does *not* tell us that, for one man, the more support sat-

isfaction he has the lower his biomedical scores will become. We are not talking about a study in which one man's scores are taken at a number of intervals over time. This is a study in which many men are measured *once*. (In fact, we are using an hypothetical example for Figure 2.1B. Research has yet to determine if social support and biomedical measures are correlated in prostate cancer patients.)

3. Social support satisfaction and coping might be unrelated. One man might be very satisfied with social support but be coping poorly. Another could be satisfied and coping well. Others may be coping well without any social support. Figure 2.1C illustrates this lack of relationship. You can see that the scatterplot does not form a shape we could draw a line through to capture that shape. Contrast this with the "cigar-shaped" scatterplots for the positive and negative correlations in Figures 2.1A and 2.1B.

FIGURE 2-1 Hypothetical Positive, Negative, and Zero Correlations

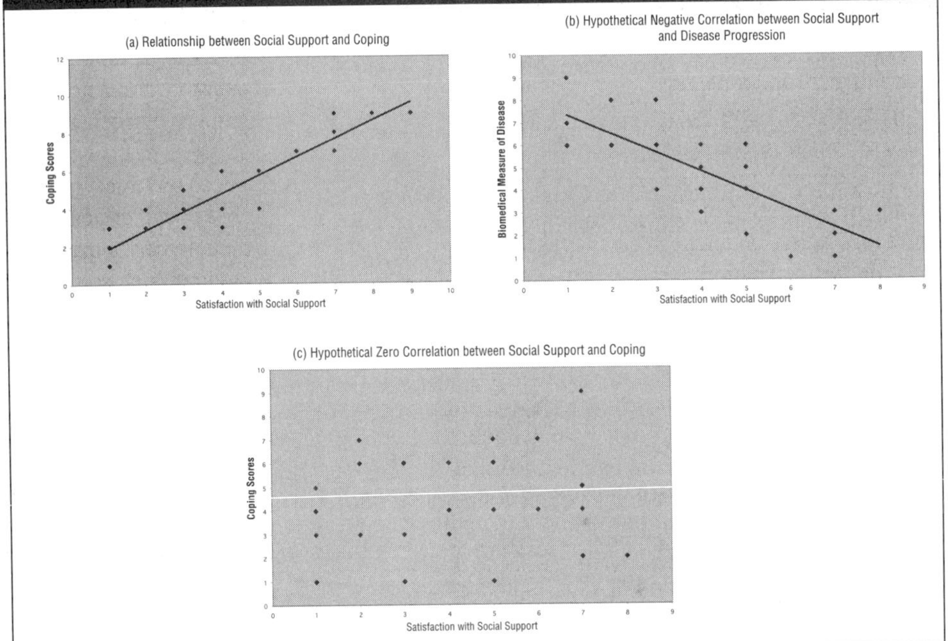

Figure 2.1a This scatterplot indicates a positive correlation between social support and coping. The line through the plot is drawn so that it comes as close as possible to all the points. Notice that the slope is positive, which is what you get with a positive correlation.

Figure 2.1b This scatterplot indicates a negative correlation between social support and disease progression. Those with higher levels of satisfaction with their social support had slower disease progression. Notice that the slope of the line of best fit is negative in this case.

Figure 2.1c This graph would indicate no linear correlation between social support and coping. Notice that it would be difficult to find one single line of best fit that could be drawn through the plot.

Correlation is expressed as a number. As we have already seen, the sign of the number indicates the direction of the relationship. The absolute value of the number, which falls between 0 and 1, indicates the strength of the relationship. Thus, a correlation of +.67 is stronger than a correlation of +.52. Similarly, a correlation of -.81 is stronger than -.43. A correlation of +.76 is the same strength as one of -.76, though they describe different types of relationships.

We can draw a line through the scatterplots in Figures 2.1A and 2.1B because the relationship between the two variables is **linear**. We would not be able to draw that line, or calculate correlations, if the relationship were not linear. For example, what if there was an *optimal* amount of social support that aided coping and any more support actually made coping more difficult? In that case, we would have a relationship like the one shown in Figure 2.2. This is called a **curvilinear relationship**. (In fact, research investigating social support and coping with other types of cancer suggests the relationship is probably linear.)

FIGURE 2-2 Hypothetical Curvilinear Correlation

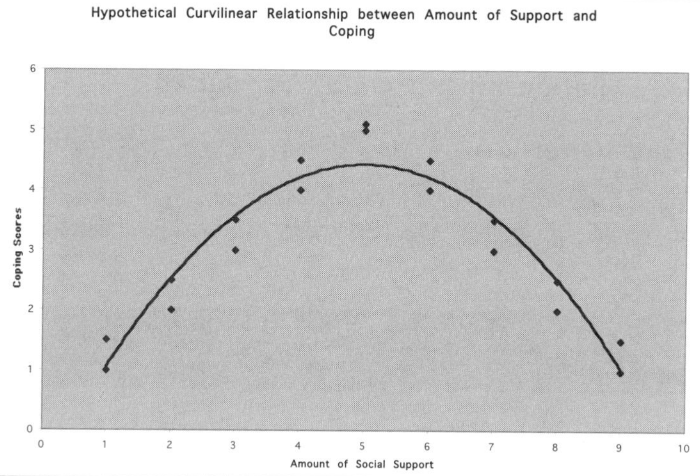

This graph shows a relationship, but it is curvilinear rather than linear. This would mean that there is an optimal amount of social support for best coping. Too little or too much would result in poor coping

Correlation and Cause-Effect Relationships

It is very important to realize that correlational research does not allow us to draw conclusions regarding the cause-effect relationship between variables. For example, if satisfaction with support and coping are positively correlated, we cannot jump to the conclusion that support *caused* improved coping. There are at least two reasons why we can't draw cause-effect conclusions from correlations. The first of these is that both causal directions are possible. While it is possible that good social support causes better coping, it is also possible that those people who are coping better are more able to seek social support. If this is the case, then coping could affect social support scores. The point is that the correlation does not give us any definitive data regarding the direction of this relationship.

The second reason we can't draw cause-effect conclusions from correlations involves the possibility of third-variable explanations. It is entirely possible that social support and coping aren't causally related at all. Instead, there might be a third variable that explains both of them and, in so doing, results in a correlation. For example, it is possible that one's income could be related to both social support and coping. People who can afford cars go to support groups and get more support than people who can't. Also, that income might be affecting coping by allowing for the purchase of other things that make life more comfortable. In other words, income is a **third variable** that may be causally related to both support and coping.

We can reduce this third-variable problem statistically by calculating what is called a **partial correlation** between support satisfaction and coping. This is a correlation between two variables that takes into account possible correlations they might have with a third variable. To do this, we "partial out" income. We can determine the extent to which support and coping are both correlated with income. When this is taken into account statistically, we can then calculate the correlation between support and coping, *independent of income*. If you read descriptions of studies that do this, they may say that they calculated a **first-order partial correlation** between social support and coping, partialling out income. "First-order" simply means that only one variable was partialled out. A "second-order" correlation means that two variables were partialled out. A "zero-order" correlation means that none were.

Testing other Relationships through Correlation

The Correlation Matrix

With a little imagination, we can think of ways to use correlational methods so that we are not restricted to one pair of variables. Our researchers may well have measured a large col-

TABLE 2-2 A Correlation Matrix of Psychosocial Variables for Prostate Cancer Patients

	Emotional Support	Info Support	Practical Support	Overall Support	General Coping	Physical Coping	Overall Quality of Life
Emotional support	1.0	.69	.81	.78	.27	.35	.40
Info support	.69	1.0	.69	.65	.20	.30	.40
Practical support	.81	.69	1.0	.77	.18	.28	.42
Overall support	.78	.65	.77	1.0	.22	.35	.39
General coping	.27	.20	.18	.22	1.0	.36	.55
Physical coping	.35	.30	.28	.35	.36	1.0	.62
Overall quality of life	.40	.40	.42	.39	.55	.62	1.0

Source: Poole et al. (1999). Adapted by permission.

lection of variables in their study of prostate cancer patients. They may also have subdivided social support and coping into subscales. For example, a person might have an emotional support score, an informational support score, and so on. They may have measured coping in terms of quality of life subscales such as physical quality of life and social quality of life. The researchers may be interested in correlations between numerous possible pairs of these variables. If they are, they can create a **correlation matrix** presenting all possible correlations. Table 2.2 presents a possible correlation matrix for this study. You can see that it allows for comparisons of all possible pairs of correlations.

Table 2.2 represents a matrix of all possible correlations among the variables. The correlations along the shaded diagonal are 1.0 because they are correlations between a variable and itself. The highlighted area in the top right corner indicates that measures of social support correlate more closely with quality of life than with coping. The highlighted area to the left indicates that measures of social support correlate quite highly with one another. This could mean that they are all measuring the same factor.

Let's look at the matrix in Table 2.2 for a moment. One of the first things you will notice is that the correlations along the diagonal are all 1.0. We have shaded these to highlight them and to divide the matrix in half along that diagonal. These correlations are all 1.0 because they represent correlations of a variable with *itself*, which, of course, will be perfect. We really only need to look at the correlations above or below the diagonal since the matrix is symmetrical. The emotional support-informational support correlation is the same as the informational support-emotional support correlation (.69).

What sorts of things can we conclude from this matrix? Let's look at the first three correlations in the General Coping column and compare them to the first three in the Physical Coping column and the Overall Quality of Life column. These correlations tell us that the measures of social support are more predictive of physical coping than of general coping (correlations of .35, .30, and .28 versus correlations of .27, .20, and .18). The correlations in the Overall Quality of Life column are higher still, indicating that social support is more predictive of quality of life than of self-reports of coping.

With the aid of computers, it is possible to produce a very large matrix of correlations. We must be careful when we do this, however. For one thing, not all pairs are meaningful. For another, the chance of getting a large correlation between two variables increases just by increasing the size of the matrix. Sweeping correlational research of this type must therefore be interpreted with caution.

Combining Variables to Form Factors

If you look further at the correlation matrix in Table 2.2, you will see that some variables that might be predictors actually correlate quite well with each other. Look, for example, at the correlations among emotional support, informational support, and practical support. They are .69, .81, and .69. Perhaps these variables can be combined somehow to form a *factor* called social support. In statistical terms, a factor is created by combining variables that correlate with one another. The correlation suggests that the variables are measuring the same thing, and that "thing" is a factor. When factors are created, through a statistical process called **factor analysis**, people's scores on that factor can be calculated by combining their scores on the variables comprising the factor.

Factor analysis has at least two important benefits. First, it improves our ability to predict outcome variables. Second, it clarifies our analysis conceptually by showing which variables fit together, allowing us to identify psychological constructs that are related to health. An excellent example of these benefits can be found in research attempting to link personality factors to cardiovascular health. In Chapter 5 in our discussion of stress and coping, we will talk about this research in some detail when we introduce the notion of the Type A Coronary Prone Behaviour Pattern.

You may have heard of the Type A pattern; we touched on it in Chapter 1. When it was first identified, the claim was that competitive, time-urgent, hostile people were at greater risk for heart disease. Factor analysis can be used in research that identifies such patterns. In the first stage of the research, people are administered a large battery of personality tests. Then, they are monitored for the ensuing years to see who develops heart disease. The numerous variables that emerge from the original personality tests are then subjected to a factor analysis, to see which predictor variables correlate with each other, or "cluster", to form factors. These factors are then correlated with coronary heart disease outcomes. If you used this method, you would discover that individual variables that measured anger and hostility would cluster together to form a factor and that this factor would be predictive of heart disease. The naming of the factor is up to the researchers. In this case, it is called "hostility." You will see in Chapter 5 that hostility is a risk factor for heart disease.

Using Correlations to Account for Variance

We have made the point that correlations do not give us conclusive information regarding cause and effect. Of course, this does not mean that they aren't useful tools in analysis. In fact, correlations can be very useful because they allow us to account for variance in some phenomenon. For example, we know that among prostate cancer patients some cope very well while others have a very difficult time and that there are many patients between these two extremes. In other words, there is *variance* among the patients in terms of coping. In our analysis, we would like to identify variables that account for this variance. Correlations allow us to do this in a fairly simple way. We can calculate the amount of variance accounted for by a variable simply by squaring the correlation between the two variables. So, if the correlation between social support and coping was .5, then we could say that social support *accounts for* 25 percent of the variance in prostate cancer patients' coping abilities ($.5^2 = .25$ or 25%).

Using Combinations of Variables to Account for More Variance

It would make sense that social support would account for a certain percentage of the variance in patients' coping abilities. However, we are still left with 75 percent of that variance unaccounted for. Other variables must account for it. Wouldn't it be helpful if we could identify some combination of variables that together accounted for as much variance in coping as possible? If you have studied correlational methods, you will know that we can create such a combination. We do this by creating a formula that combines selected variables and gives them more or less weight in the formula depending upon how much variance each accounts for alone.

From this combination of variables, we can calculate a **multiple correlation**. This is the correlation between the value our formula would predict for the outcome variable and what that value actually is. The higher the correlation, the better our formula is at predicting the outcome variable score. We can then square that multiple correlation to find out how much variance is accounted for by our combination of variables, as we did with our single correlation.

We can create a model featuring a combination of variables that serves at least two important functions. First, the model allows us to predict, with some accuracy, what an outcome would be if we knew a person's scores on the predictor variables. If the outcome variable is some biomedical measure of health, then the predictor variables become *risk factors* in our model. Indeed, this is one way that risk factors are identified in health research. Second, **multiple regression modelling**, as it is called, allows us to identify variables that account for variance in the outcome. In summary, then, this process allows us to *predict* and *explain* outcomes.

Multiple regression modelling works well when our outcome variable is a *continuum*, like age or income. But what happens when the outcome variable is a *category*? The task then becomes one of predicting if someone would belong in the category, based on their scores on the predictor variables. This situation is very common in health psychology research, because one of the more common outcome variables is mortality. This isn't a continuum. Rather, it is a dichotomous variable with only two possibilities—a person is either alive or dead. In this case, we want our formula to predict if a person would be in the category or not. This is the job of **discriminant function analysis**, a fairly common method in health psychology research. Let's look at an example.

It is very possible that one of the most important questions we could ask about our social support research with prostate cancer patients would be if social support helped predict how long they would live. To answer this question, we might start our study with a group of newly diagnosed prostate cancer patients. We would collect data from them on a number of predictor variables, such as the ones we have been talking about in this section on correlational methods—age, income, biomedical measures, social support, etc. We would then monitor these men for a period of time, say 10 years. At the end of this period, we would record which men were still alive and which were not. Then, using our predictor variables, we would create a formula that would do the best possible job of discriminating between survivors and non-survivors. The better job our formula does discriminating between these two categories, the better job it would do in *predicting* whether someone would survive 10 years if we knew his score on the predictor variables.

The accuracy of our formula would be assessed by determining the percentage of the men in our study who were correctly categorized when we plugged their predictor variable scores into the formula. For example, we would have made some valuable discoveries if we could say that our formula correctly categorized 80 percent of the men in the study as either survivors or non-survivors. Of course, we can determine the accuracy of our formula because we *know* whether the men in our study survived 10 years or not. You might wonder, then, why isn't our formula 100 percent accurate if we know this? It can't be totally accurate because it doesn't include all the variables that are related to a given category of the outcome variable. After all, we can't measure everything. A good model then, features a tradeoff between accuracy of categorization and the number of variables it contains.

We could then use this model to assess how much a newly diagnosed person was at risk for being in the non-survivor category in 10 years. With the fictitious model we have created in this example, we could be 80 percent confident that our prediction would be correct. For those men whose scores on the predictor variables (now risk factors) were such that we predicted they would be dead within 10 years, our next job would obviously be to discover interventions that would change their scores on as many of the predictor variables as possible and thus reduce their risk. For example, we would try to increase their social support, or reduce their anxiety, if these were risk factors.

In this section, we started with the relatively simple concept of correlation and built on it to explore some of its more complex uses in the form of model development. We hope you can see how valuable this is to health psychology research, because these techniques allow psychologists and others to do a better job of predicting, explaining, and, eventually, controlling health outcomes. As you can imagine, we have only scratched the surface in terms of the statistical processes involved. The main thing to understand at this point is the logic behind correlational approaches so that you could make more sense out of research papers you might read and want to critique.

EXPERIMENTAL METHOD: DRAWING CONCLUSIONS REGARDING CAUSE

Correlational methods provide a number of powerful tools for furthering our understanding of the relationship between psychology and health. There are things that these methods can't do, however. Perhaps the most obvious is that *researchers using these methods have no control over the variables they are studying*. The researchers trying to learn about social support and prostate cancer could not control the amount of support the patients receive. They can only measure it. Similarly, they could not control the type of medical treatment the men received. If we want to learn anything definitive about the extent to which variables cause certain health outcomes, we must be able to control those variables. When we control a variable and then observe changes in a specific health outcome, we can be much more confident when drawing conclusions about that variable causing the change.

The language of experimental design is somewhat different from that used in correlational research. The variables researchers manipulate are called **independent variables**. The outcome variables that are measured to determine the effects of the manipulation are called **dependent variables**. In its most basic form, then, the experimental method involves manipulating independent variables to determine their effect on dependent variables.

Independent variables most often take the form of categories. In the simplest version, one group gets the manipulation (the independent variable) and another group doesn't. The group receiving the manipulation is called the **experimental group** and the group that doesn't is called the **control group**. The control group is used as a source of comparison to measure changes that can be attributable to the independent variable because, in theory, the independent variable is the only difference between the two groups. We say "in theory" because it is practically impossible to create groups that differ in only one way.

Individuals vary in many ways. Researchers using the experimental method take these individual differences into account by using **random assignment** to determine who will be in the experimental group and who will be in the control group. In this way, individual differences in such variables as intelligence and medical history, which might not be independent variables in a given study, should be evenly divided between the two groups because people have been placed randomly in the groups.

If we are very concerned about control, we will want to conduct our research in a laboratory setting. The team investigating social support in prostate cancer would bring people into a controlled setting in which support groups were created for some of the patients and not for others. The content of the support group meetings would also have to be controlled as much as possible. The support group meetings would constitute the independent variable. The researchers could choose from a number of dependent variables, such as self-reports of coping, quality of life, or biomedical measures. The results of those coming into the lab for meetings would be compared to a control group, who would come in and spend their time in solo activities. Men would have to be randomly assigned to either the support group or solo condition, to be sure that such variables as illness stage, education level, and age were evenly distributed between the experimental and control groups.

A study of this nature is easy enough to describe, but it has its share of practical problems. First, these groups would feel more artificial than the support these men might get from family or friends, or even from support groups in their community. In fact, the more scripted or controlled the laboratory groups were, the more artificial they would feel. Yet, if they weren't controlled in terms of content, why bring men into the lab in the first place? Why not just use groups that already exist in the community?

These are important questions. In fact, we will find that certain types of experimental research does go out into the "field" and use people in real settings. Perhaps the most important benefit of the experimental design is that the men were *randomly assigned* to the groups. This way, the researchers would not have to worry about the very real possibility that certain types of people are more likely to attend support groups, as this type would represent an uncontrolled variable that could very well cause group differences. Uncontrolled variables that can affect the dependent variable are called **confounding variables**. In the experimental method, the tradeoff is clear. You reduce the number of potential confounding variables, but you also sacrifice realism.

Manipulating One Variable

In the simplest of experiments, one variable is manipulated and everything else about the experimental and control groups is kept the same. Then, if differences are noted in the dependent variable, we can say that those differences were caused by the one independent variable. If the experiment is really simple, the independent variable has only two levels. This is the case for the independent variable in the example we have been using. Men were either in a support group or they weren't—two levels only. For these studies, researchers would use a statistical procedure called a **t-test** to analyze their data. A t-test compares two means to determine if the difference between them is due to the independent variable or to chance. If the t-test indicates that the difference could be due to chance only five times or fewer in one hundred, then the results are considered to be **statistically significant**.

The t-test is actually a fairly straightforward statistic. It takes three things into account: the number of participants, the amount of variability *within* each group, and the size of the difference *between* groups. It makes sense that a difference is going to be significant if the difference between groups is large, the variability within each group is small, and the number of participants is large.

It is also possible to manipulate an independent variable such that it has more than two levels. For example, physicians might want to test three different dosages of a new medication, or psychologists might want to have support groups of four different sizes. The logic of this type of experiment is the same as for two levels. You still are concerned with the number of people in each group, the variability within each group, and the differences among the groups. However, you now need a new statistic because you have more than two groups. That statistic is called an **analysis of variance (ANOVA)** and is used to compare means among groups when there are more than two groups in the study. The ANOVA tells you if *any* of the differences between the groups are statistically significant. To determine just which ones are statistically significant, you need to chart the means and compare groups.

Manipulating More Than One Variable at a Time

In our fictitious drug study, we manipulated one variable. It is possible, however, to manipulate more than one variable in the same study. This is often done for at least two reasons. First, there is the efficiency of being able to test the effect of more than one variable while only needing one sample of people. Second, and perhaps most important, by manipulating more than one variable at a time we can learn about the relationships among those variables.

Main Effects and Interactions

In the experiments we have discussed so far, the assumption has been that one variable has a significant effect on some outcome (dependent variable). This assumes something called a **main effects model**. We say a variable has a main effect if it alone causes a significant change in a dependent variable. In a drug study, a significant ANOVA would indicate that the drug had a main effect on an outcome such as depression. Main effects certainly do occur in health psychology research, but it is much more common to find that variables *combine* to produce an effect. For example, the effects of a person's social support may combine with the amount of stress that person is experiencing to have an effect on how well the person is coping with an illness, an effect that is different from the effect of either independent variable alone. We call this combined effect an *interaction*. Research that manipulates two or more variables often assumes an **interactional model**.

Let's say we were interested in the effects of a new diet on weight control for a group of people with adult-onset diabetes. If we were using a main effects model, we would simply create two groups—one that received the diet and one that did not. We would then measure percent weight loss and compare the means of the two groups using a t-test. If we had more than one version of the diet, we would have more groups but still only one variable (diet), so we would run an ANOVA to test for differences. In either case, the assumption would be that *diet alone* affects weight.

But what if we believed that certain psychological factors *interacted* with diet to affect weight? For example, we might think that a diet is more likely to work if a person *believes* that he or she is capable of sticking to that diet. This belief, that we are capable of doing something, is called *self-efficacy* and is an important component in weight control (Brownell & Cohen, 1995). Also, self-efficacy can be enhanced by trained therapists who present cognitive interventions. Our study now becomes a bit more complex because we have moved to an interactional model.

We now have people who either go on the diet or do not, and we have people who are given the self-efficacy intervention or not. When we combine these two variables, we end up with four possibilities:

Group 1: No diet and no self-efficacy intervention. This is the control group.

Group 2: Gets the diet but no self-efficacy intervention. This is the diet-only group.

Group 3: Gets the self-efficacy intervention but not the diet. This is the self-efficacy-only group.

Group 4: Gets the diet *and* the self-efficacy training.

Clearly, we need more people for our interactional design. We now have four groups instead of two. We can represent this study quite neatly in a table such as Table 2.3. We have placed some hypothetical numbers in this table that represent percent of weight loss over a 6-month period. Let's assume that we have the same number of people in each of our four groups. With this simple table, we can assess the *main effect* for each variable and the *interaction* between them.

TABLE 2-3 A 2 x 2 Contingency Table for Diet and Self-Efficacy Intervention

Self-Efficacy	Diet	
	Not on Diet	**On Diet**
No intervention	Group 1 0%*	Group 2 4%*
Intervention	Group 3 2%*	Group 4 14%*

*Hypothetical percent weight loss over a 6-month period.

This table indicates a main effect for diet (average loss for dieters = 9%, compared to 1% for non-dieters). There is also a main effect for self-efficacy intervention (average loss for intervention groups = 8%, compared to 2% for non-intervention groups). There is also evidence of an interaction between diet and self-efficacy intervention, since the difference between the diet and no-diet groups is greater for those who received the self-efficacy intervention.

Because the numbers of people in each group are equal, we can assess the effect of diet by averaging the No Diet column and comparing it to the Diet column. When we do this, we find a *main effect* for diet alone. The diet groups averaged 9 percent weight loss and the no diet groups averaged 1 percent, regardless of self-efficacy intervention. Similarly, we can assess the effect of the self-efficacy intervention by averaging the No Intervention row and comparing it to the Intervention row. This comparison indicates a *main effect* for self-efficacy intervention. The intervention groups averaged an 8 percent weight loss compared to the no intervention groups' average of 2 percent. This means that self-efficacy intervention alone affected weight loss, regardless of whether a person was on the diet.

If there was an interaction between these two variables, this would mean that the effect of one variable depended on the level of the other variable. For example, the effect of being on the diet would be different depending on whether a person was in a self-efficacy intervention group or not. To determine if there is an interaction, we must look at individual cells of our table. When we do this for our table, we see that Group 4, who received both the intervention and the diet, did considerably better than the other three groups. The effectiveness of the diet was greater when combined with the self-efficacy intervention. In Table 2.3, this is shown by the fact that the difference between Groups 3 and 4 is greater than the difference between Groups 1 and 2. We would call this a *two-way* interaction because there are two variables involved. Our conclusion in this study would be clear. We should combine self-efficacy training with diet to help diabetics control their weight. While the data we have used for our example are fictitious, the conclusion is not. An interaction of this type is common in studies of weight control and exercise (e.g., Brownell & Cohen, 1995; Wilcox & Storandt, 1996).

Remember that this research differs from correlational research because the researchers had *control* over both variables and they *randomly assigned* diabetics to each of the four groups. In a correlational study, self-efficacy would be measured on a scale and the scores would be correlated with weight loss. Since diet is a dichotomous variable, it is better to test it using an ANOVA or t-test. You should know that there are more complex designs that actually allow researchers to combine correlational variables and manipulated ones (called multivariate analysis of variance, or MANOVA), but these are beyond the scope of our discussion.

In Chapter 1, we introduced a number of prominent theories in health psychology. Most of these theories assume an interactional model. For example, remember that the two main elements of the **theory of reasoned action** are a person's attitudes toward a behaviour and the person's beliefs regarding other people's thoughts regarding this behaviour. To test this theory, we might want to manipulate these attitudes and beliefs to determine their effect on behaviour. Our assumption would be that these variables *interact*. In other words, the effect of a person's attitude toward the behaviour will depend on their beliefs about other people's thoughts regarding the behaviour.

QUASIEXPERIMENTAL DESIGNS: TAKING OUR EXPERIMENTS INTO THE FIELD

Experimental methods using laboratory settings have the advantage of control, but the disadvantage of artificiality. It would be helpful if there was a method that allowed for control yet was conducted in real-life settings. This would increase the ability to generalize results to applied settings. This is the objective of **quasiexperimental designs**. They are called "quasi" because researchers do relinquish some control by moving to real-life settings, but since they are still manipulating variables, they are using experimental methods. These studies are sometimes called **field research**, because they are conducted in real-life settings. Correlational studies can also fit into this broad category.

Because they attempt to strike a balance between realism and control, quasiexperimental studies are challenging to carry out. Researchers talk about "noise" that enters into the data when they move to real-life settings. By "noise", they mean uncontrollable factors that can affect the results. For example, imagine asking an elderly patient to complete a questionnaire while in a waiting room at a hospital. She is accompanied by her daughter, who feels obliged to help her mother complete the questionnaire. As the researcher, you can urge her to let her mother complete the questionnaire alone. The daughter might even agree. Still, it is difficult to ensure that she will have no influence over her mother's responses. As a more extreme, yet possible, example, imagine you are having patients complete a measure of anxiety before going through a medical procedure. On one day, another patient has a heart attack in the waiting room. What do you do with the results on that day?

These examples illustrate the conundrum of field work. Life happens. On the one hand, these events get in the way of tidy data collection. On the other, it is *life* that researchers are trying to understand. Let's look now at some other specific challenges inherent in quasiexperimental designs.

Matching Groups

You will remember that, in a proper experiment, participants are randomly assigned to groups to ensure that extraneous variables such as age and IQ are equally distributed among the groups. In this way, the groups can be closely matched on most variables so researchers can attribute the cause of changes in the dependent variable to their manipulation (the independent variable). In quasiexperimental designs, researchers don't usually have the opportunity to randomly assign people to groups.

For example, they might be studying children who tend to suffer from upper respiratory infections. In other words, they get colds and coughs more than most other children do. In one actual study that focused on these children, researchers wanted to assess the effects of relaxation training on the problem (Drummond & Hewson-Bower, 1997). At first glance, this seems like a straightforward enough study. Create two groups—one that gets the relaxation training and one that doesn't—and run a t-test using upper respiratory infection scores as the dependent variable. However, these researchers weren't just interested in the effects of relaxation on infection-prone children. They also wanted to know if it could benefit healthy children as well. This introduced another variable—health status. Because of this, they now had an interactional design with four groups: (1) a group of healthy children getting the relaxation training; (2) a group of infection-prone children getting the training; (3) a group of healthy children not getting the training; and (4) a group of infection-prone children not getting the training. (As a test of your comprehension of this type of design, try drawing a two-by-two contingency table for this study like the one in Table 2.3).

Even this isn't particularly difficult. However, there is the problem of **matching groups**. The researchers cannot randomly assign children to the healthy or infection-prone groups. Therefore, they must be sure that the healthy and infection-prone children are similar in as many ways as possible. They must be matched for numerous variables, such as age, family income, family structure, and other health indicators, to name just a few. This matching procedure is logistically challenging for a number of obvious reasons. One is that it can be hard to get a large sample size if you need to find a matching control for every experimental group participant. Another is that it can be difficult to decide how many variables need to be taken into account as matching criteria, given that the list is potentially endless. The researchers need to know which variables might be potential confounds and try to match control and experimental group participants on those.

RANDOM CLINICAL TRIAL STUDIES: ASSIGNING PARTICIPANTS TO GROUPS RANDOMLY IN FIELD STUDIES

There are times when it is possible to randomly assign participants to groups even though the study is being conducted "in the field." In the study we just described, the health status of the children wasn't manipulated and randomly assigned, but the relaxation training variable was. In **random clinical trial studies**, participants are randomly assigned to treatment conditions. This eliminates the possibility that the treatment might work only because it attracted a certain type of person to it. In Chapter 3, you will read about the work of David Spiegel and colleagues. They randomly assigned women with breast cancer to either a support group condition or a control condition and discovered that the women in the support group condition significantly outlived the women in the control condition (Spiegel et al., 1989). This is an example of a random clinical trial study in health psychology.

Spiegel and colleagues' study and the Drummond and Hewson-Bower study using upper respiratory infection-prone children did not control the medical condition. Instead, like most quasiexperimental designs, they used participants who fit within their **inclusion criteria**. Inclusion criteria are those characteristics that make a person eligible for a study. These criteria represent another challenge for people doing field research. On the one hand, it is important to establish narrow enough inclusion criteria that a minimum of confounding variables are introduced. On the other, if the inclusion criteria are too narrow the researchers could be waiting a long time before they find enough people who fit them. Also, it is important to note that results of a study *cannot be generalized beyond the inclusion criteria*. For example, if your inclusion criteria stipulate that children between the ages of 10 and 12 are to be included and that they cannot have a history of other illness, then you cannot draw conclusions about younger or older children, or children who have a host of medical conditions. In Focus on Research 2.1, you will find an actual quasiexperimental study in which random assignment and inclusion criteria became major challenges.

Often, hospital staff can provide accurate "traffic rates" for the types of patients that fit a study's inclusion criteria. In other words, they can predict how many patients of that type they will treat over the course of a study. Sometimes, however, even hospital staff are surprised by what eventuates in a study. One of us was once trying to conduct a crosscultural study of men who had suffered their first heart attack. We were told that Indo-Canadian men were frequent patients in the hospital's Cardiac Care Unit. However, when we started to conduct the study, we went 3 months with only one Indo-Canadian man fitting our inclusion criteria! Hospital staff assured us that this was atypical, but we had to adjust our design nonetheless. The lack of Indo-Canadian men suffering heart attacks was good news for that community, though, and we weren't about to go out and try to induce heart attacks so we could do our research.

Even when clear inclusion criteria are established and there are lots of people who fit them, there is still considerable variability within that group of people. For example, let's go back to our study of children with recurring upper respiratory infections. Clearly, an inclusion criterion for children in that group is that they have to suffer regularly from coughs and/or

FOCUS ON RESEARCH 2-1 Too Many "Veterans" in Day Surgery

One of our graduate students is currently studying the psychological effects of two different ways children can be given general anesthetic for surgery (called anesthetic induction). In one method, children are given an injection; in the other, they are given a mask so that they breathe in the anesthetic. Like other studies we have introduced in our discussion of quasiexperimental designs, this one looks simple enough on paper. There are two groups, one gets anesthetic induction by way of injection and the other by way of a mask. Then a series of psychological tests is administered as dependent variables, perhaps before and after the procedure; perhaps some can even be administered several weeks after surgery to test for longer-term effects. A series of t-tests is then run on these psychological measures to determine the relative effects of each anesthetic induction method. However, our graduate student soon discovered that it wasn't going to be that easy.

First, there was a problem with random assignment. Interestingly, parents were often hesitant to agree to their child's participation in the study when they discovered that the decision regarding anesthetic induction method was going to be made randomly. Parents are rarely involved in this decision as a rule, and both methods are equally effective medically. But the point was that, if a study was being conducted using two different methods, one was assumed to be better than the other, and parents did not want their children to be subjected to what they thought might be an inferior method.

Then there was the problem of inclusion criteria. For reasons that make very good sense methodologically, our graduate student wanted to use first-time patients only. In other words, one of her inclusion criteria was that the child had not been given general anesthetic before. She reasoned that past experience with anesthetic induction could easily be a confounding variable. She also wanted to limit the *kind* of surgery the children were having. There is obviously a world of difference between the psychological effects of having day surgery on one's ears and having major surgery on one's abdomen. So, the graduate student decided to use first-time patients having day surgery for recurring ear infection. This all sounded very reasonable but for one unanticipated problem—children who have day surgery for ear infections often end up having this procedure done a number of times! It proved very difficult to find first-timers.

From this example, the challenges of field work become apparent. It is not uncommon to find that inclusion criteria have to be broadened to get enough participants to learn anything meaningful. Of course, this is done at the expense of control. In this study, a decision was made to include children who have previous experience with general anesthetic. Whenever the decision is made to broaden inclusion criteria, researchers must be careful to keep track of the new variables that are introduced. In this case, researchers kept track of how many previous surgeries a child had gone through, as well as the method of anesthetic induction and the child's memory of the experience. Even this has its problems, as anyone who has relied on retrospective data (i.e., data drawn from patients' memories) will tell you.

colds. But how regularly? And how severe does it have to be? No two will be identical. Also, researchers in that quasiexperiment will have no control over the children's amount of *exposure* to infection. In Chapter 3, you will read about *viral challenge studies* that attempt to reduce some of this variability. In these studies, adults are injected with a controlled dosage of a virus. Their exposure to others is then controlled through quarantine. Obviously, this method might be feasible for viruses, but not for other illnesses. For those, researchers have to contend as best as possible with the "noise" of real life.

Correlational studies also have to establish inclusion criteria. For example, a study investigating the correlation between number of visits to the doctor and children's anxiety over medical procedures would need to establish just who the children will be.

Outcome Studies: Measuring the Effects of Interventions

Some of the most valuable applications of quasiexperimental designs are found in **outcome studies**. An outcome study is designed to measure the effects (outcomes) of an intervention or program. This is a very important area of research because it measures the extent to which we can actually *do* something to improve people's health, rather than simply identifying variables that affect it. The interventions being tested should be implemented in applied field settings so that there can be some assurance that the intervention works in these settings. The outcome variables, or dependent variables, in outcome studies must be derived from the *objectives* of the intervention or program. For example, if the objective of a program is to foster total abstinence from smoking, then number of cigarettes smoked per day must be the central outcome variable. Success of the program is clearly defined in terms of the gap between the outcome measure and the objective.

It is important in outcome studies to understand the aspects of an intervention that are considered most crucial to its success and to make those aspects independent variables in the study. For example, outcome studies have been conducted to assess the effectiveness of various programs designed to prepare children psychologically for surgery. The crucial aspects of this type of intervention fit into three different categories: providing information, modelling, and giving coping skills training. Outcome studies in this area have yielded mixed results. Unfortunately, most programs feature a combination of these three categories, so researchers are unable to isolate one category. If they could, then they may be able to tell if providing information is the key to success in the program, as opposed to modelling and/or coping skills training (Whelan & Kirkby, 1998).

For a number of reasons, outcome studies can be major undertakings. First, they are often conducted after an extensive set of preliminary studies has identified the variables that need to be targeted in the intervention. Second, they are often time consuming because the interventions take time to implement and the desired outcomes are usually longterm rather than short-term. Third, outcome studies require a great deal of coordination with local agencies and hospitals. It is one thing to get permission to administer a questionnaire. It is quite another to get permission to put people through an intervention. Fourth, the most convincing outcome studies are in the form of random clinical trials, so participants must agree to be randomly placed, either in a group that is put through some "experimental" intervention or one that is denied some new and potentially beneficial one. In some ways, it is a no-win situation. Despite these challenges, there are those who have argued emphatically that outcome studies are the key to the success of health psychology as a discipline (Belar, 1997).

At some point in their research program, the researchers we introduced at the beginning of this chapter will hopefully make some discoveries about the relationships between social support and men's ability to cope with prostate cancer. Let's say that they are able to identify components of support groups that a significant number of men consider beneficial. From this information, the researchers could design an "ideal" support group program that contained as many of these components as possible. The next step would be to conduct an outcome study in which men were randomly assigned either to this group or to a control group. Perhaps there could be a third condition featuring men who attended existing groups of their choice.

WAYS OF CHARTING HEALTH-RELATED CHANGES OVER LONGER PERIODS OF TIME

Researchers working in health psychology must decide whether their work is going to be descriptive or explanatory. They must also decide whether they will use observational, case study, survey, correlational, or experimental methods. Within a number of these methods there are other basic decisions to be made. Some of these decisions arise when researchers want to learn something about how things change over time. Since this is often a goal of health psychology research, these decisions are common and important. Basically, they address two issues. In one, researchers must decide whether they are going to follow one group of people for a long period of time, or if they are going to look at a number of groups of people, each one being at a different stage of life. In the other, they must decide on the basic order of their work. Will they measure the variables they are interested in then monitor people to see how these variables affect their lives? Or will they find people in varying degrees of good and ill health and look back to see what variables might have brought them to this state? Let's take a closer look at these two issues.

Longitudinal versus Cross-Sectional Research

The first issue we identified concerned following one group over time versus looking at different groups who were at different stages. Following one group over time is called **longitudinal research**. Using numerous groups that differ according to stage is called **cross-sectional research**. For example, if our research group was interested in the ways the needs of prostate cancer patients changed over time, they could conduct longitudinal research, in which they collected data from a group of newly diagnosed men and then continued to collect data from that same group every 6 months. Alternatively, they could test a wide variety of men who varied in terms of their time-since-diagnosis. They would then group these men according to stage (in 6-month intervals) and compare groups in terms of their social support needs. This would be a cross-sectional approach.

The relative advantages and disadvantages of each approach are fairly obvious. Longitudinal research features fewer confounding variables than does cross-sectional research. This is because, in cross-sectional designs, there will be more differences between the groups than just time-since-diagnosis. Since it is impossible to randomly assign people to these groups, researchers have to do their best to keep track of these other differences like age, severity of disease, marital status, and so on by either matching their groups carefully or perhaps partialling these variables out of their analysis. On the other hand, researchers using a longitudinal approach will compare the same group of men at 6 months, 1 year, etc. While there will be some changes within the group in terms of severity of disease, marital status and other variables, the differences across time will be fewer than would be expected between groups in the cross-sectional design. Also, in the longitudinal study the group will *age together*. This means that historical events, medical breakthroughs, and so on will be timed the same for all participants.

The group that is followed in longitudinal research is called a **cohort**. Often, the main inclusion criterion is age, and so you will read about *age cohorts* in longitudinal research. In our prostate cancer example, the main criterion for the cohort was time-since-diagnosis, which is also commonly used. The National Population Health Survey calls the groups they follow longitudinally **panels**.

On the other hand, longitudinal research is much more time consuming, logistically difficult and, therefore, more expensive. It is time consuming, of course, because many health problems take a long time to develop. This is good for our health but not so good for our research. Also, people don't live their lives for the convenience of longitudinal studies. They move from one city to another, they marry and change their names, they go to jail. For these and many other reasons, keeping a cohort together can be difficult. Just ask someone who has tried to organize a high school reunion.

Of course, one of the most relevant reasons for attrition in longitudinal cohorts is that people die. Researchers doing longitudinal research need to know the circumstances of these deaths. Exactly when did they occur and what were the official causes? If you were trying to answer these questions, you would need access to death certificates and, possibly, other medical records. You can just imagine trying to contact one of your participants for his 6-month data collection in the prostate cancer study only to find that he had died. You ask his wife for the cause of death and she says, "Old age", or "He lost his will to live." When pressing these individuals for further details, such as whether the cancer had metastasized (spread), there is no guarantee that they will be forthcoming. And this lack of information can come after monitoring the patient for years. Certainly, you wouldn't give up at this point, but you can see that data collection can become very labour intensive.

This problem doesn't exist in cross-sectional research because you are only collecting data once, usually while your participants are still alive. If you include a group of deceased patients because you are interested in mortality statistics, you are now doing case study work. This means that you can select people based on the availability of their mortality data, rather than selecting people and hoping that these data exist somewhere.

It is probably fair to say that most researchers would prefer to conduct longitudinal research because the methodological advantages outweigh the logistic disadvantages. In reality, however, longitudinal research is less common than cross-sectional research because longitudinal research is so much more expensive and labour intensive. Also, much data collection in psychology is undertaken by graduate students as part of their thesis work, and health psychology is no exception. Since graduate thesis work has time constraints on it, it is not common for a graduate student to undertake a project that will take many years to complete. In health psychology, therefore, large longitudinal studies are the exception rather than the rule; because of their scientific rigour, however, they are often very influential.

Prospective versus Retrospective Research

If we wish to monitor people's health over long periods of time, longitudinal research is the ideal, though it requires rather extensive resources. However, there is a possible shortcut that could save time and effort. What if we started at the *end* of the timeline and moved *backward*? In other words, we could take people who have developed medical conditions, or who have died from them, and trace back in their history to find variables that would possibly explain how they came to have that condition. This is called **retrospective** research. Its advantages are clear in terms of convenience. Unfortunately, though, like so many shortcuts in research, there is a tradeoff between convenience and scientific rigour. Let's look at some of the problems we would have to live with if we chose a retrospective design.

First, retrospective data can be unreliable, especially if its collection relies upon people's memories. We know, for example, that our memory of the past is influenced considerably by our current mood state (McFarland & Buehler, 1998; McFarland & Buehler, 1997). This is particularly relevant for health psychology research if participants are ill when they are asked to remember their past.

Second, even if the data were proven to be reliable, we would have a problem with cause and effect. For example, let's say that our prostate cancer researchers chose a retrospective approach. They found people who were attending support groups and measured factors distinguishing them from people who didn't attend groups. Perhaps they used *discriminant function analysis* (described earlier in the chapter), in which they came up with predictor variables that distinguished attenders from non-attenders at a better-than-chance rate. Let's say they discovered that those attending support groups had a more optimistic view of their illness. Because this work must be correlational, cause and effect cannot be sorted out. The researchers cannot determine whether these men developed their optimism as a result of attending the groups or if optimistic men were more likely to attend the groups in the first place. (In fact, there is no evidence to date that optimism is even related to support-group attendance for prostate cancer patients.)

A classic example of this problem surfaces when researchers attempt to determine a possible causal relationship between mood and cancer (we will explore some of these attempts in Chapter 3). If it was discovered that cancer patients are more likely to be depressed, who would be surprised? The most logical conclusion is that having cancer makes people more depressed. If this work is to provide evidence for the opposite causal direction—that mood increases risk for cancer or makes cancer progress more quickly—it simply cannot be retrospective. Instead, it must be **prospective**. This means that the researchers must conduct a longitudinal study in which participants begin disease free or, at least, newly diagnosed. Data would be collected in the form of predictor variables at the outset of the study. If it turned out that people who scored higher on measures of depression were more likely to develop cancer, or have their cancer worsen, then we could say with some confidence that the cancer did not cause the depression (though we cannot be certain that depression caused the cancer). For this reason, large, prospective studies are very influential in health psychology. In Chapter 3, you will find that people who score high on measures of depression are more likely to have their cancer progress more rapidly than those who score low on that predictor variable.

Also in Chapter 3, you will read about research investigating possible causal links between personality and cancer. This work must be prospective in nature to be at all convincing. One of the champions of this work was the late Hans Eysenck. In one paper in which he documents a substantial portion of his work, Eysenck also outlines the problems associated with prospective research, especially when mortality is one of the outcome variables (Eysenck, 1996). Let's look at what he identifies, to see what you would have to deal with if you were interested in conducting this type of research.

First, you would need a very large sample to ensure that a large enough number of people in your study will develop the problem you are investigating. This becomes even more pressing if you want to be quite specific about the causes of death. For example, it might be too general to simply count up general cancer mortalities. There is a considerable difference between lung cancer and skin cancer, to name two cancers. They are too different to be grouped together. Yet, the more specific you want to be in your illness outcome measure, the more people you will need at the outset.

Second, if you need a large sample at the outset, what will your inclusion criteria be? You want to have some homogeneity in the sample, so you would like to specify certain ages and so on as inclusion criteria. However, it is difficult to have numerous inclusion criteria *and* a large sample. Further, how old do you want your sample to be at the outset of the study? If they are all young, then you had better be young too—it wouldn't make sense to have your participants outlive you! On the other hand, if they are old, then what of value have you learned about health risks? It is really the factors that put people at risk for premature death that are of most interest, so why have a cohort that consists of older people unless you are doing work in gerontology? Obviously, a compromise is in order. To achieve this compromise, you should have a wide variety of ages, but then you will need quite a few people at each age, so the size of your sample, which is already in the thousands, must be even larger.

Let's say that all this can be worked out and you get access to this very large group of people who meet your inclusion criteria. Now you must collect data from each of them on the predictor variables. Maybe you'll be lucky and find that this has been done for you. Perhaps these people all had a battery of psychological tests administered to them upon entrance to university or a particular job. In fact, this is how opportunistic researchers are often able to conduct large prospective studies.

In sum, it is daunting work. Nonetheless, there are people with the resources, skills, and inclination to conduct large prospective studies. You will read about a number of them in this book.

IMPORTANT CONSIDERATIONS WHEN MEASURING PHENOMENA

We have looked at a number of different types of designs in health psychology research and have seen examples of each. In this exploration, we have also tried to convey the challenges involved with each type. One thing that all these designs have in common is that they set out to *measure* something. This in itself poses numerous challenges. Have you ever wondered if some of these psychological phenomena can actually be measured? Can we really measure anxiety, satisfaction, or beliefs? Obviously, researchers in health psychology think we can, but there are a few important things to keep in mind when trying to do so.

Operational Definitions

An **operational definition** explains how an abstract concept or phenomenon is going to be measured concretely. For example, "evidence of upper respiratory infection" is an abstract concept until it has been *operationalized* in the context of a particular study. The operational definition answers the question: "How did you actually measure evidence of upper respiratory infection?" There is no single right answer to this question, though some answers are more convincing than others. When you read in Chapter 3 and elsewhere about studies that measure this phenomenon, you will discover that a number of operational definitions are used. In some studies, *self-report* is used. This means that the existence of upper respiratory infection (URI) is defined by someone complaining about the symptoms of a cough or cold. In other studies, this operational definition is considered inadequate, so researchers add *clinical diagnosis*. In this research, evidence of URI is defined as a physician's declaration that it exists. This seems fairly convincing as a definition, but we can get more rigourous still. Other studies measure mucous weight as evidence of URI. Still others use immune system cell counts.

As you read through these operational definitions, you can see that we get more and more stringent as we move from patient self-reports to biomedical confirmation. A similar continuum of operational definitions can be found in other types of health psychology research. One interesting example is *compliance*. You will discover in Chapter 7, on relationships in medical settings, that compliance is an important issue in health care. A dictionary might define compliance as a tendency to yield to another. But what does this mean in medical settings? An operational definition of compliance often uses a particular context—for example, taking medication as instructed. This moves us closer to a working definition, but we still need further guidance regarding measurement. To get this, we can go back to our continuum. We could define compliance in terms of patient self-report, or we could ask the patient to bring in his or her container of pills and we could count them, or we could do blood tests. From these examples, you can see that operational definitions are very context dependent, and the context is our research.

Reliability and Validity

Let's say that we know what we must measure and we have come up with a practical and convincing way of defining it in our study. Now we have another two important considerations. These relate to the tools that we will use to measure our variables. These tools must be **reliable**. If they are, they will give us the same reading of a consistent variable each time we measure it. A reliable friend is one you can count on to be consistent. A reliable measure in health psychology is no different.

Some measures may be perfectly reliable when administered to people of one particular culture but become quite unreliable when administered to people from another. For example, when administered to people born and raised in North America, the Health Locus of Control Scale provides quite reliable measurements of people's beliefs regarding the forces that control their health (Wallston, Wallston, & DeVellis, 1978). These forces are defined as being *internal* (I am in control), *external* (luck or fate controls my health), or *powerful other* (health professionals control my health). However, when administered to other cultures where the distinction between the internal and external is less clear, it is possible to find people scoring high on both internal and external items one time, and then low on these items if the questionnaire is administered at another time (Hart & Poole, 1995).

In addition to being reliable, our tools must also be **valid**. This means that they measure what they claim to measure. When we administer a questionnaire to measure patient satisfaction, we must be sure that it is measuring just that. Assume that our questionnaire consisted of a checklist of correct procedures, based on the assumption that patient satisfaction is derived from receiving correct treatment. We might present items like, "Took vital signs", or "Conducted thorough internal exam", and ask the respondent to tick off the items that applied to a given medical encounter. However, it is very possible that a patient would tick quite a few items and still not be satisfied. Our questionnaire would be *invalid*, because it didn't measure satisfaction, as it claimed. Instead, it measured procedural correctness, which may be quite unrelated to satisfaction.

You might be thinking that the best way to make a questionnaire valid is to ask questions very directly. So, in this case, we would simply include an item that asked people to rate, on a seven-point scale, how satisfied they were with the medical encounter. This item would have a great deal of **face validity**. This means that, "on the face of it", the item appears to be directly measuring what it intends to measure. In fact, when measuring patient satisfaction, face-valid items are probably well advised. However, remember what we said earlier in the chapter about direct and blunt items. Sometimes they put people on the defensive, causing them to provide a *socially desirable* response rather than an *honest* one. In that case, we would be measuring their desire to be viewed favourably, which would destroy the validity of our measure.

Quantitative versus Qualitative Measures

You may have noticed that virtually all of the methods described in this chapter attempt to express psychological phenomena as *numbers*. Correlations require numbers, as do ANOVAs. Surveys often yield *scores*. One exception might be the case study, in which the data may come in the form of a narrative rather than a graph or table. **Quantitative methods** attempt to express phenomena numerically. **Qualitative methods** rely on verbal descriptions. There is a fairly long tradition in psychology of striving for quantification. It has, for some time, been considered the way to make psychology a credible science. Also, it allows us to apply all those sophisticated statistical procedures we have been talking about in this chapter. However, qualitative methods, which are very common in other social sciences like anthropology, are becoming more popular in psychology. The reasons for this growing popularity are very relevant to health psychology.

Consider the following ways of asking this common question:

1. How are you today?

2. On the following 7-point scale, indicate how you are today:

1 2 3 4 5 6 7

Very poor Very good

Method 2 provides us with a number we can compare with other numbers. We can add up a group of these responses and calculate an average. We can administer the item once a week and graph the changes. This is all very convenient, but what does the number *actually mean*? If Method 2 is so informative, why don't we ever use it in daily conversation, as in, "Oh dear, I'm a 1.4 today?" By the same token, Method 1 might be far from perfect if the person answers, "Fine, thank you", as we so often do. How "fine"is "fine?" What can we do with that piece of data?

This simple example illustrates the problems associated with deciding between quantitative and qualitative methods. The question, "How are you today?" might seem trivial, but in its own way, it is a measure of quality of life, which is an absolutely vital outcome measure in health research. Indeed, the quantitative/qualitative debate is very applicable to quality-of-life measures. Physicians and psychologists alike want a quantitative quality-of-life measure. This will allow for the sorts of comparisons and other analyses we have discussed throughout this chapter. On the other hand, it is *quality* of life we are talking about, not *quantity*. With this in mind, some researchers have argued that we must allow patients to express this in their own words rather than giving them our words to respond to on a scale.

The challenge comes when we try to analyze qualitative data. We try to code it (indeed, quantify it) and summarize it. Perhaps we would be well advised to simply *report* it more often, using the person's own words. To this end, researchers are relying more on in-depth interviews and focus groups than they once did. With these methods, people get a chance to use their own words, either one-on-one with a researcher, or in groups. The upshot of this debate is that most comprehensive research programs today feature a combination of qualitative and quantitative methods. Our prostate cancer researchers would be well advised to have some open-ended questions for their participants and, perhaps, some focus group discussions in which the men could talk about what they liked and disliked about the support they were receiving.

COMMON FLAWS IN HEALTH PSYCHOLOGY RESEARCH

We have spent some time in this chapter discussing the reasons why applied research and, in particular, field research, is so challenging to conduct. Given that discussion, you won't be surprised to find that research in the field of health psychology is not without its flaws. Some of these are unavoidable. There is only so much control that can and should be exercised over people's responses. Still, there are some flaws that *are* avoidable. Let's look at some of the more common ones.

Demand Characteristics

It is entirely possible that people change their behaviour when they know they are in a psychology study. They try to assess what is expected of them and either comply with that expectation or violate it. These implicit expectations that participants hold are called **demand characteristics** (Orne, 1962). They refer to participants' beliefs regarding how they are "supposed" to respond. For example, what might be the demand characteristics when measuring patients' anxiety in a waiting room before they go in for a procedure in nuclear medicine? Possibly, a patient might think that a strong and mature person doesn't experience anxiety. Then, when you ask this patient to complete a very face-valid anxiety questionnaire that features direct-item questions like, "Do you feel tense?" the person answers, "No", because that is consistent with the perceived demands of the situation. On the other hand, the person might think, "This is obviously a study about anxiety in waiting rooms and this nice person who has asked me to complete this questionnaire is looking for anxiety, so I'll cooperate and say that I am experiencing it." Either way, the *validity* of the measure is compromised, because it is not measuring anxiety any more. Now it is measuring people's perceptions of what is expected. Demand characteristics are reduced by creating less direct measures and by assuring the participant that a wide range of responses is expected and that their responses will be kept confidential.

Placebo Effects

In medicine, a placebo is a substance that has a medicinal effect even though it contains no active ingredients designed to have such an effect. Thus, people might report a reduction in pain after taking a pill that contains salt but no analgesic. A number of explanations have been put forward for the **placebo effect**. One holds that simply *receiving attention* is medicinal. If this is true, then it poses some problems for researchers, since every experimental group in health psychology research receives attention. To account for the extent to which the effect of an intervention is due to placebo, researchers often include a placebo condition. In this condition, people are given general attention but not the specific intervention that constitutes the independent variable.

Experimenter Bias

The potential for **experimenter bias** exists when a person who knows the hypothesis interacts with participants or interprets qualitative data. It means simply that this knowledge affects participants' responses or qualitative data interpretation. It is especially problematic when the person has a *vested interest* in the outcome of the study. If a researcher believes that anxiety is a problem for people about to go through medical procedures, then he or she can interact with the participant in such a way that anxiety is either induced or at least expected. This won't necessarily be done consciously, but it can be powerful all the same.

Some of the most extensive longitudinal, prospective research investigating cancer-prone personality types has been criticized because the principal investigators did much of the interviewing that yielded the personality types (Amelang, 1997). Attempts to replicate studies substantiating the claim that there is a cancer-prone personality have often been unsuccessful. The original investigators have countered by claiming that the collection of personality data at the outset of the study must be done in a particular way for it to yield information on the cancer-prone type (Grossarth-Maticek, Eysenck, & Vetter, 1997). The reply to this claim, of course, is that the personality typing is the result of experimenter bias rather than of interviewer skill. The way to avoid experimenter bias is to, whenever possible, use people to collect data who are **blind** to the hypothesis or at least into which group a participant has been placed. In this case, "blind" simply means being unaware. We will discuss research on the cancer-prone personality in Chapter 3.

Sampling Bias

People who take part in health psychology research must consent to do so. As we will see in the next section, this is essential for ethical reasons. Nonetheless, it can result in a problem called **sampling bias**. This means that some variable or factor is shared by the people who take part in the study, which makes them somehow different from the population the researchers are studying. One form of sampling bias is quite straightforward—a researcher simply selects participants whom he or she expects to behave in ways consistent with the hypothesis (the researcher's prediction regarding results). This blatant form of bias isn't common, however. Instead, sampling bias can best be captured by the question, "Is there a certain type of person who is more likely to volunteer for the study?" The answer to this question is often "Yes", making a certain amount of sampling bias unavoidable. Consider the following example.

Hospitals often have strict rules in place governing the ways patients can be invited to take part in a study. Typically, a researcher is not allowed to be the first person to approach a patient. This way, the researcher can't pressure patients into taking part against their will. In one case, patients were shown a one-page notice providing some information about the study. If the patient was interested, he or she was asked to take the notice and wait for a researcher to come along and provide more information. The researcher knew to approach only those patients who had the one-page notice. This procedure worked very well except for the problem of sampling bias. This was because one of the variables being measured was anxiety. It became quite clear from the start of the study that people who were very anxious were not interested in talking to some researcher and filling out a bunch of questionnaires. In other studies, it is possible that people who choose to take part have "an axe to grind" regarding the hospital, or their condition, or life in general. These people might not be representative of the population being studied.

There is no simple solution to sampling bias in studies of this type. The best that can be done is to have a large sample of participants and hope that it is representative. People conducting survey research can at least use random sampling procedures in the way they send out their surveys or approach people to complete them. Still, there is the potential for bias in the sample that chooses to complete and return the surveys.

ETHICS

Psychological research is subjected to a strict code of ethics as articulated by the American Psychological Association (APA, 1992) and by committees that are part of most institutions where the research is conducted. The guidelines laid down by these organizations cover all aspects of research with human or animal participants. Let's look at two aspects that are particularly relevant to research in health psychology.

Informed Consent

Before taking part in research, a potential participant must sign a form indicating his or her consent. This consent must be **informed**, in that the person knows enough about the research to make a reasonable decision regarding participation. To this end, most consent forms today contain a general description of the research and particulars regarding what the participant will be asked to do. We have already seen an example of informed consent in this chapter when we discussed the work of the graduate student measuring the psychological effects of anesthetic induction. You might remember that, on the consent form, parents of the children who were having surgery were informed that their child would be randomly assigned to either an injection or mask induction. Even though the parents would not normally make the decision regarding induction, some chose not to take part in the study because of this random assignment. Ethically, participants (and parents if the participants are minors) must have a clear understanding of what the study will involve. If at some point during the study a participant says, "You never told me I would have to do that", then there is the real possibility that the study is unethical.

What Happens to the Control Group?

When we were describing randomized clinical trials in which people were placed in the experimental group or control group at random, did you wonder about what would become of the people in the control group who did not get the treatment? This poses a difficult ethical dilemma. If the experimental group is getting a new treatment or psychological intervention that is expected to be beneficial, then the control group is being denied that benefit, simply by virtue of the fact that they were placed randomly in the other group. To address this, studies will often make the intervention available to the control group after the study, if the intervention has proven to be beneficial.

This isn't always possible, however. The most difficult situation involves studies in which the outcome measure is mortality rates. For example, David Spiegel and his colleagues measured the effect of support group attendance on survival rates for women with breast cancer (Spiegel, Bloom, Kraemer, & Gottheil, 1989). In that study, women randomly assigned to a support group lived almost twice as long as those who were assigned to a control group. Of course, the control group women had no opportunity to reap the benefits of a support group. Nevertheless, random clinical trial studies must be conducted. Certainly, the countless women who have benefited from support groups since Spiegel's work are evidence of that.

KEY TERMS

applied research
basic research
descriptive research
descriptive statistics
explanatory research
grounded theory
inferential statistics
observational research
unobtrusive
natural observation
systematic observation
case studies
nomothetic approach
idiographic approach
double-barrelled items
counterbalancing
correlational research
positive correlation
scatterplot
line of best fit
negative correlation
linear relationship
curvilinear relationship
third variable explanations
partial correlation
first-order partial correlation
correlation matrix
factor analysis
predictor variables
outcome variable
multiple correlation
multiple regression modelling
discriminant function analysis
independent variables
dependent variables
experimental group
control group
random assignment
confounding variables
t-test
statistical significance
analysis of variance (ANOVA)
main effects model
interactional model
quasiexperimental designs
field research
matching groups
random clinical trial studies
inclusion criteria
outcome studies
longitudinal research
cross-sectional research
cohort
panels
retrospective
prospective
operational definition
reliability
validity
face validity
quantitative methods
qualitative methods
demand characteristics
placebo effect
experimenter bias
blind designs
sampling bias
informed consent

Chapter 3

PSYCHONEURO-IMMUNOLOGY

Chapter Outline

Key Questions

1. What is the relationship between our psychological states and our health?
2. Why is the study of psychoneuroimmunology so important to the work of health psychologists?
3. How does the immune system work to fend off infection?
4. How can researchers assess the effectiveness of someone's immune system?
5. What proof is there that the immune system is affected by psychological states and life circumstances?
6. What are the biological mechanisms linking these psychological states to our immune system?

Lori's last exam was scheduled for December 11. She was flying home the next day. Lori was really looking forward to being home for a while, but she expected she would spend the first few days with a bad cold or maybe the flu. You see, Lori was a third-year student who was experienced with final exams and flying home. Every year she got sick when she went home.

Was there something about being home that made Lori sick? That didn't seem likely. She got along well with her family and loved her parents' cooking. Maybe it was the airplane. She had heard about "bad air" on planes. But Lori played university volleyball and flew with the team all the time without ever getting sick.

Could it be the exams? That seemed more likely, since Lori often got sick right after April finals too, and she didn't fly home until mid-May. Lori finally concluded that writing exams somehow affected her immune system.

Lori is not alone. Many university students get sick either during or just after exams. Indeed, research has shown that immune system functioning suffers during exam time (e.g., Glaser et al., 1993). Glaser and colleagues measured immune-system functioning in medical students one month before an exam period and then again on the last day of that exam period. They found significant declines in a number of indicators of **immunocompetence**—the extent to which our immune system is functioning properly to ward off microorganisms that invade our bodies.

This research raises a number of important questions for students of health psychology. How is immunocompetence assessed in studies like this? What biological mechanisms link a psychological state like stress to immune-system functioning? How strong is this link? These are some of the key questions addressed by **psychoneuroimmunology** (PNI), which is the study of the relationship between psychological states and the functioning of the immune system. The link between the two is provided by the central nervous system.

The term "psychoneuroimmunology" is best understood by dividing it into its three component parts. Our psychology ("psycho") affects nervous-system functioning ("neuro") which, in turn, affects our immunity to disease ("immunology"). In this chapter, we will study the immune system and learn how research has discovered a link between this system and a number of psychological states. Let's begin with an explanation of why PNI is so important to health psychology as a discipline.

THE IMPORTANCE OF PSYCHONEUROIMMUNOLOGY TO HEALTH PSYCHOLOGY

In Chapter 1, we traced the development of health psychology from its roots in the study of biofeedback and behavioural medicine. Many of the people participating in this early development cautioned that, while health psychology held considerable promise, it would be essential to avoid extravagant and unsubstantiated claims regarding what was known and what could be achieved in terms of improving health through psychological interventions. One very important piece of the puzzle not yet found in those days was empirical proof that psychological states were directly linked to biological processes. Psychoneuroimmunology provides that piece.

Not only does PNI research provide much needed information linking psychology and health, it also provides data in a form that makes sense to people whose training is biomedical in nature. As such, PNI research represents an invaluable bridge between social scientists and health care providers. It thereby increases the credibility of health psychology in the eyes of health care providers.

When David Spiegel and colleagues discovered that women attending breast cancer support groups had average survival rates that were almost twice that of women who were not randomly assigned to such groups, people in the medical community sat up and took notice (Spiegel, Bloom, Kraemer, & Gottheil, 1989). The next step is to identify a biological mechanism that explains this link between social support and survival; this is the job of PNI research. We will return to Spiegel's work in Chapter 4 when we discuss health promotion programs designed to encourage people to provide mutual support for each other. The justification for pouring millions of dollars into such promotion programs will be strengthened by PNI research.

This research must be interdisciplinary in nature. It features teams consisting of people with a knowledge of the biology of immune functioning and others with an understanding of psychosocial factors and the ways they are measured. These partnerships move health psychology forward in constructive directions and make psychoneuroimmunology a vital area of study.

AN INTRODUCTION TO THE IMMUNE SYSTEM

The immune system is designed to monitor the invasion of microorganisms in the body and prevent their spread and growth by eliminating them. **Microorganisms** come in many different forms. In terms of the immune system, the relevant forms include bacteria, viruses, parasites, and fungi. These invading microbes are called **antigens**. The term "antigen" is generally used to refer to any microorganism that is foreign to our physiology. If these antigens have the potential to cause disease, they are called **pathogens**.

Put simply, the immune system is our guard against infection and the growth of cells associated with disease. The infection, if confined to a defined site, is called **localized infection**. If it remains in one area but send toxins to other parts of the body, it is called a **focal infection**. If it spreads to affect a number of areas of the body at once, it is called a **systemic infection**.

The immune system's first line of defence is the skin and mucous. Most antigens are stopped here. This is why people who suffer serious burns are at much greater risk for fatal infection. The skin's ability to prevent the invasion of large numbers of dangerous pathogens is compromised, and the internal components of the immune system aren't able to deal with such a massive invasion.

To understand the workings of these internal components of the immune system, you must know that the system does its job by producing cells that are designed to attack antigens and eliminate infected cells. An understanding of the immune system, therefore, involves an understanding of the nature of these cells and the jobs they perform. In this section, we will provide a basic introduction to these cells and the work they do. From this explanation, you will then be able to make sense out of research in psychoneuroimmunology that assesses the number of these cells and the efficiency with which they carry out their work.

Once our immune system has detected an antigen, it acts in one or more ways to eliminate it. This action can be **specific** or **non-specific** in nature. As the terms imply, specific immunity refers to protection against a particular antigen. This immunity is acquired some time after birth and is the result of prior exposure to the antigen, either by having contracted the disease or by receiving an inoculation that presents the body with a non-toxic dose of the antigen. This is called acquired immunity.

Specific immune function is the result of acquired immunity. There are three hallmarks to this functioning: memory, specificity, and tolerance (Seymour, Savage, & Walsh, 1995). **Immune-system memory** means that certain immune system cells have the ability to adapt to an antigen and, as the term implies, remember the antigen when it encounters it again and work to eliminate it. Not only will it recognize the antigen, it will also react much more explosively upon this subsequent exposure to it. If you have had chicken pox, you probably won't get the disease again. This is because your immune system has a *memory* for the virus causing chicken pox. It is for this same reason that we are more susceptible to certain diseases when we travel to exotic destinations. We increase our chances of encountering a pathogen (in the drinking water, for example) for which we have no memory. By contrast, the water doesn't bother the locals, because they have cells (B lymphocytes) that have a memory for the pathogen, and they produce the antibody to deal with it before it causes any trouble. We can help prevent problems by getting inoculations before we travel. These present the body with small dosages of a given pathogen so that we can produce some antibodies and develop a memory for the pathogen. That way, if we do encounter the pathogen when travelling, our immune systems can produce cells quickly and deal with it while we lie on the beach.

Specificity means that this cell will not only remember this antigen, it will respond to *this antigen* only. Having chicken pox does not make you immune to the mumps. **Tolerance** means that these cells will not react to the body's own cells—what is called "the self", in the language of immunity. Instead, immune cells react only to antigens, which are recognized as "non-self."

Non-specific immunity differs from specific immunity in that it relies on a system we are born with. It works in a number of different ways. In one process, white-blood cells (called "phagocytes") consume antigens. This process is called **phagocytosis** and has four stages: (1) attachment to the antigen; (2) ingestion of the antigen; (3) killing the antigen; and (4) digestion of the antigen (Seymour et al., 1995).

In another process, the immune system creates chemicals (called **antimicrobial substances**) that kill antigens. One result of these processes that can often be seen by the naked eye is inflammation. An infected cut will usually become inflamed because fluids carrying white blood cells enter the area, making it red as the fluids build up. In other words, inflammation is one indication that an immune system is working.

These specific and non-specific forms use two different processes to do their work. In one, called **humoral immunity**, cells called **B lymphocytes** produce antibodies that attack antigens. It is these B lymphocytes that produce antigen-specific antibodies for specific, acquired immunity. Thus, we have antitetanus antibody, for example. A particular kind of B lymphocyte, called **memory B cells**, develops a "memory" for a specific antigen after being exposed to it and acts only on that antigen by producing antibodies and immunoglobulins. The production of these antibodies is sometimes referred to in the literature as **seroconversion**.

An important point to realize is that the process involved in humoral immunity takes time. In fact, it takes B lymphocytes five or more days to generate specific antibodies (Maier, Watkins, & Fleshner, 1994). Fortunately, in most cases the immune system generates antibodies at a rate that is faster than the antigen can multiply.

You may wonder why the body doesn't just keep an ample supply of these specific antibodies on hand for immediate response to the antigen. The answer is that there are many millions of different antigens and the body can't keep a plentiful stock of the antibody required for each. Instead, it keeps a small stock of each and relies on the B lymphocytes to generate an ample number when called upon to do so, which is what takes the time. Fortunately, memory B lymphocytes allow this process to occur more quickly if we are re-exposed to the antigen.

To fully understand research in PNI, you need to know a bit more about the work of these lymphocytes. For example, B lymphocytes need help to produce antibodies. This help comes from **T lympocytes** called, conveniently, **helper T cells**. These helper cells produce substances called interleukins that speed the division of B lymphocyte cells. When you read PNI research, therefore, you will encounter references to things like interleukin-1 or interleukin-2 production as measures of immunocompetence. These helper T cells are also referred to in the literature as CD4. Humoral immunity also needs an "off switch" so that antibodies aren't produced unnecessarily after the antigen has been destroyed. This is the job of **suppressor T cells**. These cells are sometimes referred to as CD8. You can see, then, that B cells and T cells work together to maintain our humoral immunity.

The other type of immune-system work is called **cell-mediated immunity**. This features "cells battling cells" rather than sending antibodies to do the work. In this process, other T lymphocytes secrete chemicals that kill antigens and infected cells. The cells involved in cell-mediated direct attack are called **cytotoxic T cells**.

Lymphocytes, then, are important components of the immune system. They include B cells, T cells, and **natural-killer (NK)** cells. Natural-killer cells have the specific job of "seeking and destroying" cells that are infected, cancerous, or altered in some other way. The rapid and efficient production of lymphocytes is essential to **immunocompetence**—the effective functioning of the immune system.

HOW IMMUNE-SYSTEM FUNCTION IS MEASURED IN PSYCHONEUROIMMUNOLOGICAL RESEARCH

One of our main objectives in presenting this section on measuring immune-system function is to help you develop a familiarity with the language used in PNI research. Without this familiarity, PNI research can be very confusing to read. With this objective in mind, we have included a focus on the *language* of PNI research as well as the *processes* involved in assessing immune-system function.

You will remember from our discussion of research methods in Chapter 2 that the *dependent variable* in an experiment is the variable we measure to determine if our treatment or manipulation has had any effect. In PNI research, dependent variables take the form of measures of immunocompetence. The manipulation, or *independent variable*, is usually some psychological state. This can be naturally occurring, as was the case with Lori's exams in our opening example, or it can be experimentally induced by putting people through stressful experiences or presenting them with stimuli that will elicit positive moods such as happiness.

We know that immune-system function involves the production and activity of specific cells. It stands to reason, then, that we should measure immunocompetence by somehow counting the number of these cells and by subjecting them to antigens to see how well they work. This is, indeed, the basic approach to measuring immunocompetence in PNI research. It sounds simple, but it is actually quite complex.

There are many reasons for this complexity. First, there are a number of places throughout the body where immune-system cells are located, such as the tonsils, appendix, small intestines, spleen, and bone marrow. This makes it difficult to just go to the source and measure activity. Instead, we must assess cellular activity in the bloodstream or mucous. Second, there are a variety of forms this cellular activity can take, which operate independently of each other. So it is possible that a psychological state might influence one aspect of immune functioning and not another. This means that researchers must assess a number of immune-system cellular functions to ascertain the potential impact of a situation or mood state. It also means that two studies assessing the impact of the same psychological variable, such as exam stress, might come to different conclusions depending on which aspect of immune functioning is being assessed—that which fights off colds or that which kills tumour cells, for example.

Counting Cells to Measure Immunocompetence

You have learned that immune-system function is dependent upon the system's ability to produce, or *proliferate*, cells to do its work. We have also said that one simple way of measuring immunocompetence is to count these cells (typically white blood cells) as they exist in the bloodstream. This cell counting is called an **enumerative assay** and is common in PNI research. In studies using cell counts, you will see lymphocyte measures taken from blood samples, counting such white blood cells as NK, T, and B cells. Researchers look for two things in these counts: (1) a minimum number of cells for adequate immune function; and

(2) a balance between various cell types, such as different types of T cells (Herbert & Cohen, 1993).

In general, the better the immune system functions, the higher these counts are. Studies using cell counts will often report lower cell counts in blood samples taken from groups that have been exposed to a stressor, such as an exam.

Functional Tests of Immunocompetence: Measuring Cells in Action

Counting cells can be informative, but it would be even better if we could assess the immune system *at work*. This is what **functional tests of immunity** do. You will remember that the immune system functions in both humoral and cell-mediated ways. In the former, antibodies are produced. In the latter, cells work directly to destroy invading cells. Functional tests assess both of these ways. Most studies test either humoral or cell-mediated immune functioning; few test both (Cohen & Herbert, 1996).

We can perform these functional tests inside the body, though this can be difficult at times because it is hard to localize the sites of the immune system. However, we can also measure cell functions by *removing* them from the body and incubating them with other cells to see how the immune-system cells respond. Functional tests performed on cells outside the body are called *in vitro* tests. Those performed inside the body are called *in vivo* tests.

In vitro tests of immunocompetence start with a blood sample that is combined with a substance called a **mitogen**. A mitogen is a substance that stimulates immune-cell activity as though the immune cell were acting against an invading cell, or antigen. Three of the most common mitogens used in PNI research are concanavalin A (Con A), phytohemagglutinin (PHA), and pokeweed mitogen (PWM).

So, when you read a PNI study, you might encounter language like this: "People whose interactions with others were less confrontational showed greater lymphocyte proliferation in response to PHA." Translated, this means that blood samples were taken from people who differed in the amount of confrontation they experienced in their interactions with others. Those samples were incubated with PHA. From this, it was discovered that blood taken from people whose interactions were less confrontational produced more lymphocytes when put with PHA. Other studies using this general design might substitute Con A or PWM as the mitogen, or they might run a number of tests (or assays, as they are sometimes called) using two or more different mitogens. In these studies, you will see data reported separately for each mitogen.

Natural-killer cell activity is also measured through *in vitro* techniques. Remember that NK cells perform a "seek and destroy" function. With this in mind, NK cell activity is measured by exposing NK cells to diseased cells, usually tumour cells. For this reason, PNI research linking psychological variables to cancer often measures NK cell activity.

After exposure, NK cells are assessed in two ways. In one, proliferation is measured through cell counts taken after the introduction of tumour cells. In the other, NK cell *effectiveness* is assessed by measuring the destruction of the tumour cells. In PNI literature, this is often called an **NK cell cytotoxic activity assay**. This process of killing tumour cells is called **NK cell lysis** because to *lyse* a tumour cell means to destroy it. For these reasons, PNI researchers, especially those dealing with cancer, will talk of "a decrease (or increase) in NK cytotoxic activity", or "a significant effect on NK cell lysis." It is important to note that

NK cells aren't the only immune-system cells capable of cytotoxic activity. However, they are the most commonly measured in PNI studies involving cancer. When reading this type of research, look for data reporting cytotoxic activity or cell lysis. It will provide evidence for a link between psychosocial factors and cancer.

There are also a number of *in vivo* functional tests of immunocompetence. Let's look at two of the more common types. One takes advantage of the fact that almost everyone carries herpesviruses. The other uses injections of small dosages of antigens.

Herpesviruses are somewhat unique in that, once you have been exposed to one, you carry it with you for life. Of course, that virus usually stays in such small quantities that you don't experience any symptoms, but it is there all the same. There are many different types of herpesviruses, from cold sores to Epstein-Barr virus (EPV).

One reason why you don't have to spend much time worrying about herpesviruses is that your immune system does the worrying for you. It produces antibodies (Ab) whose job it is to "flag" herpesviruses for destruction, thus keeping their numbers under control. Herpesviruses will multiply when the immune system is suppressed, thus creating the need for more Ab. Therefore, we can determine immunocompetence by measuring Ab. Be careful when you read studies that use this measure, though. The more suppressed the immune system, the more herpesviruses, and thus the more Ab. This means that, when herpesvirus-specific antibodies are being measured, the *higher* the Ab count, the *poorer* the immune-system function.

This is an indirect measure of immune functioning, because we are relying on the existence of herpesviruses that exist naturally in most people. Another approach would be to introduce another type of antigen into the body and measure the specific Ab activity meant to deal with that intrusion. In these studies, small quantities of an antigen are introduced by injection. After this is done, there are two ways to measure immune-system activity. In the simplest, the skin is observed at the site of the injection. If the immune system is working properly, there should be swelling and redness. Remember that inflammation is a sign of a properly functioning immune system.

The second way involves counting antigen-specific Ab produced in response to the injection. This can be done through blood samples or mucous secretions, measured most often in the saliva. One antibody commonly measured in the saliva or mucous is called sIgA, which stands for *secretory* or *salivary immunoglobulin A* antibody. Because it exists in saliva and mucous, it represents one of the body's first lines of defence against antigens (Tomasi, 1971).

But measuring salivary sIgA isn't always as easy as it sounds. What happens when we want to measure sIgA levels during times of stress? For many people experience "dry mouth" at these times—they don't produce much saliva! Interestingly, the immune system compensates for this somewhat and produces greater concentrations of sIgA protein. However, some have argued that this isn't a good measure of immunocompetence, since protein levels aren't the same as antibody counts (Stone et al., 1987).

These, then, are other *in vivo* tests that measure Ab production to assess immunocompetence. Be careful when you read these studies, though. It is easy to get confused regarding the meaning of Ab counts, because they have opposite meaning depending upon whether the count is herpesvirus-specific or is in response to an injection. In herpesvirus studies, higher Ab counts indicate *immunosuppression*. An increase in that virus comes about because of suppression of the immune system. This means that an increase in Ab has come about because of a *poor* immune system that can't keep herpesvirus counts down. In the case of injection studies, more Ab indicates *better* immunocompetence. In these studies, the antigen is introduced into the body. This means that Ab is being produced by a *competent* immune system that is dealing with an invading antigen.

Methodological Issues in the Measurement of Immune-System Function

As you read through the preceding section on measurement, did you wonder just *how* these blood samples were taken, and *when*, given that the independent variable in much PNI work is often stress related? Can we casually draw blood from someone who is in the middle of an argument with his wife or studying for final exams? Hardly. In PNI research, a sophisticated knowledge of measurement techniques and biological processes is needed. Measurement of immune functioning requires skill and is intrusive. Certainly, conducting research in psychoneuroimmunology is not without its challenges. Let's take a look at some of them.

Short-Term versus Longterm Effects

In PNI research, an important distinction must be made between short-term and longterm effects. In laboratory research, it is common for a participant to be subjected to an acute stressor, which is to say one that is immediate in its duration and proximity. The effects of this **acute stressor** are then measured through blood samples that are taken just before, just after, and then again some time (minutes to hours) after the stressor has been introduced. Studies of this nature measure the quick reactivity of the immune system. As we will see in the next section, when we look at specific studies in PNI, short-term changes in immune-system function occur quite commonly in the face of these acute stressors. This leads to the conclusion that our immunocompetence fluctuates over the course of a day that features ups and downs or what have been called "daily hassles." It remains to be determined, however, whether these short-term fluctuations actually increase our susceptibility to disease.

Not all psychological variables occur on an acute basis, however. Trait anxiety, job stress, marital problems, loneliness, and many other facts of life are *chronic*, or longterm, in nature. Their effects are more like a constant hum than a single blast. Psychoneuroimmunological research designed to measure the effects of chronic stressors cannot rely on well-controlled laboratory environments. Instead, field research must be conducted that studies people exposed to these stressors and compares their immune functioning to those who are not exposed. It is much more difficult to ascertain definitive cause-and-effect relationships in these studies, because there are so many other variables in field work that cannot be controlled for.

One reason to emphasize the short-term versus longterm distinction is that some research has found that immune-system function is actually temporarily *improved* in the face of acute stressors. The body reacts with what Hans Selye (1976) called **resistance**, a set of physiological responses that allow the person to deal with the stressor. The question is, do these short-term responses take their toll on the immune system in the long run? Most researchers in the field would say that they do. Conversely, it is possible that some events, such as expressing emotion, might show detrimental short-term effects on immune functioning but still result in improved functioning over the longterm. The important point here is that short-term immunologic effects of some psychological variables may be *opposite* to longterm effects.

Immune-System Function Takes Many Forms

As we mentioned earlier, there is no single accepted measure of immunocompetence. This is because the immune system does its job in a variety of ways, from humoral to cell-mediated processes. Also, the nature of the immune system's work differs depending on the nature of the antigen. Not only that, but external factors and the internal states accompanying them will have different effects on the immune system depending on what those factors are. Finally, as is the case with all biological systems, there are individual differences among all of us regarding the ways our bodies respond to these factors.

For example, stress might result in the suppression of immune functioning in one person such that he or she becomes more susceptible to upper respiratory infections, such as colds and coughs. For another, the suppression might be less overt but nonetheless problematic. It might take the form of compromised NK cell activity, thus making the person more prone to the growth of tumours.

For these reasons, PNI studies often report a multitude of dependent measures. This makes the work more difficult to wade through if you are a student of the field, but it also makes it more valid in that multiple measures increase the likelihood that an effected immunologic process will be identified.

Statistical Significance versus Clinical Significance

In Chapter 2, we introduced the notion that data might be statistically significant without being clinically or socially significant. We also explored the possibility that data can have clinical or social significance without being statistically so. This notion is very relevant to measurement and data analysis in PNI studies when we try to determine if an aspect of the immune system has been affected by a person's psychology.

When we say that some aspect of immune functioning has been *affected*, what exactly do we mean? In terms of PNI research, we usually mean that, when two or more groups of people are compared on immune-system function measures such as the ones we have described in this section, the difference in cell count or cytotoxic activity is different enough to say that it did not occur by chance. You will remember from Chapter 2 on research methods that this means the results are said to be *significant*. By this, we mean that they are statistically significant—there is a less than one-in-twenty chance that the differences we detected would occur without the manipulation. When this is applied to PNI research, it means that some psychological factor brings about *real* immunologic effects.

This is scientifically important, but is it *clinically* important? In other words, do the differences resulting in statistical significance actually mean that people are more or less likely to *get sick*? Or are the differences, though statistically detectable, actually too small to affect our susceptibility to illness? These are very important questions for PNI research, because it is entirely possible that our statistical tests are more sensitive to cellular differences than our bodies are.

In a concise review of some important PNI research, Kiecolt-Glaser and Glaser (1995) observe that, "Considerable evidence has accumulated demonstrating psychosocial or behavioral modulation of immune function. However, relatively few studies have simultaneously shown actual health changes in individuals with immunological alterations" (p. 269). In other words, there are studies showing that psychosocial factors can make us sick or well, and others showing that these factors can affect the immune system at the cellular level. What we need more of are studies that do *both*—measure symptoms and immune functioning concurrently. In this way, studies can show clinical effects and immune function changes that can be cited as the cause of those effects. You will note in our upcoming discussion of PNI research that a number of studies, especially more recent ones, do this.

Such studies are difficult to carry out, in part because of the short-term versus longterm distinction we discussed earlier in this section. If we want to measure the clinical effects of acute stressors, we must be patient, because people don't develop upper respiratory infections right before our eyes. On the other hand, if we want to link immunocompromise to illnesses such as cancer that take a relatively long time to develop, then we must take our measurements regularly, on a longitudinal, prospective basis. This means that we must start with participants who are well, follow them over a long period, take regular assays, and compare the results for those who get sick and those who do not. This work isn't impossible to do, but it is expensive, intrusive, and fraught with all the problems of longitudinal work in the form of extraneous variables that can account for health differences.

One way to get around these problems is to expose healthy people to antigens and psychological factors in the same study. Then we can observe progression in terms of symptom display while we monitor immune functioning. In studies that follow this approach, volunteers are exposed to a cold virus or similar pathogen, and disease course is monitored for a two- or three-week period following exposure. During that time, some volunteers go through a life event of interest, often something like an exam period.

Who would volunteer for such a study, you may ask. The most common answer is medical students. Of course, we must be careful when generalizing results of a study in which usually young and healthy medical students are injected with a controlled dosage of a cold virus. All the same, you can see the rationale for such a design, given that it helps answer concerns the regarding clinical significance of PNI research.

Psychoneuroimmunological Procedures are Expensive and Intrusive

The assays required for PNI research tend to be costly. Further, blood samples are often taken, which few participants are entirely nonchalant about, especially when they are taken in conjunction with such things as difficult problem-solving tasks or discussions with one's spouse (e.g., see Kiecolt-Glaser, Glaser, Cacioppo, & Malarkey, 1998).

In addition to the obvious limitations imposed by expense and intrusion, there is also the problem of obtaining data on test-retest reliability. It would seem reasonable to expect normal day-to-day fluctuation in immune-system function, regardless of whatever experimental manipulations a study might introduce. These fluctuations means that *reliability*, the extent to which a measurement device can be expected to obtain repeatable and thus trustworthy readings over a series of identical trials, is important to assess in PNI work. It is also difficult to assess, however, because the procedures are expensive for the researcher and less than convenient for the participant.

With this in mind, a number of studies have attempted to assess the test-retest reliability of a number of PNI research procedures. These studies have generally come to the conclusion that the reliability of most measures varies from being acceptable to quite good (see Uchino, Cacioppo, & Kiecolt-Glaser, 1996, p. 519, for a concise review).

Despite the problems that can be associated with PNI research, investigators have persevered to find ingenious solutions and produce very important work. In the next section, we will look at some of this work in detail to develop a sense of what is known in the fascinating study of the relationship between psychological states and physical health.

RESEARCH IN PSYCHONEUROIMMUNOLOGY: PROVIDING EVIDENCE FOR A BIOLOGICAL LINK BETWEEN PSYCHOLOGY AND HEALTH

In the following overview of PNI research, we have organized the studies according to psychological factors. You will notice that some are acute in nature. Examples include such things as mood and state anxiety as well as short-term stress. Others are more chronic or longterm. Examples of these include personality factors (such as cynical hostility, coping styles) and social support. As you read through the summary of these studies, keep in mind the methodological issues discussed in the previous section. Also, we have tried to select studies that are not only representative of the field of PNI but that also use dependent measures and terminology consistent with that which we introduced earlier in this chapter. If you get confused at any point as you read this section, try referring back to our explanations in the section entitled, "How Immune-System Function is Measured in Psychoneuroimmunological Research."

The Effect of Stress on Immune Functioning

In the example we presented to open this chapter, you read about Lori, a university student who got either a cold or the flu regularly just after final exams. The assumption in this example, as far as PNI is concerned, is that the stress of exams increased Lori's susceptibility to these illnesses by having a compromising effect on her immune system. In fact, a large number of studies have looked at immune functioning in students before, during, and after exam time (e.g., Jemmott et al., 1983; Jemmot & Magloire, 1988; Kiecolt-Glaser et al., 1984; McClelland, Ross, & Patel, 1985). The general finding is that symptom complaint goes up and that cellular measures of immune response indicate immunosuppression at these times.

We have devoted Chapter 5 to stress and coping and so will not go into a great deal of detail at this time regarding the nature of stress. Our purpose here is to link stress to disease using PNI research. To do this, though, we need at least a working definition of stress. For this purpose, we will use a simplified version of the definition forwarded by Lazarus and Folkman (1984), who define stress as an aversive condition in which the demands of a situation are perceived to be greater than our ability to cope with them.

The study of the relationship between stress and disease may have been initiated in 1964 with the publication of a study by Solomon and Moos entitled, "Emotions, Immunity and Disease: a Speculative Theoretical Integration." Since that time, a large number of studies have linked various types of stressors to a wide variety of diseases.

In the laboratory, volunteers have been exposed to acute, short-term stressors such as making speeches or doing mental tasks under time pressure. At the same time, their immune functioning was monitored. Using designs such as these, researchers can learn about the immediacy with which a stressor can affect immune functioning. Such studies have discovered that, while it may take days for the immune system to react to an antigen, it takes as little as 5 minutes for a stressor to inhibit the ability of the immune system to respond effectively (Herbert et al., 1994). Laboratory studies have also shown that the effect of stressors on immune functioning is stable over time for a given individual, leading to the conclusion that there are dispositional or personality factors that influence the extent to which a stressor affects immunity (Marsland et al., 1995).

In addition to laboratory studies of the effects of acute stressors, other work has investigated chronic, longterm stress as it occurs in real life. Boscarino (1997) conducted a 20-year follow-up of 332 Vietnam veterans who had presented symptoms of post-traumatic stress disorder (PTSD). He compared their health to 1 067 veterans who did not suffer from PTSD. Post-traumatic stress disorder was reasoned to be evidence of severe stress exposure.

Boscarino discovered that the veterans who had suffered from PTSD were signficantly more likely to suffer from a wide range of medical problems, including circulatory, digestive, musculoskeletal, and metabolic ailments. The worst problems were nervous-system disorders, which PTSD veterans were 2.47 times more likely to suffer from than non-PTSD vets, and non-sexually transmitted infectious diseases, which they were 2.14 times more likely to contract. Two aspects of this study are most impressive. First, Boscarino controlled 14 other factors that could account for increased susceptibility to illness, including substance abuse, hypochondriasis, age, and smoking history. This greatly increases the likelihood that the higher odds of suffering from this wide variety of illnesses is attributable, in large part, to the effects of the stress exposure. Second, the long range of the follow-up (20 years) demonstrated that severe stress exposure can have longterm effects, either by lingering or by compromising the immune system for long periods.

Other studies have demonstrated the potential longterm effects of stress on immunity. For example, a study of people living near the Three Mile Island nuclear disaster site almost ten years after the accident found more antibody to herpes viruses than those living elsewhere in a demographically matched control-group (McKinnon et al., 1989). (Remember that increased antibody to herpesvirus is a result of an increase in herpesvirus numbers, indicating immunocompromise.)

Another study measured the stress involved with hospitalization and correlated it with *in vitro* and skin sensitivity (inflammation) measures of immune-system function (Linn, Linn, & Jensen, 1981). Upon admission to hospital, 75 patients were asked to complete a symptoms checklist that included a measure of anxiety. They were also asked to estimate their stress on a 10-point scale. To test immunocompetence, blood samples were taken to assess antibody counts and lymphocyte proliferation to the mitogens PHA, Con A, and PWM (see "How Immune System Function is Measured in Psychoneuroimmunological Research", above). Three skin sensitivity tests were also conducted. Finally, patients were asked to use a 6-point scale to assess their health over the past 6 months.

Scores on the anxiety measure were significantly correlated with poorer self–assessments of health and less lymphocyte responsiveness to PHA and Con A (but not PWM). Anxiety was not related to antibody counts. Interestingly, anxiety was associated with greater skin sensitivity. These findings remind us of the need to collect multiple measures of immune response in PNI research, since some are affected negatively, some positively, and some not at all by hospital-related anxiety. Nevertheless, this study indicates that stress can interfere with hospital treatment and recovery, given its effect on some aspects of immune functioning.

In another study of real-life stressors and their effect on general health and the immune system, Kiecolt-Glaser and colleagues (1987a) took multiple measures of immune functioning from women who were recently divorced or separated (within the past year). They found that these women had significantly poorer functioning on five of the six immune-system measures compared to women who were neither divorced nor separated. In a subsequent study of men, it was found that those who initiated the divorce reported better health than those whose partner had initiated it (Kiecolt-Glaser et al., 1988).

It is clear from this collection of work that stress affects health through the immune system, both in acute and immediate ways as well as on a longterm basis. Let's now look at specific illnesses to learn more about the extent to which stress can be a factor.

Stress and Upper Respiratory Infection

Many people doing research in PNI believe that, of all the medical conditions that are either brought on or worsened by stress, **upper respiratory infection (URI)** might be the most prominent. Upper respiratory infection refers to a collection of common illnesses such as colds, coughs, flu, and bronchitis. This is the category that Lori from our opening example would fall into. If you have ever developed sniffles and sneezes or a nagging cough during or after exams, you may well have been a walking demonstration of the well-established relationship between stress and URI.

In an early study, people were tracked for 6 months and asked to report stressful life events and daily hassles, the two most commonly identified sources of stress in our lives (Graham, Douglas, & Ryan, 1986). At the same time, these volunteers were monitored for URI episodes. It was discovered that those people experiencing high levels of life-event and daily-event stress suffered more and longer bouts of URI than those people who were not having to deal with stressful events.

Field studies such as this one are important because they are clearly applicable to the realities of our daily lives. However, they also feature less than optimal experimental control. For example, we can get self-report measures of the intensity of the stress being experienced, but we can't control the event. As such, we can't know for sure whether we are dealing with the kind of events most people would find stressful, or if we have a volunteer who is particularly vulnerable to stress. Is the variable a *situational* one that might affect most people the same way, or is it a *dispositional* one that can only be generalized to certain types of people? Some might argue that it doesn't matter. Rather, if a person reports stress, then there is stress—stress is seen as an entirely subjective experience. In support of this view, we know that immune functioning clearly fluctuates with self-reports of stress, so it must be a valuable way of assessing stress for the purposes of PNI research.

It is the case that some people are more prone to stress than others. From the perspective of PNI, we should be able to learn something about them and the effects of stress by studying their URI experiences. This is just what was done by La Via and his colleagues (1996). They studied 14 people with generalized anxiety disorder. As the term implies, this disorder is typified by excessive worry and apprehension about a wide variety of aspects of one's life, such as work, family, and social contacts. This worry persists for at least 6 months.

People with generalized anxiety disorder experience greater impact from stressful events, or in the language of stress research, their **stress-intrusion scores** are high. La Via and his team measured stress intrusion in these 14 people using the Impact of Events Scale. To measure immune functioning, they took *in vitro* measures of lymphocyte activity and kept track of the number of URI-related sick days the people reported. They began by confirming that the people with generalized anxiety disorder had higher stress-intrusion scores. The researchers then discovered that the anxiety group had less lymphocyte activity and more sick days than a control group. In fact, the anxiety group averaged 24.8 URI sick days in a 12-month period, compared to only 9 days among the non-anxious control participants. Finally, they showed that lymphocyte activity was correlated with URI sick days ($r = .44$) and with stress intrusion ($r = .33$).

There is another potential problem that we need to address concerning field studies, though. In studies of this type, researchers lose control over the amount of antigen participants are exposed to. For example, it might well be that, in times of stress, people turn to others for help, thus increasing their exposure to people who might be infected with cold or flu viruses. This would mean that stress increased the likelihood of URI, not because of immunosuppression, but because of increased exposure to others who were infected.

One way to solve this problem is to conduct studies that measure immune activity and URI symptoms concurrently, as La Via did. Studies of this nature also address the problem we discussed earlier in this chapter regarding the distinction between statistical and clinical significance. If a study found URI symptoms without evidence of immunosuppression, we might be inclined to look more closely at exposure rates to explain the result. It is also possible that we could find statistical evidence of immunosuppression but no URI symptoms. In this case, we would be left with at least two possibilities: (1) that the suppression of immune function was too small to increase susceptibility to actual disease, or (2) that the person wasn't exposed to a URI virus when susceptible.

A study of medical students during their exam schedule yielded results that are open to either of these interpretations, underscoring the importance of measuring immune function and URI symptoms at the same time (Deinzer & Schüller, 1998). Forty-two medical students writing exams were compared to twenty-four who were not writing. Stress measures were taken for both groups well in advance of the exam schedule, 3 days prior, just after the exam, and 4 days after written exams. A similar pattern was followed for the same students when they completed their oral exams. Deinzer and Schüller also kept track of the amount of time these students spent studying and the number of breaks they took. To measure immune functioning, daily saliva samples were taken to measure sIgA, and symptom questionnaires were also completed daily. Salivary immunoglobulins are an important line of defence against URI.

Over the course of the study, students writing exams showed a progressive reduction in sIgA concentration from baseline to pre-exam to post-exam for both written and oral exams. This reduction was negatively correlated with study time—more studying was related to worse sIgA concentration. It is interesting to note that this effect persisted for 6 days following the exam. This finding causes problems for other studies that have used post-exam immune function measures as baseline comparisons. These studies are prone to the incorrect conclusion that immune function was unaffected by exam writing because immune cell levels were the same just after and a few days after writing. However, that may well be because the poor levels hadn't returned to baseline yet.

There is more to report from the Deinzer and Schüller study, though. Remember that they also had the medical students complete symptom questionnaires. It was discovered that there were no differences in URI symptom reporting for students writing and those not writing, even though there *were* significant differences in their sIgA concentrations. Could it be that sIgA concentration changes were too small to increase susceptibility to URI, or is it that medical students, when studying, hole up in their rooms and thus avoid contact with infected others? Or are there better ways to measure URI-related immonocompetence than sIgA concentration? These questions remain unanswered, though this study makes it clear that immune functioning and symptoms must be measured concurrently.

Another way to gain even more control over antigen exposure is to do laboratory experiments in which volunteers are given controlled dosages of viruses and have their course charted over a period of time. It is this technique that was used by Cohen, Tyrrell, and Smith (1993) (see Focus on Research 3.1). In this study, volunteers were given one of five respiratory viruses or a placebo by way of nasal drops in dosages intended to simulate those occurring in natural, person-to-person transmission. Not only was exposure controlled via the nasal drops, participants were also quarantined alone or with one or two others for the duration of the study. As you know from reading the details of the study, cold symptoms flourished more in people who had experienced more stressful life events prior to participating in the study.

FOCUS ON RESEARCH 3-1: A Virus Up Your Nose

Sheldon Cohen, David Tyrrell, and Andrew Smith (1993) have studied possible links between negative life events, perceived stress, negative affect, and susceptibility to the common cold. The purpose of this study was to test the hypothesis that stress affects URI through the immune system. A secondary purpose was to eliminate the possibility that the link between stress and URI was due solely to increased exposure to viruses. Field studies in which people's stress levels are measured while they are being monitored for the development of upper respiratory infection (URI) have the advantage of *external validity*, which means that the results can be generalized to real-life settings more confidently because the studies were conducted in these settings. The downside to these studies, though, is that control is relinquished. For example, researchers don't control the intensity of the stress-inducing stimulus, nor do they control exposure to viruses that cause URI. Researchers doing field work aren't so concerned about controlling stress-inducing stimuli because the researchers consider stress to be a subjective phenomenon that is best measured by self-report rather than by stimulus intensity. The same situation can be considered stressful to one person but not another. It is the *perception* that matters concerning stress, not some objective measure of the stimulus that brought on the stress.

Controlled exposure to antigens is another matter. It is very possible that stress causes people to either seek out the company of others or hide away from them. In either case, exposure to viruses is significantly affected. For this reason, a number of studies have adopted a methodology whereby they intentionally expose volunteers to controlled dosages of URI-related viruses. These are called **viral challenge studies**.

In one viral challenge study, 394 participants ranging in age from 18 to 54 years were exposed to one of five respiratory viruses or a placebo (a saline solution that had no effect on disease). Viruses were administered by way of nasal drops in dosages intended to approximate those encountered in person-to-person exposures. To further control exposure, participants were also quarantined from 2 days prior to exposure to 7 days after, such that they were either alone or with one or two other participants. They were given daily clinical examinations for URI symptoms from 2 days prior to exposure to 6 days after. Blood samples were taken 2 days prior to exposure and then again 28 days after exposure to assess specific antiviral IgA and IgG. Body temperatures were taken twice daily and mucous weights were calculated. Three measures of stress were included: (1) number of major stressful life events in the past 12 months having negative impact; (2) perception that current demands exceeded coping resources; (3) current negative emotion. Numerous other variables were controlled for, including demographics, health behaviours, health status prior to the study, and some personality variables.

No placebo subjects developed symptoms. Of those reporting a higher number of stressful life events, 44 percent displayed URI symptoms. This compared to 33 percent of those reporting a low number of stressful events. These rates were unrelated to health behaviours. Perceived current stress and current negative emotions were not related to URI symptoms. The blood sample data showed immunocompromise for people who perceived more stress overall. More specifically, people reporting stressful life events had significantly elevated body temperatures after exposure to the virus.

The authors concluded that, while perceived current stress and negative emotion might influence other aspects of our health, it is the major difficult events in our lives that appear to make us more susceptible to developing upper respiratory infections when we are exposed to them. The viral challenge approach used in this study proves that this increased susceptibility can't be explained solely by increases in exposure to virus at times of stress.

Thus far, we have assumed that stress works alone to influence URI. Referring back to some of the language you learned in Chapter 2 on research methods, you will see that our discussion of stress has assumed a *main effects* model. However, we know that, while main effects models allow us to isolate a factor to determine its unique contribution to illness, they also represent oversimplifications of the realities of health and well-being. Stress rarely works in isolation. Instead, it *interacts* with other factors such as social support, demographics, and personality.

In recognition of this, Turner Cobb and Steptoe (1996) conducted a study using an *interactional model* to measure the relationship between stress and URI. In addition to measuring stress, they also measured social support, coping style, and aspects of the family environment. Their particiipants, 107 adults ranging in age from 18 to 65 years, kept a respiratory daily diary over the 15 weeks of the study. When participants reported symptoms indicating URI, they were given a clinical exam to confirm the diagnosis.

Stress was measured in three ways: (1) a list of major stressful life events was made for the 12 months prior to the study and again at the end of the 15 weeks of the study; (2) a summary of daily hassles was recorded at the end of each week of the study; and (3) general perceived stress was measured weekly. Social support was measured at the beginning and end of the study, as was participants' tendency to cope by confronting or avoiding stressful situations (using something called the monitor/blunter scale). Finally, family environment was assessed at the end of the study.

Three variables were associated with the 29 people who experienced at least one clinically verified URI episode during the 15 weeks of the study. These were stressful life events 12 months prior to the study, daily hassles, and an avoidant coping style. In terms of interactions, it was found that these three factors combined to increase susceptibility to URI. Social support interacted with stress in an unpredicted way. Support lowered susceptibility to respiratory illness for people low in stress but not for those high in stress. This contradicts the belief that social support kicks in as a buffer when stress gets too high. This study adds to our knowledge of the interactions that exist when stress is associated with URI. However, because there were no direct measures of immune-system function taken, we cannot be sure if the URI episodes were a function of immunosuppression or of increased exposure.

It is worth noting that a least one study has found that *positive*, rather than negative, life events increased vulnerability to URI (Evans, Doyle, Hucklebridge, & Clow, 1997). University students were asked to complete the Life Experience Survey as well as other measures such as personality and stress experience. They were then monitored for just over 6 weeks for URI episodes, which were verified with body temperature readings. It was discovered that it was positive life experiences that were most closely related to URI, independent of personality measures or health-related behaviours. This may mean that we need to consider the effect of *any* major event, not just the negative ones, when conducting PNI research.

If stress makes people more susceptible to URI, can we then reduce that susceptibility with interventions that reduce stress? The answer may well be "Yes." After ascertaining that a sample of 45 children with recurrent URI problems had lower levels of sIgA, almost twice as many stressful experiences, a greater proneness to stress, and more signs of emotional disturbances than a group of 45 healthy children (Drummond & Hewson-Bower, 1997), researchers gave both groups of children relaxation sessions. They discovered that children with and without URI problems produced increased sIgA concentrations after these sessions (Hewson-Bower & Drummond, 1996).

What, then, can we conclude about the extent to which stress puts us at risk for upper respiratory infection? Certain types of stress do affect specific aspects of immune functioning. In particular, major life event stress, like Lori's exams, often results in immunosuppression. If the timing of this is such that a person is also exposed to a respiratory virus, then it is likely that the person will get sick. These stressful events don't all have to be recent, though they probably have an additive effect if a bunch of them "pile up" over time.

How do we decrease our risk of URI in these cases? One way is to reduce stress. We will talk about that in detail in Chapter 5. Another is to minimize exposure to respiratory viruses during or after major stressful life events. This simply isn't practical, though. For one thing, a person's first priority at these times isn't to avoid a cold. It is coping with the stressor and its aftermath. For another, we often cope with these stressors by seeking the support of others. It would be highly unwise, if not downright neurotic, to avoid this support because it might mean catching a cold!

Stress and Autoimmune Diseases

The immune system of people with autoimmune diseases becomes their own worst enemy. It produces antibodies that attack the body's own tissue. In other words, the system fails at one of its hallmarks—*tolerance*. A number of diseases fit this category. Some of the better-known diseases include rheumatoid arthritis, insulin-dependent diabetes, and multiple sclerosis.

Does stress put someone at greater risk for contracting these diseases or suffering more once they have contracted them? Research indicates that stress does have both these effects (Homo-Delarches et al., 1991).

On a more positive note, Cohen and Herbert (1996) reviewed a collection of studies indicating that cognitive-behavioural training has been proven reasonably effective in reducing the symptoms of rheumatoid arthritis (Bradley et al., 1987; O'Leary et al., 1988; Radojevic, Nicassio, & Weisman, 1992). This training usually includes relaxation training and other strategies that would be considered stress reducing. As such, these studies lead to the conclusion that, at the very least, stress makes arthritis worse (as it does with most medical conditions). What we don't know is just what is going on in the immune system that might be affected by stress in such a way that antibodies become more likely to turn against the body's own tissue.

Stress and Cancer

If you were to look up stress and cancer in the health psychology literature, you would find a large number of studies. Not surprisingly, however, most of these studies tend to discuss stress brought on by cancer rather than cancer brought on by stress. There are some researchers who have provided notable exceptions, however. One is David Spiegel, who presents a convincing argument that the immune system can be used to explain how stress can affect cancer. Another is Hans Eysenck, who has developed theories relating personality and illness. We'll begin by presenting Spiegel's reasoning.

In our explanation of how the immune system works, we pointed out that natural-killer (NK) cells were primarily responsible for seeking out and destroying abnormal cells. This function makes NK cells crucial in the body's ability to remain cancer free. We also know from numerous *in vitro* studies that NK cell activity is affected by psychological factors. Among these factors, the relationship between stress and NK cell activity has been clearly established (Herbert & Cohen, 1993). This relationship invites an investigation of the effects stress can have on cancer incidence and progression.

David Spiegel and colleagues (1998) reviewed the literature on the impact of major life stressors on the progression of cancer. The results are somewhat mixed. Two studies found a positive relationship between severe adverse life events and cancer growth. In one (Ramirez et al., 1989), breast cancer patients with relapse had experienced significantly more of these events than had a group of matched patients who were in remission. In fact, patients who had experienced a family death or job loss were more than five times as likely to have had a relapse. In the other study (Geyer, 1991), women who had seen a physician to have a breast lump diagnosed were monitored for 8 years after. It was found that stressful life events were more common among women who developed malignancies.

On the other hand, a study of 204 breast cancer patients found no relationship between severe life events and relapse (Barraclough et al., 1992). In contrast to the Ramirez study, Barraclough used a prospective design, in which stressful events were measured *before* rather than *after* relapse.

These mixed findings indicate that the progression of cancer is not always adversely affected by major life stressors. Spiegel and colleagues (1998) also point out that the cause-effect relationship between immune-cell activity and cancer progression isn't one-way. In addition to the fact that compromised immune systems put the body at greater risk for tumour growth, it is possible that the presence of cancerous cells may bring on immunosuppression. Nevertheless, given the potential role of NK cells in the process, further investigation is certainly warranted. Indeed, Spiegel and colleagues (1998) conclude that, "The role of stress in immunosuppression and tumor progression may be central to *potentiating* existing tumor rather than *initiating* primary carcinogenesis" (p. 679). In other words, stress may worsen existing cancer but not make a person more susceptible to getting it.

Hans Eysenck spent much of the latter part of his very distinguished career studying the relationship between psychological factors and two types of disease—cancer and coronary heart disease. Much of this work focused on personality factors that Eysenck believed put people at risk for these health problems. However, he was also interested in the possible role stress might play as a risk factor in cancer development. Eysenck's interest in this isn't surprising, since there is a close relationship between our personalities and our tendency to perceive situations as being more or less stressful.

For example, Eysenck and colleagues (1989) identified a number of personality types that were hypothesized to be at varying degrees of risk for illness. Type I, as it is called, is typified by the belief that happiness is determined by nearness to an object or person that is highly valued emotionally. Any situation that prevents this nearness is very stressful (Grossarth-Maticek, Eysenk, & Vetter, 1998). So, Type 1 people are more prone to stress (not to mention hopelessness and depression). It is the contention of Eysenck and his colleagues that Type 1 people are more susceptible to cancer. We will be discussing the relationship between personality and cancer later in this chapter. At this point, it is worth noting that this work also implicates stress as a risk factor.

The Effect of Mood on Immune Functioning

Our body's physiological responses to stress may be adaptive in the face of the stressor, but in the long run, they compromise our immune system and put strain on other functions. All of this comes about because of the *arousal* associated with stress. But what about those times when we are depressed or sad or lonely? Rather than being over-aroused, we feel down, uninspired, maybe even hopeless. What effect, if any, do these feelings have on our immune system?

When reviewing research in this area, you will find that a number of terms appear to be used interchangeably to describe the independent variables. "Mood" and "affect" are probably the most common. Some psychologists consider *mood* to be a transient or short-term experience of emotion. A person's mood may fluctuate over the course of a day. Indeed, psychologists talk about *mood states* as opposed to traits, which are much more stable. In general conversation, when we call someone "moody" we are referring to short-term swings in emotional experience and expression.

Mood is also used in a more general way, however. The Diagnostic and Statistical Manual of Mental Disorders (DSM-IV) refers to mood disorders, one of which is depression, which can last for long periods of time. There are other psychologists who prefer to use the word *affect* when they are referring to longer-term emotional phenomena; they call depression an *affective disorder*. Our purpose here is not to resolve this debate. It is, rather, to make you aware of the interchangeable use of these terms when health psychologists investigate the effect of emotion on immunity.

We have seen in our discussion of stress and immunity that so-called "major negative life events" affect immunity. One reason for this is that these events are stressful. But there is often another reason. These events can also elicit strong, unpleasant emotions, like depression, sorrow, anger, grief, and helplessness. A clear example of such a life event is the death of a loved one. Most health psychologists believe that coping with a seriously ill loved one brings on *stress*. Coping with the death of that person, on the other hand, brings on *negative mood*. This is why studies often measure immune functioning of a caregiver when the loved one is very ill and then again if the loved one dies.

Using a design of this nature, Irwin and colleagues (1987) measured immune functioning in three groups of wives: (1) wives whose husbands were in good health; (2) wives whose husbands were being treated for lung cancer that had spread to other parts of the body; and (3) wives whose husbands had died from lung cancer up to 6 months previously. They discovered that this third group was the most depressed and also had the poorest immune functioning. A similar study of men whose wives were dying of breast cancer found that lymphocyte proliferation was better for pre-bereavement husbands than among those in the group whose wives had died (Schleifer, 1983).

These studies indicate that depression is generally not good for the immune system. Longitudinal work supports this conclusion. Having discovered that almost 25 percent of hospital patients had abnormally high depression scores, a group of researchers set out to measure the relationship between this depression and mortality. They measured depression in 454 people when they were admitted to hospital (Herrmann et al., 1998). These 454 people (with an average age of 56.8 years) were then monitored for the next 22 months. Fifteen percent of them died. The strongest predictors of mortality were then identified through statistical analysis. Some of the results were not surprising.

Herrmann and colleagues found that age was the single best predictor of mortality. Next was principle diagnosis—that which brought them to the hospital in the first place. Highest mortality rates were found for oncology (cancers) and hematology (blood disorders) patients. The number of diagnoses was the next best predictor. Then came the depression scores that were taken upon admission. When the other factors were controlled for, it was discovered that people scoring high in depression were over three times as likely to die as those scoring low (see Figure 3.1).

FIGURE 3-1 Depression and Mortality

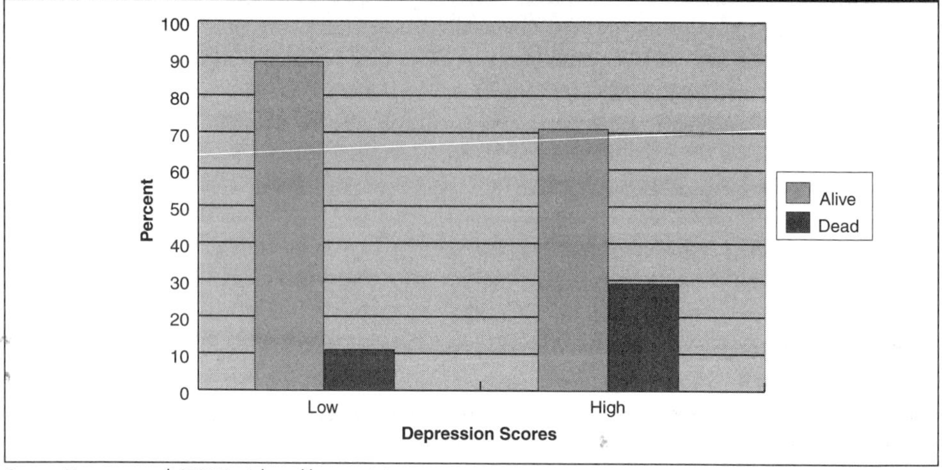

Source: Herrmann et al. (1987). Adapted by permission.

Patients who scored high on a measure of depression were more than three times as likely to die within the next 22 months.

Depression increased mortality risk for all types of patients, regardless of their age or sex. However, depression had its strongest impact on patients with cardiopulminary disease, which is consistent with research showing that depression increases mortality risk after myocardial infarction (heart attack) (see for example, Lespérance, Frasure-Smith, & Talajic, 1996). Herrmann and colleagues also found that depression increased mortality risk for patients with hematological diseases and cancer, which contradicted earlier studies that did not find a relationship between depression and cancer survival (e.g., Richardson et al., 1990).

These studies linking mortality rates and mood provide an important first step, but they do not measure immune functioning, and so we can't conclude from them that the link is due to immunocompromise. Other research has shown that certain components of the immune system fluctuate along with mood. It has been argued, for example, that the relatively short life of sIgA makes it more susceptible to daily fluctuations in mood (Stone et al., 1987). To test this, people were monitored for just over 8 weeks. Three times per week they completed checklists of adjectives describing mood. Their responses were divided into positive and negative moods. Two weeks prior to all this, they started to ingest a harmless antigen. It was discovered that negative moods suppressed immune function and positive moods improved it (see Figure 3.2). (Remember that sIgA is more often associated with the prevention of upper respiratory infection rather than of cancer.)

Stone and colleagues obtained similar findings a number of years later when they monitored mood and immune function over a 12-week period (Stone et al., 1994). However,

FIGURE 3-2 The Relationship between Daily Mood and sIgA Production

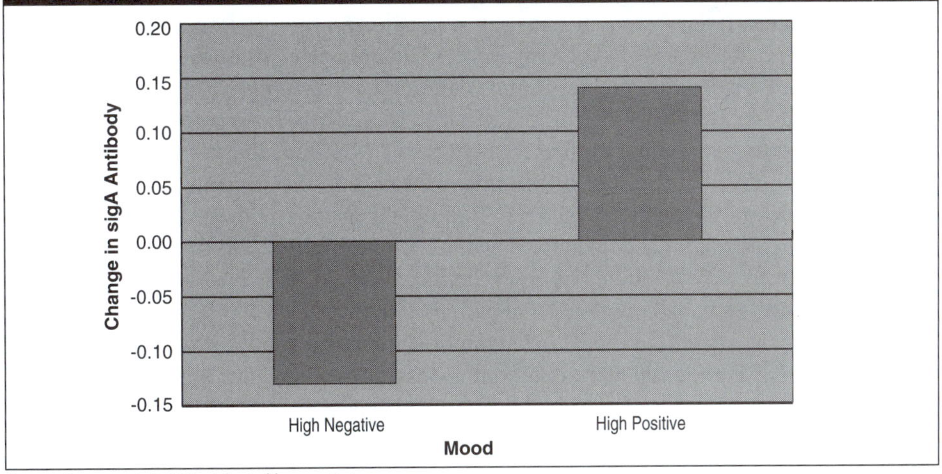

Source: Stone et al. (1987). Adapted by permission.

when people are asked to *summon up* mood in a laboratory setting by recalling positive and negative events, the results are different. In one study, it was discovered that such recollection caused immunosuppression regardless of whether the recalled event was positive or negative (Knapp et al., 1992). In another, actors depicting emotions from scripts showed lymphocyte response to PHA that was consistent with the work of Stone and his colleagues. Those depicting positive moods had greater proliferation of lymphocytes than those depicting negative moods (Futterman et al., 1994). To further complicate matters, Evans and colleagues (1993) found an opposite relationship between mood and sIgA secretion. Greater secretion was associated with *negative* moods.

The contradictions among these studies could be due to the different ways that mood was defined and induced as well as to the different ways immune functioning was measured. Whatever the case, it is clear that mood does generally affect immune functioning. Let's move now to look at specific disease conditions to see if mood is related to them through immunosuppression.

Negative Mood and Upper Respiratory Infection

One of the conceptual problems encountered when studying negative mood is that it can be difficult to distinguish between mood and personality characteristics. In other words, we must be clear that we are dealing with a "person who is down" rather than a "downer of a person." In the language of psychology, we are talking about a distinction between **states**, which are short-term conditions, and **traits**, which are enduring characteristics. This distinction might be particularly relevant if one of your dependent measures was symptom reporting, because increased reporting could just as easily be an indication of chronic complaining as it is of genuine symptom experience.

A study by Cohen and colleagues (1995) made the distinction between state and trait-negative affect, which was an important contribution to our knowledge of the relationship between mood and immunity. In this study, the term "negative affect" is a catch-all phrase for a number of affective states. Four were assessed in this case: anxiety, anger, depression, and fatigue. The main purpose of the study was to sort out the relative contributions of state and trait-negative affect to the experience of cold and flu. By "experience", we mean both the objective existence of symptoms and the self-reporting of them.

At the start of the study, blood samples were taken to establish baseline measures of specific antibody levels. The participants were then exposed to either a cold or influenza virus by way of nasal drops (another viral challenge study). Measures of state and trait-negative affect were also taken at the start of the study. To do this, participants filled out a scale called the Profile of Moods States (POMS). They did this twice—once for how they have felt in the past 24 hours (state) and once for how they felt generally (trait) (the two administrations of the POMS were separated by a few hours).

When these steps were completed, the participants were quarantined in hotel rooms for the duration of the study and their URI symptoms monitored daily. This monitoring was done in two ways. First, nasal secretions were assessed for weight and amount of infection. Second, participants gave self-reports of symptoms. These reports were given for 7 consecutive days following exposure to the virus. Finally, a second blood sample was taken 4 weeks after exposure to the virus.

Seventy-two of the 86 participants developed URI as confirmed by mucous analysis and blood tests. The question was: to what extent were symptom severity and frequency related to negative affect? The answer is interesting, because it underscores the importance of drawing a distinction between state and trait affect. Both state and trait-negative affect were correlated with symptom reporting; however, *only state-negative affect was correlated with objectively confirmed symptoms*. This means that higher state-negative affect at the outset of the study predicted the actual symptoms a person would experience upon exposure to a virus. It also means that people high on trait-negative affect reported symptoms that could not be verified objectively.

You see now why we have to make the distinction between personality and state in this work. Interestingly, people who scored high on trait-negative affect didn't start complaining about symptoms until they actually started experiencing some. They therefore weren't simply inventing them. Instead, their *cognitive bias*, as it is called, took the form of a *misinterpretation* of sensations once they started to feel the symptoms of a cold or the flu. The authors suggest that this misinterpretation is due to an inability to accurately discriminate between real symptoms and other sensations, rather than to an oversensitivity to actual URI symptoms.

At least three important points must be noted concerning the design of this study. First, the authors demonstrated statistically that state and trait-negative affect are different things. Second, in their design they did not correlate antibody proliferation with symptoms. This means that we can only infer that the high state-negative affect people had compromised immune systems, though it is arguably a reasonable inference in this case. Third, this study used a *prospective* design, starting with healthy individuals and charting their course. This is important because the relationship between mood and URI is bidirectional (Hall & Smith, 1996). Most of us would admit that our mood isn't at its best when we have a cold or the flu, so studies in this area must start with people who are healthy.

Negative Mood and Cancer

At the beginning of this section on negative mood, we showed that depression was a significant predictor of a number of illnesses, including cancer. Here, we will take a closer look at the relationship between such negative moods as depression, hopelessness, and pessimism on the risk that a person will get cancer or that people with cancer will survive the disease for shorter lengths of time. Of course, all research in this area must be prospective in nature. A diagnosis of cancer is depressing for most people. As such, we know about that causal direction. What we need to know is the extent of the other direction—the impact of depression in causing or accelerating cancer.

Prospective studies in this area, therefore, take one of two forms. In one form, researchers begin with cancer-free people, measure their levels of negative mood, then monitor them for cancer onset. In the other, people with cancer have their moods assessed, and then the *progression* of their cancer is monitored. In this latter type of study, researchers have to be careful to control for type of cancer and severity at the outset of the study to be able to make meaningful comparisons among people regarding survival.

Interest in the relationship between mood and cancer progression was fuelled back in the 1960s when Arthur Schmale identified what he and George Engel called the "giving up-given up" complex (Schmale & Engel, 1967). This referred to the accelerated rate of decline they observed in cancer patients after these patients gave up hope for survival. Again, cause and effect can be difficult to sort out in these cases. Not so, however, for a study published some 15 years later, in which cancer-free participants were monitored for 17 years to assess the extent to which depression predicted cancer deaths (Shekelle et al., 1981).

In this large prospective study of male employees at the Western Electric Company, over 2 000 cancer-free men were administered a battery of psychological tests, including the Minnesota Multiphasic Personality Inventory (MMPI), in the 1950s. The MMPI is a comprehensive measure that is often used in the diagnosis of psychological disorders. Its subscale that measures depression provided the main independent variable for this study. Once the study began, the men were given annual physical exams for each of the next 11 years. Then, 17 years after the start of the study, mortality statistics were collected on the sample.

Overall, 4.1 percent of the men had died of cancer over the course of the study. It was discovered that men who showed evidence of clinical depression on the MMPI were 2.3 times as likely to have died of cancer at some point in the 17 years covered by the study (see Figure 3.3). This effect was independent of age, cigarette smoking, use of alcohol, family history of cancer, occupational status, or type of cancer contracted. Further, depression was not related to any other cause of death. These results were replicated in another follow-up at the 20-year mark (Persky, Kempthorne-Rawson, & Shekelle, 1987).

More recently, researchers have discovered that pessimism, independent of depression, is related to survival among younger people (between the ages of 30 and 59) who already have cancer (Schulz et al., 1996). Participants in this study were receiving palliative radiation treatment for either recurrent or metastasized cancer. **Palliative treatment** is designed to relieve suffering but is not expected to lead to a cure or remission. To be included in this study, however, a patient needed a life expectancy of at least 1 year. Even with this inclusion criterion, 80 patients died within the 8-month follow-up of the study. It was discovered that, for patients aged 30 to 59 years, pessimism was a significant predictor of mortality, regardless of type of cancer (see Figure 3.4).

FIGURE 3-3 Cancer Deaths Over a 17-year Period Categorized by Presence or Absence of Pre-Cancer Depression

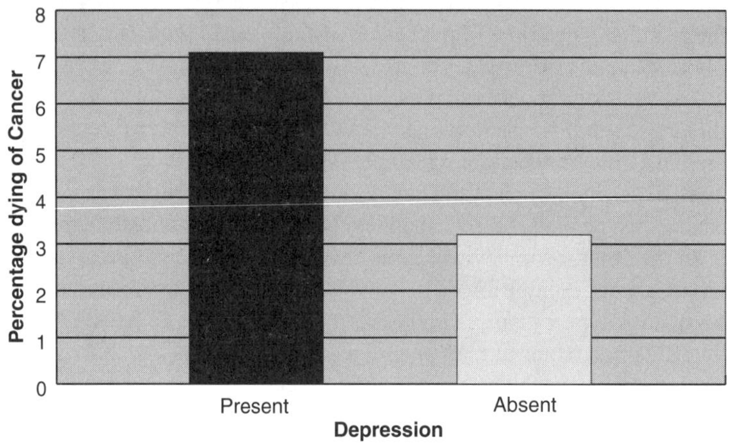

Source: Shekelle et al. (1981). Adapted by permission.

In a 17-year prospective study, physically healthy men who showed signs of clinical depression at the start of the study were 2.3 times more likely to die of cancer.

Here again we run into the difficulty of distinguishing between a psychological state and a personality trait. We all feel pessimistic from time to time (state) but that doesn't mean that we are *pessimists* (trait). The distinction between state and trait is not made in this study, though the authors present a convincing explanation for why pessimism would be worse among younger rather than older cancer patients, implying a state rather than trait perspective. The important point here is that this study does not lead to the conclusion that pessimists are more likely to get cancer. First, the design did not begin with cancer-free participants. Second, pessimism was conceptualized more as a state than a trait.

Other studies have reported a relationship between feelings about the future (such as pessimism and hopelessness) and cancer-related outcomes (e.g., Everson et al., 1996). However, these studies have not taken concurrent measures of immunocompetence, and so we are left to speculate on the extent to which the immune system is involved when negative mood is implicated in cancer. Still, there is evidence from other studies linking immune function and depression that makes it reasonable to speculate that the immune system is, indeed, involved.

In one such study, people with major depression had lowered lymphocyte proliferation in the presence of mitogens (Kerepcic et al., 1995). In another that is perhaps more relevant to cancer, 24 people with major depression were shown to have lower natural-killer cell activity (NKCA) than a group of non-depressed people who were matched on other variables (Kook et al., 1995). (Remember that NK cells are important in the identification and destruction of cancerous cells.) Interestingly, this same study found that NKCA activity increased when the depressed people were treated with an antidepressant.

FIGURE 3-4 Pessimism Scores for Survivors and Non-Survivors of Cancer by Age

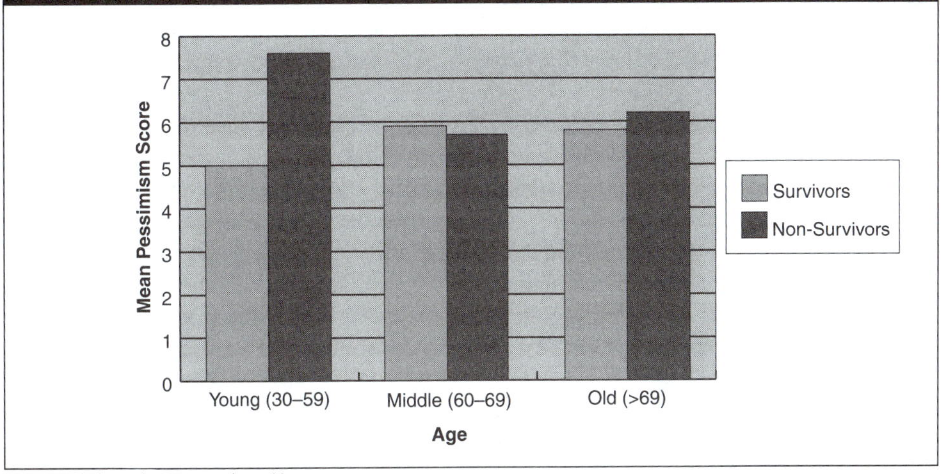

Source: Schulz et al. (1996). Adapted by permission.

Younger patients who had survived with recurrent or metastasized cancer had significantly lower pessimism scores than those in that age group who did not survive.

In summary, it is safe to say that depression and other negative mood states are related to cancer mortality in that these states are associated with increased risk of contracting cancer and of dying from it once it is contracted. It is also likely that immunocompetence provides one explanation for these increased risks. However, we must remember that negative mood states are related to a number of other behavioural phenomena that can affect the experience of cancer, especially its progression. People who are experiencing depression or hopelessness are less likely to follow medical regimens and to generally take care of themselves. Also, they tend to sleep poorly and have less energy (Jenkins, 1996). So it would be an oversimplification to say that negative mood compromises the immune system and that is the sole reason why negative mood is associated with increased risk concerning cancer. Whatever the reasons, there is no doubt that health psychologists, counsellors, and others working in a psychosocial capacity with cancer patients must pay close attention to patients' moods and work to help patients be optimistic and hopeful. As for those who are cancer free, optimism and hope are always healthy states to practise.

Negative Mood and Heart Health

In general, the immune system is not as commonly associated with heart health as it is with infection or cancer. As we saw earlier in our discussion of research investigating negative mood, it is often the case that mood is studied as an *outcome* rather than a *cause*. In this vein, researchers have suggested that depression deserves more attention as an underdiagnosed problem for people with heart problems such as myocardial infarction or cardiovascular disease (e.g., Musselman, Evans, & Nemeroff, 1998). Still, there are some prospective studies indicating that negative mood, depression in particular, is a risk factor for heart disease and related mortality.

One large study measured depression and hopelessness in over 2 800 adults of various ages and then monitored their health for an average of just over 12 years. Over that period, 189 of the participants died from heart disease. When these people were analyzed, it was concluded that depressed affect elevated a person's risk of fatal heart disease by 1.5 times and severe hopelessness by 2.1 times (Anda et al., 1993).

Another prospective study followed over 3 700 adults who were over the age of 70 years at the start of the study. These researchers made a distinction between what they called new depression and chronic depression. Newly depressed participants were those who were depressed at the outset of the study but had not been either 3 or 6 years before. Chronically depressed participants were depressed at the outset *and* at either 3 or 6 years before. It was discovered that for men, new depression (but not chronic depression) increased the risk of contracting heart disease and dying from it. In fact, it was concluded that newly depressed older men were twice as likely to have a cardiovascular disease event than were men who were either chronically depressed or not depressed at all (Penninx et al., 1998).

As has been the case with much of the research discussed in this chapter, it is important to remember that mood is correlated with a number of other factors that can influence heart health. For example, depression and age are correlated and, of course, heart health is related to age. This means that we must statistically control these correlated risk factors so that we can conclude that depression affects risk, *independent of other risk factors*. Both these studies on depression and risk of heart disease did that.

From this work, we can conclude that depression is a risk factor for heart disease. However, these studies do not implicate the immune system as a way of explaining this risk. Indeed, the most common reference to the immune system in relation to the heart comes in discussions of heart transplants and the body's attempts to reject a new heart. Given that the role of the immune system is to seek out and destroy "non-self" entities, it is not surprising to find that the immune system must be repressed just following transplantation.

Negative Mood and HIV Infection

Given what we know about the general effects of mood on the immune system and that AIDS is a disease of that system, it stands to reason that we should investigate the effects of negative mood on HIV infection and AIDS. There have been a few fairly large studies in this area, but the results have been quite contradictory.

Burack and colleagues (1993) measured depression in a group of 277 HIV-positive men. They then tracked T-helper cell activity in these men over a period of 5 years (T-helper cell activity is an important predictor of prognosis for people who are HIV positive). The depressed men showed a significantly greater decline in this cell activity than the non-depressed men did. There was no relationship between depression and the onset of HIV or mortality, however. Lyketsos et al. (1993) studied over 1 700 men to find that depression was *not* linked to T-helper cell decline over an 8-year period. In a review of these two studies (Kiecolt-Glaser and Glaser, 1995), it was pointed out that the men in the Lyketsos study started with a lower baseline T-helper level than did the men in the Burack study. This suggests the possibility that depression affects only those who have a relatively high T-helper cell count.

To test this possibility, the Burack data were reanalyzed by dividing the men into high and low T-helper baseline cell counts. When this was done, it was discovered that depression affected the men whose cell counts were initially high but not those whose counts were initially low. So it may well be that depression affects HIV-positive individuals more when their T-helper cell counts are relatively high.

The negative moods accompanying bereavement can also have an affect on the disease progression of people who are HIV-positive. It has been suggested, however, that *grief* from the loss of an intimate partner to AIDS has a different effect on the immune system than *depression* does (Kemeny, 1994). While depression affects those T-helper cells we were talking about earlier for non-bereaved men, depression doesn't have this affect for men who are in the process of grieving over a loss.

In a review of all this work on negative mood and HIV status, it has been pointed out that these studies didn't measure daily fluctuations in mood and immune function. Instead, they looked at longterm effects of depression that was only measured once at the outset of the study. We don't know if immune system status fluctuates more with daily mood variations for those who are HIV-positive. It may be argued, though, that the most important measures for these people are those involved with disease progression over longer periods of time rather than with day-to-day changes.

We do know that some interventions intended to help elevate mood have had encouraging effects on HIV-positive individuals. For example, a group of men were randomly assigned to an aerobics class 5 weeks before they were to receive notification regarding their HIV status. Compared to a group of men who had not been assigned to these classes, the exercisers who found out they were HIV-positive showed less anxiety and depression as well as less NK cell decline. All exercisers, whether they turned out to be HIV-positive or not, showed an increase in T-helper cell counts compared to non-exercisers (LaPerriere et al., 1991).

What can we conclude from this work on mood and HIV status? It does appear that depression affects disease progression in the form of T-helper cell counts, for men who have initially higher counts. It also looks like exercise is one way of fighting the effects that depression can have in these cases.

Personality and Immune Functioning

In other parts of this chapter, we made reference to the effect of psychological *states* on the immune system. We have contrasted that with *traits*, which refer to stable characteristics that do not vary from situation to situation. We will now look more closely at this notion of "trait", as in personality trait. In this section, we will explore the extent to which certain *types of people* have differing levels of immune functioning. We can then extend this exploration to draw conclusions regarding the likelihood that certain types of people are more susceptible to certain illnesses.

It should be remembered that the states we have already discussed, stress and mood, are closely related to personality. The difference is that, when we talk about **personality** in psychology, we are talking about a person's collection of attributes and behavioural tendencies that are consistent over time and across a variety of situations. Personality isn't a fleeting thing. As we mentioned earlier, there is a difference between occasionally feeling pessimistic and being a pessimist. Indeed, there are social psychologists who believe that people don't actually behave consistently enough across situations to warrant belief in personality as a psychological concept. Regardless of debates about the true nature of the construct of personality, it stands to reason that there are some things about us that are enduring and distinctive. And it is also possible that these things affect our health by way of the immune system.

CASE 3-1 Two Different Reactions to a Diagnosis of Cancer

Jack and Craig had never met. They were sitting across from one another, leafing through magazines in a waiting-room at the cancer clinic. Both had recently found out that they had prostate cancer. The news had been upsetting for both men. However, from the moment when their respective family physicians told them the news, each had reacted quite differently. In this case study, we will describe these different reactions and speculate on the effect they might have on the progression of the disease for each man. We will base our speculation on what we know from PNI research with cancer patients.

Both men were in their early 60s. Both were happily married. Jack kept in close contact with his two children, who were both married and had children of their own. Craig didn't hear from his children much since they had started lives of their own. He saw them at major holidays and that was about it.

The most significant difference between the two men was in the way they had taken the news that they had cancer. Jack was upset, of course, but he considered himself to be relatively young and determined. He went to the library and took out books on prostate cancer to learn more about the disease and what his options were. He also checked out the Internet for information. He felt thankful that he wasn't in very much pain at this point and was confident that he could handle the treatment and that it would work.

Craig responded differently. When he was told he had prostate cancer, he suddenly felt very old. He had heard of others who had the disease and they were all in their 70s and 80s. He felt bitter that he had contracted a disease that put him in such an infirmed category. He decided that this would be the way his life would end—prematurely and terribly. Sure, he would go through with the treatments, but he had no confidence that they would work. He was convinced that his quality of life was about to fall apart permanently and that there was nothing that could be done about it. Soon, he began to feel depressed much of the time.

Other aspects of these men's lives were different as well. When Jack came home from the doctor and told his wife his diagnosis, she had said that the two of them were going to grow old together and that was that. She maintained an upbeat attitude and helped Jack through the times when he got discouraged or was in discomfort. Jack's friends and neighbours responded the same way.

Craig had a different experience. His wife had been devastated by the news that her husband had cancer. They had both just retired and they had plans to travel and enjoy life. Now, in her mind, all of those plans would come to nothing. When Craig would get depressed, he was difficult to be around. At these times, his wife would leave him alone. Craig didn't have many friends, and those he did have he felt awkward around now because he felt that he had a horrible disease that made him different from them.

If it were the case that Jack and Craig were at the same stage of illness when they were diagnosed, and that they we similar in all other aspects of their health, PNI research findings would suggest a more favourable prognosis for Jack. He has an optimistic attitude and he believes in the efficacy of the treatment. These cognitions help him avoid getting depressed, and depression has been shown to accelerate cancer progression. Jack also has a strong support system in the form of family, friends, and neighbours. This support is associated with better survival rates for cancer patients.

Craig is on a much less encouraging course. His depression has the potential to suppress his immune system to the extent that his cancer could worsen over time. This, of course, would only depress him more. Somehow, this cycle needs to be broken and Craig needs to get help for his depression. His social support network isn't strong, which is another disadvantage for Craig. He needs to change his thinking in this regard as well. Perhaps if he gave his friends more of a chance, they could be more supportive of him and this would help him feel less depressed. Also, as hard as it may seem for him, Craig needs to be a more positive companion for his wife. For her part, she needs to persevere through the difficult times brought on by Craig's depression and try to maintain an optimistic and positive approach to his treatment and their future together.

It's not that Jack and his family are "better people." Craig's response and that of his wife are perfectly understandable. However, though their responses are understandable, they are not going to help Craig. They must try to make changes in the way they are reacting to Craig's illness. All of this is easier said than done. Fortunately, there are counsellors who specialize in helping families cope with illness. We emphasize the need for such counselling here, because an improvement in Craig's mood and thinking will likely increase the competence of his immune system and thus better the chances of his survival, not to mention his overall quality of life.

There has been a great deal of work investigating general relationships between personality and health. There has been much less, however, looking specifically at personality and immunity. Cohen and Herbert (1996) have reviewed studies assessing the effects of two related coping strategies, **repression** and **denial**. People displaying these traits ignore distressing events or deny that such events exist or that negative emotions are being felt. Remember that for a coping strategy to be part of one's personality, it has to be used *consistently*. Studies linking repression and denial to the immune system have demonstrated that the effects differ depending on the way denial and repression are assessed and which immune functions are being considered.

For example, when repression was assessed by way of a personality questionnaire, it was associated with suppression of immune function as defined by an increase in herpesvirus antibody (Esterling et al., 1993). (Remember that an increase in herpesvirus antibody means that herpesvirus is proliferating in the body, which is a sign of immunosuppression.) On the other hand, a study of gay males about to be tested for their HIV status showed a *positive* correlation between amount of denial and proliferation of lymphocytes to PHA (Antoni et al., 1990). Other studies have shown that breast and cervical cancer patients who respond with denial have better survival rates that those who feel helpless or unemotional (Greer, 1991).

Why do these studies produce conflicting results? One explanation focuses on subtle differences between the ways repression and denial were operationalized. In the study by Esterling and colleagues, repression was assessed as a general personality trait. In the other two studies, denial was assessed as an active process in the face of real threats (possible HIV-positive status and cancer). We may be able to conclude from these studies that the general tendency to push unwanted thoughts and emotions out of consciousness is problematic in terms of controlling herpesvirus. In contrast, the active attempt to deny the existence of a threatening situation or condition may stave off a sense of helplessness or depression and, as such, be good for our immune response, at least in the short-term.

Personality and Upper Respiratory Infection

Research to date has failed to find a link between personality characteristics and susceptibility to upper respiratory infection (URI). Posse and Haellstroem (1998) measured *alexithymia*, people's tendency to interpret arousal in purely physical terms without feeling the emotion others would associate with that arousal. This tendency was unrelated to URI or other diseases such as asthma, gastrointestinal diseases, or cardiovascular diseases. Similarly, other researchers have found no relationship between sex-role orientation (masculine, feminine, or androgynous) and self-reports of URI (Shifren, Bauserman, & Carter, 1993).

Personality and Cancer

You can imagine how compelling it would be to explore the possibility that certain types of people are more likely than others to get cancer. A number of people have taken on this exploration; most notably, Eysenck and Grossarth-Maticek. They studied over 1 000 Jewish concentration camp survivors, comparing their mortality data to 367 Jewish people who had no connection with concentration camps (Grossarth-Maticek, Eysenck, & Boyle, 1994). They discovered that mortality rates for cancer and coronary heart disease were more than twice as high for concentration camp survivors. The authors argued that the concentration camp experience changed those people in permanent ways and that these changes, independent of general life stress, age, or sex, accounted for the increased mortality rates.

From this and other studies like it, Grossarth-Maticek and Eysenck formulated what has been called the **diathesis-stress model** of illness. A diathesis is a factor that predisposes someone to illness. The illness will result when people with this predisposition are exposed to conditions that combine with the diathesis to compromise health. In this case, the experience of being in a concentration camp engendered certain personality characteristics that, when combined with stress, put a person at greater risk for cancer. The personality characteristics constituted the diathesis.

Just what are these personality characteristics? They include such things as consistent feelings of helplessness or hopelessness as well as suppression of emotional expression. This combination was identified as Type 1 by Grossarth-Maticek, who also identified five other personality types in his research. Each of these types was associated with a different health outcome. Type 1 was predictive of contracting cancer in longitudinal studies. These types were based on a number of fairly complex criteria, including feelings regarding valued people and objects (Grossarth-Maticek, Eysenck, & Vetter, 1988). For example, a person might feel great stress if he or she can't get near to this object or person.

This research has come under considerable criticism, however (Amelang, 1997). Methods of data collection have been reported inconsistently in a variety of papers, so that it is unclear just how questionnaires were administered to such large groups of people (over 5 000) or what specific criteria were used to place people in one of the six personality types. In spite of this criticism, the search for the "cancer-prone" personality continued.

After the work of Grossarth-Maticek and colleagues, Eysenck presented what he called the **Type C personality**. This cancer-prone personality was analagous to the Type 1 category. Consistent with the diathesis model, Eysenck has asserted that the Type C personality doesn't cause cancer in and of itself. Rather, it *interacts* with other factors, such as smoking, to yield a risk factor that is much more toxic than smoking alone. More recently, Eysenck hypothesized that the immune system was involved in these personality-cancer links. In particular, he has cited evidence to suggest that cortisol is the biological link between repressed emotion and immunocompromise relevant to cancer (Eysenck, 1996).

Social Support and Immune Functioning

To this point, our exploration of psychological factors has focused on the level of the individual. We don't exist in isolation, however. What role does our social network play in our ability to maintain effective immune functioning? Are some people healthier than others because of the nature of their social world? There is a mound of evidence indicating that one's social network can have a profound impact on one's health, both in terms of staying healthy and recovering from illness or surgery. In the late 1970s, Berkman and Syme (1979) presented data showing that what is called "all-cause mortality rates" are twice as high for people who are socially isolated. This risk ratio was similar to that for cigarette smokers.

It is not an exaggeration to claim that social isolation is as unhealthy as cigarette smoking for many people. Further, there are a number of studies showing that the immune system is involved when it comes to the beneficial effects of social contact. Cohen and Herbert (1996) review research demonstrating these effects as well as the detrimental effects of being alone.

Some of these studies measure **social support** rather than social isolation. You will find that we mention social support a number of times throughout this book. For example, you will encounter the concept again in Chapter 4, when we talk about health promotion. Social support tends to be viewed in terms of social resources; specifically, a collection of interpersonal resources we have at our disposal to help us avoid or cope with difficult times in our lives. It takes a number of forms, including emotional support, informational support, and tangible or practical support (also called instrumental support).

Glaser and colleagues (1985) and Kiecolt-Glaser and co-investigators (1984) found that medical students who reported higher levels of loneliness showed lower NK activity, higher herpesvirus antibody, and lower proliferation of cells in response to PHA; all of these indicate immunosuppression. More recently, Glaser and colleagues (1992) found that medical students who reported higher levels of social support produced more hepatitis B antibodies after a hepatitis B injection. Esterling and colleagues (1994) looked at social support and immune functioning in people who provided care for a seriously ill loved one. They found that lower levels of emotional and tangible support were associated with lower NK cell activity. This was regardless of whether they were still providing the care or if the loved one had died. Other studies of caregivers have come to similar conclusions regarding the relationship between social support and immune functioning (e.g., Kiecolt-Glaser et al., 1991).

Of course, it is possible that this suppression is caused by the negative affect that accompanies loneliness rather than by being deprived of anything that social contact might directly provide. To test this possibility, Thomas and colleagues (1985) controlled for psychological distress when they measured the extent to which elderly people had relationships that allowed them to confide in others. They found that those who reported having such relationships showed a better proliferation response to PHA. This was unaffected by psychological distress. Similarly, Baron and colleagues (1990) found that spouses of patients with cancer showed better NK cell activity and proliferation in response to PHA if they had good levels of emotional and instrumental support. This relationship existed independent of any depression the spouses might have been experiencing.

We must also remember that social support can come in the form of organized *support groups*. Participants in these groups might gain a number of benefits beyond emotional support, however. For example, information, relaxation training, and stress management techniques are often part of the program. It can be difficult, therefore, to isolate which factor, or combination of factors, is having an effect on the immune system in these cases.

Social Support and Upper Respiratory Infection

Little research currently exists in this area. Two studies by Julie Turner Cobb and Andrew Steptoe (1996; 1998) have looked at family dynamics and social support as predictors of URI in adults and children. Family dynamics weren't operationalized so much in terms of social support as they were in terms of family structure and rigidity. It was found that URI is more common in families featuring a more rigid structure. In terms of social support, children with higher levels of support were less likely to suffer URI as a result of stressful life events.

Social Support and Cancer

More work has been done investigating the link between support and cancer. For example, Levy and colleagues (1990) found that female cancer patients who reported higher levels of emotional support had higher levels of NK cell activity. Other research suggests that this immunological advantage translates into better survival rates. Goodwin and fellow researchers (1987) found that married cancer patients had better survival rates than did patients who were not married. Similarly, Hislop and colleagues (1987) and Waxler-Morrison and co-investigators (1991) found that longer survival from breast cancer was associated with being married and having support from friends, relatives, and neighbours. Maunsell, Jacques, and Deschenes (1995) also found that married women and women with confidants lived longer after being diagnosed with breast cancer. On the other side of the equation, Reynolds and Kaplan (1990) found that women who were socially isolated had twice the risk of contracting hormone-related cancer.

Social Support and Autoimmune Diseases

The effects of social support on immune-system status for HIV-positive men have been investigated in at least two studies. In one, Goodkin and colleagues (1992) studied 62 symptom-free HIV-positive gay men. They found that NK cell activity was greater for men who were low in stress and who reported higher levels of social support. Here is another example of social support working for people low in stress but not for those experiencing high levels of stress (see reference to Turner Cobb and Steptoe in the "Stress and URI" section, above.) Again, this seems to contradict the notion that social support is most useful as a buffer against high stress. This is an interactional design, so we can't simply conclude that only people low in stress have good social support. In this study, there was also a group who reported high social support and high stress. For them, however, social support did not affect NK cell activity.

In another study, Theorell and colleagues (1995) looked at changes in T-helper cell counts in 48 HIV-positive men over a 5-year period. They found that social support did have a significant effect on these counts but that it took time for that effect to be realized. Figure 3.5 shows that there was little difference between the high- and low-support men in the first 2 years of the study. However, after that, the men with low support showed a much more dramatic decline in T-helper cell counts. Remember that these cells are considered to be important in the prognosis of people who are HIV positive.

FIGURE 3-5 Decline in T-Helper Cell Counts Over Five Years for HIV-Positive Men with High or Low Social Support

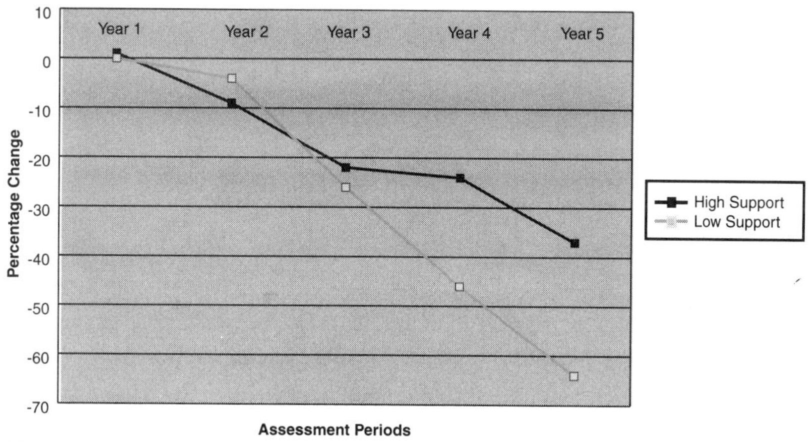

Source: Theorell et al. (1995). Adapted by permission.

What can we conclude, then, from these studies on social support and immune function? While the effects on immunity aren't as striking as those for stress, social support is clearly beneficial to health. This is especially true for people who are low in stress to begin with. It is also worth investigating further the possibility that the effects of social support are more significant over longer time periods rather than in short bursts.

PROPOSED BIOLOGICAL MECHANISMS TO EXPLAIN WHY PSYCHOLOGICAL STATES AFFECT THE IMMUNE SYSTEM

We have reviewed many studies indicating that psychological states and traits can influence our immune system in a variety of ways. This influence increases or decreases our susceptibility to a range of medical conditions and helps or hinders our ability to cope with these conditions once we have them. An important question remains to be answered, however. Just how does our biological makeup allow for this influence? Maier, Watkins, and Fleshner (1994) put it succinctly when they said, "Obviously, psychological factors cannot directly contact white blood cells..." (p. 1009).

There have been a number of mechanisms postulated to explain this, with most of them involving the autonomic nervous system. This system includes parts of the brain such as the hypothalamus and pituitary gland as well as other glands throughout the body that regulate certain vital functions such as heart rate and respiration. As the name implies, the autonomic nervous system tends to work without our conscious control; life is demanding enough without having to remember to take every breath. The system has two divisions—one that stimulates the system when stressors are introduced (the sympathetic division) and one that returns it to a more balanced, calm state (the parasympathetic division).

It has been discovered that elements of the immune system are receptive to neurotransmitters and neurohormones (substances released by the nervous system and glandular system) (McDaniel, 1996). In particular, the immune system is affected by **glucocorticoids**, which are substances released by the adrenal glands upon stimulation from the sympathetic division when we are under stress. We also know that lesions to the hypothalamus affect immune functioning (see Maier et al., 1994 for a review of this research).

Also, there are nerve pathways that stimulate parts of the immune system. Therefore, pathways exist, both in terms of glandular secretion of hormones and neurological stimulation, that provide the opportunity for brain activity to influence immune functioning. Since psychological states such as the ones we have discussed in this chapter affect brain activity (and are affected by that activity), we now have a biological pathway linking these states to immune functioning. It is also worth noting that immune-system activity can, in turn, influence nervous-system functioning. For example, substances produced by lymphocytes affect brain activity in areas such as the hypothalamus (McDaniel, 1996).

At least two important conclusions can be drawn from these discoveries. First, the system most actively involved in stress responses (the sympathetic division of the autonomic nervous system) has direct links to the immune system. This provides some explanation for the relationship between stress and immune functioning. Second, numerous psychological conditions produce different patterns of responses within the central nervous system, which is connected to the immune system through hormones and nerve pathways. It stands to reason that these different patterns of responses would have different effects on immunity.

Certainly, the research we have introduced in this chapter documents a wide range of immunologic responses to psychological conditions.

Following this reasoning, it has been hypothesized that people whose sympathetic divisions are more reactive would be more likely to experience immunosuppression when under stress. This has been called the **reactivity hypothesis** (Cacioppo et al., 1998). In support of this hypothesis, it has been shown that people who show higher levels of cardiovascular reactivity also show the greatest immune changes when in stressful situations (Kiecolt-Glaser et al., 1992; Manuck et al., 1991; Sgoutas-Emch et al., 1994). We are talking here about people whose heart rate and other autonomic functions require less stimulation to kick into "fight or flight" mode. This explains immunologic changes in the face of acute stressors. Kiecolt-Glaser and Glaser (1995) speculate further that chronic stressors have lasting effects on cardiovascular reactivity that bring about the same susceptibility to stress-related immune changes. They suggest that people whose sympathetic division is particularly reactive might be at greater risk for infectious disease. In times of stress, the body must make a priority decision. Does energy go into combating the stressor or fighting off antigens? The answer is that we give priority to the stressor. For those who react more markedly to those stressors, their immune functioning may be further compromised, on both a short-term and longterm basis.

One final question remains. What is the adaptive advantage of a biological system that places greater priority on fight or flight responses than on fighting off disease? Our ancestors required biological resources to deal with immediate concerns in the form of fight or flight responses. It did them little good to be free of upper respiratory infection if their very survival was in jeopardy. Disease control wasn't a priority. Further, when under attack it is advantageous to inhibit inflammation due to injury, so the immune system has to be temporarily suppressed. Today, we might argue otherwise, but we are living with the vestiges of our ancestors' biological priorities.

FUTURE DIRECTIONS FOR PSYCHONEUROIMMUNOLOGICAL RESEARCH

Given the importance and complexity of PNI research, there is much to do in the future. At least three directions have been suggested for this research (Maier et al., 1994):

1. We need to know more about which psychological factors affect which specific aspects of immune functioning. We must be careful not to jump to generalizations such as, "Stress compromises immune function." We need to know more about the relative timing of stressor, immunosuppression, and antigen introduction. Exactly when are we most susceptible to disease?
2. More research is needed that includes disease as an endpoint while concurrently measuring immune functioning.
3. It is important to remember that psychological factors affect other aspects of biological functioning that can, in turn, affect health (e.g., fatigue). We need to learn more about the interaction between these factors and immune functioning.

KEY TERMS

immunocompetence
psychoneuroimmunology
microorganisms
antigens
pathogens
localized infection
focal infection
systemic infection
specific immunity and acquired immunity
non-specific immunity
immune-system memory
specificity
tolerance
phagocytosis
antimicrobial substances
humoral immunity
B lymphocytes
memory B cells
seroconversion
helper T cells
interleukins
suppressor T cells
cell-mediated immunity
cytoxic T cells
natural-killer (NK) cells
immunocompetence
enumerative assay
functional tests of immunity
mitogen
NK cell cytotoxic activity assay
NK cell lysis
acute stressor
resistance
upper respiratory infection (URI)
stress intrusion scores
viral challenge studies
states and traits
palliative treatment
personality
repression
denial
diathesis-stress model
type C personality
social support
glucocorticoids
reactivity hypothesis

Chapter 4

HEALTH PROMOTION

Chapter Outline

Key Questions

1. What are the goals of health promotion?
2. How has health promotion developed in Canada?
3. How can the principles of psychology be applied to improve health promotion efforts?
4. What was the ParticipAction Program and how effective was it?

A group of twelve teenagers is sitting around a table. They are watching a 60-second videotape. On the tape, another group of teenagers is standing around in a playground. A few are smoking cigarettes. Gradually, one of the teens on the tape begins to turn into a cigarette, much to the shock and horror of her friends. Fortunately, though, this terrible transformation has helped them see the error of their ways. They throw away their cigarettes and start playing basketball. When they do, their friend morphs back to her old self.

After watching this tape, the group sitting around the table is asked to comment on it. They have been brought together as a focus group to provide insight into the impact of video campaigns such as this one. The teens say that they are insulted by the video. They find it demeaning and ineffective. They highly doubt if this approach would make them or their friends quit smoking.

This is discouraging. Millions of dollars have been invested in the production and airing of this 60-second piece. Yet, if the focus group is to be believed, it will do nothing to reduce the number of teenagers who smoke.

The feedback provided by that focus group reminds us that health promotion is no easy task. **Health promotion** refers to strategies intended to maintain or improve the health of large populations. The World Health Organization defines health promotion simply as "the process of enabling people to increase control over, and to improve, their health" (Ottawa Charter for Health Promotion, 1986). Yet, even with this seemingly straightforward definition, the fact that health promotion takes so many forms—from smoking-cessation programs to patient education, public awareness campaigns, and political activism—makes it difficult to state in concrete terms just what health promotion is.

Health promotion strategies, like the quit-smoking campaign in our opening example, are often undertaken at a federal level of government. These strategies are virtually always experimental and large and their effectiveness is difficult to measure directly. Further, the challenges inherent in changing attitudes and behaviour on such a large scale are daunting. Yet, even with all these potential problems, effective health promotion is essential to our well-being.

Health promotion is also practised at an international level. The World Health Organization (WHO) has a Health Promotion Department working at political and sociological levels to improve the health of the world's citizens. A good example of one of their initiatives is the program called *Healthy Cities*. Its objectives are to put health on the agenda of decision-makers, build support for local public health action, and develop local participatory approaches to health and environmental issues (WHO web site, 1999, www.WHO.org). Canada has played an active role in the WHO health promotion initiatives and has developed its own health promotion strategy. Let's look at the development of this work in Canada then describe the Canadian strategy in some detail. In so doing, you should get a general sense of what health promotion entails.

THE DEVELOPMENT OF HEALTH PROMOTION IN CANADA

Canadian governments have actually been in the business of health promotion since the 1700s. Back then, the main task was *regulatory* in nature, coming up with rules of operation for hospitals and regulations regarding sanitation. In the early 1900s, with this regulation firmly in place, the focus could be shifted to *education* of the general public regarding the value of proper sanitation (Badgley, 1994).

In the first half of the 1900s, provincial health promotion programs were started in Ontario (1921), Manitoba (1929), Québec (1943), and Newfoundland (1949). National programs followed, for example, *ParticipAction*, aimed at increasing Canadians' activity levels (started in 1971), the *Hole in the Fence* program, to curtail drug use (started in 1973), and *Dialogue on Drinking* (started in 1976).

Other examples of health promotion programs in Canada include the Prince Edward Island Heart Health Program, which started in 1990, the Sun Smart campaign in Alberta, and Health Communities in British Columbia. Later in this chapter, we will take a more detailed look at some of the more prominent programs in Canada.

In Canada, successful health promotion as we now know it has been a clearly stated goal of federal governments since at least the mid-1970s. The kick start came in 1974 from then Minister of Health and Welfare Marc Lalonde's paper, *A New Perspective on the Health of Canadians*. In it, he identified lifestyle as an important factor in health and well-being and, as such, an important target for health promotion and education.

In 1986, then Minister of Health and Welfare Jake Epp published *Achieving Health for All: A Framework for Health Promotion* (Epp, 1986). In it, Epp referred to the World Health Organization's definition of health promotion and applied it to Canada. Most important, in that paper Epp presented a framework that has guided health promotion and related research in Canada ever since.

We present this framework in Figure 4.1. By studying its categories, you will get a feel for what health promotion is all about. Notice the scope of the goals. Everyone in the country should find some relevance in the framework. Notice also the implications regarding locus of responsibility. Any health promotion program places the responsibility for good health on the individual rather on than medical staff or medical facilities.

Consistent with this is the World Health Organization's reference to *control* in its definition of health promotion. Also, note that self-care and mutual aid are cited as health promotion mechanisms in the Canadian framework. In other words, one goal of health promotion is to encourage people to look after themselves. Another is to encourage them to look after each other. A cynical view of these goals might suggest that they represent ways in which the government is shirking its responsibility to look after us. The reply to that cynicism is that there are limits to how much a government can do today to look after its citizens.

FIGURE 4-1 Canada's Framework for Health Promotion

Aim	Achieving health for all		
Health challenges	Reducing inequities	Increasing prevention	Enhancing coping
Health promotion mechanisms	Self-care	Mutual aid	Healthy environments
Implementation strategies	Fostering public participation	Strengthening community health services	Co-ordinating healthy public policy

Source: Epp (1986).

In fact, some authors have argued that if health promotion is to be truly effective, it must be a *social movement* rather than a *government edict* (Labonte, 1990; O'Neill, Rootman, & Pederson, 1994). In other words, the real promoters of healthy choices must be the general public. For example, we know we are getting somewhere in terms of health promotion when parents won't start the car until every child's seatbelt is fastened. Another example of success can be found in the number of community-initiated programs that have been started independent of federal or provincial mandates.

Labonte (1987) provides a three-level framework for successful community-oriented health promotion. His analysis provides a useful taxonomy of health promotion and is very reminiscent of the biopsychosocial approach introduced in Chapter 1.

The first level identified by Labonte is **medical**. This is disease-based and the goal is disease *treatment*. For example, a community might develop a program to help people recover from heart attacks or devote funding to finding a cure for cancer. The second level is **public health**. This is behaviour-based and the goal is disease *prevention*. A good example of a behaviour-based intervention would be the promotion of safe sex, or drinking-driving counterattack programs. The third level is **socioenvironmental**. At this level, the orientation is toward social change and public health policy. Examples include such things as legislation to reduce poverty or school board policies to provide lunches for school children.

Admittedly, one goal of health promotion at the governmental level is to save those governments money on health expenditures. In Canada, where health care is socialized, total health expenditures will have topped $80 billion in 1998. That amounts to over $2 500 per person in 1 year. The public sector's share of that is $55 billion per year (Canadian Institute for Health Information, 1998). When we consider that a great deal of that money is spent on treating conditions that are preventable, we can see why health promotion is important from a fiscal as well as a medical perspective.

In addition to being tragic and traumatic, serious illness is expensive. It is not surprising, then, to find an emphasis on health promotion in Canada today. People who study health at the sociological level of the biopsychosocial approach will argue that saving money and saving lives often amount to the same thing in that they are affected by the same strategies.

These strategies focus on prevention more than a cure, and they feature messages that are intended to affect self-care behaviour, usually through attitude change. Let's take a closer look at Canada's health promotion framework now to develop an understanding of what forms these strategies can take.

The Goals of Health Promotion in Canada

In Chapter 1, we traced the major topics of health psychology as they have developed over the years. As we work through Canada's framework for health promotion, you will see that a number of these same topics receive attention. Look for potential applications of research on coping, social support, and stress reduction as examples. You will also see that the level of emphasis is far broader than the purely biological. In keeping with the biopsychosocial approach, you will find elements in the framework related to individual psychology (e.g., self-care), sociology (e.g., strengthening community health services), and geography (e.g., healthy environments).

Health Challenges

When Canadians think of their health care system, they are more likely to think of its equity rather than its inequity. It is, after all, a system designed to promote and provide equal access for all. The truth, however, is that inequities do exist in the Canadian health care system. These inequities may be based on differences in geography, culture, age, education, income, or labour-force status, to name a few. For example, about 50 percent of men living in the poorest neighbourhoods in Canada will live to age 75, whereas almost 70 percent of men from the richest neighbourhoods will reach this age (Report on the Health of Canadians, 1996). Let's look at some other examples of inequity taken from various issues of the Statistics Canada publication, *Health Reports*.

How far do you live from your family physician? The answer to that question may depend, in part, on what area of the country you call home. In 1993, 90 percent of people living in Canada's large cities (one million or more people) lived less than 5 kilometers from the nearest doctor. By contrast, only 56 percent of people from rural areas had a physician that close. Not surprisingly, if you live in Canada's far north, the nearest doctor is likely much further away. Two-thirds of the people living between the 65th and 69th parallel are more than 100 kilometers from the nearest physician (Ng, Wilkins, Pole, & Adams, 1997). A country as vast and geographically varied as Canada must deal with health promotion challenges that would be much less pressing in smaller countries.

Even with socialized medicine in Canada, the higher one's income the better one's health tends to be (Manga, 1993). The same is true for education level, which is also related to general health (Manga, 1993). It has also been found in the province of Québec that infant mortality rates are higher among delivering women with lower levels of education (Chen et al., 1998). Health-related education is a fundamental goal of health promotion.

It is obvious that our health changes as we age. Still, we need to know about the specific nature of those changes and also about the ways in which our health-related needs change (Chen & Wilkins, 1998). This is a particularly important health-promotion challenge given the growing percentage of people in Canada who are over the age of 65 years. It is estimated that this number will exceed 3.5 million people, or 12 percent of the population, by the year 2001 (Statistics Canada). Age-related health concerns are not restricted to our seniors, however. We know that our adolescent population has its own set of health promotion issues as well. Central among these are risk-related behaviours such as cigarette smoking (Chen & Millar, 1998). As we saw in the example that opened this chapter, it is the job of health promotion to affect these behaviours.

The nature of people's occupations can be another source of health-related inequity. This is due, in part, to the differences in stress levels associated with various jobs (Wilkins & Beaudet, 1998). We also know that certain risk-related behaviours vary from occupation to occupation. For example, in 1994 and 1995, 43 percent of people working in construction, transportation, or mining smoked cigarettes daily. By comparison, only 18 percent of people in so-called "white collar" occupations smoked every day (Gaudette, Richardson, & Huang, 1998).

These inequities are prime targets for health promotion programs. The question is, what sorts of behaviours must be promoted to foster constructive change in people's health? The framework presented in Figure 4.1 attempts to answer this question, as does the following section on **health promotion mechanisms**.

Health Promotion Mechanisms

How can we best meet the health challenges laid out in the framework in Figure 4.1? This is the central question for people working in health promotion. The framework provides three answers: (1) people must be encouraged to look after themselves; (2) people must be encouraged to look after each other; and (3) we must make our environments healthier by reducing pollution, improving safety, etc.

As we review these health promotion mechanisms, notice again where the *locus of responsibility* is placed—squarely on the shoulders of the citizen. Remember that this is a key assumption of the health promotion process. Spending money encouraging people to look after themselves costs considerably less and results in better quality of life than having the government look after them. It has been estimated that obesity alone costs the Canadian health care system over $1.8 billion a year in the treatment of obesity-related medical problems. The most prevalent of these are high blood pressure, Type II diabetes, and coronary artery disease (Birmingham et al., 1999). About one-third of all Canadians are obese, as defined by having a body mass index of 27 or greater, so you can imagine the saving in money and health problems if at least some of those people could be convinced to manage their diets in a healthier way.

Hence the rationale for an emphasis on **self-care**. When we talk about self-care, we are talking about such things as exercise, diet, risk behaviours, voluntary screening, and regular medical checkups. Effective health promotion programs have measurable effects on these behaviours and, consequently, the general health of Canadians.

In the late 1940s, the province of British Columbia became one of the first places in the world to introduce regular screening for cervical cancer (Wardle & Pope, 1992). The test used in this screening is called a **Pap test** or **Pap smear**. When compared to screening tests for other kinds of cancer, the Pap is considered to be among the most effective. By "effective", we mean that it is an accurate early detection strategy that has significantly helped reduce cervical cancer mortality rates (Paraboosingh et al., 1996). In spite of this, older women, who are more at risk for cervical cancer than are their younger counterparts, do not receive Pap tests as often as they should (Lee, Parsons, & Gentleman, 1998).

The Canadian Pap test data illustrate a truism in health promotion—the work never ends. To be sure, there is tangible success. For example, it is now the case that the majority of women in Canada have Pap tests. In 1994 and 1995, 84 percent of women between the ages of 40 and 49 had received a Pap test in the last 3 years. At the same time, 8 percent of that age group had *never* had a Pap test (Lee, Parsons, & Gentleman, 1998).

The very large topic of smoking cessation also fits in the self-care category. Quit-smoking campaigns, therefore, are a major concern for people working in health promotion. It has been estimated that, in the year 2000, close to 47 000 people in Canada will die from tobacco-related diseases (Ellison, Mao, & Gibbons, 1995). This number can be lowered substantially if current smokers can find a way to quit smoking, but that is easier said than done.

In spite of what we know about the dangers of cigarette smoking, health promotion in this particular area of self-care runs into problems brought on by social pressure and addiction. Attempts to simply frighten people away from cigarettes have been discouragingly unsuccessful (Becker & Janz, 1987; Sutton & Eiser, 1984). The relative ineffectiveness of this approach obviously makes health promotion more difficult. It isn't enough to parade grim statistics or blackened lung tissue in front of people to make them avoid smoking. Programs must involve much more than simple appeals to fear. Later in this chapter, we will look more closely at the use of fear appeals and what must be added to them.

Improving self-care among citizens is a fundamental objective of any health promotion program. Having said this, we must also acknowledge that people do not live in isolation from one another. In addition to looking after ourselves, we must also look after each other. We have a responsibility to family, friends, loved ones and, for that matter, society as a whole when it comes to health and safety. This responsibility is highlighted in the Canadian framework with the promotion mechanism called **mutual aid**.

A large body of literature in health psychology supports the framework's inclusion of mutual aid as an important promotion mechanism. The general conclusion of this literature is that it is just plain healthy to have other people around (for a review, see House, Landis, & Umberson, 1988). Mortality rates are lower in communities featuring a high level of social integration. Close-knit communities are healthier.

Health psychologists are very interested in **social support**—that collection of interpersonal resources we have at our disposal to help us avoid or cope with difficult times in our lives. Social support is remarkably beneficial. Research indicates that strong support systems reduce the likelihood we will suffer from ill health and that they promote quicker recovery rates when we do get sick (Kulik & Mahler, 1989).

In fact, social support has been shown to affect survival rates among cancer patients. In a well-known study by David Spiegel and colleagues, breast cancer patients were randomly assigned to either a year of weekly support group meetings or routine medical care (Spiegel, Bloom, Kraemer, & Gottheil, 1989). Patients in the support groups survived an average of 36.6 months, compared to control group patients who survived an average of 18.9 months. A number of other studies have also documented the beneficial effects of social support on people's ability to cope with cancer and survive it (for a review, see Blanchard et al., 1995).

We will be referring to social support a number of times in this book. For example, it is a very important resource when coping with stress, which we will go into detail in later in

Chapter 5 on stress and coping. Also, as we have mentioned, social support is a critical factor in people's ability to cope with serious illness, which we will return to in Chapter 11.

It is important to know that social support doesn't always "just happen." Some people benefit from it more than others do. And social support comes in a number of different forms, some of which are easier to promote than others. Let's look at factors that affect the amount of support a person might receive, in an attempt to determine specific goals of health promotion strategies in the area of what Canada's framework calls mutual aid.

Perhaps the most important point to make at the outset of this exploration is that social support is related to other elements of Canada's health promotion framework—most notably "Reducing Inequities." For example, seniors living on low incomes have less support than their more affluent counterparts. We also know that as people get older, their number of unmet needs in terms of health-related personal assistance goes up (Chen & Wilkins, 1998).

To understand how health promotion can be used to help reduce these inequities, we must divide social support into two general types, based on the source of that support. First, there is **naturally occurring support**. This is the support we find from friends, relatives, coworkers, and others in our own social networks. If you have just had triplets, you might have friends or family over to help out with meals or household chores or to look after the babies so you can get some sleep. This would be an example of naturally occurring support.

The other kind of support might be called **agency-provided support**. This is support that is provided by agencies and organizations formed to fill the void when naturally occurring support is either lacking or unavailable. Imagine that you had those triplets after just moving to a new city where you didn't know a soul. You might be relieved to find that there was a triplet's support group in that city. This would be a group made up of people like yourself who help each other and find community resources to provide further help.

When we study social support in the context of serious illness, we find that many people who are seriously ill don't have many people "like them" who share their illness. For example, wives of prostate cancer patients can be loving and extremely supportive, but they can't have had prostate cancer. For this reason, prostate cancer support groups are popular among men who want information and empathy that can only come from other patients. This is another important reason for agency-provided support.

Now let's get back to the role of health promotion. What is its main job here? In terms of mutual aid, health promotion campaigns must encourage the creation of support groups and attendance at them. This is especially true for segments of our population in which support is less available and for people who have illnesses or other health problems and whose ability to cope can be improved by spending time with others who are in a similar situation.

We have just seen that social support can be categorized in terms of its source. Social support can also be categorized by its type (House, 1981). For example, we can receive **practical support**, sometimes called *tangible support*, which includes help with the demands of daily living—getting meals, rides to doctor's appointments, mowing the lawn, and so on. Also, there is **informational support**, which could include such things as being made aware of treatment options, typical recovery times from treatment or injury, or what to do to speed recovery. Finally, there is **emotional support**. This is provided by people who take the time to understand our fears and frustrations, who help calm us during anxious times, who help bring our moods up, or who distract us from our worries.

When we know the types of support that people need, we can do a better job of promoting that support. To develop an appreciation for this, imagine how you would respond

if you found out that a close friend had just been diagnosed with cancer. You mi
exactly what to do. On the other hand, because this is a thankfully rare thing to hav
tend with, you might feel awkward. Do you call your friend right away or do you
you call, what do you say? What should you do? These are difficult questions that c par-
alyze us.

But what if we knew that people who have been diagnosed with cancer need practical, informational, and emotional support? This might help us answer those difficult questions and make it easier for us to provide support. Perhaps your friend needs a ride to an appointment. Maybe kids need rides to school. Or perhaps there is something your friend needs to know that you might be in a position to find out. In terms of emotional support, maybe you just need to be there to listen. The point is that we can educate people through health promotion such that they are aware of these ways of providing support. Further, we can promote the clear benefits of providing this support. In Chapter 11, you will find further data from studies proving that mutual aid—social support—is of tremendous benefit to people with serious illnesses. For now, it is important to know that good health promotion programs can increase the likelihood that such support is forthcoming and that it will be effective because it will match people's needs (Cohen & McKay, 1984).

By examining Canada's health promotion framework, you will see that mutual aid isn't the only element for which social support is relevant. Consider also the two implementation strategies of *fostering public participation* and *strengthening community health services*. While these strategies clearly require the involvement of professionals from a variety of segments of the health care system, they also require the participation of the general public. Support groups obviously grow out of public participation and they are often offered through community health services facilities.

In this section, we have used Canada's health promotion framework to provide some examples of the challenges faced by people working in health promotion and the jobs that must be done. The number of health promotion programs that could be mounted in a country as vast and varied as Canada is virtually infinite. However, when we use the framework, we can consolidate this number to a very manageable set of jobs. We must find ways to promote self-care and mutual aid and we must reduce health-related inequities. These goals are not unique to Canada. Indeed, they are common to health promotion programs worldwide.

IMPROVING HEALTH PROMOTION BY APPLYING PRINCIPLES OF PSYCHOLOGY

Now that we know what the main goals and challenges are for health promotion in Canada, let's look at the ways psychology can be used to help achieve these goals. To do this, we will draw on the major theories of health psychology, introduced in Chapter 1. We will also look closely at theories taken from social psychology.

Prominent Theories in Health Psychology Applied to Health Promotion

Much of health promotion is targeted at people's thinking. The assumption here is that one way to change behaviour is to change the beliefs relating to that behaviour. This line of reasoning is very consistent with the **health belief model**, the **theory of reasoned action**, and the **theory of planned behaviour**, all of which were introduced in Chapter 1.

Recalling those theories, you will remember that people's beliefs regarding their vulnerability to a threat and the effectiveness of a given course of action to reduce that threat are of central importance. In addition, it is important that people place a high value on their health. Because of their importance to health-related behaviour, many health promotion programs are designed to affect these beliefs and values.

Health promotion programs, then, provide information regarding the likelihood that someone might suffer a health problem (vulnerability information) and how that person can reduce that likelihood (information regarding efficacy of preventative behaviours). Prominent theories in health psychology provide other types of content for health promotion as well. For example, the theory of reasoned action and the theory of planned behaviour both make reference to the fact that people weigh the potential *costs* and *gains* of a given behaviour before adopting it. With this thinking in mind, health promotion programs geared toward physical activity, such as Canada's Vitality program, which grew from the well-known ParticipAction Program, focus on the gains rather than the costs of exercise. They emphasize the fun of exercise, not the fatigue that may result. These programs make the point that physical activity can be convenient, uplifting, and healthy. In so doing, they target people's beliefs regarding cost and gain.

As you can see, the theories of health psychology are called upon to form the foundation of health promotion programs. It is also the case that these programs rely on *social psychology*. This is because health promotion involves *persuasion*, which is a social phenomenon. Let's look at what social psychology has learned about persuasion and then apply this knowledge to health promotion.

The Social Psychology of Health Promotion

Persuasion is the attempt to change people's attitudes and beliefs. An **attitude** is a cognition in which a person *evaluates* some target. Attitudes involve words like *good* or *bad*, and verbs such as *like* or *dislike*. Given this definition, health promotion programs attempt to change attitudes when they try to persuade people that low-fat diets are *good*, and that people should *like* them. We might call this *health advertising*.

In Chapter 1, we defined a "health belief" as something we think to be true concerning our health. More generally, beliefs are our personal encyclopedias on the world. They are the things we consider to be factual and *believable*. Beliefs are different from attitudes in that they are not evaluative in nature. For example, we might hold the *belief* that yogourt contains less fat than ice cream and this belief might cause us to *like* yogourt. Liking yogourt is the attitude. In the language of social psychology, this belief leads to a positive attitude toward yogourt.

Health promotion programs try to affect what people believe to be true and what they *like* and consider *good*. Over the years, social psychologists have conducted extensive research on persuasion (for a detailed review, see McGuire, 1985). Well-proven principles have emerged from this research that can be applied to health promotion. Several examples follow.

The Elaboration Likelihood Model of Persuasion

Research investigating people's attitudes toward political candidates has discovered that there are basically two routes through which these attitudes are influenced (Petty & Cacioppo, 1981). One way, called the **central route**, refers to the use of logic, facts, and reason. Political campaigns using the central route present statistics and logical arguments in favour of a given candidate or, perhaps, in opposition to a candidate. Health promotion programs using this route will also present statistics and medical facts.

The second way is called the **peripheral route**. This involves an appeal to emotion and general impression. Political campaigns using this route will focus on the looks and charisma of the candidate. Health promotion campaigns using the peripheral route feature healthy-looking people or show the potential horrors resulting from risk behaviour.

Research in social psychology shows that some people are influenced more by central routes and others more by peripheral routes. This means that health promotion campaigns must cover both bases. Statistical presentations, which make use of a central route, must also be packaged well to appeal to people who are more influenced by peripheral routes.

A number of studies have applied the elaboration likelihood model to health promotion. In the area of AIDS prevention, for example, it has been suggested that there might be problems with programs focused exclusively on providing facts. People may become overloaded with information; they need to have it packaged in ways that arouse constructive emotional responses (Mulvihill, 1996; Helweg-Larsen & Collins, 1997). A similar suggestion has been made regarding substance abuse prevention programs for college students (Scott & Ambroson, 1994), the point being that a peripheral route must be adopted in such a program because most college students don't see substance abuse as being a pressing issue in their lives.

Fear Appeals: An Example of Health Promotion by the Peripheral Route

One fairly obvious application of the peripheral route is the use of what are called **fear appeals**. The term is self-explanatory. The assumption, of course, is that we can change people's behaviour by presenting frightening accounts of what will happen to them if they continue a given behaviour (for example, smoking) or if they don't adopt a behaviour (for example, dental hygiene).

There is considerable theoretical support for this assumption. For example, a main component of the health belief model is *perceived threat* and *personal vulnerability*. Fear appeals are designed to intensify people's beliefs regarding this threat and the extent to which they are vulnerable. In fact, long before the health belief model came along learning theorists predicted that, under the right circumstances, fear would motivate behaviour change (Hovland, Janis, & Kelley, 1953).

Hovland and colleagues' **drive-reduction theory** argues that we are driven to reduce the tension brought about by deprivation or other states we have an aversion to. According to this theory, fear appeals should work because we are driven to reduce fear, and when we are successful, the behaviour that we use is reinforced. In other words, it becomes part of our repertoire because it was instrumental in reducing the fear. This seems straightforward. All we should have to do with our health promotion messages is arouse fear and then supply recommendations for behaviours that will reduce that fear. So why don't fear appeals always work? Drive-reduction theory also has an answer for that question.

It turns out that if the fear arousal is *too high*, the person will respond in ways other than the recommended behaviour. There are a number of reasons for this, but the main one is that very frightening messages present situations and outcomes that appear to be so awful that we don't think we can deal with them effectively no matter what we do. As a result, the recommended behaviour looks ineffective in comparison to the potentially catastrophic nature of the threat. For example, can I prevent the devastating effects of cancer by eating broccoli? In answering this question, many people would see a mismatch in strength between the threat and the behaviour and so remain uninfluenced. They carry on with their old behaviour because the high-fear message makes the situation look too hopeless to do anything about anyway.

A similar view holds that fear messages must strike a balance between *tension* and *energy* in order to be effective. Up to a certain threshold, fear messages should increase a person's energy for constructive action. Beyond that threshold, however, tension arouses anxiety that depletes that energy and reduces the likelihood that the person will respond in a constructive way (Henthtorne, LaTour, & Nataraajan, 1993).

There are other reasons why high-fear messages often don't work. For one thing, we lose confidence in our ability to carry out recommended behaviours when we are afraid. To illustrate this, ask yourself the following question: How reassuring are instructions on how to employ a backup parachute in the event that the main chute doesn't open? Imagine yourself listening to these instructions. How confident would you be that, in the event that you were plummeting to earth under the full force of gravity, you would be able to carry out those backup instructions? Or would you be too afraid to remember the instructions and carry them out correctly? Confidence levels vary from person to person under such circumstances. Concerning health promotion, we might affect people's confidence in their ability to perform self-examinations for cancer if we portray cancer in particularly frightening ways. This may be why 54 percent of women who were sent a reassuring letter listing "encouraging facts" about breast cancer made an appointment for a mammogram, whereas 42 percent made an appointment after receiving an anxiety-arousing letter listing "worrisome facts." Interestingly, only 38 percent made an appointment when they received a standard letter listing no facts at all (Kendall & Hailley, 1993).

The point of these explanations is that the effectiveness of fear appeals depends very much on people's *responses* while frightened. This makes the fear-appeal approach very tricky. Perhaps the best analysis of the various types of responses to fear appeals comes from what is called the **parallel response model** (Leventhal, 1970). According to this model, recipients of fear-arousing messages focus on either *fear control* or *danger control* or some combination of the two. Put simply, people who focus on **fear control** are not likely to change their behaviour in constructive ways. Instead, they will engage in what more recently has been called **emotion-focused coping** (Folkman & Lazarus, 1985; Folkman et al., 1986; Lazarus & Folkman, 1984). The main goal in this response to the message is to reduce the discomfort of a situation without trying to change the situation itself.

There are a number of possible responses stemming from a fear-control motive. People who respond to fear appeals in this way are more likely to *deny* their personal vulnerability to a threat by saying something like, "This is a really awful thing, but it won't happen to me." They are also more likely to *minimize* the threat by thinking, "This really can't be as bad as people say it is." They tend to be *inattentive* when the message is presented and they will avoid thinking about it afterward. Finally, they might engage in *source derogation*, in which they discredit the source ("They don't know what they're talking about") or dislike the source ("My school counsellor is always such a downer—nothing but doom and gloom messages"). For a more detailed review of these responses, see Eagly and Chaiken (1993).

None of these responses leads to constructive change, which is the goal of health promotion. On the other hand, **danger control** will. This is a form of **problem-focused coping**, in which the person attempts to alter the situation or create conditions in which stress and danger are reduced (Lazarus & Folkman, 1984). There are two important things to note about danger control. First, it usually leads to constructive change when the danger is health related. Second, danger control can proceed *without fear*. In fact, as we saw earlier, fear might inhibit danger control if it is too strong.

In terms of health promotion, danger control usually takes the form of *risk reduction*. From this perspective, you can imagine the wide range of behaviours that fit in the category of danger control. Wearing a seatbelt, exercising, and practising safe sex are all examples of danger control behaviours. The key, then, in fear appeals, is to encourage danger control instead of fear control.

When can we expect a person to respond with fear control and when can we expect danger control? Leventhal's parallel response model doesn't answer this important question; Kim Witte's **extended parallel process model** does (Witte, 1992). Witte's model extends the work of Leventhal by postulating a relationship between the amount of fear presented in a message and the nature of the person's response. Witte argues that low-fear messages stimulate neither fear control nor danger control, since neither fear nor danger appears to be an issue. In contrast, high fear messages will stimulate fear control. They will also stimulate danger control if the message is accompanied by an effective *behavioural recommendation*.

Even with the presentation of these workable suggestions, some people will focus primarily on fear control. This is largely due to the habitual coping strategies of the person receiving the message. We will look more closely at coping styles in Chapter 5 in our discussion of stress and coping. The important point to learn now is that fear appeals differ in their effectiveness, partially because of the different coping approaches adopted by the receivers of the appeals. It is also true, though, that some of the effectiveness of a fear appeal is determined by the strength of the fear message. If the fear is too high, then fear control often becomes the person's first priority, which doesn't lead to constructive change, especially if the high fear is not accompanied by a clear suggestion for reducing the threat. Moreover, high fear reduces people's concentration and processing ability, so they might not be particularly receptive to the suggestion anyway (Christianson, 1992).

As you might expect, there are quite a few published studies that test the effects of fear appeals in health promotion programs. Let's look at some of them in an attempt to draw some final conclusions about the use of fear appeals.

One study in Holland presented Dutch adolescents with anti-smoking messages that varied in a number of ways, one being the severity of the fear component. How did adolescent smokers respond to the more severe messages? As predicted by the parallel response model, almost half were defensive rather than receptive. In other words, they engaged in fear control (van Wel & Knobbout, 1998). Just over half the adolescents in that study, though, expressed a desire to quit smoking. The question is whether that desire would be translated into action, or danger control.

In a study of AIDS-related public service announcements, it was discovered that fear-arousing announcements were more effective than humourous, erotic, or fact-based messages in increasing the intention to use condoms. This effect was greater for women than for men (Struckman-Johnson, Struckman-Johnson, Gilliland, & Ausman, 1994). Another study using AIDS-prevention messages concluded that people must have a strong sense of self-efficacy regarding the recommended behaviour for the fear appeal to work (Witte, 1994). In other words, we must make a distinction between **response efficacy**, which is our perception that the threat-reducing suggestion will work, and **personal efficacy**, which is our belief that we are able to carry out the suggestion (Beck & Frankel, 1981).

If people believe they are capable of carrying out the recommended behaviour, they will focus on danger control rather than fear control. This also means that the message must enhance personal efficacy at least as much as it arouses fear. In the case of AIDS prevention, we can present messages that emphasize the terrible consequences of being HIV positive (i.e., fear appeal), but we would be better off to put more emphasis on how people are very capable of greatly reducing the risk (i.e., personal efficacy).

What can we conclude from our analysis of fear appeals as a health promotion strategy? Clearly, messages that do nothing more than frighten people without providing suggestions of ways to reduce the fear are likely to be counterproductive. In fact, messages that arouse a great deal of fear probably won't work even if we do accompany them with suggestions for prevention. On the other hand, if we arouse moderate amounts of fear and accompany that with recommendations on ways to reduce the threat and a convincing argument that these ways are within the capabilities of the people receiving the message, then we increase our chances of success. "Success" in terms of health promotion means that people will pay attention to our message, remember it, and behave in ways that are consistent with it by reducing health risks and increasing well-being. (For detailed advice on using fear appeals in health promotion, see Hale & Dillard, 1995).

The Application of Other Social-Psychological Principles to Health Promotion

We know that we are more likely to be influenced by messages the more often they are repeated (Zajonc, 1968). Advertisers have known this for decades, as is evidenced by the number of times we will see the same commercial in a 30-minute television program. Slogans take advantage of the repetition effect because they are repeated in every different ad that appears in a given campaign. Health promotion campaigns could take greater advantage of slogans, as advertisers do. Imagine the effect if a health promotion campaign had come up with the phrase, "Just do it."

Of course, advertising campaigns are far more than just repeated words and phrases. We must also consider who is saying those words. When we adopt a central route, we want to use people who are very credible, which is to say that they are seen as being knowledgeable and believable. Not surprisingly, research has shown that sources perceived to be credible tend to be more persuasive than non-credible ones (Birnbaum, Wong, & Wong, 1976). If we are mounting an anti-smoking campaign, for example, we might want to put a physician on camera. If it is a drinking and driving counter-attack program, we could use a police officer who is often first on the scene of motor vehicle accidents.

If, on the other hand, we are using a peripheral approach, we will be concerned about the *attractiveness* of our speaker, or we might want to pick someone who is famous. This is why anti-drug abuse campaigns use professional athletes as speakers.

Good health promotion campaigns use both credible and popular speakers. As an example, imagine that you had been asked to design a program to reduce the incidence of drinking and driving at high school graduations. Sixteen percent of teenage males and seven percent of teenage females report that they drink and drive (Health Canada, 1995), and that number may well go up at graduation celebrations. Your counterattack programs for high schools, aimed at affecting the drinking and driving behaviour, would be most effective if they combined messages from motor vehicle accident victims (because they are highly *credible*) and school presidents (because they are *popular*).

Social psychologists have also learned that the nature of the *audience* must be taken into account when planning persuasive pitches. For one thing, it is important to know whether the audience is initially in favour of your position or against it. If the audience is in favour of your position, then it is best to present only one side of an argument or message. For example, if you are trying to increase the exercise rates of a group of ex-athletes, you would only have to talk about the virtues of staying active. Presumably, this audience would be in favour of the idea of exercise at the outset but might need some encouragement to adopt a plan that would get them back to their old activity levels.

If, on the other hand, you were talking to people who had never been very active, it is more likely they had considered and adopted some beliefs about the downside of exercise, making them initially less in favour of your pro-exercise position. In this case, your pitch must address both sides of the argument—specifically, the pros and cons of exercise. Of course, when addressing the cons you must refute them or, at least, minimize them. For example, you could acknowledge that exercising takes time, but not an inordinate amount of time, to realize tangible benefits.

Why must we present these two-sided programs to this type of audience? Again, the answer comes from social-psychological research in persuasion. It turns out that, if you fail to acknowledge the cons when presenting a message to an audience that is not initially on your side, they tend to generate counterarguments to your one-sided pitch (Greenwald, 1968; Osterhouse & Brock, 1970). In fact, they will be doing this instead of paying attention to your pitch! Can you remember ever being presented with a one-sided argument by someone you disagreed with, all the while thinking of rebuttals that started with the words, "Yes, but..."?

Following this principle, health promotion campaigns must acknowledge that quitting smoking isn't easy, that the first few days of an exercise program may seem too tiring, that such a program must be planned out to accommodate busy schedules, and so on. If these sorts of realities are not dealt with, many people will simply bring them up on their own as justification for resisting the program.

In addition to the audience's initial position, a health promotion program must consider that audience's *knowledge level*. When talking to small audiences, people in health promotion can make educated guesses about an audience's knowledge level. However, this is much more challenging when planning national campaigns. How much do people know about heart anatomy, for example? Early research found that people's knowledge of medical terminology was poor (Samora, Saunders, & Larson, 1961). A more recent update of that study showed that knowledge had improved somewhat, but not impressively so. People were presented with 50 medical terms to define. Only two of 224 adult participants were able to define all 50. This for a sample in which 71 percent had postsecondary education (Thompson & Pledger, 1993).

Obviously, Canadians vary tremendously in their knowledge of medical language and procedures. For this reason, good health promotion campaigns must be basic enough to include as many people as possible without insulting anyone's intelligence. This can be a tricky balance to achieve.

Complicating the issue of knowledge is *literacy*. In Canada in 1994, 62 percent of Canadians could meet everyday reading needs, but 2.9 million adults could not deal with most everyday written material because of inadequate reading skills (Canadian Survey of Literacy Skills, 1994). More recently, it has been discovered that there are regional differences in literacy. Using a five-level scale and testing people in the official language of their choice, a large study of literacy in Canada discovered that 18 percent of people in Ontario and the western provinces were reading at the lowest level, Level One. This compares with 25 to 28 percent in Québec and the Atlantic provinces. In this case, "Level One" means that a person can probably read the instructions on a medicine bottle well enough to determine dosages, but more intricate instructions would not be comprehended (Jones, 1996).

In addition, there are people in Canada who are not fluent in English or French. According to Statistics Canada census figures, over 450 000 people in Canada cannot understand spoken English or French. That figure represents 1.6 percent of our population. In British Columbia, 2.6 percent of the population cannot understand spoken English or French. Effective health promotion campaigns for these segments of our population must be either highly visual or multilingual.

Poole and Ting (1995) discovered that Indo-Canadian maternity patients scored lower on tests of knowledge of hospital procedures, baby care, and self-care than did Euro-Canadian patients. Language barriers are cited as a significant reason for these differences. It is also worth noting that, in the large suburban hospital where this research was conducted, none of the maternity nursing staff was Indo-Canadian, yet at least a quarter of the patients were. It is clear, from studies such as this, that patient education and health promotion will be more effective when presented in a person's native language and, preferably, by people of the same cultural background.

In summary, we have seen that theories of psychology can and must be applied to the design and implementation of health promotion campaigns. When we consider these theories, we develop a greater appreciation for the complexities of health promotion. Changing the minds and behaviour of large groups of people is no easy task. The good news is that people who can be convinced to change their behaviour often come to endorse that behaviour and go on to carry out health promotion for others.

A classic example of this is the wearing of seatbelts. Just before it became the law to wear a seatbelt when driving in Sweden, a survey showed that the majority of Swedes were opposed to wearing them. One year after seatbelt legislation had been introduced, the survey was conducted again, and it was found that the majority of people were in favour of wearing seatbelts. How many people in Canada who were driving when seatbelt legislation came into being were initially opposed to it, only to become the very people we referred to earlier in the chapter—who wouldn't start the car until their children were buckled up?

Therefore, as difficult as health promotion is, there is reason for optimism. Let's now look at some of the major health promotion programs in Canada that have made a difference to our nation's health.

THE PRECEDE-PROCEED MODEL

It would be very helpful if people working in health promotion had a theoretical framework that would help them in the planning of their programs. Not only would this provide structure and direction for the planning process, it would also provide a set of criteria by which an existing program could be assessed. This is exactly what the Precede-Proceed Model (Green & Kreuter, 1991) does. The model was designed as a way to facilitate and analyze health promotion programs from the planning stages through their implementation and impact.

There are two key attributes to the model. One is the identification of stages involved in planning, implementation, and evaluation of health promotion programs. The other is the identification of causal pathways among the components that are the concern of health promotion. Table 4.1 presents the model. The "precede" phases of the model relate to the planning of health promotion programs. The "proceed" phases relate to the implementation and evaluation of that program. By examining Table 4.1, you can see that the model has an element of symmetry that helps clarify it conceptually. We begin by moving from right to left across the top of the model then proceed by moving from left to right across the bottom. In so

TABLE 4-1 The Precede-Proceed Model of Health Promotion Planning, Implementation, and Evaluation

				← **PRECEDE**
Phase 5 Administrative and policy diagnosis	**Phase 4** Educational and organizational diagnosis	**Phase 3** Behavioural and environmental diagnosis	**Phase 2** Epidemiological diagnosis	**Phase 1** Social diagnosis
Health promotion	Predisposing factors			
Health education	Reinforcing factors	Behaviour and lifestyle	Health	Quality of life
Policy regulation organization	Enabling factors	Environment		
Phase 6 Implementation	**Phase 7** Process evaluation	**Phase 8** Impact evaluation	**Phase 9** Outcome evaluation	
PROCEED →				

Source: Green & Kreuter (1991). Adapted by permission.

doing, we end up where we started, with a focus on health and quality of life. Let's walk through the phases of the model to develop an appreciation for its logic.

We begin in Phase 1 by diagnosing quality of life. If there are no problems here, there is really no need to continue with our health promotion plan. However, there are always problems because there is never a case in which an entire population is disease, disability, or accident free. In Phase 2, we would conduct an epidemiological diagnosis. This means that we would identify patterns of health and illness in our population. In terms of causation, the model assumes that these health patterns affect quality of life. Phase 3 requires a diagnosis of behavioural and environmental factors that explain our epidemiological data. We are now beginning to create a causal pathway from behaviour and environment, to health, to quality of life. In Phase 4, we assess factors affecting behaviour and environment. What biological, psychological, or social factors influence behaviour? (This should remind you of the biopsychosocial model.) What factors affect environment? In the final phase of planning, Phase 5, we would devise programs and policies meant to create optimal environments that are physically healthy and reinforce healthy behaviours.

Now we are ready to "proceed", which is to say implement our plan and evaluate its effects. In Phase 6, we would implement our education programs, new health policies, environmental regulations, and so on. These may take advantage of some of the psychological theories we discussed earlier in the chapter. To assess the effectiveness of these programs, we would first enter the Process Evaluation phase (Phase 7). At this point, we would evaluate the extent to which our programs were affecting the factors that predispose people to healthy behaviour and reinforce that behaviour. In addition, we may also be trying to bring about conditions that foster improvements in people's physical environments. In Phase 8, we assess impact by measuring changes in behaviour, lifestyle, and environment, both pre- and post-program. These changes should, in turn, bring about better health and, ultimately, better quality of life. This brings us back to where we started.

A good example of all this would be a program that was designed to increase the physical activity levels of senior citizens (Frankish, Milligan, & Reid, 1998). This program would stem from the diagnosis that health-related quality of life was influenced by behaviours and lifestyles that were active rather than sedentary. The next step (Phase 4) is to identify factors that would predispose a person to activity and other factors that would reinforce it. Now we are ready to design a health promotion program that takes advantage of psychological theory to bring about these factors. When we move in the "proceed" direction, we would implement our program and evaluate the extent to which it brings about predisposing and reinforcing factors, like community events and norms that favoured active living (Phase 7). Next we would evaluate the extent to which these events actually had an impact on the seniors' behaviour and, more generally, their lifestyles: were people being more active? (Phase 8). Finally, we would need to determine whether the seniors' health improved and, as a result, their quality of life.

The Precede-Proceed Model has been tested in over 600 published studies, making it the most widely tested model of its kind. One of the advantages of the model is that it works in conjunction with any other model or theory of health promotion design. For example, in Phase 5, planners could use the health belief model as their guide, trying to educate people about their vulnerability beliefs and beliefs regarding the efficacy of the behaviour in question. The model has been criticized for being too individually oriented, with its emphasis on behaviour and lifestyle (Luschen, Cockerham, & Kunz, 1996). An expanded model might take the social and cultural context of that behaviour into consideration.

ASSESSING THE EFFECTIVENESS OF HEALTH PROMOTION PROGRAMS ON POPULATION HEALTH

Health promotion programs are labour-intensive initiatives that can be expensive. It is important, therefore, to find ways to assess their effectiveness. Research on health promotion is conducted at major universities across Canada. These research centres have joined forces to form the Canadian Consortium for Health Promotion Research. This consortium is coordinated through the Centre for Health Promotion in the Faculty of Medicine at the University of Toronto. The various partners in the consortium have devised research methods for assessing the impact of health promotion programs in their geographic areas and across the country.

Assessing the effectiveness of health promotion programs can be a difficult task because, as we have stated, it is hard to find direct measures of the impact of something as large-scale as a health promotion program. One of the places in Canada conducting research on health promotion programs and on population health in general is the Institute for Health Promotion Research (IHPR) at the University of British Columbia (UBC). The IHPR consists of faculty members from the Division of Health Promotion and Preventive Medicine in UBC's Faculty of Medicine (Department of Health Care and Epidemiology), research associates, postdoctoral fellows, and graduate students.

The IHPR conducts research on a wide range of health promotion topics. For example, they evaluate health education materials that attempt to encourage women to increase their daily intake of calcium. They assess the factors affecting policy makers' use of research in population health and health promotion. Researchers also assess the implementation of health goals on a national level. Others have evaluated a chronic disease self-management program in the Yukon.

One of the comprehensive studies undertaken at the IHPR concerns smoking cessation. Researchers conducted an extensive analysis of the very large collection of studies in this area in an attempt to identify the cessation techniques that were most effective and that had impact on the greatest number of people. They then calculated the impact of these techniques on people in British Columbia. There are at least two statistics of interest in this work. One assesses the *effectiveness* of a given strategy, reported in terms of the percentage of people using the strategy who were able to stay off cigarettes for at least 6 months. The other measures the *popularity* of a strategy, defined in terms of the number of people reporting that they tried it.

Basically, there were four types of strategies identified in the literature review. There is unaided self-care, most commonly known as "cold turkey." There is nicotine-replacement therapy, both prescribed and over the counter. There are behavioural interventions such as those implemented by psychologists and counsellors. And there are inpatient treatment programs that people check into. The most popular method by far is unaided self-care. It is also the least effective, with only three percent of the people using this method abstaining for 6 months or more. This combination of popularity and ineffectiveness is important to those working in health promotion.

Nicotine-replacement therapies were found to have a 14 percent effectiveness rate. In the early stages of their use, they were only available by prescription. The IHPR review of the literature indicated, though, that subsequent over-the-counter versions had the same effectiveness rates. However, this does not mean that physicians can't play important roles in encouraging smoking cessation. Also, the IHPR researchers do not recommend the use of nicotine replacement therapies with adolescents.

Behavioural methods were much less prevalent than nicotine-replacement therapies or unaided self-care. However, they were much more effective, with 24 percent of participants staying off cigarettes for 6 months or more. The most effective method was inpatient treatment, with an effectiveness rate of 32 percent. However, compared to other methods, use of this approach is rare. In conclusion, then, this review of the literature on smoking cessation found that the most effective methods were the least commonly used.

Health promotion programs are most often initiated by governments, whether at the federal, provincial, or local level. Assessing the impact of these programs can be difficult, since it is hard to establish a direct causal link between a major program on something like heart health and morbidity or mortality statistics. There are many other factors affecting cardiovascular health that cannot be controlled for. Nevertheless, it is possible to get some useful, if indirect, measures of a program's effectiveness by looking at health statistics before and after the program's implementation.

AN ANALYSIS OF THE PARTICIPACTION PROGRAM

The ParticipAction program was created in 1971. Its goals included raising the awareness of Canadians regarding the benefits of a healthy lifestyle, providing courses of action that are healthy and doable, and motivating Canadians to engage in these actions. In the late 1990s, ParticipAction changed its name to Vitality. Many elements stayed the same, such as the television segments with Hal and Joanne.

The people working in the ParticipAction program believe that it has had a significant impact on the activity levels, and thus health, of Canadians. This belief is somewhat difficult to test empirically, not just because of the problems we mentioned regarding the identification of direct causes but also because little data exists assessing the activity levels of Canadians before ParticipAction came into being.

The first large-scale assessment of Canadians' activity levels came in 1981 with the Canada Fitness Survey. At that time, 56 percent of Canadians over the age of 9 years described themselves as being physically active. That description, of course, is open to a wide variety of interpretations regarding what it is people are doing when they are being active. Nevertheless, the most common forms of activity included walking and jogging. The 1981 survey also found that people said they had increased their participation in other activities, such as cross-country skiing.

Canadians were surveyed again in 1985. At that time, it was reported that 54 percent of the population over the age of 14 years exercised for at least 15 minutes three or more times a week (Stephens, 1988). By 1990, that number had dropped to 48 percent (Stephens, 1993). The National Population Health Survey in 1996 and 1997, using the same criteria (exercise for at least 15 minutes, three or more times per week), reported that 57 percent of the population fit in the category of regular exercisers (Statistics Canada). These fluctuations in the activity levels of Canadians don't correspond with any documented increases or decreases in health promotion programs such as ParticipAction or its more recent version, Vitality.

Perhaps of more concern is the number of people over that time period who would be classified as *sedentary*, meaning they exercise either never or less than once per week. In 1985, just over one-quarter of Canadians over the age of 14 (27 percent) were sedentary (Stephens, 1988). By 1990, that number had risen to 31 percent, or nearly one in three (Stephens, 1993). In the 1996/97 National Population Health Survey, the number who reported rarely exercising had dropped to 22 percent. These fluctuations follow the same pattern as that found in regular exercisers—a drop in activity in the late 1980s followed by an increase in the early 1990s.

At the very least, these survey results indicate that health promotion work aimed at Canadians' activity levels is a never-ending challenge. Even with over 25 years of health promotion in this area in the form of ParticipAction and Vitality and with the general hoopla surrounding fitness in the latter half of the twentieth century, one in five Canadians rarely exercises (Statistics Canada) and one in three is considered obese (Birmingham, 1999).

KEY TERMS

health promotion
medical level
public health level
socioenvironmental level
health promotion mechanisms
self-care
pap test
mutual aid
social support
naturally occurring support
agency-provided support
practical support
informational support
emotional support
persuasion
attitude
central route to persuasion
peripheral route to persuasion
fear appeals
drive-reduction theory
parallel response model
fear control
emotion-focused coping
danger control
problem-focused coping
extended parallel process model
response efficacy
personal efficacy

Part 2

IMPORTANT TOPICS IN HEALTH PSYCHOLOGY

Chapter 5

STRESS AND COPING

Chapter Outline

Key Questions

1. Before you read further take some time to write down your definition of the two terms used in the title of this chapter, "stress" and "coping." What do these terms mean to you?
2. What are the major sources of stress in your life at present? Remember, that to be

a major source of stress it does not necessarily need to be a major event such as a car accident; it may involve something less significant, although important to you, such as having recently received a speeding ticket.

3. What are the coping strategies you use most frequently in your life? It is important to remember that it will be obvious to you that some of these strategies are more appropriate or more effective than others are.
4. Each one of us tends to have characteristic behavioural responses that indicate stress is overwhelming us. Typical behaviours include: nervous tics, nail biting, accident proneness, unusual mannerisms, absent mindedness, increased alcohol consumption, changes in eating and sleeping patterns, and inappropriate emotional reactions. Take a moment to think about the signs that indicate stress is beginning to get the best of you.
5. What do we mean when we use the term "fight or flight" response?

It is thousands of years ago and a young man wakes in the morning to prepare for the coming day's work. He is well rested, as he fell asleep the previous night with the setting sun and slept uninterrupted until the warmth of the new day woke him. He is a hunter and, after a leisurely breakfast, he goes forth, with spear in hand, in search of prey. He is excited and optimistic, as he has a feeling that today he will be successful. However, as he crosses the brow of a hill he unwittingly disturbs a large tiger feeding on a freshly killed deer. It appears to be very angry at being disturbed during its breakfast and moves aggressively toward the hunter. The hunter has little time to prepare himself. There is no opportunity to flee and so he prepares to fight the advancing animal. His body immediately begins to respond to this stress in a manner designed to allow him to optimize his skills as a hunter. He experiences a pounding in his chest as his heart beats faster and his blood pressure rises, increasing the blood supply to the areas that need it. Muscles in his arms and legs tense in preparation for action. His breathing is rapid, providing more oxygen to his system. He grits his teeth, his pupils are dilated and all is senses are heightened. His emotions race in anticipation of the battle ahead, and he vacillates rapidly between fear and excited anticipation. Perspiration covers his body but most noticeably on the palms of his hands and the soles of his feet. He is only minimally aware that this improves his grip on the spear and his bare feet cling to the smooth rock beneath him. He is ready. Suddenly the tiger turns and walks away, perhaps intimidated, but we will never know. The young hunter slumps to the ground, exhausted and relieved. Although it seems like a long time, he realizes that only a short time has passed. He goes in search of a cool, mountain stream in which to wash the sweat from his body and quench his thirst. After doing this he will get back to his work.

It is many, many years later and a young business executive is awakened by his alarm. He hits the "doze" button but it just won't go away and his relief lasts only 10 minutes. He snaps to attention, realizing that he is already running late. He was out until 11:30 last night at a social function and, although he understands that it is important for his work, he wishes he had not had so much to drink and had got home earlier. He rushes to shower and shave and in his haste cuts his chin badly. Blood from the cut stains the shirt he had planned to wear and the replacement he finds is not a good colour match, but there is nothing he can do. Almost ready to leave, he bends to tie his shoes and breaks a lace. After a series of loud curses he decides to change shoes, although again the match is poor. Leaving his apartment, he runs to his car through heavy rainfall only to discover that he left his briefcase back inside. When he returns to his car he realizes that someone has snapped off his car aerial during the night. Once on the road he aims for Starbuck's for his morning dose of caffeine, the first thing he will ingest today. He arrives to a long lineup but he knows that the alternative, a commute without coffee, is not an option he would even consider. This is the first of approximately 20 cups of coffee he will have today and he wants it to be a good one. His impatience is visibly obvious and he curses under his breath at the woman in front of him who doesn't know the difference between a "latte" and a "mocha" and has the audacity to order a pound of ground coffee beans as well. As he leaps back into his car, grande latte and chocolate croissant in hand, he spills coffee on his pants. A heavy rush hour is endured by riding the bumper of the car in front and yelling at those around who seem oblivious to his sense of urgency. His cellular phone appears to be glued to his ear. Periodically, he has to slam his brakes on in order to avoid rear-ending the vehicle ahead of him. He has difficulty finding a parking spot and, after running through the rain again, arrives at his office 45 minutes late for an important meeting. His boss tells him not to bother coming into the meeting and suggests, in a somewhat sarcastic manner, that he should attend instead to some of the accumulated work on his desk. As he curses again, he pours himself another coffee and sneaks a jelly donut from a box in the coffee room. Sitting down to his desk he is aware that his heart is racing, he is sweating profusely, his jaw is clenched, he is grinding his teeth, his breathing is rapid and shallow, and he feels a muscle-tension headache beginning. He is angry, frustrated, and worried by the boss' response to his lateness. His confidence has been shattered, and he is having difficulty focusing on the tasks in front of him. His motivation for his work has decreased dramatically. He longs to return home and curl up in his bed but knows this is not a possibility if he wants to keep his job. There is nowhere to go. The abundance of sweat on his hands and feet will not find expression in the gripping of a spear and a sureness of step on smooth rocks. Rather, it results in embarrassingly sweaty palms and socks that give off an increasingly unpleasant smell as the day progresses. The tiger in front of him is made of paper.

ISSUES OF DEFINITION

In this text, we provide many definitions for the terms we use. We do this to ensure clarity and consensus with regard to the meaning of the concepts presented. Many of these terms are highly objective, and there is considerable agreement concerning the correct definition for a particular term. For example, when we speak of "aerobic exercise" and "anaerobic exercise" there is clear consensus as to how to use these terms appropriately. However, with regard to **stress** and **coping** this is just not the case. At the beginning of this chapter, we asked you to write down how you would define both these terms. If we were to compare your definition with those of others reading the same chapter, we would expect that there would be considerable variation in the meanings given both these terms. Individual definitions would be highly personalized and reflect the uniqueness of a particular individual's life experiences.

This dilemma is reflected in observations made by Brannon and Feist (1999). They compare the concept of stress to that of love; everyone appears to know what the latter term means, the role it plays in their lives, and they are sure they know when they feel it. We have a common sense understanding of both terms, and when someone indicates they are feeling stressed we can identify with what they are feeling because we believe we have experienced similar feelings. Many of us would identify ourselves as being "experts" in the field. We have attained a high level of competency through one of the acknowledged avenues by which this can occur, experience. We clearly seem to understand the term, and yet it is unlikely that two individuals would provide us with the same definition.

A similar ambiguity exists with regard to how we define coping. To say we "cope with stress" is a highly individualized statement that will again reflect the variability of human experience. It is obvious that there is no "right" way to cope with stress; there are different ways. My stress is not your stress, and my coping strategies are not yours. We do not experience stress in a similar way. What stresses me does not stress you and vice versa. The questions are many. Is all stress a bad thing, or should positive events such as getting married or having a child be viewed as stressful? How much more stressful is it to lose a close relative than to receive a speeding ticket? Is it true that we are living in a more stressful world today that that of 100 years ago? Do we all react to the same stress in the same manner?

Similar questions exist with regard to coping. Are the strategies one person uses to cope applicable to another individual's world? Can particular coping strategies actually increase the stress we experience? Why do we continue to use coping strategies that appear to be quite ineffective? It seems we are describing two phenomena that appear to have meaning only in the eye of the beholder, like love. Given the number of times we use both these terms in our description of our daily activities, it is remarkable how little consensus exists as to how to define them.

Our opening examples remind us that stress and coping are concepts that have existed throughout time. Only recently, however, have they been the subject of research and systematic efforts at conceptualization. What we are struggling with here is what Smith (1993) has described as **stress literacy**. He considers this to be an issue of considerable importance, as the alternative is confusion. He suggests that the "popular culture provides volumes of conflicting bits of stress wisdom" (p. 5) and provides numerous examples. For example, is it better to face your problems or ignore them? Do we perform better when we are "psyched" up or when we are relaxed? The contradictions are many, and Smith suggests that the first step in the process of "stress literacy begins with a useful definition of stress" (p. 6).

One might expect that, in the empirical world, this issue would be somewhat clearer; however, even in that context considerable confusion seems to exist regarding these two terms. Haan (1993) addresses this concern directly. She believes that those involved in the investigation of stress and coping are "handicapped by a lack of consensus on the meaning of these terms. The concept of stress is used and understood by laypersons, but its scientific study has proven difficult" (p. 256). Haan also suggests that this same level of controversy and confusion is attached to the meaning of coping. She suggests that if we would acknowledge "that our knowledge of stress arises from common, shared understandings and not from objective reality, the insight would be liberating" (p. 260).

The extent of this confusion and discontent in the field has led to discussion as to whether the concept of stress is worth retaining (Pearlin, 1993). Pearlin believes that the very nature of stress dictates that it can be many things and that it is a diffuse, multidimensional phenomenon that cannot be reduced to one thing. Our efforts should be directed toward examining the interconnections between its multiple dimensions. It is this process that is proceeding slowly, as it requires an interdisciplinary focus that will be difficult to bring about. He laments that "firmly and actively engaged in his chosen research, each investigator is convinced that the manifestation of stress that he is examining represents 'real' stress" (p. 305). However, Pearlin is convinced that we should continue to work on the concept of stress but do so in an interdisciplinary fashion. It will be interesting to observe whether or not the kind of paradigm shift he considers necessary occurs in the near future.

Aldwin (1994), while acknowledging that some researchers have described stress as an amorphous concept that should be abandoned, argues that the term need not be applied in an inappropriate way. She writes that "stress refers to that quality of experience, produced through a person-environment transaction, that, through either overarousal or underarousal, results in psychological or physiological distress" (p. 22).

In this context, it is important to consider the opinions of those most identified with the field. Hans Selye, the originator of the term stress in its present form (see Box 5.1), defines stress as "the nonspecific result of any demand upon the body, be the effect mental or somatic" (1993, p.7). He also recognizes that, for most people, stress is viewed as a negative experience that equates it with "distress." The concern here is that this will lead to the assumption that it is something to be avoided. To counter this position, he coined the term **eustress** to reflect a positive, yet stressful, experience. The similarity to the word *euphoria* is clearly intentional. It is a state of physical and psychological well-being that is associated with increased motivation and the acceptance of challenge. The ultimate expression of this positive state is found in the title of the book by the Canadian physician Hanson, *The Joy of Stress* (1986). Selye argued that what is essential is a sense of balance; that we function best when stress is used to produce an optimal level of arousal. The implication is that too little stress can be as harmful as too much, that distress can result from being over- or under-stimulated. Selye wrote that, "Stress is the spice of life" (1974, p. 83).

Lazurus and Folkman (1984) have provided us with a description of both stress and coping that has received wide acceptance in the field. Stress is described in terms of a relationship that exists between a "person and the environment that is appraised by the person as taxing or exceeding his or her resources and endangering his or her well-being" (p. 21). An individual's cognitive appraisal of their situation will determine the level of stress they

Box 5-1 A Great Canadian

Hans Selye has been described as "the grand master of stress research and theory." Although born in Vienna in 1907, Selye lived and worked in Montreal for 50 years until his death in 1982. He first used the term "stress" in 1936 to describe the non-specific result, either mental or physical, of demands placed on the body. It is interesting to note that close to 40 years later, Selye indicated that if his English had been better at the time, he would probably have chosen the word "strain" to describe this response. He had taken the idea of stress from the field of physics where it describes the force exerted by one body against another. The response to this tension is strain and, as what Selye was describing was a response, he acknowledged that he probably should have used this term. Rather than correct him, we have adjusted our definition to fit his model. To get a sense of how completely we have done this, you might try to substitute the word "strain" for "stress" and experience how awkward this feels even though it may be more appropriate. For example, how does "I feel so strained today", "the strain of life", "it strains me to be around him", "this has been a very strainful experience for me", or "this really strains me out" sound to you?

Selye initially observed a consistent pattern of responses in work he was doing with rats when these animals were exposed to diverse noxious stimuli. He called this a "stereotypic response", which he had first become aware of in human patients some 10 years earlier (the "general adaptation syndrome" or "biologic stress syndrome") and for which he now had experimental evidence. He also identified an initial "alarm reaction" in which the organism's defences were activated. If the organism survived this initial attack, Selye identified an adaptive phase or rebound effect that occurs, which he called the "the stage of resistance." Eventually, if the demands on the organism were of sufficient severity or length a "stage of exhaustion" occurred.

In 1956, Selye published his best-selling book, *The Stress of Life*, in which he translated the concept of stress for the layperson. Seyle dedicated his life to the study of stress and wrote over 1 700 articles and 39 books on the topic. He was a scientist, trained as both a physician and an endocrinologist. He served as a professor and director of the Institute of Experimental Medicine and Surgery at the University of Montreal. In addition to these responsibilities, Selye served the non-scientific world through texts such as that mentioned above and *Stress without Distress* (1974), which he wrote to help us better understand the impact of the stress response on humans throughout the lifespan. He was made a Companion of the Order of Canada, the highest honour this country can bestow upon an individual. He has been described as a "Canadian resource to the world."

will experience. Coping is defined as "constantly changing cognitive and behavioral efforts to manage specific external and/or internal demands that are appraised as taxing or exceeding the resources of the person" (p. 141).

Central to our understanding of stress are the contributions of Walter Cannon. In 1939, he introduced the concept of **homeostasis**, which describes the body's attempt to maintain a stable internal state. This is a dynamic physiological response on the part of the body to the demands of the environment. The body seeks balance, and stress presents a challenge to homeostasis. A major contribution by Cannon has become a part of our everyday language, as it was he who articulated the **fight or flight response**. As we implied in Question Five at the beginning of the chapter, most of us are familiar with this term and use it without hesitation in our daily lives. The fight or flight response involves a complex autonomic reaction in preparation for emergencies. The sympathetic nervous system and hormones secreted by the adrenal glands interact in an adaptive response developed through evolution. It is this response that allows us to cope with threats from the attacks of a threatening world. In the vignette we presented at the start of this chapter, we observed two individuals, separated by thousands of years, responding to threat in their world with essentially the same physiological response. Clearly, the options available to them were quite different as a function of the point in history at which they found themselves.

Cannon (1939) expressed concern over the implications for physical illness through the continuous activation of the fight or flight reaction in response to the chronic pressures and demands of the contemporary world. One might argue that the term "fight or flight" may still be appropriate to describe a bodily response. However, the actions implied by this phrase may not be appropriate given the restraints often imposed by the contemporary world. In fact, to engage in either of these responses for many of us living in today's world could have disastrous consequences. As our young businessman found out, neither response was acceptable. He could not fight or flee. He had to sit at his desk while his body experienced the same responses as his ancient brother. The stomach churns, the muscles tighten, the heart pounds, the blood pressure soars, the teeth grind, hyperventilation occurs, sweat flows, and the emotions run wild. It is not difficult to understand how the continual stimulation of this response could eventually result in physical illness.

Rice (1999) describes three distinct meanings attached to stress. The first has to do with external causes. These are the environmental demands placed upon us that cause us to feel stressed. As such, these should be described as stressors, rather than stress. It is in response to these external stressors that we invoke coping strategies to reduce their impact. The second meaning of stress is concerned with subjective responses and refers to the interpretive mental state of the individual. It allows us to react cognitively to diminish, augment, or distort the impact of external events. We can create our own stress. This intuitive sense that it is somehow "all in our minds" has been expressed by writers and philosophers throughout history.

Just for fun, we present the following. Epictetus said some two thousand years ago that, "Humans are not disturbed by events, but by the view they take of them." Shakespeare wrote in Hamlet that, "There is no such thing as good or bad, but thinking makes it so." Milton suggested in Paradise Lost that, "The mind is its own place, and in itself can make a Heaven of Hell, a Hell of Heaven." Mark Twain commented, "I am an old man and have known a great many troubles—but most of them never happened." Finally, Woody Allen observed, "Life is full of miserableness, loneliness, unhappiness; and it's over too quickly." You might want to create your own list of quotes showing that stress is a state of mind.

Rice (1999) points out that even though we are describing an internal state, we frequently use physical terms to explain the impact of stress. We speak of being on the "edge" of a breakdown, of feeling the "weight" of the world, of not being sure that we can cope with "the pressure" or of "exploding" if we are exposed to any more stress. The third definition of stress focuses on the body's physical response to events in the manner described by Selye and Cannon. As previously described, stress imposes a physiological challenge, which if prolonged can result in a negative state or, alternatively, an improved capacity to cope physiologically (Rice, 1999).

THE PHYSIOLOGY OF STRESS

There are two major components of the physical response to stress: the **nervous system** and the **endocrine system**. The nervous system comprises two divisions, the **central nervous system** and the **peripheral nervous system.** The former is composed of the brain and the spinal cord. The latter is made up of the somatic nervous system and the autonomic nervous system, which is further divided into the sympathetic and parasympathetic nervous systems. The physiology of stress features a highly complex response that begins when an individual perceives stress. As we have discussed, the brain makes no distinctions in this regard. Perceived threat, whether actual or imagined, results in the brain alerting the body to mobilize its coping resources.

This response begins with the **hypothalamus**, which is located in the central core of the brain. It initiates the stress response in both the nervous system and the endocrine system. The hypothalamus helps maintain homeostasis in the body through its many regulatory functions. It controls activities like eating, drinking, and sexual behaviour, all of which are greatly affected by stress. The activities of the hypothalamus increase arousal in the sympathetic nervous system in the form of the previously described fight or flight response (Cannon, 1939). The physiological changes we described in the initial vignette now occur. The heart beats faster and blood pressure increases at the same time as peripheral blood vessels, in areas such as the hands and feet, constrict to ensure sufficient blood supplies for the brain and skeletal muscles. Stored fats and glucose flow into the bloodstream to provide fuel for necessary actions. Respiration rate increases and the bronchial tubes dilate to help increase oxygen flow for the metabolism of fuel. Pupils dilate to allow more light to enter the eyes and improve vision. The efficiency of the process is demonstrated when non-essential activities, such as digestion, decrease.

As a part of this response, the hypothalamus causes the **adrenal medulla**, located above the kidneys, to secrete catecholamines, which contain the hormones adrenaline and noradrenaline. Catecholamines affect the response of the sympathetic nervous system, and the level of these two hormones increases with the severity of the stress. Adrenaline has a powerful impact on heart function and blood pressure. Presumably, it is this experience which finds expression in the phrase "adrenaline rush." It is interesting that this phrase is usually viewed in positive terms as something that people seek. We even go so far as to ascribe an addictive quality to it by describing some individuals as "adrenaline junkies", people who purposefully seek the physiological "high" that adrenaline brings. When we think of such individuals, we envision a crazed sensation seeker involved in extreme activities that presumably initiate the fight or flight response and the flow of adrenaline. It is interesting to note that the action of adrenaline and noradrenaline is different. The former is fast acting and increases with mental stress; the effect of the latter is more prolonged and increases with physical activity (Rice, 1999).

Also involved in the stress response is the **limbic system** of the brain, which adds an element of *emotion* to the response that goes beyond the identified dimensions of fight or flight. The experiences associated with the limbic system include aggression, anger, fear, anxiety, sexual arousal, and pain. The **reticular formation** is a complex system running through the middle of the brain stem that performs several functions in the stress response. It serves as a communication network that filters messages between the brain and the body. This is most important when we consider the impact that the brain's perception of psychosocial stressors can have on physical systems in the body. The reticular formation receives input from all of the sensory systems and can influence which sensory information is processed or blocked.

Such selectivity results in increased efficiency in the system, which can become apparent to us in quite dramatic ways. For example, in high-arousal situations we may find ourselves remarkably able to selectively attend to a specific task while ignoring irrelevant distractions. A basketball player, given the opportunity to win a game by sinking a last-second foul shot, is able to focus his attention on the front rim of the hoop. He is not distracted by the noise of the crowd and the purposeful movement of those behind the basket, who will go to considerable extremes in an attempt to get his attention to waiver. We find that during an exam we can block all distractions and become completely absorbed in the task. Parents notice that they are able to selectively attend to the sounds of their children above all other noises. We develop confidence in our ability to motivate ourselves to attend to what we need to and ignore the rest. The reticular formation also serves an important role in modulating the brain's levels of arousal or alertness in preparation for action.

In contrast to the sympathetic nervous system, the **parasympathetic** component of the autonomic system is activated by the hypothalamus to re-establish homeostasis in the system and promote the reconstructive process following a stressful experience. It is associated with a relaxed state in which the heart rate slows and blood pressure drops. Muscle tension decreases and respiration is slow and easy. In essence, the fight or flight response is neutralized.

The endocrine system responds to stress more slowly than does the nervous system, but the effects associated with it can persist for weeks. The **pituitary gland**, which is located in the brain close to the hypothalamus, is described as the "master gland" because of its controlling effect on other glands. Most of the hormones secreted by the pituitary gland have an indirect impact on stress. The most important of these is adrenocorticotropic hormone (ACTH), which acts on the adrenal glands and is eventually involved in the release of up to 30 stress hormones (Smith, 1993).

The **adrenal cortex** secretes glucocorticoids and mineralocorticoids. One of the former is cortisol, an important stress hormone that provides energy to the system through the conversion of stored protein and fats to glucose. If stress is prolonged, glucocorticoids can adversely affect the body's ability to resist disease and recover from injury. Cortisol levels are often used as an index of stress. Aldosterone is a mineralocorticoid that is important in the regulation of minerals in the body that assist the body to act during stress by increasing blood pressure.

The **thyroid gland** functions in the stress response to produce thyroxine, which increases the release of fatty-acid fuels that are metabolized in the stress process. Elevated thyroxine levels increase blood pressure and respiration rate. Mental processes are also affected, in that individuals feel more anxious or agitated. The **pancreas**, which lies close to the stomach, secretes insulin and glucagon as a function of blood sugar levels. The former serves to decrease blood sugar by storing it, whereas the latter stimulates increases in blood sugar, which is an energy source during stress.

The indication is that the autonomic nervous system responds rapidly in response to stress and the endocrine system somewhat slower, although its impact usually continues for much longer periods of time. Acting together, these two systems provide a physiological response to stress which can be both adaptive and potentially maladaptive. We will now turn our attention to Selye's model of stress, which is concerned with physical responses to stress in the environment.

The General Adaptation Syndrome

Initially, Selye conducted research on laboratory animals. He observed that animals exposed to chronic stress demonstrated physical distress that included organic pathology and ultimately death. This work and that of others, such as Brady's work on executive monkeys (Brady, Porter, Conrad, & Mason, 1958), resulted in Selye's conceptualization of the **General Adaptation Syndrome** (GAS) (Selye, 1956). This is a three-stage response of the body to stressors. In the initial phase, the body goes into alarm as it mobilizes its defences against the stress. This involves many of the processes involved in the fight or flight response. As our own experience will confirm, this acute response is often enough to allow us to deal successfully with the impact of a stressor and to allow homeostasis to be re-established.

If a source of stress moves from acute to chronic, the body enters the second phase of adaptation, which Selye called **resistance**. Here the body mobilizes its resources over an extended period of time. Initially, the individual will appear as normal. If the stress continues for too long, however, the body's resources are depleted and resistance decreases. The result of longterm neurological and hormonal changes can be what Selye described as **diseases of adaptation**. These include problems such as cardiovascular disease, hypertension, peptic ulcers, bronchial asthma, and increased risk of infection.

The body's resources to resist stress are clearly finite. Eventually, if the stressor is too severe or continues for too long, the body enters what Selye called **exhaustion**. This is an endpoint at which the body's ability to resist the stressor breaks down, possibly resulting in death if a return to homeostasis is not possible.

Criticisms of Selye's theory centre on its narrowness, suggesting that it is concerned only with physical responses to stress and does not take into account psychosocial factors influencing the human stress response. Part of Selye's emphasis is felt to derive from his initial work with animals, and his critics suggest that he neglected those cognitive processes unique to humans (Brannon and Feist, 2000).

Other biologically based models have been proposed to explain our ability to resist the impact of stress. One concern relates to genetic influences that may predispose an individual to be at increased risk for specific diseases or to display vulnerabilities or reductions in resistance that may expressed under certain conditions. Closely linked to this is the **stress-diathesis model** that examines the interaction between the environment and heredity. The issue is often expressed as *nature versus nurture*. There may be predisposing factors present in an individual that may or may not be expressed depending on the presence of specific precipitating factors. The model proposes that an individual who possesses a high level of genetic predisposition may never display signs of the predisposed problem if they are never exposed to the precipitating stress. It also implies that high levels of stress may extend the limits of invulnerability even in those who are genetically robust. There is a sense of adaptability to the model. It makes us think of phrases that relate to a "survival of the fittest" mentality. The implication is that stress forces an individual to adapt and evolve or run the risk of being selected out. Certainly many of us, when we consider our own vulnerability to disease, are quick to blame or applaud our genes. We boast to others that we will never develop cardiovascular disease no matter how much we abuse our body through environmental stressors such as a poor diet or lack of exercise, as we are blessed with "good genes." We develop an inappropriate sense of invulnerability. The stress-diathesis model (or diathesis-stress model, as Grossarth-Maticek and Eysenck call it) is also discussed in Chapter 3 in our examination of psychoneuroimmunology.

COGNITIVE TRANSACTIONAL MODELS

The impact of Selye's work on the popularization of the idea of stress and on our understanding of it can't be underestimated. It's hard to imagine where we would be today without the contributions he made to the field. He brought us a long way in a very short time. However, as we indicated previously, his theory may be limited in its reliance on physiological processes in the context of an animal model of behaviour. In this regard, it fails to take into account those higher level cognitive abilities that are distinctly human and allow us to interpret our vulnerability to a particular stressor both now and in the future. Compared to Selye's model, **cognitive transactional models** of stress hold more appeal for psychologists. As indicated by the definition provided by Lazarus and Folkman earlier in this chapter, these models emphasize the relationship existing between an individual and their environment and the appraisal the individual makes of their situation. Personal **cognitive appraisals** determine whether or not an event will be perceived as stressful. These are based on an individual's unique social learning history. Also of relevance here are temporal concerns, as what is psychologically or physically threatening at one time may not be at another. The most influential cognitive transactional model of stress is that of Lazarus and his colleagues, which we will now examine in more depth.

Lazarus and Folkman (1984) indicate that the process of cognitive appraisal is "largely evaluative, focused on meaning or significance, and takes place continuously during waking hours" (p. 31). They distinguish between three kinds of appraisal influencing the coping process: **primary appraisal**, **secondary appraisal**, and **reappraisal**. Lazarus and Folkman acknowledge that these are somewhat unfortunate terms, as one form of appraisal (e.g., primary as compared to secondary) is neither superior to nor precedes the other.

Primary appraisals are concerned with the initial evaluation of a situation. Three kinds of primary appraisal are identified: **irrelevant**, **benign-positive**, and **stressful**. The first involves a cognitive process by which an event is appraised to have no implications for the individual's well-being, it is simply irrelevant and requires no response. Benign-positive appraisals involve outcomes appraised to be positive and that may increase well-being. They are associated with pleasurable emotions such as happiness, joy, or love. The only demand benign-positive appraisals place on the individual is the awareness that these feelings will end.

There are three types of stressful appraisal: **harm/loss**, **threat**, and **challenge**. Harm/loss appraisals involve significant physical or psychological loss such as might be experienced in a serious illness or the loss of one's job. Threat involves the anticipation of situations of harm or loss. When an individual has experienced harm/loss, threat is involved, as it has implications for the future. Perceptions of threat allow one to anticipate and prepare for the impact of an event. Challenge appraisals involve events perceived to be stressful, but the focus is one of positive excitement and anticipation of the potential for growth contained in the situation. Having to speak in front of a class may be perceived as very threatening by a person with anxiety about public speaking and as an opportunity to test one's public-speaking abilities in a meaningful situation by an individual who has worked on these skills. Clearly, threat and challenge may be experienced in the same situation. The latter individual may experience some threat in the speaking opportunity, which is expressed in the form of anxiety and some fear, however the dominant emotions are confidence and anticipation. The overall emotional tone is positive and the individual actively employs available resources to prepare to meet the demands imposed by the presentation.

Secondary appraisal is concerned with a person's evaluation of his or her ability to cope with a situation. After the initial evaluation of the nature of the event, which is *primary appraisal*, options are considered. As Lazarus and Folkman (1984) make clear, this is not simply an intellectual exercise. It is "a complex evaluative process, that takes into account which coping options are available, the likelihood that a given coping option will accomplish what it is supposed to, and the likelihood one can apply a particular strategy" (p. 35). They point out that this is very similar to the distinction Bandura (1985) makes between outcome and efficacy judgments. In his work on self-efficacy, Bandura states that, "Efficacy and outcome judgments are differentiated because individuals can believe that a particular course of action will produce certain outcomes, but they do not act on that outcome belief because they question whether they can actually execute the necessary activities" (p. 392).

The interaction between the secondary appraisals of coping options and the primary appraisals of the situation determines the emotional reaction to the event. If the consequences of an event are important to the individual, considerable stress may be experienced if they believe they do not have the ability to cope with the event; a state of helplessness may result. Conversely, *challenge appraisals* are more likely to result when an individual feels in control of the situation, even if this means overcoming extreme adversity. We are all aware of individuals who, when faced with a devastating situation such as an illness or loss of a relationship, articulate their efforts to cope in very positive ways. They describe the challenge of *confronting* through their own behaviour what others would perceive as overwhelming odds. They know they may not ultimately have an outcome others would consider desirable, but they focus their attention on elements of the situation that are under their control. For example, they may talk of the challenge of coping with pain, either physical or psychological, to the best of their ability while recognizing that there are elements of the situation that are outside of their control and will have to run their course. Even though a situation may appear hopeless they search for challenges.

Reappraisal is a continuous experience in which existing appraisals are changed or modified on the basis of new information. In reality, there is no difference between the two. Reappraisal simply follows an earlier appraisal of an event and results in a new appraisal; we can all identify with this process. What may vary is the direction the appraisal may take. For example, an irrelevant situation may now be perceived in terms of threat, or a harm/loss situation may now be appraised as a challenge. Lazarus and Folkman (1984) also identify what they call a *defensive reappraisal*. They describe this as a self-generated coping strategy in which an attempt is made to reinterpret past events more positively, or to view current threats or losses as being less threatening.

Also of importance in the cognitive appraisal process is the concept of **vulnerability**, which reflects the adequacy of an individual's resources (Lazarus and Folkman, 1984). This is a concept which, like so many in this area, is defined in the context of a relationship. With regard to physical issues it is possible to think of vulnerability only in terms of resources. A physical injury can increase vulnerability to further injury. However, deficiencies in resources will result in a psychological vulnerability only when it threatens that which is valued by the individual. Therefore, an individual may have resource deficiencies but not experience vulnerability, as the deficiencies do not threaten areas that are important to them.

This model also identifies **person** and **situation** variables that influence appraisal. The impact of these variables is in the determination of the salience of an event, an individual's understanding of the event, the consequence of an event, and, ultimately, the outcome of a particular encounter (Lazarus and Folkman, 1984). Person and situation variables are interdependent and involve transactions between the individual and their environment. The person variables of importance are **commitments** and **beliefs**. Commitments are concerned with what is important to an individual. They influence appraisal by determining the importance of a particular encounter and will affect the choices made to achieve a desired outcome. They interact with concepts discussed within the context of primary appraisal, such as challenge, threat, benefit, or harm, to determine whether an individual will engage in or avoid an encounter. Beliefs are pre-existing notions that determine the meaning given to the environment. They can be both personal and cultural. Their impact, which is often difficult to observe, is most obvious when there is a sudden change in the belief system.

Numerous properties of situations influencing the appraisal process have been identified. **Novelty** is concerned with an individual's previous experience with a situation. **Predictability** identifies characteristics of the environment that can be learned or discerned. A preference for predictability is indicated, as it allows an individual to prepare for an event and therefore reduce the stress involved. Of more relevance to appraisal, particularly in humans, is the concept of **event uncertainty**, which involves issues of probability. The observation is that high levels of uncertainty can be extremely stressful. Temporal situational factors are considered important in stress appraisal. **Imminence** concerns the interval during which an event is being anticipated. It is usually the case that the more imminent an event, the more intense the appraisal. **Duration** refers to the period during which a stressful event occurs. The implication is that the longer the duration, the more stressful the event.

This is reminiscent of Selye's General Adaptation Syndrome, discussed above, in which the duration of stress plays an important role—continued exposure to stress compromises resistance and leads ultimately to exhaustion. **Temporal uncertainty** is concerned with the stress involved in *not knowing* when an event will occur. A final concern here relates to the *timing* of stressful events in the context of the life cycle. This suggests that there are appropriate or "usual" times for events to occur in one's life. If these expectations are violated, it may result in the event being appraised as more stressful by some individuals. We have a sense of an order that we move through in our lives, and this master "daytimer" allows us to develop expectations and prepare for events. When the timing is wrong, normal life events become sources of stress. We can all think of life events that have affected us, and others, in this way. It may be the couple who has children later in life. There is the athlete whose athletic career was brought to an abrupt and expected end due to injury. Or perhaps it is the middle-aged individual who is finally able to attend university after 25 years in the workplace.

The model developed by Lazarus and his colleagues views stress as a complex, dynamic process in which an individual's experience of stress is determined by their own unique cognitive appraisal of the event and their coping abilities.

PERSONALITY IN STRESS AND COPING

The possibility that personality is related to stress and coping is very appealing. Given the stable, enduring qualities attached to personality characteristics, the possibility is raised of being able to predict and hopefully intervene to reduce risk if a particular disposition or set of personality traits is found to predispose an individual to a specific disease. There are several possibilities as to how such a model might work (Rice, 1999). One suggestion is that a specific personality profile can cause a specific disease to develop, as is the case with Type A personality and coronary heart disease. A second possibility is that a particular disease process may result, after the fact, in a particular personality profile. This would be the situation when depression results following diagnosis of a serious illness. The third possibility is that personality affects or filters the response to an illness, as might occur in response to a particular disease. One individual receiving the news of a serious illness may respond in an optimistic and active manner compared to another who responds passively and pessimistically. In the fourth possibility, personality interacts with the disease process in a feedback loop that affects the individual's physiology and may influence the disease process itself. Ultimately, the question centers on whether there are a set of personality traits that predict addictive behaviours such as smoking or alcohol use, or disease processes such as cancer or coronary disease.

The most extensively studied personality type in this regard is the **Type A behaviour pattern**. This set of behaviours was first identified by two cardiologists, Friedman and Rosenman, in 1974. They described an individual they saw frequently in their medical practice who they felt was at much higher risk for cardiovascular disease. Such an individual displays a sense of time urgency, is impatient, is very competitive, and can be aggressive and hostile. This is a person who does not relax. He or she displays behavioural characteristics such as rapid, explosive, clipped speech, frequent interruptions of another speaker, speech hurrying techniques (e.g., nodding the head while another person speaks), vehement reactions to time impedance, emphatic one-word responses, and the pointed finger to emphasize speech.

One of the authors has identified two favourite Type A behaviours. The first is the individual who makes his or her way to the parking lot with briefcase, books, and all other belongings in one arm (usually the left, if the individual is right handed) with the car key waiting poised in the other hand. Their left hand becomes numb and painful with the weight it is carrying as they zero in on the lock of their car at a distance of some 600 yards. It's as if they can't tolerate the idea that they wouldn't be ready to open the door the moment they arrive at their car. They can't spare the extra time it would take if they distributed their load evenly between both arms then had to reach into their pocket for the car key.

The second individual is responsible for weight-sensitive coffee dispensers being designed. This person comes to the office or departmental coffee room only to discover, much to their frustration, that it is empty and that a new pot needs to be brewed. After cursing the world, he or she quickly changes the filter and adds the water and coffee. After all this, they are not prepared to allow the entire pot to fill as they are only concerned with their own cup. Their efforts to extract only a cupful can result in spilled coffee spitting off a hot base. However, the coffee machine industry designed the weight-sensitive base that stops the flow of coffee if the pot is removed during brewing. The implication is that these individuals can't spend the time to allow a coffee pot to fill and that we are prepared to support such impatience.

Individuals such as these stand in comparison to Type B individuals, who give the impression of being relaxed and calm, are less competitive, are not overly reactive to time impediments, and rarely display hostility. Very strong empirical support has emerged for the suggestion that Type A behaviours are linked to an increased risk for coronary disease. Indeed, this set of behaviours has been identified as a risk factor for all forms of morbidity (Yakubovich, Ragland, Brand, & Syme, 1988). However, some inconsistencies in the findings have led to a search for the toxic core of Type A behaviours. This work initially identified the components of hostility and anger to be the crucial elements. Wright and colleagues (1988) expanded it to describe a multicausal pathway that identifies Type A behaviour in combination with family history, lifestyle risks, anger directed inward, and anger directed outward as being the core risk factors. Being able to identify the risk factors increases the likelihood of designing successful interventions that may be able to modify or eliminate the destructive behaviours. This could involve a variety of activities ranging from making philosophical decisions about one's lifestyle, training in relaxation techniques, to specific behavioural management programs. The latter are designed to help people learn to do things like retrain emotions such as hostility and anger, take control of their environment through techniques like time management, engage in problem solving, begin an exercise program, develop communication skills, and manage their diet.

You might find it relevant at this point to read Peter's Story in Chapter 12 of this book. Peter is an example of an individual who would have been described as a Type A individual prior to having a heart attack. After surviving this scare he became involved in a hospital-based behavioural retraining program and has made significant lifestyle changes that have resulted in remarkable improvements in his health.

There is some evidence that the patterns responsible for Type A behaviours are established early in childhood and exert their influence over time. There is a sense in which many of these behaviours are, in part, learned responses to demands placed on individuals by the environment. One of the consequences of this behaviour pattern is that it is usually rewarded in the workplace and is often associated with success. Type A people tend to get more things done, accumulate more credits, and are more likely to be promoted, although the consequences of this obsession with success may ultimately be life threatening. The emphasis is placed on the retraining or learning of adaptive behaviours to replace those that are maladaptive, that is, making conscious decisions to change behaviour.

It is interesting to note that programs designed to change maladaptive behaviours are not usually described in terms of coping but instead reflect the other side of the relationship. They are usually described as being programs in "stress management." This suggests that it is easier to sell the concept of *stress* than of *coping*. The term "stress management" permeates our culture to such an extent that it is hard to think of it being otherwise. We are taught to "manage" our stress rather than to cope. This sounds like an active, dynamic, even aggressive response to the situation by which we will overwhelm the stress. Coping, on the other hand, suggests a more passive, reflective stance. We might go so far as to suggest that the term stress management is reflective of a Type A behavioural approach whereas coping is a Type B position. To say that one is going to a stress management workshop implies that you are still in control of your situation and are learning techniques to help you maintain your position. A workshop in coping suggests that things have deteriorated for you and you are seeking help. We could imagine a response to the comment that one is taking a stress-management workshop to be, "That's great", whereas if it was a coping workshop the question would be, "What's wrong?"

COPING

This discussion of the Type A behaviour pattern and its modification provides us with a nice transition into a discussion of specific coping behaviours. Earlier in the chapter we discussed different views of the stress and coping process. Here we will summarize our position with respect to coping as part of that dynamic. Sarafino (1998) does this nicely. He states that as individuals engage in coping behaviours in an "effort to neutralize or reduce stress, coping activities are geared toward decreasing the person's appraisal of or concern for this discrepancy. Thus coping is the process by which people try to manage the perceived discrepancy between the demands and resources they appraise in a stressful situation" (p. 133). It is clearly the case that these efforts may not necessarily improve the person's situation. As Rice (1999) points out, it has not always been clear whether we are talking about the process or outcome of coping. He cites research by Rudolph, Dennig, and Weisz (1995) that identifies three components of coping. They distinguish between a **coping response** and a **stress response**. The former is an intentional physical or mental act that is initiated in response to a stressor. It can be directed toward either external events or internal states. The latter is defined as "any response that reflects a spontaneous emotional or behavioral reaction to stress, rather than a deliberate attempt to cope" (p. 329). The objective of a coping response, which is usually to reduce the impact of stress, is described as a **coping goal**. The specific or actual outcomes of a coping response are called **coping outcomes**.

Lazarus and his colleague suggest that coping can serve two functions (Lazarus & Folkman, 1984). One, **problem-focused coping**, is concerned with changing the situation by defining the problem, looking at alternative solutions, evaluating the implications of the alternatives, and choosing the best one to act on. It is a rational approach and in this way is similar to problem solving. However, it also includes solutions that are inward focused as well as those directed at the environment. In our daily existence we use problem-focused coping strategies frequently as we take action to reduce the demands placed upon us. A student who feels overwhelmed with assignments may seek out the professor to discuss how he or she can reduce the impact of their workload. As part of this process, they might focus on what material to study, using time management to plan their study time more efficiently and reorganizing their approach to prepare for the exams.

Emotion-focused coping is concerned with controlling the emotional responses to an event. This often consists of cognitive processes such as avoidance or minimization that are intended to decrease emotional distress. This could also involve situations in which the attempt is to increase emotional intensity, as might occur in preparation for action in an athletic competition. Some forms of emotion-focused coping change nothing about the objective situation. They only change the manner in which an event is perceived and, as such, constitute reappraisal. One's emotional response to a situation can be regulated both through behavioural and cognitive strategies. For example, exercise, the emotional support of a relative, or watching television may serve as a distraction from a problem. They are not forms of reappraisal, although they may lead to it. Cognitive strategies are intended to change the way we think about a situation. There is a tendency to use emotion-focused coping when the individual believes there is nothing that can be done to change the stressful situation. It is indicated (Lazarus & Folkman, 1984) that problem-focused and emotion-focused coping strategies can be used at the same time and can either facilitate or impede one another in the coping process.

In their efforts to cope with stress, people call upon the **personal resources** available to them to help reduce the potential for stressful events and to help them cope with stressful situations as they occur. These are resources that we all possess to some degree, but the question is how effective they will be for a particular individual's situation.

The first of these personal resource mechanisms is **social support**. We discuss social support on a number of occasions in this book. In times of stress we have all experienced the benefits of social support received from friends, family, and institutions such as the church, social agencies, and the health care system. As an example, it is reported that 80 percent of Americans believe prayer can have a positive impact on the course of an illness (Levin & Puchalski, 1997). We are also aware that we ourselves provide assistance to family and friends when they are stressed—we turn to others and they to us. It is an expectation of the human condition and, as a first line of defence, it is a highly effective and widely used resource. You may recall from Chapter 4 that social support takes different forms. **Emotional support** focuses on feelings of being cared for and loved; **informational support** is concerned with the advice and information made available to us concerning a particular event; **tangible support** is concerned with the direct aid or services we receive to assist us in coping with stress. Each of these forms of support will be more relevant at different times in the coping process. However, it is clearly the *perception* of social support rather than the *objective situation* that is most important (Coyne, Aldwin & Lazarus, 1981).

Social support is felt to exert its effect on stress in one of two ways (Cohen & Wills, 1985). The **stress-buffering hypothesis** suggests that social support has an indirect effect and acts as a buffer to protect individuals from the negative effects of stress. This means that when an individual is exposed to stress, the social support they receive from others serves to buffer and therefore reduce the impact of the event. Social support has its effect between the event and the recipient or between the response to the stress and the outcome. This means that the effect of social support should be most noticeable at higher levels of stress and that it will have little impact on the effect of stress at lower levels. Alternatively, social support may have effects that are independent of stress and serve to enhance an individual's general sense of well-being and self-esteem. This may increase one's sense of control, decrease anxiety, and increase health-promoting behaviours.

The impact of social networks may be to reinforce health behaviours. Such effects would be expected to directly provide a sense of control over both low and high levels of stress. Whether we view social support as having an indirect buffering effect or a direct impact on stress seems to be a function of how one measures social support. A direct effect of social support emerges if it is measured by the extent of an individual's social support network, whereas the indications that social support serves as a buffer to stress depends on the specific social-support function being measured.

Kaplan, Sallis, and Patterson (1993) suggest that more complex models will ultimately be required to explain the relationship between social support and the impact of stress. One possibility is a direct-effect model incorporating the functional effects of the social support system (which may affect health either positively or negatively). The investigators state, "We would expect that close, caring relationships would play a stronger role in reinforcing health behavior and in enhancing use of the healthcare system. At the other extreme, social isolation might contribute to disconnection with services, poor nutrition, and inadequate responses to emergency" (p. 145). It is clear that social support is a risk factor. For example, with regard to cardiovascular disease social support is reported to be as important a risk factor as concerns such as cigarette smoking, diet, and physical activity (Kaplan, Sallis, & Patterson, (1993).

Another factor that may influence a person's ability to cope with stress is their sense of **personal control**. To the extent that an individual feels they are in control of their situation, the impact of stressful events will be reduced. Alternatively, to feel that a situation is out of control and that there is nothing that can be done can be very aversive and extremely stressful. Recently, during the cold of the Canadian winter, one of the authors of this text found himself sliding down an ice-covered hill in a car over which he had absolutely no control. His pumping of the brakes produced no response. The hill was sheer ice and the vehicle had turned sideways, so that he could not control its direction. As he approached the bottom of the hill, he thought he might have to jump out of the car if it went over the edge into the ravine below. Fortunately, the wheels bumped against a small ridge at the edge of the road and the car stopped just short of the cliff. The futility of his attempts to control the vehicle, and the realization that there was nothing he could do, produced the fight or flight response we discussed earlier in this chapter. His response was flight. Approximately 10 minutes later, he had stopped shaking and recovered sufficiently to be able to leave his car and ask some people to help him push it onto the lawn of a nearby house, where he left it until the next day. He walked home, as this was something over which he had control. Remembering the event, what is most salient for the author is the helplessness associated with the loss of control.

As Bandura (1985) has indicated, one's sense of controllability can be achieved either behaviourally or cognitively. In the former, people take actions to reduce the impact of stressful events, whereas in the latter they believe that if stressful events occur they can be controlled. Bandura points out that it is important to distinguish between these two forms of controllability, as the relationship between actual and perceived coping efficacy is often not perfect. He states: "There are many competent people who are plagued by a sense of inefficacy, and many less competent ones who remain unperturbed by impending threats because they are self-assured of their coping capabilities" (p. 440).

Behavioural control has been demonstrated to greatly reduce the impact of stressful events. To have behavioural control over an event increases one's sense of predictability, which reduces stress. With regard to cognitive control, it has been demonstrated that individuals who believe they can effect control over stressful events will be less affected physiologically and behaviourally than those who believe they have no personal control over the situation.

Social support and personal control are personal resources that increase one's ability to cope with stress. However, at times such resources are unavailable or insufficient to cope with high levels of stress. At these times, it is often necessary to seek the assistance of techniques that have been specifically developed to help people cope with stress either directly or indirectly. It is important to recognize that these are techniques that are considered adaptive, compared to strategies such as alcohol or drug use that, although effective in the short-term, are not adaptive and ultimately increase stress. Although these are coping techniques they are, as noted in our discussion of the Type A behaviour pattern, quite frequently identified with the label **stress management techniques**.

Some of the most widely used and effective interventions against stress are the various **relaxation techniques** that have been developed throughout history. These are strategies based on a very simple principle, that we can not be relaxed and tense at the same time. It is the antidote for the fight or flight response. Whereas that response is under the control of the sympathetic nervous system, the relaxation response is under the control of the parasympathetic nervous system. In this relaxed state, the heart slows, blood pressure drops, breathing is slow and easy, muscle tension decreases, blood flow shifts, and we notice warmth in the hands and feet. This response, described as a **hypometabolic state**, is the opposite of the fight or flight response, which is a **hypermetabolic** response. These responses reciprocally inhibit one another. One of the implications of the inhibitory process is that we may be able to gain some control over the autonomic nervous system, which has been described as an involuntary system outside of volitional control. Demonstrations of physiological control by highly trained yogis coming out of India posed an interesting challenge to these assumptions. A series of studies carried out by Western scientists on some of these individuals further expanded our understanding of physiological control.

East and West: Now the Twain Shall Meet

Since the mid-1960s, Western society has shown an increased interest in Eastern philosophies and meditative disciplines. This enthusiasm, shared by many, has largely focused on techniques designed to promote psychological and physical well-being; it therefore forms an important component of the stress and coping literature. As part of this interest in things "Eastern", many have been intrigued by accounts of abilities or powers often difficult for us to comprehend (Brunton, 1972; Murray, 1980; Yogananda, 1946). In the "Yoga-sutras" of Patanjali, written in the fourth or fifth century A.D. (Woods, 1966), lengthy discussion is given to how one can attain "supernatural powers." In his translation of these writings, Woods states that, "These supernatural powers are to be accomplished by constraints. And constraint is the combination of fixed-attention and of contemplation and of concentration" (p. 205). Brunton, in a book first published in 1934, describes his travels to discover a "secret" India. He speaks of a culture described under the generic term of "Yoga" that "proffers benefits to mankind as valuable in their own way as any proffered by the Western sciences. It can bring our bodies nearer the healthy condition which nature intended them to possess; it can bestow one of modern civilization's most urgent needs—a flawless serenity of mind" (p. 6).

More recently, Naranjo (1971) describes how our concern for personal development has caused us to "turn a respectful gaze to the wisdom of the remote past and to the wisdom of the East that we once thought obsolete and superceded" (p. 3). The philosopher Harvey

Cox suggests that the "mystics and contemplatives have served as the guardians of that uniquely human realm called interiority" (1973, p. 93). He believes that our renewed interest in this realm represents a survival instinct intended to turn our attention from without to within.

Our fascination with these traditions is significant, as it has caused us to question our understanding of the mind-body interaction. Our ability to control bodily functions was challenged by reports of individuals who made claims such as being able to control or even stop their heart, to survive lengthy pit burials, to regulate their body temperature, or to permit penetration of the skin without bleeding. It is quite reasonable to suggest that it was these early investigations that provided the foundation for many of the stress-management techniques we practise today. Techniques such as biofeedback and many of the secular relaxation strategies we use today are firmly rooted in the belief that we can regain control of physiological variables previously thought to be outside our control.

Therese Brousse was a pioneer in this field. She took a crude, portable electrocardiograph to India in 1935 to record attempts by yogis to achieve voluntary control of cardiovascular activity. One of her published records indicates that for one individual heart potentials and pulse waves, recorded from the radial artery, decreased almost to zero and remained there for several seconds. Over 20 years later, Wenger, Bagchi, and Anand (1961) returned to India with more sophisticated equipment to record cardiovascular activity in four individuals claiming to be able to slow or stop their heart. One of those investigated included the subject previously investigated by Brousse.

It was clear from the investigators' results that these individuals did not directly control the functioning of their heart; rather, evidence suggested that they used striate muscle control to produce changes in circulatory patterns. The indication was that these yogis used a technique called the Valsalva maneuver, which involves an increase in muscle tension in the abdominal and thoracic muscles, closure of the glottis, and development of intrathoracic pressure. The effect is to interfere with venous return to the heart, so that heart sounds are diminished and masked by muscular sounds, and the radial pulse seems to disappear. The increased sophistication of the equipment in the study by Wenger and colleagues indicated that normal cardiac activity continued to occur. The results Brousse had reported were an artifact of the crude recording techniques she used and did not take into account the impact of the Valsalva maneuver. It is interesting to note that although these individuals did not stop their heart, they did demonstrate a remarkable level of muscular control. Can you imagine how many bets you could win at a party if you were able to make your radial pulse disappear and gave the "appearance" of having stopped your heart?

Anand and China (1961) carried out a similar investigation with three yogis who claimed to be able to stop their heart. Rather than supporting their claim, the electrocardiogram (EKG) indicated that their heart rate actually increased while the yogis held their breath and for a short period following. This finding is supported by accounts of research done on Swami Rama, a yogi with 40 years experience, at the Menninger Foundation (Luce & Peper, 1971). Physiological recordings indicated that when Swami Rama "stopped" his heart, his heart rate actually increased to approximately 300 beats a minute over a period of 17 seconds. This sudden atrial fibrillation, a dangerous cardiac condition that prevents the necessary volume of blood from being pumped to the body, would normally render a person unconscious and, if continued, would soon lead to death. Apparently the Swami was intrigued by this result, as he indicated that when he did this he experienced a "fluttering" in his chest. It is also reported that he was able to produce a temperature difference of 10 degrees between two spots on his hand.

An interesting extension of this work was done by Anand, Chhina, and Singh (1961a) who conducted experiments on Sri Ramanand Yogi while he was sealed in an air-tight box for two periods of 8 and 10 hours. The data indicated that he was able to reduce his oxygen intake and carbon dioxide output over his requirements under basal conditions. His average oxygen utilization while in the box was 13.3 liters per hour as compared to a basal requirement of 19.5 liters per hour. Even when breathing air with decreased oxygen and increased carbon dioxide content, his heart rate did not increase, nor did his respiratory activity increase or deepen. The electroencephalograph (EEG) indicated brain waves suggestive of early stages of sleep, despite there being no evidence that he actually slept.

The use of EEG measures is also of interest here as it provides us with an indication of an ability to maintain attention without being distracted. Anand, Chhina, and Singh (1961b) used EEG to attempt to assess the assertion that during meditation highly trained yogis are oblivious to external stimulation. They examined four such individuals and found that they were indeed able to achieve this state. The yogis did not demonstrate the expected blocking of the EEG alpha wave in response to stimulation during meditation. Two of the subjects kept their hands immersed in cold water for 45 to 55 minutes with no apparent discomfort. During this experience, they displayed persistent EEG alpha wave activity, which is associated with a state of wakeful relaxation. Swami Rama, while at the Menninger Foundation, experimented with EEG recordings and is reported to have produced alpha and theta waves with ease. The latter are slow waves associated with sleep states. He is also said to have entered a state he called "yogi sleep", which appeared, on the basis of the EEG, to be much like deep sleep. He was able to repeat, almost verbatim, statements made to him during this state upon awakening 25 minutes later. Lucia and Peper (1971), commenting on these findings, stated that, "Our idea of a 'normal' EEG is based upon the particular, limited, habitual use that a person makes of his brain. Swami Rama's agile and controlled transitions from one state of consciousness to another would, no doubt, be considered abnormal" (p. 43).

It is this final point that is important. As indicated earlier, this research raised questions as to what is normal or what our physiological and psychological limitations really are. When we think of stress and coping, we often think of physiological and psychological processes that are out of our control. It is our opinion that research such as that just described has considerable historical significance as it resulted in the development, over a very short period of time, of highly effective techniques oriented more to the Western mind and lifestyle. The impact of these on our ability to regain control of our lives and effectively cope with stress has been profound.

Relaxation

There are many different forms of relaxation. The most popular of these is **Progressive Muscular Relaxation (PMR)**. It originated with Jacobson in the 1930s, who spent the next 50 years of his life developing the technique. The literature abounds with the many variations on Jacobson's original relaxation strategies, with the most widely cited being that of Bernstein and Borkovec (1978) (we have provided you with the opportunity to practise this technique through instructions provided at the end of this chapter). Autogenic training is an imagery-based relaxation technique developed in Europe by Schutz and Luthe (1959). As a result of his interest in transcendental meditation, Benson developed a secular form of meditation, which he stated was based on achieving the "relaxation response" (1975). Although there are many different relaxation techniques, they share many similar features. To a large extent they require a quiet, undisturbed setting, where the person can sit passively, usually with eyes closed and allow the muscles to completely relax. It is of major importance that patterns of deep, rhythmical breathing be observed, although variations on the breathing are often used.

Systems of **meditation** have been used throughout history to reduce stress. There are literally thousands of different forms of meditation practised throughout the world. Again, they usually share common features such as positioning and attention to the *process* of thought rather than its *outcome*. There are differences in approach, particularly as many of these forms of meditation are based on religious belief systems. The system that has most influenced Western culture has been **transcendental meditation (TM)** a technique of meditation introduced by Maharishi Mahesh Yogi in the late 1950s. He adapted a system of meditation developed initially for monastic practice to the life of the householder, thereby making it more acceptable to the Western lifestyle. To practise the technique, individuals are "initiated" into the system by a trained teacher then encouraged to practise it twice daily. An international organization supports those involved in the technique, with follow-up courses and training. An aspect of TM that has been most important is the extensive body of empirical research that has accumulated regarding the efficacy of the meditative practice. Although there are concerns about some of the research methodology, a consistent picture emerges, indicating that the practice of TM has a beneficial physiological and psychological impact on an individual, and that its benefits accrue with time (Dillbeck & Orme-Johnson, 1987; Alexander et al., 1994). In the context of this chapter, techniques such as this have important implications for stress and coping.

Biofeedback is another technique that has received significant attention with regard to the possibility of modifying physiological processes. It involves the recording of physiological measures through electronic instruments and providing the individual with immediate information or feedback concerning their physiological state. The implication is that, given the new excitement about humans been able to control physiological processes, this feedback would allow individuals to exercise conscious control over aspects of their physiology and presumably make beneficial alterations where necessary. The enthusiasm for this procedure came from several areas. One was the interest in the control of autonomic activity such as that observed in India, described earlier. Another was similar to this in that it examined practitioners of Zen in Japan (Hirai, 1974; Kasamatsu & Hirai, 1963; 1966).

The main observation here was the control of electroencephalography (EEG), which many of these individuals displayed and which was considered to be indicative of states of consciousness. It was hoped that biofeedback could be used to hasten one's ability to attain these states, particularly as they relate to the experience of relaxation and perhaps "higher" states of consciousness. This thinking encouraged the research of individuals such as Kamiya (1968; 1969), which suggested that this was indeed possible. Another line of research was that of Miller and DiCara who reported that laboratory animals were able to achieve control of the autonomic responses, specifically cardiovascular activity, through reinforcement by way of feedback (Miller, 1969; Miller & DiCara, 1967).

A wave of enthusiasm resulted for the development of biofeedback technology and physiological control of variables such as muscle tension, heart rate, blood pressure, brain wave activity, and skin temperature. For example, electromyography (EMG) has been widely used to record and modify muscle tension in specific muscle groups in the body. Specifically, this might be used to decrease muscle tension in the frontalis muscle in the forehead as it relates to muscle tension headache or to increase muscle tension in a particular muscle group as a part of the rehabilitation process. Temperature control of blood flow has been examined in the context of migraine headaches and Raynaud's disease (Blanchard & Haynes, 1975; Green, Green, & Walters, 1972). Using temperature thermistors attached to the fingers, individuals with conditions such as these are encouraged to raise the temperature in their fingers as a strategy for causing blood to flow into the hands and increase levels of relaxation. The initial enthusiasm for biofeedback was considerable, given the implications for cardiovascular disease in our culture. However, the improvements observed were clinically disappointing and less effective than other strategies (Blanchard & Young, 1978).

The initial enthusiasm for biofeedback has been tempered by realistic evaluations of its efficacy. It has been disappointing, particularly given the promise the technique held for teaching people to regain control of their physical and psychological state and thereby effect important changes in their lifestyle. The effects of the procedure have been attributed to placebo or non-specific effects (Simkins, 1982). It appears that many of the effects attributed to biofeedback have more to do with the general state of relaxation, or the relaxation response, experienced during the procedure than the specific feedback provided.

Behaviour Therapy and Cognitive Therapy

Within the context of the field of behaviour therapy and cognitive behaviour, a wide array of strategies have been developed that have direct relevance for coping with stress. Some of these strategies will be discussed here. For example, Wolpe (1958) developed the technique of **systematic desensitization** to help people cope with fear and anxiety. It is based on the principle of reciprocal inhibition between the sympathetic and parasympathetic nervous systems and recognizes that anxiety and relaxation are incompatible responses. The individual is initially trained in a relaxation technique such as we have discussed above. They are then asked to construct an anxiety hierarchy consisting of a list of relevant events that elicit anxiety, ranked in order of increasing levels of anxiety. The client is then asked by the therapist to imagine or visualize these events from the least to the most anxiety-arousing situation. The technique assumes that imagining the feared event results in significant anxiety for the individual, which you no doubt have had personal experience with. Our ability to create high levels of stress as a function of our thinking is a fundamental principle underlying our discussions in this chapter. How many times have you uttered the phrase, "It wasn't nearly as bad as I had imagined it would be?" When we imagine ourselves dealing with fears, we often think in terms of all possibilities, from the best to the worst. When the worst does not occur, we are relieved. Through exposure to the feared situation we have entered into the process of *desensitization*. At the point at which the anxiety attached to imagining a particular event becomes unpleasant, the individual is encouraged to use the relaxation component to decrease arousal. The process of pairing these two inhibiting responses can lead to a significant reduction in the stress associated with the situation, whether it be undergoing a medical procedure such as an MRI or an injection, flying on an airplane, giving a public talk, or writing an exam. It is clear that a crucial component of this process is the repeated exposure to the feared situation, which ultimately leads to fear reduction (Newman et al., 1994).

Modelling is another procedure that can be used effectively to reduce stress associated with fear-provoking situations. Bandura (1985), who has described this process in detail, points out that most human behaviour is learned through the observation of models. We acquire cognitive skills and new behaviours through observing others. The influence of a model can serve to instruct, inhibit, disinhibit, facilitate, enhance environmental effects, and arouse emotions. Individuals can learn to cope with stressful situations by observing models. The process is very similar to that of desensitization in that observing a model coping with a situation well encourages a similar response in others.

In **participant modelling**, the individual observes a model coping with the anxiety-evoking situation. The individual is then encouraged to imitate the model and engage in the behaviour themselves while receiving reassurance from the model (Ritter, 1968). The model may also be presented symbolically through videos or films. This procedure has been used very effectively by Melamud and her colleagues to help reduce children's anxieties concerning hospitalization and medical procedures (Melamud & Siegal, 1975). It has also been applied to adults in preparation for the stress of aversive medical procedures. Bandura indicates that modelling is an effective intervention because it increases the individual's sense of self-efficacy (1995).

In **cognitive restructuring**, maladaptive, stress-producing cognitions are identified and replaced with ones that are more appropriate. The most well-known approach to cognitive restructuring is based on the work of Ellis, who developed *rational emotive behaviour therapy* (REBT) (Ellis, 1962). Ellis believes that it is our beliefs about events, not the events themselves, that create stressful emotional reactions. The sequence proceeds in the following manner: an event occurs, it is interpreted irrationally, and negative emotions and inappropriate behaviours occur. Ellis has identified specific logical errors that form the basis of this irrational thinking, such as over-generalization, catastrophizing, and absolute thinking. To reduce the stress of the experience, it is necessary to identify the thoughts that are based on irrational beliefs, challenge the irrational beliefs, and replace them with thoughts based on rational beliefs. Rational emotive behaviour therapy has been used effectively in stress-related situations such as anxiety, anger, fears, and depression as well as in addressing behavioural concerns such as Type A behaviour and obesity.

The work of Beck is similar to that of Ellis in its identification of distorted cognitions and helping of people to modify them (Beck, 1963, 1976). Beck describes his approach as *cognitive therapy*. Although it was initially developed to treat depression, it has now been applied to a wide variety of psychological problems. It differs from REBT in that it encourages people to identify dysfunctional beliefs through a process of hypothesis testing. These hypotheses are then tested through a process Beck calls "collective empiricism" to test the validity of the individual's dysfunctional beliefs.

The final behavioural technique we will consider here is based on the work of Meichenbaum and is appropriately called **stress inoculation training** (Meichenbaum, 1977). This is a package of procedures designed to help people cope effectively with stressful events. Initially, individuals are asked to examine how they conceptualize stressful events and to realize that they can be reconceptualized in less stressful ways. They are encouraged to view coping as a process in which they can prepare for, confront, and cope with stressful events. In the second phase, they learn and rehearse coping strategies such as relaxation training, problem solving, and self-reinforcement. In the third phase, this reconceptualized approach, both cognitive and behavioural, is applied to relevant situations. This can be done initially through imagery and role-playing and then applied in a gradual fashion to increasingly higher levels of stress. Like so many cognitive and behavioural strategies, stress inoculation training has been applied with success to a wide variety of problems within the health psychology realm.

In concluding this discussion of behavioural and cognitive strategies, we present an example in Box 5.2 of dealing with a medical crisis that combines the use of many of these strategies. The model itself is presented by DiTomasso and Kovnat (1994).

As we bring this chapter to a close, we thought that after speaking so much about stress and coping, we should give you the opportunity to experience the benefits of relaxation for yourself. So, read on.

Box 5-2 Medical Crisis

Crisis is described as a situation in which an individual perceives a stressor as being insurmountable. In the medical situation, crises can occur in a manner that is biologically certain or as the result of random events. For some of these events, it is possible to prepare in some ways, but for others it is unreasonable to dwell on their possibility. When they occur, we will often find ourselves totally unprepared to deal with the threat and loss of control such events result in. The manner in which a crisis is precipitated is considered important in determining how stressful it will be. Factors include: type, number, timing, and nature of the event (DiTomasso & Kovnat, 1994, p. 329). The cognitive factors that will determine how stressful a crisis will be include those we are familiar with: unrealistic beliefs and assumptions, cognitive distortions, biased recall and perception, self-efficacy, lack of information, and the cognitive triad identified by Beck, which includes a negative view of self, world, and future (p. 330). The behavioural factors that will influence the stress of the crisis are: lack of coping strategies, negative coping, lack of social support, and the inability to access support (p. 331).

In response to the crisis, DiTomasso and Kovnat describe a number of cognitive-behavioural interventions that can be used to help a patient cope. They include: forming a working relationship with the patient, identifying the disturbing aspects of the crisis, emphasizing the patient's strengths, setting mutually acceptable goals, identifying dysfunctional cognitions, emphasizing realistic thinking, using graduated task assignment, using behavioural rehearsal, inoculating the patient against negative factors, setting homework assignments, and providing reinforcement (p. 332). As DiTomasso and Kovnat point out, medical training has historically focused on the physical components of crisis; as a result, physicians are not prepared to deal with the psychosocial concerns of their patients. It is only recently that we have become concerned with the implications of the severe stress experienced by individuals in such crisis situations. The cognitive and behavioural interventions described here are clearly important in the coping process.

The Relaxation Responses: A Personal Guide

You can have someone else read the procedure to you, you can make your own tape of it or you can commit it to memory and take yourself through it. We'll provide you with a general overview and the specifics of the technique. It's based on the original procedure developed by Jacobson in the 1930s and subsequently modified by Bernstein and Borkovec (1973) and Bernstein and Given (1984). The basic principle upon which the procedure is based involves learning to identify the sensations associated with muscular tension and relaxation through learning to tense and then relax different muscle groups in the body. It's important to realize that learning relaxation skills is like learning any other skill—no one else can do it for you, it's not a matter of desire, it's a skill that needs to be learned. This means learning the technique and practising it. If you do it you will learn it, if you don't, you won't.

You will be asked to tense the specific muscle group initially to become aware of what muscle tension feels like and to be able to compare it to the experience of relaxation. As well, if the muscle group is tensed prior to relaxation a greater reduction in muscle tension will occur upon relaxation.

You should rest in a comfortable position such as in a recliner chair or lying down with support for your head and spine. Do not cross your legs or arms, and try to minimize body movements. You should close your eyes so as to be less aware of your external surroundings and loosen any tight items of clothing. During the relaxation session, you should breathe slowly and regularly. Each muscle group should be tensed for 5 to 7 seconds and relaxed on cue for 30 to 40 seconds. If you have a tape of the procedure or someone is guiding you through it, a cue word such as "tense" can be used to signal the beginning of the tension phase and "relax" to signal the relaxation phase.

It's also important to remember that the tension phase need not be extreme and should not involve any pain to the muscle. If you feel the tensing of a muscle could cause pain or cramping, shorten the period of tension. You only need to tighten the muscles, not strain them. At the beginning of the relaxation phase, you should focus your attention on the sensations attached to the reduction in tension and the increase in relaxation in the muscles.

On tapes it's common to have statements at the beginning of the relaxation phase such as, "Allow the muscles to relax completely", or "With every breath the muscles relax more completely and more deeply." It's usual to relax each muscle group twice, although it's not inappropriate to continue the tension/relaxation sequence in a particular muscle group several times until a desired depth of relaxation is obtained. There are many variations on the sequence and methods used; the following is one example. As you practise and develop your relaxation skills, it's important to remember that you do not need to "try" to relax, you just let it happen. You are not being evaluated, and increased effort is not the key to success. Rather, you need to take a passive stance, let go, and enjoy the experience.

1. Dominant hand and forearm: make your hand into a tight fist, then relax.
2. Non-dominant hand and forearm; make your hand into a tight fist, then relax.
3. Dominant upper arm: bend your arm at the elbow and bring your hand toward your shoulder, then relax.
4. Non-dominant upper arm: bend your arm at the elbow and bring your hand toward your shoulder, then relax.
5. Forehead: raise your eyebrows and wrinkle your forehead, then relax.

6. Eyes: close your eyes tighter than they are, then relax.
7. Lower face and jaws: clench your teeth and tighten the corners of your mouth, then relax.
8. Shoulders: raise your shoulders as if to touch your ears, then relax.
9. Chest: take a deep breath and hold it, then relax.
10. Abdomen: tighten the stomach muscles, then relax.
11. Legs one: point your toes downward, away from your body, then relax.
12. Legs two: bring your toes upward, toward your body, then relax.
13. Scan your body for residual tension: if tension is experienced in a muscle group, repeat the tension/relaxation sequence for that muscle group.
14. Take some time to enjoy the feelings of relaxation in your body.
15. You can end the session by counting backwards from five to one, becoming more alert as you count down. When you get to one, open your eyes.

The procedure will take approximately 30 minutes. You should practise the technique regularly for optimal effectiveness; twice a day would be ideal. When you begin to learn a relaxation procedure, it's best to do so in a setting that is quiet and comfortable, where distractions are minimal, and in which you are not likely to be disturbed. This may require some preparation on your part, but it will make it easier to focus your attention on learning the technique. As you become more skilled at relaxation, you'll want to generalize the learning experience to those places in your life where relaxation is most relevant (e.g., your workplace, a performance activity, social situations). Also, as you become more familiar with the relaxation experience, as indicated by greater levels of relaxation both during and outside of the relaxation sessions, you can cut out the tension phase of the sequence and focus only on the relaxation of the muscle. Increased familiarity with the sensations of relaxation will make it unnecessary for you to have the feeling of tension to compare them to.

With time, you'll be able to combine muscle groups in obvious ways. For example, the four-group procedure involves the following groups: (1) hands and arms; (2) head; (3) chest, shoulders, and abdomen; and (4) legs. This will reduce the time of the procedure to under 10 minutes. Eventually, you should be able to achieve a relaxed state through recall. This means that you simply recall the sensations of the relaxed muscle groups together with a cue word such as "relax" or "let go." This is usually combined with deep breathing to achieve a state of relaxation in a shorter period of time. Ultimately, this relaxed state should be achievable simply through a countdown (e.g., from 10 to 1) in combination with your breathing. When you have arrived at this level, you have achieved the desired skill level. You should continue to practise and use the skill to maintain it. You have now developed a powerful resource for coping with stress.

KEY TERMS

stress
coping
stress literacy
eustress
homeostasis
fight or flight response
nervous system
endocrine system
central nervous system
peripheral nervous system
hypothalamus
adrenal medulla
limbic system
reticular formation
sympathetic
parasympathetic
pituitary gland
adrenal cortex
thyroid gland
pancreas
general adaptation syndrome (GAS)
alarm
resistance
diseases of adaptation
exhaustion
stress-diathesis model
cognitive transactional models
cognitive appraisals
primary appraisal
secondary appraisal
reappraisal
irrelevant appraisal
benign-positive appraisal
stressful appraisal
harm/loss appraisal
threat appraisal
challenge appraisal
vulnerability
person variables
situation variables
commitments as person variables
beliefs as person variables
novelty
predictability
event uncertainty
imminence
duration
temporal uncertainty
Type A behaviour pattern
coping response
stress response
coping goal
coping outcomes
problem-focused coping
emotion-focused coping
personal resources
social support
emotional support
informational support
tangible support
stress-buffering hypothesis
personal control
stress management techniques
relaxation techniques
hypometabolic state
progressive muscular relaxation (PMR)
meditation
transcendental meditation (TM)
biofeedback
systematic desensitization
modelling
participant modelling
cognitive restructuring
stress inoculation training

Chapter 6

COMMUNICATION IN MEDICAL SETTINGS

Chapter Outline

Key Questions

1. What factors influence our perception and interpretation of symptoms?
2. Why do people delay in seeking medical care?
3. How have researchers conceptualized physician-patient relationships?
4. What patient and physician characteristics lead to poor communication?
5. How widespread is patient non-adherence?
6. How can we improve patient adherence to medical advice?
7. Does patient adherence lead to better health outcomes?

Lynn is visiting her physician, primarily because she has been recently experiencing a lot of stomach problems. However, this isn't Lynn's only complaint. In addition to her stomach problems, Lynn hasn't been sleeping, she has more blemishes on her face than usual, and her mother has recently been diagnosed with adult-onset diabetes. Lynn is quite concerned about her. Upon visiting her physician, Lynn decides she will present her symptoms, in order of ease of describing them. Lynn states, "My face has been worse than usual lately, I haven't been getting enough sleep, and I've had a lot of butterflies in my stomach these last few weeks." Lynn doesn't bother to mention her concern about her mother to the physician because she already has a lot of issues to discuss and knows the physician can't possibly cure her mother during this visit. Lynn's physician assumes the "butterflies" aren't really an issue because Lynn has downplayed this symptom and hasn't reported any pain in her stomach. He also assumes Lynn hasn't been getting enough sleep because she has been busy lately. Finally, the doctor decides that the reason Lynn has visited is because she is seeking help for her "worse than usual" face. He provides her with a prescription for a topical ointment and sends her on her way. The main reason for Lynn visiting her physician, her upset stomach, is never discussed.

Compare Lynn's visit with her physician to the more positive visit experienced by Alexander and his parents to the emergency ward.

Alexander is an 18-month-old toddler who just loves to run. However, running is a relatively new talent and he sometimes forgets a few required details, such as looking where he's going! After a head-on collision with the corner of a kitchen cupboard and a resulting gash on his forehead, his parents take him to Emergency to get his cut sutured. As expected, there is a wait before Alexander can see a doctor. Once Alexander sees the doctor, the stitchwork begins. The physician seems to realize it is a very stressful situation for the young family. Mom and Dad are told how to care for the laceration and all their questions are answered. They are allowed to stay in the room to lessen Alexander's anxiety, and when the suturing is complete Alexander is given a "rubber glove balloon." He is also rewarded with a popsicle. Although Alexander isn't interested in the popsicle right now, Dad makes sure it doesn't go to waste.

Most people can recall both positive and negative experiences they have had with physicians. Lynn's experience exemplifies a situation where a patient isn't completely satisfied with the outcome of a visit with a physician. In this case, Lynn didn't have all of her concerns addressed during the physician-patient interview. Indeed, her primary concern, stomach problems, wasn't even mentioned by her physician. In contrast, it is obvious that Alexander, or at least his parents, were very satisfied with their interaction with the emergency room physician. From the moment Alexander arrived at Emergency, it was obvious why he was seeking treatment. Treatment was provided for Alexander and his parents had all of their questions answered.

Communication was a major contributing factor to the satisfaction both Lynn and Alexander's parents felt with the treatment they received from their physicians. A breakdown or lack of communication between patient and physician resulted in a somewhat negative experience for Lynn (the physician did not comprehend the main reason for her visit). However, communication about Alexander's injury was more straightforward. Therefore, there was less chance for miscommunication to arise, with a positive experience resulting.

Communication is central to the physician-patient relationship. In this chapter, we will discuss how both physician and patient behaviours contribute to faulty communication. As well, we will outline the impact communication has on physician-patient relationships, medical adherence, and health outcomes. However, before we begin our discussion of communication and related factors, we must consider the factors that lead one to seek medical advice.

PERCEIVING AND INTERPRETING SYMPTOMS

How do we decide when to seek medical advice? How do we know whether we are ill or not? Clearly, Alexander's parents knew they should seek medical care for their son. The cut on his forehead and the dripping blood were fairly obvious clues. But what was the determining factor that led Lynn to seek medical advice? Many of her symptoms are sensations that people experience every day. For example, people often have blemishes on their skin and most people do get stomach aches from time to time. But they don't seek medical advice each and every time one of these "symptoms" arises. At what point should a person seek medical advice?

Perceiving symptoms is not as easy as it may seem. People have difficulty deciphering and even noticing some symptoms. For instance, people seem to have difficulty assessing highly visible external symptoms, such as whether a mole-like lesion is melanoma (Miles & Meehan, 1995). Therefore, it is not surprising to learn that people also have difficulties accurately assessing their internal states. For example, people's estimates of their own heart rate are not well correlated with physiological indices (Pennebaker, 1983). Partly as a result of these inaccuracies, there is considerable variability regarding when an individual will seek medical advice.

Certainly, there are individual differences in the perception of symptoms. Have you ever noticed how some people seem to "carry on" no matter what, whereas others seem to adopt the sick role the instant they are faced with a minor impediment (something even as small as a paper cut). Some of these individual differences are constant over time. That is, some people are consistently more likely to notice a symptom than others are. Indeed, some individuals pay more attention to their internal states than others do (Pennebaker, 1983; Pennebaker, 1994). This does not necessarily mean that these people are more accurate in their interpretation of sensations; in fact, they may overestimate changes in their bodily functions, such as heart rate and nasal congestion.

Stressful periods in people's lives can precipitate or aggravate the experience of symptoms. In Chapter 3, we discussed the influence stress has on our immune system. People who have experienced a great deal of stress are more vulnerable to illness. It follows that people who believe they are more likely to contract an illness will attend more closely to their bodies. This inward focus of attention may lead them to interpret stress-related physiological changes, such as accelerated heart rate or breathing, as symptoms of illness (Cameron, Leventhal, & Leventhal, 1995).

Our current mood affects our ratings of our health (Salovey et al., 1991). People in a good mood view the world and their own health more positively than do those in a bad mood. We have all had days when we were in such a good mood that we didn't notice the various aches and pains that would normally be an aggravation. Yet we have also had days when we have been in a bad mood and seemed to notice every discomfort, no matter how minor. Research backs up these experiential observations. People in a good mood report fewer symptoms and fewer illness-related memories. In contrast, people in a bad mood report more symptoms, are less likely to believe that any behaviours they engage in would relieve symptoms, and assume they are more vulnerable to future illness (Salovey et al.; Leventhal et al., 1996; Stegen et al., 1998). One study (Croyle & Uretsky, 1987) found that inducing a temporary bad mood in participants led them to judge their health more negatively and to report more symptoms than was the case for participants put into a good mood. Along these same lines, another study, in which participants kept a diary of symptoms and moods, found that bad moods were a consistent trigger for the reporting of symptoms (Verbrugge, 1985).

Situational factors also influence whether a person will recognize a symptom. When the environment is exciting or demands a great deal of attention or concentration, people are less likely to notice internal symptoms (Pennebaker, 1994). Internal symptoms are also likely to go unnoticed when an individual is engaged in physical activity. In contrast, an individual in a boring or otherwise uninteresting environment will likely notice physical symptoms. Pennebaker (1983) relates many findings that are consistent with this view. For example, "Individuals are more likely to notice itching or tickling sensations in their throats and emit coughs during boring parts of movies than during interesting portions" (p. 191).

There are also age differences in the reporting of symptoms. Elderly people frequently complain of physical symptoms that prompt them to seek medical intervention. There is evidence to suggest that normal age-related bodily changes are perceived by older people as illness symptoms (Haug, Musil, Warner, & Morris, 1997). Other researchers have suggested that the trend of increasing symptoms as one ages may be partially due to decreased cognitive performance that some adults experience as they age (Frisoni, Fedi, Geroldi, & Trabucchi,

1999). In other words, mild cognitive impairment is associated with the perception of poorer body functioning. These studies suggest that older adults may over-report their symptoms. However, a study of cancer patients discovered that older adults were less likely than younger adults to notice cancer symptoms (Mor et al., 1990). Thus, the issue of age differences in the recognition of symptoms is quite complex. We must acknowledge this complexity while at the same time bearing in mind the likelihood that older adults do experience more symptoms than younger adults.

In summary, symptom recognition depends on individual differences in attention to one's body as well as transitory situational factors that alter the direction of one's attention. When attention is directed inward, symptoms are more likely to be recognized. On the other hand, when attention is directed outward, by physical activity or a distracting environment, symptoms are less likely to be noticed. Age differences as well as our current mood also influence symptom recognition.

Once a symptom is perceived, it must then be interpreted. How a symptom is interpreted is influenced by a number of factors, including prior experience with the symptom. If, for example, your mother and your siblings have had their appendixes removed, you are more likely to consider appendicitis whenever you experience pain in your lower abdomen. Other people, who do not share this family history, would likely consider other causes for the pain before contemplating problems with their appendix.

A symptom's meaning is influenced by how common it is within a range of family, friends, acquaintances, and even within one's culture (Croyle & Hunt, 1991). Symptoms that are perceived as commonplace are generally considered to be less serious than more rare or unusual factors (Croyle & Ditto, 1990). As strange as it may seem, the simple fact that a symptom or condition is widespread may lead people to attach little significance to it.

Cultural factors affect how quickly and what kind of symptoms are recognized and reported (Klonoff & Landrine, 1994). For example, one study compared the symptom recognition reported by Anglos and Mexicans (Burnum, Timbers, & Hough, 1984). The researchers reported that Mexicans were more likely than Anglos to report symptoms that occurred frequently. In contrast, Anglos were more likely than Mexicans to report only those symptoms which they experienced infrequently. Another study (Alonso et al., 1998) noted that there are crosscultural differences in the reporting of vision problems. Specifically, cataract patients in Canada and Spain were less likely to report trouble with their vision than Danish or American patients. These reports could not be accounted for by either clinical or sociodemographic factors.

In considering the symptoms that people report, we also need to include the role of learning. In a very real sense, we learn how to experience symptoms. Therefore, it is likely that people in different cultures receive different "lessons" in the experience of symptoms. At a very young age, children are taught both directly and by example which symptoms are important and which are trivial. A parent's concern over a fever and seeming unconcern over a superficial cut provide a child with powerful cues about which symptoms to attend to and which to ignore. One study documenting the role of learning in symptom experience comes from a survey of adult nursing students and their mothers. Whitehead, Busch, Heller, and Costa (1986) discovered that a mother's reaction to menstrual symptoms when her daughter was an adolescent was closely related with the daughter's experience of menstruation as an adult. When mothers displayed menstrual distress or took on a sick role during menstruation, daughters reported significantly more menstrual symptoms and were more likely to take time off or seek help for those symptoms compared to daughters whose mothers did not respond to menses with distress.

Our families contribute to our interpretation of symptoms in other ways as well. We often consult our family and friends to help us interpret the meaning of a symptom. These advisers form a **lay referral system**, an informal network of non-practitioners who offer their own interpretations long before any medical treatment is sought (Freidson, 1961). People in the lay referral system provide advice when the person mentions the symptoms, requests an opinion, or even if he or she simply looks sick. The friend or relative responds with personal views of what the symptom is likely to mean: "Connor and Liam both had rashes like that. It turned out it was a reaction to the new brand of bubble bath their Mom had bought" (c.f. Croyle & Hunt, 1991). The friend or relative provides advice about seeking medical attention: "Parker's temperature was getting quite high and he ended up having convulsions. You'd better call your doctor." They may also recommend various home remedies, such as, "Soak a wool sock in boiling water and vinegar and then wrap it around your neck, your sore throat will be gone in no time" (e.g., Stoller, 1984). They may also suggest consulting another lay referral person: "Allister had the same problem. You should give him a call."

The advice provided by the lay referral network varies in its usefulness. At times, it is good. For example, a study conducted at the Children's Hospital in Montreal determined that mothers who consulted their lay referral system about their child's symptoms were less likely to take their children to the emergency department unnecessarily. Although much of

CASE 6-1 Delay in Seeking Treatment

One day after Dean returned from a 4-hour bike ride, he noticed that one of his testicles was quite sore. He thought the sensation was odd, but he quickly rationalized that he had just spent a considerable amount of time in the "saddle" and that this was likely responsible for his discomfort. The discomfort did not completely go away but Dean, an aspiring professional cyclist, continued to spend a large amount of time on his bike. About a month later he was thinking about his testicular soreness again. He realized that the discomfort just wasn't subsiding. He vowed to visit a physician the next chance he got. Unfortunately, he was off to Dijon, France in 2 days to try out for a professional cycling team and would likely have to wait until he returned to Canada before he could visit the physician. Three weeks later Dean returned to Canada. He hadn't experienced much discomfort when he was in France because he had been quite caught up in the excitement of fulfilling his dream of getting paid for doing what he loved—cycling. Back home, in his own environment, he became aware that his discomfort was becoming more intense. Obviously, there was more wrong with him than simply spending too many hours training. He was extremely anxious as he made an appointment to see his family physician. The next day he visited his physician. This visit led to a number of medical tests to aid the physician in making a diagnosis. The physician felt it was likely that Dean had testicular cancer. Subsequently, this diagnosis was confirmed and the prognosis was not good. Dean was told that he had only a 50-50 chance of surviving.

the advice provided by the lay referral network is helpful, lay persons are far more likely than health professionals to recommend actions that worsen the condition or delay the person's use of appropriate and needed treatment.

SEEKING MEDICAL CARE

When do people seek medical care? The answer to this question is more complex than simply stating that people visit their physician when they have experienced one or more symptoms. In spite of the fact that 75 percent to 90 percent of the general population at any given time experience symptoms that could be considered clinically relevant, only about one-third of them seek medical care (DiMatteo, 1991). Studies of illness behaviour indicate that when a person seeks help is a function of the specific nature of the symptoms experienced as well as of their social and personal needs.

Perhaps the most obvious determinant of when a person seeks help is the type of symptoms experienced. Symptoms that are new, unexpected, painful, disruptive, highly visible, or affect highly valued parts of the body are interpreted as more serious and are particularly likely to lead the person to seek medical care (Eifert et al., 1996; Safer, Tharps, Jackson, & Leventhal, 1979; Turk, Litt, Salovey, & Walker, 1985). If one's symptoms are recognizable from past experiences and are believed to be unimportant or explainable, such as muscle aches after an athletic competition, they will probably be ignored. However, if the symptom interferes with daily activities such as job performance or participation in athletic events, medical care is usually sought. Symptoms also gain a person's attention if they attack a highly visible part of the body such as the face or eyes, or one that is particulary salient to the individual (such as the heart, for a person whose father died of heart disease) (Safer et al., 1979). Above all, the symptom that leads a person to seek medical care most quickly is the experience of pain. Few of us enjoy pain and as a result we will attempt to eliminate the painful experience as fast as possible (Turk et al., 1985).

Delaying Medical Care

Dean was lucky. He won his battle against testicular cancer and lived to cycle another day. However, his odds of survival would likely have been better if he had not delayed so long in seeking medical advice. Delay in seeking diagnosis and treatment is clearly linked to increases in morbidity and mortality of cancer patients (Ramirez et al., 1999; Richards et al., 1999). Perhaps Dean would have sought medical care sooner if it was more obvious that his symptoms required medical treatment. In medical emergencies, such as when someone sustains a severe injury, people often seek help in a matter of minutes or hours. Referring back to Alexander, the little boy with the cut on his forehead, we can assume that his parents wasted no time in getting him to the hospital as quickly as possible.

Other emergency situations are more ambiguous. Most heart attack victims initially attribute their symptoms to such conditions as gas pains, ulcers, gallbladder diseases, or even the common cold (Gentry, 1979). Patients suffering from a myocardial infarction, more commonly referred to as a heart attack, typically arrive at the hospital or into the care of paramedical staff at some point between less than one hour and several days after the onset of their symptoms. Most often the time from onset of symptoms to the initiation of medical help is between two and one-half and four hours. Yet, only about 10 percent of that time is used by heart attack victims for transportation. Studies show that heart attack victims spend about 65 percent of that time trying to decide whether their symptoms require medical treatment. Even after they have correctly attributed the symptoms to a serious condition, such as a heart attack, people will waste a substantial amount of time before taking direct action to receive treatment. In fact, 25 percent of the time between onset of symptoms and arrival at the hospital is spent doing unnecessary things such as calling the family physician (who would automatically tell the patient to go directly to the emergency department of the clos-

FIGURE 6-1 Stages of Delay in Seeking Treatment for Symptoms

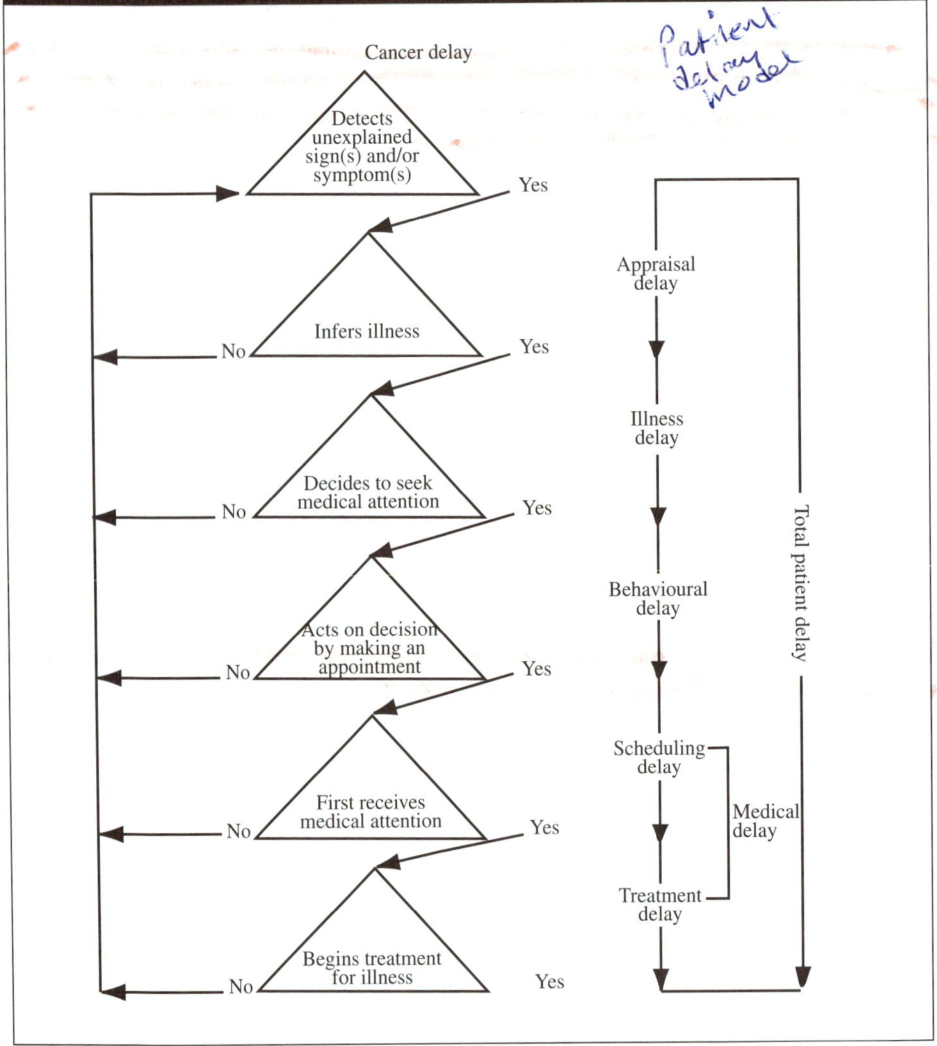

Source: Andersen, B.L., Cacioppo, J.T., & Roberts, D.C. (1995). Delay in seeking a cancer diagnosis: delay stages and psychophysiological comparison processes. *British Journal of Social Psychology*, 34, 33–52. Reprinted by permission.

est hospital), preparing to go to the hospital (gathering clothes and personal items), and washing up.

What is responsible for such delay? Researchers have attempted to answer this question. In doing so, they have developed a model to outline different stages of delay. Researchers refer to **patient delay** as the period between an individual's first awareness of a symptom and treatment for that symptom. Total patient delay occurs as a sequence of stages (Andersen, Cacioppo, & Roberts, 1995). As the diagram in Figure 6.1 illustrates, the stages are: (1) **appraisal delay**, which is the time it takes for a person to decide that a symptom is a sign of illness; (2) **illness delay**, which is the time between recognizing one is ill and deciding to seek medical care; (3) **behavioural delay**, which is the time that elapses between the decision to seek medical care and the person acting on this decision by making an appointment; and (4) **medical delay** (scheduling and treatment), which is the interval between the person making an appointment and first receiving medical care.

Safer, Tharps, Jackson, and Leventhal (1979) conducted an early study identifying stages of delay in seeking medical care. These researchers interviewed 93 patients who were waiting to see a physician at a hospital clinic or emergency room. They assessed patients' reactions to their symptoms and determined at what point these patients first interpreted their symptoms as illness, when they decided to seek medical care, and when they actually did take steps to bring the problem to a medical professional. Not surprisingly, those who demonstrated the least delay were those who were in the greatest pain. The total delay in seeking care was significantly longer for patients who currently had other problems in their lives (such as a troubled marriage), who had read about their symptoms, who were older, and who had waited for the symptoms to go away. Moreover, the best predictor of illness delay was whether the person had a new or old symptom. Patients were apparently more likely to see an old symptom as normal and to tolerate it for a long period of time before deciding to seek medical care. Somewhat understandably, patients who imagined they were severely ill and imagined negative consequences of being ill also had lengthy illness delays. It follows that people who believed they could not be cured also delayed treatment.

The findings of the previous study (Safer et al., 1979) should be interpreted somewhat cautiously because of its methodological limitations. First, because the study included only persons who actually sought medical care there is no way to generalize conclusions concerning delay to those persons who had a symptom but did not seek treatment. Second, the study uses retrospective data. This is particularly important, because the patients were asked to recall and specify the point at which they first noticed the symptom, whey they first felt they were ill, and when they decided to seek treatment. Because the patients are asked to remember this information rather than report it as it was happening, there may be inaccuracies in the information. A prospective study, in which the participants maintain a diary of their symptoms and their appraisals of those symptoms, would be a more effective way of studying delay behaviours.

Recent research investigating delay behaviours has focused almost exclusively on cancer patients. Studying this population's delay behaviour is most appropriate because, as previously mentioned, delays in treatment for cancer have a significant influence on the patient's survival rate (Ramirez et al., 1999; Richards et al.,1999). A meta-analysis of 12 studies estimated that 34 percent of women with breast cancer symptoms delay seeking medical advice for 3 months or more (Facione, 1993). Both prospective (e.g., Andersen et al., 1995) and retrospective research reveals that appraisal delay (the time during which individuals are attempting to discern their bodily state and make an inference about an illness) accounts for the majority of the total delay time.

In her review of the literature, Facione (1993) reports that both high and low levels of fear are associated with longer delays in women with breast cancer symptoms. In this case, fear refers to many things, including fear of doctors and hospitals, cancer, embarrassment, chemotherapy, disfigurement, pain, loss of femininity, and loss of control, to name but a few. Presumably, if you have tremendous fear of a diagnosis of cancer because of all the associated repercussions you will delay behaviour to circumvent dealing with these issues (Facione & Giancarlo, 1998; Lauver, Coyle, & Panchmatia, 1995; Timko, 1987). On the other hand, if you have very little fear you may not be motivated to seek medical advice.

Social influences may also affect delay behaviour. Many women expect that if they are diagnosed with breast cancer their male partner will abandon them (Facione & Giancarlo, 1998). Yet, a number of studies reveal that marital status is unrelated to delays by patients (e.g., Ramirez et al., 1999). Unfortunately, there is support for the hypothesis that role responsibilities influence delay behaviour (Facione, 1993; Facione, Giancarlo, & Ingram, 1999; Lauver, Coyle, & Panchmatia, 1995). Women report that devoting time and attention to the needs of others, taking time to make domestic arrangements prior to the biopsy, demands associated with summer and school holidays, work-related demands, caring for other ill family members, and the temporary presence of others in the home receive priority over discovered breast cancer symptoms.

Studies investigating the relationship between race, delay in seeking medical advice and delay in obtaining medical treatment have reported mixed results. Some studies report few or no differences between races in delay seeking medical care (e.g., Coates et al., 1992; Lauver, 1994). However, other studies point to the fact that there are significant racial differences in delay in seeking care (Facione, 1993). It is not surprising that minority American populations such as African-Americans delay longer before seeking medical care, given that this group tends to utilize health care services less, regardless of their degree of illness (e.g., Blendon, Aiken, Freeman, & Corey, 1989). Facione and Giancarlo (1998) examined narratives of minority American women. The narratives were told by 80 Anglo-, Latina-, and African-American women who participated in 1 of 16 community focus groups in San Francisco. The researchers discovered that one reason women do not seek medical treatment for breast symptoms is their fear of deportation. Another reason is they fear that they will be refused treatment due to poverty. Other studies in the United States (e.g., Facione, 1999; Dennis, Gardner, & Lim, 1975) have also reported that minority women lack the money to pay for health care services. Coates and colleagues (1992) conclude that the difference in time from symptom recognition to medical consultation is unlikely to account for the large racial differences in survival rates of breast cancer patients. Because the Canadian health care system strives to provide coverage for everyone in the nation, we would expect that the patient's economic level would not be a factor in delaying treatment behaviour. Another factor that has been considered in delay behaviour is the age of the patient. Age is often reported as having an effect on patient delay. Ramirez and colleagues (1999), Richards and colleagues (1999) and Sainsbury, Johnston, and Haward (1999) all report that older age is associated with longer delay by breast cancer patients. Unfortunately, these investigators have not utilized the stages of delay model provided by Andersen and colleagues (1995), outlined in Figure 6.1. However, these studies do divide the time between onset of symptoms and start of treatment (total delay) into two main phases: delay by patients,

CASE 6-2 One Surgeon's Story: Invincible or Denial?

What accounts for the behaviour of a 37-year-old male surgeon who was diagnosed as having a malignant, non-Hodgkins lymphoma (cancer of the lymph nodes)? Jorge delayed defining his symptom as that of a possible serious illness even though he was trained to identify the importance of such symptoms in his patients.

One morning, Jorge noticed a small lump on his jaw while shaving. He found the lump curious, but he was convinced he was invincible so it certainly wasn't anything he was going to worry about. As a general rule, physicians have a unique ability to think of themselves as invulnerable to the ailments and misery that they are exposed to each day. Jorge was in complete denial and he ignored the lump. As time when by, the lump slowly enlarged and he casually showed it to his physician friends. He thinks they said not to worry but he really can't remember. Finally, at a dinner party one night, a woman with no medical training asked, "What is that thing under your jaw?" Jorge, still believing all was well, set up an appointment with a surgeon. He underwent surgery, 5 months of radiation treatment, and has lived to tell his story (Shlain, 1979).

defined as time between onset of symptoms and time of first medical consultation; and delay by providers, which is any delay between first medical consultation and start of treatment. Analysis based on this definition of delay reveals that older women are more likely to engage in patient delay than are younger women. However, younger women experience more delay by their health care providers (Ramirez et al., 1999). Based on the results from the study conducted by Richards and colleagues (1999), we can conclude that the health care providers were less likely to delay treatment of the older women because the older women were at a more advanced stage of cancer (likely resulting from their delay in seeking medical advice). Fortunately, delays by providers "do not seem to be associated with decreased survival in patients presenting with breast cancer" (Sainsbury et al., 1999, p. 1132).

It is interesting to note that a different population of older patients, those with colorectal cancer, were less likely to notice symptoms than younger adults. Once these symptoms were noticed, however, the older adults were less likely than younger adults to delay seeking medical attention (Mor et al., 1990). Another study (Marshall & Funch, 1986) investigating patient delay among colorectal patients reported no age differences in delay but did report gender differences. Women were more likely than men to delay seeking care for both cancer of the rectum and cancer of the colon. A study (Mor et al., 1990) of lung cancer patients found no age differences in delay behaviour. It may be that the nature of the illness determines whether there are age differences in delay behaviour. Future research is required to confirm this assertion and to determine whether women are more likely than men to exhibit delay behaviour across all illnesses.

In summary, we can conclude that there are a number of factors which contribute to patient delay, including characteristics of the symptom, age, gender, race, societal role obligations, and psychological attributes such as fear. Even physicians who are familiar with illness symptoms and know the importance of treating these symptoms promptly are not exempt from patient delay; consider the behaviour of Jorge, described in Case Study 6.2. An additional factor contributing to people's decisions about using medical services is the quality of the relationship they have with their physicians. This important relationship is the topic of the next section.

PHYSICIAN-PATIENT INTERACTION

Onions (1986) defines a patient as, "A sufferer, one who is under medical treatment, or a person to whom something is done" and a client as, "One who is under the protection or patronage of another, a dependent." There is some controversy about what the most appropriate term is for referring to people who are receiving health care. In fact, the authors of this text had a somewhat lengthy discussion on this issue during the preliminary stages of writing this book. In this era of political correctness, we wanted to use the most appropriate term. A review of the literature discovered a plethora of opinion but little research on the issue.

A single North American study on this topic was conducted in Vancouver, British Columbia (Wing, 1997). This study includes the responses of 101 people who were attending a back-pain clinic. Each person was presented with a short letter. The letter was addressed "Dear Friend" to avoid introducing the terms "client" or "patient." It was very short, stating that, "There is an interesting discussion in hospitals at this time about the term that we use for people we try to help" (p. 288). Patients were then asked to indicate if they prefer the term "client" or "patient." To avoid selection bias for the first option, the letters with "patient" first and "client" first were alternated. The overwhelming majority of respondents (74) stated a preference for the term "patient." Nineteen respondents preferred "client", and the remaining eight had no preference.

The results obtained by Wing are similar to those reported in other studies. A New Zealand study found that 87 percent of visitors to a hospital on an outpatient basis preferred to be called "patients" (Elliot & White, 1990). Similarly, a study conducted in Australia discovered that 84 percent of patients and their companions attending outpatient departments preferred the term "patient" (Nair, 1998). There appear to be no sex differences in this preference. However, a slight trend was noted in the preference for "patient" in older age groups (Nair, 1998). Clearly, the preference, at least in these settings, is that most people wish to be called "patient."

An issue that has been, and should be, a concern to health care professionals is whether one's attitudes and behaviours are shaped (especially adversely) by the use of a particular term for the people they help. Imrie (1994) suggested that using the term "patient" provides a reminder to health care professionals that those who are being helped do suffer. Moreover, Atkinson (1993) implied that the term "sufferer" has a passive connotation. Certainly, the reference to passiveness is what may lead people to disagree with being referred to as a "patient."

Although there are concerns related to the use of the term "patient" , there are also concerns as to the possible results of using the term "client" instead. Raphael and Emmerson (1991) identify a number of points to consider before adopting the term "client." These include: (1) denial that the person has an illness or that certain treatments may be necessary (e.g., insulin for diabetics); (2) implication of effective choice of treatment and responsibility for remuneration, two conditions that cannot be met in all disease states and economic situations (e.g., a man with paranoid schizophrenia, dangerous to himself and society, has no insight or ability to make decisions about treatment that, although associated with risks, may control the condition); and (3) lack of the special elements of care and compassion implicit in the term "patient."

Undoubtedly there are arguments for the use of both terms. However, rather than throw out the word "patient" perhaps it is better to accept a shift in the term's meaning. We may best heed the logic of a participant in Nair's (1998) study, who remarked, "There is nothing in a name, provided there is care" (p. 593).

Basic Models of Physician-Patient Interaction

It has been suggested (Kasl, 1975) that the crucial element in the typical relationship between a patient and health care practitioner is probably not the exchange of information but the nature of their relationship. A classic article in the field of health psychology was written by Thomas Szasz and Marc Hollender in 1956. In this article, Szasz and Hollender outline three basic models they believed characterized the nature of the physician-patient relationship.

The **active-passive model** occurs when the patient is unable to participate in his or her own care and to make decisions for his or her own welfare because of their medical condition. For example, when a patient has a severe injury or is in a coma the physician is responsible for providing care and making decisions on behalf of the patient; obviously, the patient is not in a position to provide any input. Consider the following example:

> Dennis gashed himself with a knife while camping in the bush. He was trying to cut a rope. When the knife finally went through the rope, it kept right on going into Dennis' leg, where it severed an artery. The blood was spurting out. His buddies placed him in the back of their pickup truck and sped down the highway toward the nearest town. They drove as fast as they could. They were just too far away from civilization to call an ambulance, and every moment counted. By the time they reached the hospital, Dennis was unconscious. A few seconds after they arrived at the hospital emergency ward, Dennis was placed on a gurney and wheeled to the operating room. A few seconds later, Dennis' clothing was ripped off and the severed artery was found and tied. At the same time, others were working to find a vein that had not collapsed in order to put in an intravenous line. Others were ensuring that he was getting enough oxygen. The entire emergency room staff worked with skill and speed. Dennis, who was unconscious, could neither participate nor fight their efforts.

The **guidance-cooperation model** applies when the patient seeks advice from the physician. The patient answers the questions that are asked but the physician is responsible for determining diagnosis and treatment. In essence, the physician is responsible for the thinking and decision-making. This model would likely be followed if a person had an infection or a sprain. Consider the following example:

> Henry was told by his physician to, "Take one of these little pills three times a day. If you do what I tell you to, you will be just fine." Henry was convinced that asking the physician questions would be challenging physician authority" , so he simply nodded in agreement. Henry was to take the medication to control his hypertension. However, he couldn't seem to remember to take the pills. This may have been due to the fact that he didn't feel sick (hypertension is often referred to as "the silent killer") or because he had never been told exactly what the medication would do.

In the **mutual-participation model**, the patient has more responsibility than in the other models. In this model, the physician and patient make joint decisions about every aspect of care, from deciding what diagnostic tests the patient should undergo to the choice and implementation of treatment. Input and responsibility are shared equally by the physician and patient. The two work together in a partnership. Here's an example:

> Patient: I don't know how I'll be able to eliminate caffeine from my diet. That will be quite a challenge, especially if there needs to be an immediate reduction in my caffeine consumption.
>
> Physician: What do you think you'll be able to manage? Can you try to reduce your caffeine intake a little bit everyday?
>
> Patient: I can try but it won't be easy. And, you don't just mean reducing coffee drinking, do you? You also mean reducing the amount of chocolate I consume. I think I'm going to be pretty grumpy over the next while, perhaps you should warn my partner.
>
> Physician: Is there anything you can think of that I might be able to do to help you?
>
> Patient: Tell me again exactly why this is necessary. Also, is there anything else I should be doing to help my medical condition?

Do you think this scenario characterizes a typical interaction between a physician and patient? Or, does the patient in this scenario seem unusually assertive? According to some researchers, assertiveness and active involvement on the part of the patient are the precursors of an effective partnership with the physician. The mutual-participation model is seen as the ideal relationship between physician and patient. However, the typical physician-patient relationship is viewed as one in which the physician possesses a greater degree of power than the patient.

Power is an issue that we will return to later in the chapter. For now, let's continue with our discussion of physician-patient relationship models. Szasz and Hollender (1956) were the first to provide a theoretical model of the physician-patient relationship; however, they were not the last. Other models have been put forth over the years (e.g., Emanuel & Emanuel, 1992), but until recently none have used empirical techniques to determine whether patterns of interaction style in the physician-patient relationship correspond to the theoretical approaches found in the literature.

Roter and colleagues (1997) used audiotape analysis to describe communication patterns in 537 patients seen at 11 outpatient, private, and group primary care settings in the U.S. and Canada. Their analysis revealed five distinct communication patterns. The first, **narrowly biomedical** communication patterns, were characterized mainly by biomedical talk (e.g., "The medication may make you sleepy"), closed-ended medical questions (e.g., "Are you in pain when you walk?"), and very little discussion of psychosocial topics (such as problems of daily living, issues regarding social relations, feelings, and emotions). The narrowly biomedical pattern occurred in 32 percent of the visits. The second pattern was described as **expanded biomedical**. This pattern also includes numerous closed-ended medical questions but has more moderate levels of biomedical and psychosocial exchange for both physicians and patients. This pattern was common to 33 percent of the visits. The third pattern, **biopsychosocial**, reflects a balance of psychosocial and biomedical topics. The biopsychosocial pattern occurs in 20 percent of visits. The **psychosocial** pattern was the fourth pattern identified by Roter and her colleagues. This pattern includes substantially more psychosocial exchanges than the previous patterns. An example of such an exchange is, "It is important to get out and do something on a regular basis. The recreation centre is a great place to find the company of other seniors." Eight percent of visits are considered psychosocial. The final pattern was coined **consumerist**. This pattern of communication also represented eight percent of visits. The consumerist pattern suggests the use of the physician as a consultant who answers questions rather than one who asks them.

It is somewhat difficult to compare the model proposed by Roter and colleagues (1997) with that proposed by Szasz and Hollender (1956) because of the different terminology that is used in describing the models. However, it is clear that both models are placed on a continuum where, at one end, the patient has little involvement in the decision-making process or in contributions to the interaction and at the other end is at least on par with the physician in guiding the interaction. Szasz and Hollender stated that the mutual-participation model was "essentially foreign to medicine." Now, more than 40 years have elapsed and this statement no longer seems to be true. Roter and colleagues' study suggests that while collaborative models do not predominate, they are certainly evident in primary care practice.

Is the collaborative model the most preferred model of physician-patient interaction? According to patients in Roter and colleagues' (1997) study, the collaborative model, or in Roter's terminology the "psychosocial pattern", is preferred, at least by patients. Somewhat surprisingly, physicians were especially satisfied with the consumerist pattern, reporting that these visits made good use of their time. Patients were moderately pleased with these interactions, though they didn't receive the highest patient satisfaction ratings. Inasmuch as the patients who engaged in this pattern of communication were younger than others, there may be a cohort effect, suggesting that younger generations of patients will be "consumerist" in their relationships with physicians. In Roter and colleagues' study, the consumerist pattern only occurred in a small proportion of visits. We might speculate that this pattern will increase as younger cohorts get older and develop more chronic conditions and therefore become more frequent users of health services. The patterns least preferred by both patients and physicians were the biomedical patterns. Biomedical patterns of communication were used most often by younger, male physicians and by those physicians interacting with patients who were more sick, were older, and had a lower income.

Physician-Patient Communication

Information-Giving

People differ in how much they would like to participate in their medical care, for example, by making decisions about their treatment. To participate in these decisions, patients need information. Physicians provide information to their patients about a number of things, including the patient's diagnosis, possible causes of the problem, and methods of treatment. Information-giving is a very important element of the physician-patient interview, and it has been stated that, "Patients tend to be more dissatisfied about the information that they receive from their physicians than about any other aspect of medical care" (Waitzkin, 1985, p. 83). Yet, when questioned about the amount of time they believed they spent giving information to their patients, physicians drastically overestimated the amount of time they were engaged in this task. Specifically, in an average 20-minute interview physicians predicted that they spent approximately 9 minutes giving information to their patients. In reality, the physicians spent an average of 1 minute giving information to their patients.

Waitzkin (1984; 1985) has asked physicians to rate each patient's desire for information and the helpfulness of giving information. Completing a questionnaire based on the same scale, patients rated their desire for information and the benefits of this information. Patients reported wanting to know almost everything and felt that this information would be extremely beneficial. Physicians, on the other hand, underestimated the patients' desire for information 65 percent of the time, and only 6 percent of the time did they overestimate their particular patient's desire for information. Physicians also reported a much lower belief in the benefits that this information would have for patients.

Faden and colleagues (1981) examined the attitudes of neurologists and their epileptic patients regarding the issue of disclosure of information. They found that patients preferred to receive detailed disclosure of almost all risks associated with medication, even those that were quite rare. Physicians, however, said they were likely to disclose only those risks with a high probability of occurrence. Physicians felt that disclosure of information about drugs would decrease compliance. In contrast, the patients felt that disclosure would improve their compliance.

A number of studies have demonstrated that physicians sometimes choose to withhold information from their patients in an attempt to protect their patients from worry. For example, family doctors who had made a diagnosis of Parkinson's disease, a degenerative nerve disorder, were very concerned about protecting their patients (Pinder, 1990). Specifically, the physicians had difficulty deciding how, when, and whom to tell and deciding just how much information to share about the patient's diagnosis and prognosis. The physicians tended to be positive and overly optimistic. For instance, they avoided detail about medications, were low-key about side effects, and did not explore the problems of longterm use of anti-Parkinsonian medication. On the other hand, most patients wanted to be given as much information as possible, including information about their medication and its side effects.

Participation

Although the vast majority of patients would like to be informed about what their illnesses are and how to treat them, some want more details about the illnesses, self-administration of treatment, and involvement in decisions than others do (Krantz, Baum, & Wideman, 1980). Elderly patients, more often than young adult patients, prefer that the health profession make health-related decisions for them (e.g., Woodward & Wallston, 1987). Knowing patient preferences is invaluable. It appears that providing the amount and type of participation patients want in their health care enhances the patient's adjustment to and satisfaction with medical treatment (Auerbach, Martelli, & Mercuri, 1983; Martelli, Auerbach, Alexander, & Mercuri, 1987). Moreover, patients who report a preference for assuming an active role in their treatment tend to recover faster than those who prefer an inactive role (Brody et al., 1989; Mahler & Kulik, 1991).

Patients differ in the amount of participation they want regarding their health, just as health professionals differ in the involvement they are likely to bestow. As we might predict, some physicians are more inclined than others to share their authority and decision-making, even among their colleagues (Eisenberg, Kitz, & Webber, 1983). It is interesting to note that patients seeing physicians of their own race rate their physicians' decision-making style as more participatory than when the race of the participants is not the same (Cooper-Patrick et al., 1999). What happens in the physician-patient relationship when the patient prefers a different level of participation from the physician than that which the physician is willing to give? A large-scale survey conducted by Marie Haug and Bebe Lavin (1981) asked both patients and physicians to describe their own attitudes and behaviour pertinent to the participation of patients in health care. Information obtained from the respondents led to three conclusions. First, although both the patients and the physicians expressed the opinion that patients should participate in activities and decisions regarding their health, neither behaved accordingly very often. Second, when the patient wants a high level of involvement but the physician wants to take complete responsibility, conflict can be expected. In this situation, the patient either finds, or is told to find, another physician. Third, when a patient prefers that the physician takes full responsibility but the physician expects the person to participate, both may feel uncomfortable. In this situation, the physician may assume responsibility or the patient may switch to a physician who will take more control.

Together, this research indicates that a mismatch between the patient's and the physician's ideas regarding participation can be detrimental to their relationship. Further, as we will discuss in more detail in the next chapter, mismatches of this type will frequently result in an increase in stress experienced by patients during medical procedures (Miller & Mangan, 1983). When determining how much information and involvement to provide each patient, health professionals clearly need to consider the needs of the patient (Kindelan & Kent, 1987).

General Patient Satisfaction

Considering the needs of the patient is certainly an important component of a physician's role. In the introduction to this chapter, we stated that most people can recall both positive and negative experiences they have had with physicians. When people talk about their negative experiences, they often cite the physician's hurried manner, insensitivity, lack of responsiveness, apparently faulty diagnoses, or useless treatment. However, most people can also provide details of an interaction with a physician that was exemplary. Patients praise physicians who take their time and answer all their questions. In fact, most of the positive attributes patients recount include personal factors about the physician. Patients show a strong preference for practitioners who have a warm and expressive emotional style as compared with those who remain emotionally neutral (e.g., Thomas, 1987; DiMatteo, Linn, Chang, & Cope, 1985).

Patient satisfaction with medical care is primarily a function of the quality of the physician-patient relationship. A particularly important consequence of this is that patients often judge the competence of a physician by their emotional satisfaction with care as well as by the degree of confidence their physician demonstrates (Ben-Sira, 1976; Ben-Sira, 1980; Johnson, Levenkron, Suchman, & Manchester, 1988). For example, a warm, confident, friendly practitioner is often judged to be both nice and competent, whereas a cool, aloof practitioner will likely be judged less favourably and thought of as both unfriendly and incompetent (Buller & Buller, 1987; DiMatteo, 1979; DiMatteo et al., 1985). The result is that when patients are satisfied with the emotional aspects of their care, they are more likely to want to return to that physician and are more likely to keep future appointments (DiMatteo,

Hays, & Prince, 1986; Ross & Duff, 1982). When the patients are dissatisfied with the emotional aspects of their care, they are more likely to "doctor shop", going from one physician to another until they find one that suits them. In reality, technical quality of care and the manner in which it is delivered are unrelated (e.g., Gough, 1967). In Canada, most complaints by the public about physicians deal not with clinical competency problems but with communication problems (Simpson et al., 1991; Richards, 1990).

Patient Satisfaction, Communication, and Malpractice Claims

Patient dissatisfaction and poor communication between patients and physicians may lead patients to file malpractice suits against their physicians (Levinson, 1994). Malpractice suits do occur in Canada with some frequency. In 1997, 1 399 malpractice suits were launched (in the same year, 108 trials took place). The connection between poor communication and complaints is evident in the Complaints Committee's reports of the College of Physicians and Surgeons of Ontario (CPSO). In 1978, the Committee stated, "Inadequate communications between MDs and patients or patients' families is still the underlying cause for most of the problems that the CPSO is asked to investigate" (cited in Stewart et al., 1999, p. 25). These concerns were reiterated in both the 1995 and 1996 Annual Reports of the Complaints Committee (CPSO, 1995; CPSO, 1996).

As we have already mentioned, patients have preferences and expectations about their interactions with physicians. The physician's awareness of the patient's expectations during a visit are critical in achieving effective communication. And, only with effective communication are patients likely to be satisfied with their medical care (Williams, Weinman, Dale, & Newman, 1995; Stewart et al., 1999). A number of studies have revealed an association between poor communication and malpractice claims (Hickson et al., 1992; Hickson et al., 1994; Vincent, Young, & Phillips, 1994). The most frequently identified communication problems were inadequate explanation of diagnosis or treatment and patients feeling ignored. However, physicians misleading patients, not understanding patient and family perspectives, devaluing patient and family views, as well as patients feeling rushed or deserted were also linked to malpractice claims. Although the combination of a bad outcome and patient dissatisfaction is said to be "a recipe for litigation", when patients and their families feel the physician was caring and compassionate malpractice suits happen less frequently (Levinson, 1994).

A study conducted by Levinson and colleagues (1997) took a somewhat different approach than previous research to identify specific communication behaviours associated with malpractice claims. Physicians and surgeons were randomly selected from the data bases of companies providing malpractice insurance in Oregon and Colorado. Ten routine office visits were audiotaped for each of the 124 participants. Analysis of the conversations revealed significant differences in communication behaviours between physicians who had and those who had not been subjected to malpractice claims. "No-claims" primary care physicians gave more orienting statements about the flow of a visit (e.g., "First I will examine you, and then we will talk about your condition"), laughed and used more humour, used more facilitating comments (e.g., asking opinion and checking understanding), encouraged their patients to talk, and spent more time with their patients (18.3 vs. 15 minutes). Roughly half of the physicians were primary care physicians and the other half surgeons. Levinson and his colleagues found no behaviours to distinguish between claims and no-claims surgeons.

Undoubtedly, there is a link between communication, patient satisfaction, and malpractice claims. Although researchers have documented a number of components of poor communication possibly responsible for this link, further research is required to explain some of the anomalies (e.g., between physicians and surgeons). While studies investigating the link between communication problems and malpractice claims began relatively recently, research exploring more general communication problems during the physician-patient consultation began decades ago. Let's now turn our attention to some of this more general research.

Physician Behaviours Contributing to Faulty Communication

Having exchanged introductions and established initial rapport, the next step is to determine what issues the patient wishes to discuss. What is their agenda for the consultation? Why have they come today? These are questions that cannot be addressed unless the practitioner listens to the patient. In a landmark study (Beckman & Frankel, 1984), physicians were found to interrupt their patients after only 18 seconds! In recent years, this behaviour has improved only slightly; now patients are given 23 seconds to speak before they are interrupted (Marvel, Epstein, Flowers, & Beckman, 1999).

Research (Beckman & Frankel, 1984; Marvel, Epstein, Flowers, & Beckman, 1999) clearly demonstrates that even minimal interruptions to patients' initial statements can actually prevent other concerns from being mentioned at all or can make important complaints arise late in the consultation. By asking patients to provide further comment on any one problem, patient options are restricted and they are prevented from expanding on other information. The patient is in fact faced with a practical problem when the physician interrupts. For example, the patient may have mentioned headaches but is interrupted before he or she can mention having experienced recent palpitations and marital problems. "Tell me more about your headaches" or, worse, "Where do you get the pain?" restricts the discussion to the headaches and limits both the patient's options and the efficiency of the interview as a whole.

Allowing the patient to complete their opening statement without interruption should not be a difficult task for practitioners, as patients usually take less than 60 seconds to do this. In Beckman and Frankel's (1984) research, not a single patient took longer than 150 seconds to complete their opening statement, even when encouraged to continue. Yet, only 28 percent of the time are patients given the opportunity to finish their explanation of concerns (Marvel, Epstein, Flowers, & Beckman, 1999). When patients are interrupted, they are afforded the opportunity to return to, and complete, their opening statement only two percent of the time (Frankel & Beckman, 1989).

Physicians seem to assume that the first complaint the patient mentions is the only one the patient has. However, patients express three concerns per office visit on average (Kaplan et al., 1995; Stewart et al., 1986). Further, the serial order in which patients present their problems is not related to their clinical importance; the first concern presented is no more likely than the second or third to be the most important, as judged by either the patient or the physician (Beckman & Frankel, 1984).

To make matters worse, it is also true that patients and physicians do not always agree on the nature of the patient's chief complaint (Starfield et al., 1981; Burack & Carpenter, 1983). If you remember Lynn from the beginning of this chapter, you will recall that her major complaint was not addressed by her physician. Lynn's primary reason for visiting her physician was to determine what was causing her stomach problems. However, this is not the first symptom that Lynn described to her physician, because she also had some other concerns. Lynn left the physician's office still wondering what was responsible for her stomach ache. Stewart, McWhinney, and Buck (1979) discovered that 54 percent of patients' complaints were not elicited during the medical interview. Similarly, Maguire and Rutter (1976) found that few senior medical students managed to discover the patient's main problem during the medical interview. These findings are shocking and have led researchers to devise interview methods that improve communication during the physician-patient interview (e.g., Silverman, Kurtz, & Draper, 1998).

BOX 6-1 **Do You Know What these Medical Terms Mean?**

The following 10 medical terms were used in Thompson and Pledger's (1993) study of patients' understanding of medical jargon. Match the terms with the definitions given below:

1. ______malignant	6. ______benign
2. ______incubation	7. ______chronic
3. ______acute	8. ______cyst
4. ______abscess	9. ______suture
5. ______diuretic	10. ______edema

A. A localized collection of pus in a cavity formed by the disintegration of tissue.
B. The accumulation of excess fluid in a fluid compartment.
C. Persisting for a long time.
D. The provision of proper conditions for growth and development.
E. Having severe symptoms and a short course.
F. Not recurrent: favourable for recovery with appropriate treatment.
G. An agent that promotes urine secretion.
H. A closed sac or capsule containing liquid or a semisolid substance.
I. A joining together of separated tissue or bone, or material used to achieve this joining.
J. Any condition that, if uncorrected, tends to worsen so as to cause serious illness or death, e.g., cancer.

The answers are provided below. Did you obtain a perfect score? If you had been asked to define each of the terms rather than simply fill in the blanks with the provided answers, do you think you would have scored as well?

1-J, 2-D, 3-E, 4-A, 5-G, 6-F, 7-C, 8-H, 9-I, 10-B

Medical Jargon

Another contributing factor to poor communication in the physician-patient interview is the physician's use of **medical jargon** and technical language. For example, the term *splenomegaly* conveys a considerable amount of information to health professionals. Splenomegaly describes an enlargement of the spleen, which is a large gland-like organ situated in the upper left side of the abdomen that breaks down red corpuscles. But splenomegaly means more than just spleen enlargement. The term splenomegaly is applied to a condition marked by hypertrophy (enlargement) of the spleen with progressive anemia (reduction below normal in the hemoglobin, the volume of packed red blood cells) and no evidence of leukemia or disease of the lymph glands (DiMatteo, 1991). Of course, once the patient asks the physician for the meaning of splenomegaly, he or she is likely to need the physician to explain the explanation! Test your knowledge of common medical terms by attempting the quiz in Box 6.1.

A classic study (Korsch, Gozzi, & Francis, 1968) revealed that more than half of mothers reported being confused by the terms pediatricians used during a consultation that had just taken place. Why do physicians use medical jargon when talking to patients? There are a number of reasons.

One reason physicians use medical jargon is because they tend to overestimate the amount their patients can understand. A number of studies have tested patient knowledge of medical terminology (McKinlay, 1975; Samora, Saunders, & Larson, 1961; Thompson & Pledger, 1993) In a typical study, physicians and nurses make lists of medical words that they believe patients understand. When these same words are presented to patients, surprisingly few can define the terms accurately. For example, in the study conducted by Thompson and Pledger (1993) less than half of the patients could define the words abscess, tumour, diuretic, or cyst adequately. Moreover, even simple, everyday words in a medical context can be ambiguous (Hadlow & Pitts, 1991). For example, Mazzullo, Lasagna, and Griner, (1974) showed that 52 percent of people thought that a medication prescribed "for fluid retention" would cause fluid retention.

Another reason practitioners use medical jargon when speaking to patients is because patients may interpret the sophisticated vocabulary of the physician to represent intelligence on the part of the physician. Perhaps they feel that they will be better "taken care" of by a physician who is obviously competent.

A somewhat more cynical view as to the reason for the use of medical jargon was provided by the famous heart surgeon Dr. Michael DeBakey: "Most doctors don't want their patients to understand them! They prefer to keep their work a mystery. If patients don't understand what a doctor is talking about, they won't ask him questions. Then the doctor won't have to be bothered answering them" (Robinson, 1973). Another famous physician, Howard Waitzkin (1985), explained, with great amusement, that if you wanted to forestall any additional questions from the patient you could simply connect the term "itis" (meaning "inflammation of") to whatever organ was troubled (for example, "stomachitis").

More commonly, however, health professionals may use medical jargon with their patients because they simply forget that their patients do not share the same medical vocabulary. Quite simply, practitioners have spent a number of years in medical school learning this vocabulary, they use it when speaking with their colleagues, and they naturally use the same vocabulary with their patients.

On the other hand, if health providers are aware that patients may not understand medical jargon they may go to the opposite extreme and engage in baby talk and simplistic explanations. One example (Toynbee, 1977) of baby talk comes from a surgeon who said to an elderly man, "We're just going to pop you into the operating theater to have a little peep into your tummy." Toynbee noticed that the term "pop" was used quite frequently in the hospital by many of the hospital staff. Another physician said, "Nurse, would you just pop off her things for me? I want to examine her." Nurses also had people "popping" in many places. Patients were popped in and out of washrooms and wheel-chairs, into and out of hospital gowns, beds, and bandages (Toynbee, 1977).

To remedy difficulties arising from the use of medical jargon and baby talk, practitioners should engage in **non-discrepant responses** or provide **multilevel explanations** when speaking to their patients (Waitzkin, 1985). Providing a non-discrepant response involves the health professional responding to the patient using the same sophistication of vocabulary that the patient used when asking his or her question. For example, if a patient asks about her "lump" , the physician might reply by saying we have to remove part of the lump to determine if there is cancer in it. When the practitioner provides a multilevel explanation, he or she uses medical jargon in the explanation but follows this by explaining the medical jargon using everyday language. Using multilevel explanations educates the patient in medical terminology. "We'll have to conduct a biopsy to determine if the tumour is malignant. In other words, we'll have to remove the lump to determine if there is cancer in it." Let us conclude by saying that the use of medical jargon by health professionals is appropriate if it is explained to the patient or if the patient is already familiar with the terminology.

Time Factors

Another factor thought to limit a physician's ability to communicate effectively is the time available for the consultation (Roland et al., 1986). In our discussion of communication issues linked to malpractice claims, we mentioned that if patients felt rushed they were more likely to file a suit. Stewart and colleagues (1999) reviewed the literature pertaining to communication and time and maintained that, "The literature is not clear on this subject perhaps because communication is defined and measured in many different ways" (p. 26). Two themes exist in the literature: first, that communication style (positive/negative) was not affected by the length of the consultation; and second, that the length of time available affected the nature of the discussion. Let's explore each of these themes in more detail.

A number of studies indicate that a longer consultation is not required to communicate effectively with patients. Arborelius and Bremberg (1992) reported that positive consultations took less time than negative consultations. In this study, a positive consultation was defined as one where both physician and patient had a positive impression of the consultation; whereas a negative consultation was one where both parties had a negative impression of the consultation. Further, during positive consultations, more time was devoted to patient ideas and concerns. Another study (Greenfield et al., 1988) evaluated an intervention to improve information-seeking skills of the patient. The total volume of the conversation between experimental group patients and their physicians was greater than in control group patients, yet there was no corresponding change in the length of the visit. What occurred by introducing this intervention was a more active interchange, but not a longer visit. Henbest and Fehrsen (1992) reported that consultations that were the most **patient-centred** did not take longer than those that were less patient-centred. Patient-centred approaches tend to include more open-ended questions by the physician, such as, "Can you describe when the pain is most severe?" compared to **doctor-centred** approaches in which physicians tend to ask questions that require only very brief answers. Referring back to Roter's (1997) classification of physician-patient relationships, we would say that patient-centred approaches most closely resemble psychosocial patterns of communication, whereas doctor-centred approaches are more similar to biomedical patterns. You may remember that patients tended to prefer the psychosocial pattern and that both patients and physicians liked the biomedical pattern the least. Another study (Clark et al., 1998) found that physicians who were educated about communication issues were rated more favourably by their patients' parents than physicians who did not take part in the education program. This occurred even though, on average, the physician reported spending less time with them. A trend toward lower patient satisfaction with longer visits has also been shown in other studies (e.g., Hornberger, Thorn, & MacCurdy, 1997).

In contrast, the results of some studies indicate a more thorough communication requires longer consultations. Some studies (Hornberger et al., 1997; Marvel, 1993) concluded that there is a tradeoff between increasing the length of the consultation, the goals of the physician, the goals of the patient, and the many and varied issues professional organizations counselling physicians deem as important. Howie, Porter, Heaney, and Hopton (1999) surveyed patients at the end of the consultation with their physician and reported that patients were more satisfied on a number of dimensions after a long consultation than a short one. A more favourable response was provided for 17 of 33 questions (e.g., "Did the doctor give you a chance to say what was really on your mind?") when the patient had participated in a longer consultation with their physician.

Patient volume has also been related to the length of consultation and patient satisfaction (Zyzanski, Strange, Langa, & Flocke, 1998). Patients visiting high-volume physicians were less satisfied with their interaction than those patients visiting moderate- or low-volume physicians. The patients of high-volume physicians reported less follow-up on patient problems, less attention to patient responses, and felt they were provided with less adequate explanations.

Other factors have been mentioned in the literature as leading to difficulty in physician-patient communication. Certain topics were described by physicians as being more difficult to discuss, such as alcohol use (Arborelius & Thakker, 1995), stress (Russell & Roter, 1993), and communications related to particular parts of the anatomy (Larsson, Johanson, & Svardsudd, 1994). Also, some patient characteristics were reported as causing communication difficulties. These characteristics include the socioeconomic status (Bain, 1979) and age of the patient. In particular, physicians had more problems communicating with teenagers (Jacobson, Wilkinson, & Owen, 1994) and the elderly (Pereles & Russell, 1996). These communication difficulties may affect the length of the consultation.

Patient Behaviours Contributing to Faulty Communication

Lack of Information-Seeking Behaviours. Given patients' desire for information from their physicians, we would expect that they might request additional information during the medical interview. However, patients do not engage in many information-seeking behaviours when communicating with their physicians (Beisecker & Beisecker, 1990). Svarstad (1974) discovered that when patients did not understand some of the terms used by their physicians, only 15 percent of the time did they admit this to their physicians. In a study conducted by Tuckett, Boulton, and Olson (1985, cited in Silverman, Kurtz, & Draper, 1998),

76 percent of the patients said that they had specific doubts or questions during the interview that they did not mention to the physician. When asked why they did not ask the physician questions, patients gave the following reasons: (1) it was not up to them to ask questions, express doubts, or behave as if their view was important (36%); (2) they were afraid of being less well thought of by the doctor (22%); (3) they were frightened of a negative reaction from the doctor (14%); (4) they were too flustered or hurried to ask coherently (27%); (5) they doubted that the doctor could tell them any more at the moment (22%); (6) they forgot or were waiting until next time to ask, when they would be more certain of what they thought was reasonable to ask (36%); and (6) they feared the truth (9%).

Many patients are reluctant to ask questions. In the following real-life example, you can see how it would be beneficial to ask for an explanation of terminology. The day after a mother had given birth to her baby, the nurse entered the mother's room and asked her if she would like to have her child circumcised. Not knowing what the term "circumcised" referred to but not wanting to ask, the mother readily agreed. After all, the mother thought, if the nurse is asking if I want this for my child she must think it will be beneficial. The mother replied, "Yes", she would like her child circumcised. A short while later, the nurse returned with a bewildered expression on her face and exclaimed, "You've got a girl!" (In case you weren't sure, a circumcision is a surgical procedure sometimes performed on baby boys or young boys to remove the foreskin from the penis.)

There are many instances when the patient attempts to understand medical jargon on their own, with varying degrees of success. You may indeed get some very strange answers to the question, "What was your diagnosis?" The following diagnoses are all very serious, but the patient's terminology might bring a smile to your lips.

The incorrect names that patients settle on may be simple, meaningless sound-alikes, but they might tell us more about how the patients view their medical problems. For example, the patient with sickle cell (sick-as-hell) anemia likely does feel extremely ill. The patient who claims the ophthalmologist saw "Cadillacs" (cataracts) in his eyes probably assumes the doctor's income to be quite high. The patient who reports she has been referred to a "groinocologist" (gynecologist) has chosen an anatomical reference to aid her understanding (DiMatteo, 1991).

Remembering. Sometimes the patient does not understand all the information the health care practitioner has provided. At times, this may be due to the patient not understanding the medical terminology. However, even when the patient understands all the terminology, he or she may not remember everything the health care practitioner stated. In a review of the literature, Ley (1988) notes that in the hospital setting patients remember approximately 60 percent of the information they are told. When Tucket and colleagues (1985) looked more closely at the information patients recalled, they found that only 10 percent of patients could not remember all of the key points they had been told. That is, most patients could remember the gist of what they heard even if they could not remember all of the little details.

Patient anxiety contributes to patients' inability to remember information from a medical interview. Specifically, when people are anxious they find it difficult to concentrate and process incoming information. Again, this is true even when patients understand the information that they are being told. The following is a description provided by one physician about her experience when she was told she had cancer. She said that even though she knew exactly what her physician was telling her, as soon as she got the "news" , she phased out. She began thinking about what this would mean in terms of all the adjustments she would have to make in her life, whether she would survive, etc., and in doing so she didn't hear another word her physician said to her.

Many factors accounting for poor communication between physicians and patients are correlated with patient adherence to treatment regimens. In the words of Moira Stewart and her colleagues at the University of Western Ontario, "Patient-doctor communication and patient adherence are inexorably linked because the interaction provides the context within which the recommendations to be complied with are delivered" (1999, p. 27). Let's take a closer look at the topic of adhering to medical advice.

ADHERING TO MEDICAL ADVICE

Traditionally, medical professionals have used the term **compliance** to refer to the degree to which patients carry out the behaviours and treatments that physicians and other health professionals recommend. But because the term compliance is interpreted as reluctant obedience, many health professionals prefer the term **adherence** (although some use the terms interchangeably). What does it mean to adhere to medical advice? Although we may immediately respond to this question by saying that to be adherent we take medication as a physician has prescribed, adherence is much more than that. To adhere to the advice of a health professional, we may be maintaining healthy lifestyle practices, such as eating properly, avoiding stressful situations, getting enough sleep and exercise, abstaining from smoking, limiting our intake of alcohol, as well as carrying out other behaviours that promote good health. If we do not follow the advice of our health professional, we are said to be **non-adherent**.

How prevalent is the problem of non-adherence? This question is actually more difficult to answer then one might first assume (Turk & Meichenbaum, 1991). For instance, failure to adhere may occur for any of the different types of medical advice just outlined (e.g., abstaining from smoking or taking medication as prescribed). People can violate each of these types of advice in many different ways. That is, patients may fail to take their medication as prescribed. However, this may mean that the patient might take medication in the wrong amount, at the wrong time, or discontinue the medication before the prescribed recommendation was complete.

Creative non-adherence is a particularly interesting form of non-adherence (Weintraub, 1976). This kind of adherence is intentional and involves modifying or supplementing the recommended treatment regimen. These alterations are often based on private theories about a health problem and its treatment. For example, the patient may decide that particular symptoms meriting treatment were ignored by the health professional; he or she may then augment the treatment regimen, perhaps including over-the-counter medications or home remedies that interact with prescribed medication in unpredictable, even dangerous ways (Kaplan, 1990). Sometimes, however, these modifications are useful. For example, some patients are thought to have a better idea of how to control their blood glucose level than their health care provider does. Similarly, parents who adjust their child's asthma regimen can control asthma better than if they precisely follow a prescribed regimen. The reason for this is that there are often fluctuations in the severity of asthma (e.g., seasonal variability) and the parents can adjust the treatment in response to their child's needs.

Assessing Adherence

To determine how prevalent the problem of non-adherence is, we must be able to assess it. There are at least five methods researchers can use to measure patient adherence: (1) ask the health professional; (2) ask the patient; (3) ask other people; (4) count pills; and (5) examine biochemical evidence (DiMatteo & DiNicola, 1982; Turk & Meichenbaum, 1991). One of the easiest methods of measuring adherence is to ask the health professional who works with the patient to estimate it. Generally, though, health professionals overestimate their patients' adherence and are also poor at estimating which patients adhere better than others. Often, the accuracy of the estimates provided by health professionals is only slightly better than chance (Blackwell, 1997). Another simple approach to measuring adherence is to ask the patient. However, patients also tend to overestimate their adherence, perhaps because they know they should follow "doctor's orders." Asking either health professionals or patients to report adherence is a very subjective process and may be biased by lying and wishful thinking. The same bias may result when family members are asked to monitor the patient.

More objective measures of patient adherence include pill counting and biochemical tests. Pill or quantity accounting involves counting the remaining medication in the dispenser. This amount is compared to the amount that should remain at this point in the treatment regimen to determine if the patient has been following directions. However, even if the right quantity of medication is found, the patient may not have been compliant. We would not know if the patient took the medication at the right times, in the correct amount, or if, wanting to please the health professional, they simply discarded some of the medication. Some researchers (e.g., Cramer et al., 1989) have instilled microprocessors in the lids of pill containers so that a record can be made of when the pill bottle was opened. Biochemical tests can be conducted, for example, on the patient's blood or urine to determine if the patient has ingested recently. This method of assessment is both time consuming and expensive. In addition, there are problems with this technique resulting from individual differences in absorption and metabolism of drugs. We should also point out that biochemical tests do not measure the degree of adherence; the presence of a drug simply identifies that the patient ingested some amount of the drug at some time. It does not indicate that the patient took the proper amount at the proper time.

Frequency and Cost of Non-Adherence

Despite the difficulties in assessing adherence, we can attempt to assess the prevalence of non-adherence. In general, the rate of non-compliance with medical or health advice is approximately 50 percent (e.g., Haynes, McKibbon, & Kanani, 1996). Robin DiMatteo (1994) reported that at least 38 percent of patients do not follow short-term treatment plans (e.g., completing a prescription for medication), and as many as 43 percent do not adhere to recommendations for longterm treatment (e.g., taking hypertensive medication). Moreover, over 75 percent of patients are unwilling or unable to follow suggested lifestyle changes such as exercising regularly or eating a low-fat diet. It is interesting to note that health professionals have many of the same problems with adherence as patients do (O'Brien, 1977).

The cost of non-adherence is considerable. A report prepared for the Pharmaceutical Manufacturers Association of Canada (Coambs et al., 1995) estimated that non-adherence costs Canadians between seven and nine billion dollars a year. We should point out that this study incorporated a very narrow definition of non-adherence: failing to adhere to physicians' instructions regarding the self-administration of medication. The dollar figure cited above includes both direct and indirect costs associated with medication non-adherence. The direct costs resulted from excessive hospital expenditure (e.g., people admitted to hospital due to non-adherence of prescription medications), excessive nursing home expenditures (medication non-adherence is the single most important reason for residence of elderly patients in nursing homes), and excessive treatment costs of ambulatory care (e.g., additional visits to a physician). The indirect costs were attributed to reduction in worker productivity due to sick days taken, less efficient work due to illness, and costs associated with premature death.

As you can see, non-adherence occurs frequently. The monetary costs of non-adherence are enormous. Perhaps more important, the personal costs due to non-adherence are also immense. If you believe that non-adherence results in people becoming sick or even dying, you are quite right. Ordinarily, we might assume that people act in a way that serves their own best interests. However, the frequency of non-adherence suggests that this is not true. Why, then, do people fail to adhere to medical recommendations? Although researchers are not completely sure how to answer this question, they have discovered a number of factors that are linked to non-adherence. These factors are outlined in the next section.

What Factors Predict Adherence?

Characteristics of the Treatment Regimen

Some medical recommendations require patients to change *longstanding habits*. For example, a physician may suggest that a patient go on a restricted diet, stop smoking cigarettes, begin a program of regular exercise, or avoid stressful situations. These changes can be thought of as lifestyle changes. Certainly, some patients will adhere to these recommendations, particularly if they are at a high risk for serious illness (Pederson, 1982). It is more likely, though, that people will not make these lifestyle changes (e.g., Turk & Meichenbaum, 1991).

Complexity of the regimen prescribed also plays a role in non-adherence. When you are told, "Take one of these pills after meals, one of these other pills every eight hours, two of these pills at bedtime, and these pills as needed" you will likely have some difficulty following the "doctor's orders." As you might predict, the greater the variety of medications one must take, the more complex the schedule, the more likely people are to make an error, thereby failing to adhere to the medical regimen (Haynes, 1976; Cramer et al., 1989).

Surprisingly, little evidence exists that unpleasant *side effects* lead to non-adherence. Although intuitively we would assume if someone didn't like a treatment he or she would discontinue it, this does not appear to be the case. Instead, it appears that most people who engage in non-adherence do not consider side effects to be a very important factor (Masur, 1981).

As mentioned previously, the longer the *duration* of the treatment the less likely people are to adhere to it. Haynes (1976) described several studies comparing adherence rates to the length of treatment and concluded that in most cases, non-adherence increases as duration of therapy increases. We should point out, however, that most longterm treatment programs are for illnesses that have no visible symptoms, such as hypertension. Understandably, people are less motivated to adhere to a treatment if there are no apparent symptoms to indicate they are unwell.

As mentioned above, people are less likely to adhere to medical recommendations if they do not perceive symptoms of illness. It follows, then, that *severity of an illness* will not lead to adherence unless symptoms are noted by the patient (Haynes, 1976). The more obvious a symptom is, the more likely people are to adhere to treatment. Perhaps this is one of the reasons why a person's experience of pain predicts adherence (Becker, 1979).

Personal Characteristics of the Patient

The association between adherence and age is very complex. Adherence can either increase or decrease with age, depending on the specific illness, the timeframe, and the treatment regimen prescribed. Some research has revealed a curvilinear relationship between age and adherence. In a large-scale, longitudinal study (Thomas et al., 1995) investigating colorectal cancer screening, those who adhered best were approximately 70 years old; the worst adherers were younger than 50 years of age or older than 80. Another study (Park et al., 1999) found a surprising pattern of medication adherence in arthritis patients. This study found an age-related cognitive decline among participants. Yet, the older participants actually adhered to their treatment regimen better than middle-aged patients. A busy lifestyle associated with middle age was found to be more of a determinant of non-adherence than cognitive functioning.

Adherence rates are also related to the age of a child. Both cancer patients and diabetic children are more likely to adhere to treatment regimens at younger ages (e.g., until about 9 years of age) (Jonasson et al., 1999; Manne et al., 1993). These results may be explained by the increasing responsibility children assume for their medical treatment as they get older (LaGreca & Stone, 1985). It is likely that before the age of 9 years a child's medical treatment was the sole responsibility of the parent.

Researchers have found very few *gender* differences in overall adherence rates. Some differences do emerge, however, when we look at adherence to specific medical recommendations. For instance, women seem to be better than men at adhering to dietary restrictions (Laforge, Greene, & Prochaska, 1994) and taking medication for mental disorders (Sellwood & Tarrier, 1994). In contrast, there seem to be few gender differences in taking antihypertensive or diabetic medication (e.g., Monane et al., 1996). There are also few gender differences in establishing and maintaining an exercise program (Emergy, Hauck, & Blumenthal, 1992).

Cultural differences in adherence rates have also been noted. Most often when cultural differences appear, they occur when the patient is from a culture that does not believe in modern medical recommendations, preferring their own tribal healers (DiNicola & DiMatteo, 1984). A recent study (Sanderson et al., 1998) documented ethnic differences in adherence to cardiac procedures. Fewer African-Americans adhered to the treatment regimen compared to Caucasians. Interestingly, these researchers noted that compared to Caucasians, fewer African-American patients recalled physicians recommending the cardiac procedures. If procedure recommendations were recalled, no ethnic differences were found in adherence rates. This finding emphasizes the need for effective communication in the physician-patient consultation.

Physician Characteristics

As we might predict, patients' adherence improves as confidence in their physician's competence increases (Gilbar, 1989). However, you may remember that the physician who is perceived with positive attributes, such as kindness, is more likely to be perceived as competent than someone judged less favourably. It follows that people are more likely to adhere to medical recommendations if their physician is viewed as warm, caring, friendly, and interested in the welfare of patients (DiNicola & DiMatteo, 1984). When physicians exhibit a good bedside manner by making eye contact, smiling, and even joking and laughing, patient adherence improves.

Physician-Patient Interaction

Earlier in the chapter, we outlined a number of elements inherent in physician-patient communication and physician-patient relationships that influence patient adherence. For instance, if the patient does not understand the instructions (e.g., due to the use of medical jargon), does not ask questions to clarify the instructions the physician provides, or does not remember those instructions, adherence is not possible. If a physician's expectations and a patient's expectations about what role each party should play in the interaction differ, patients are less likely to follow the physician's medical recommendations. In the next section, we will see how the element of social influence in the physician-patient relationship can be used to increase a patient's medical adherence.

Improving Patient Adherence

Social Influence in the Physician-Patient Relationship

In any interaction, people influence one another. This is certainly true in the physician-patient interaction. During the physician-patient interview, the physician attempts to influence the patient, but at the same time the patient attempts to influence the physician. The ability to influence someone or shape their beliefs, attitudes, or behaviours is called "social power" (Raven, 1974; French & Raven, 1959). Social psychologist Bertram Raven (1974) has described six forms of social power: informational power, reward power, coercive power, expert power, legitimate power, and referent power. Each of these forms of social power is illustrated below with examples in which the physician, Dr. Code, attempts to influence the patient, Mr. Watson. Mr. Watson is 48 years old, overweight, and is suffering from hypertension. His treatment regimen involves adherence to a low-sodium diet, weight loss, moderate exercise, and antihypertensive medication twice a day. Currently, Mr. Watson is not following the treatment regimen proposed by Dr. Code. That is, Mr Watson has not altered his diet, he rarely exercises, and he takes his medication when, in his words, "he remembers."

Informational power is based exclusively on the content of the communication. Physicians have a large amount of knowledge that they can present in an attempt to influence the patient. In this form of social power, it is the information or the facts presented that may lead to social influence. "Mr. Watson, your cholesterol level, 235, puts you at risk for a heart attack. With your uncontrolled blood pressure, that risk is increased 500 percent," said

Dr. Code. We hope that the facts Dr. Code has presented to Mr. Watson will persuade Mr. Watson to change his beliefs and his behaviour. Mr. Watson will follow the physician's advice because he is trying to avoid a heart attack, and the facts suggest that he needs to alter his behaviour to avoid one. Thus, there is nothing about the physician that leads the patient to change his behaviour; any behaviour change is solely the result of the information that the patient has been presented with. Informational power is independent of any social factors related to the physician. The remaining forms of social power are socially dependent. That is, social influence results from something about the health care practitioner or about his or her relationship with the patient.

Reward power stems from the health care practitioner's ability to mediate rewards. Rewards can be either tangible (e.g., money, free drug samples) or intangible (e.g., approval, praise, time, availability). "Mr. Watson, I would be very pleased if you could make a commitment to take your medication as I've prescribed and to, at least, reduce the salt in your diet." In this instance, if the patient changes his behaviour and does what the physician has advised he has done so because he wants his physician to think highly of him. The patient is attempting to attain the reward, in this case praise. Although the patient may also report other factors he believes are responsible for his behaviour change, a primary factor responsible for the behaviour change is the reward.

Coercive power stems from the health care practitioner's ability to mediate punishment for failure to comply. Although punishments can take the form of a physical threat in some interactions, or the threat of a monetary fine in others, in the practitioner-patient relationship the punishment is limited to the practitioner withholding praise or services. "Mr. Watson, if you can't follow the treatment plan I've suggested, I'm afraid I won't be able to treat you anymore."

Expert power stems from the patient's belief that the health care practitioner has knowledge and skill pertaining to health matters. "That's right Mr. Watson, there is a lot of research looking at how one can reduce the risk of heart attacks by lowering blood pressure. The researchers all agree that the best course of action is for the patient to lose weight, if they are overweight, and to take medication to reduce high blood pressure. That is what you need to do. If you can fit exercise into your schedule you should do that as well. I'm very familiar with this research, you really need to trust me on this one."

Legitimate power stems from the patient's belief that a health care practitioner can make medical demands of him or her. Obviously, we expect those demands to be in the best interest of the patient. While such power is ultimately backed up by coercive power, if the patient has respect for the physician no coercion is necessary. "Mr. Watson, as your physician, I suggest you follow the treatment plan I have outlined for you."

Referent power stems from the patient's desire to identify with a particular person or group. The person or group the patient desires to identify with does not need to be the influencing agent, the health care practitioner. "Mr. Watson, I know you are aware that your friend, Mr. Gilbert, also has problems with his blood pressure. Mr. Gilbert has been able to stick with the treatment plan we devised." In this example, Mr. Watson may be motivated to be as compliant as his good friend, Mr. Gilbert. More commonly, however, the health professional practitioner acts as referent. "I find it very hard to find time to exercise too. My schedule seems so hectic. Yet, I do exercise at least three times a week and I certainly feel better as a result." Of course, the health care practitioner can only use him or herself as a referent if the patient has a desire to be like him or her in some way. To have referent power, the target of influence must perceive the practitioner to be likable, benevolent, admirable, and accepting. The referent power is derived from the patient's own desire to model his or her behaviour after the person or group. The person's motivation comes from the social-emotional aspect of the physician-patient relationship.

Usually, the health professional will use a number of kinds of social power, in combination, at any given time. Rarely would the health professional use only one form of power in any single communication with the patient. As mentioned in previous chapters (see Chapters 1 and 4), it is important that people perceive themselves as having personal responsibility or control over their own health behaviours. When health professionals use expert, legitimate, coercive, or reward powers to influence their patients, the patients will likely attribute their compliance to external incentives. Consequently, the patients will be less likely to perceive themselves as having personal control over their behaviours. According to Brehm (1966), if people feel that they lack personal control they feel **reactance**, a psychological state that motivates them to regain a sense of control and restore their lost freedom. This type of reaction may help to explain why patients sometimes act against what appears to be in their own best interests by quitting treatments before they are completed. For example, cancer patients have been known to quit their chemotherapy treatments before they have been completed. Rodin and Janis (1982) suggest that the use of expert, legitimate, coercive, and reward powers might be beneficial for patient compliance in the short-term, but in the longterm the use of these forms of power might be detrimental.

Rodin and Janis (1982) suggest that the use of referent and informational power will promote internalization. **Internalization** involves the patient changing his or her existing pattern of beliefs to accommodate the beliefs advocated by the health care practitioner. Thus, internalization leads a patient to perform a behaviour even when the patient no longer feels under the scrutiny of a health care practitioner. It is expected that the same circumstances that promote internalization also increase patients' feelings of personal control because the patients perceive themselves to be acting on the basis of internal, self-motivated norms and goals. Therefore, referent and informational power may be the best forms of power for health care practitioners to use.

In the first phase, which Janis has labelled, "Establishing Referent Power," the practitioner attempts to build up motivating power. This is accomplished by the practitioner encouraging the patient to disclose personal feelings and problems. When the patient engages in self-disclosure and the practitioner responds in a warm and accepting way, a relationship characterized by cohesiveness and trust is formed. This trusting relationship then results in increased self-esteem of the patient and increased adherence to the practitioner's recommendations.

The second phase of Janis' model is entitled, "Using Referent Power." During this phase, the practitioner uses his or her power to motivate the patient to engage in the requisite behaviour change. If the desired behaviour is to lose weight, the practitioner may help the patient to set realistic goals for changes in eating behaviour and lifestyle. Providing the patient with information regarding behaviour change and medical regimens is thought to be more effective after referent power has been established. There are many studies suggesting that providing information about a medical regimen without first establishing referent power is not likely to lead to patient adherence (e.g., Blackwell, 1972; Wilson, 1973). In this phase, the practitioner attempts to prepare the patient for the potential discomforts and difficulties that will arise with the patient's behaviour change.

"Maintaining Referent Power" comprises the third phase of Janis' model. In this phase, the goal of the practitioner is to promote further internalization of the recommended behaviour changes for the patient. This is important, as the practitioner and patient will likely have less contact once the desired behaviour change is established. For example, if someone has successfully given up smoking or achieved a desired weight, they are likely to cease or greatly reduce contact with their practitioner. Patients whose chronic diabetes has been stabilized, for example, have been found to stop following their treatment regimen after several months when they no longer have regularly scheduled appointments with their physicians (Kasl, 1975). To maintain one's medical regimen, Janis (1983) suggests that appointments between health professionals and patients be reduced gradually over time and that, if possible, periodic contact should be maintained.

Over the last couple of decades, the patient has asserted more power in the physician-patient relationship. One reason for this is, perhaps, the increased level of education attained by people in Western society. The average person is better informed now than ever before about health. It is interesting to note that models of physician-patient relationships did not include a profile wherein the patient dominates until relatively recently. Roter and colleagues (1997) model of communication noted that young patients often choose to interact with their physicians by controlling the consultation (e.g., asking the majority of questions). Whatever the cause of this change, it may necessitate health professionals to alter their style of social influence to maintain patient adherence. Moreover, there are additional strategies available to improve patient adherence.

Educational Strategies

Educational strategies to improve adherence are abundant. Health education is thought to fill the gaps in patient understanding about the need for following medical recommendations (Coambs et al., 1995). Types of patient education vary considerably and include package inserts, written information sheets to reinforce verbal instructions, one-on-one counselling, small group sessions, lectures, demonstrations, and mailed information. In Canada, health education is provided by hospital-, clinic-, community-, worksite-, and privately-based programs. As well, pamphlets and brochures are readily available to supplement and reinforce verbal instructions (Coambs et al., 1995).

Behavioural Strategies

Behavioural strategies may be somewhat effective in increasing patients' motivation to adhere to their treatment regimens (DiMatteo & DiNicola, 1982; Miller & Stark, 1994). Providing *prompts and reminders* to serve as cues may encourage patients to perform recommended activities. These cues may include notes posted at home, reminder phone calls from a clinic, or even certain forms of drug packaging (e.g., some medications now come in dispensers with dated compartments or other built-in reminders). *Tailoring the regimen* so that activities in the treatment are fitted to habits and routines in the patient's daily life may also help. For example, taking medication is easiest to do if it is tied in with another activity such as brushing one's teeth in the morning. *Self-monitoring* is another way to encourage patient adherence; the patient keeps a written record of regimen activities, such as monitoring one's resting heart rate or documenting foods eaten during the day. *Contingency contracting*, whereby the patient and health professional (or parent, if the patient is a child) negotiate a series of treatment activities and goals as well as rewards that will apply based on the patient's fulfillment of these activities, can also help. For example, "A diabetic child and his or her parents may enact a contract that specifies a particular reward for each day the child does his or her insulin injection without argument" (Miller & Stark, 1994, p. 81). The child may choose the reward, for example, a bedtime story or a special game. These techniques have a clear advantage in that the patient must actively participate in their design and execution (Turk & Meichenbaum, 1991). Further, the patient can for the most part carry out these strategies without assistance.

Social Support

Social and emotional support can provide much needed motivation for patient adherence, particularly when the regimen is longterm or requires lifestyle changes (e.g., Peck & King, 1985). Family and friends can provide positive encouragement about the treatment activities and help to ensure they occur. Social support can also be provided by self-help groups, patient groups, and organizations established to help with specific health conditions. Patients who receive encouragement, inspiration, reminders, and aid in carrying out the regimen are more likely to comply than those who do not.

Unfortunately, research evaluating these strategies is not encouraging (Haynes, McKibbon, & Kanani, 1996; Roter et al., 1998). The strategies appear to have a fairly weak effect on patient adherence. However, the more comprehensive the program of intervention, the more effective the outcome. Roter and colleagues contend that the most powerful interventions include combinations of all three strategies—educational, behavioural, and social or affective. Haynes, McKibbon, and Kanani, from McMaster University, conclude that little evidence exists that adherence can be improved. Moreover, complex, labour-intensive intervetions are "not very effective despite the amount of effort and resources they consumed" (p. 386).

HEALTH OUTCOMES

How important is it to adhere to medical recommendations provided by health care professionals? This is another question that is not easy to answer. By not adhering to treatment regimens, people increase their risk of developing health problems or of prolonging or worsening their current illnesses. Approximately 20 percent of hospital admissions are thought to result from patient non-adherence to medical recommendations (Ley, 1982). One study documented that both male and female heart patients who did not adhere well to medication recommendations were almost three times more likely to die in the next year than those who adhered fairly closely (Gallagher, Viscoli, & Horwitz, 1993; Horwitz et al., 1990).

Other studies have not shown a strong positive relationship between loyal adherence and improved health. Haynes and colleagues (1996) reviewed more than 1 500 studies on adherence to medication and concluded that it does not generally lead to better patient health. Other researchers have conducted longitudinal research and found that after four years compliant patients were not much more improved on a variety of disorders than were non-adherent patients. Before we take these results as "gospel", we must understand that there are a number of factors to consider. First, this study relied on self-reports of adherence and, as mentioned earlier, there are a number of problems inherent in this form of data collection. Second, it may have been that the participants did not completely understand the recommendations. Third, it may be that four years is not enough time to observe the results of non-adherence. Finally, other factors including heredity and environmental conditions may have had an influence on the course of the illnesses.

Perhaps another avenue to be explored in determining the effectiveness of adherence is the possibility that complete adherence may not be necessary. Perhaps there are only certain levels of adherence that are required to obtain health benefits. If this is the case, it may explain why there are few differences between those who adhere completely and those who do not adhere. For example, consuming 80 percent of the medication prescribed has been described as the minimum rate of adherence necessary to effectively treat hypertension (Epstein & Cluss, 1982). Non-adherence that is unhealthful might then be defined as "the point below which the desired preventive or therapeutic result is unlikely to be achieved with the medication prescribed" (Parrish, 1986, p. 456).

In summary, non-adherence appears to be a fairly common phenomenon. There are a number of factors associated with non-adherence, including: poor physician-patient communication; complexity and duration of the regimen; age, gender, and race of the patient; and affective characteristics of the physician. Several strategies have been created to increase adherence to medical regimens (e.g., educational and behavioural strategies) but researchers question their effectiveness. Further, researchers have been unable to find a significant benefit to high levels of adherence. However, it may be that more moderate levels of adherence contribute to health benefits, thereby eliminating the likelihood of finding differences between high- and low-level adherers.

KEY TERMS

lay referral system
patient delay
appraisal delay
illness delay
behavioural delay
medical delay
active-passive model
guidance-cooperation model
mutual-participation model
narrowly biomedical communication pattern
expanded biomedical communication pattern
biopsychosocial communication pattern
psychosocial communication pattern
consumerist communication pattern
medical jargon
non-discrepant responses
multilevel explanations
patient-centred approach
doctor-centred approach
compliance
adherence
non-adherent
creative non-adherence
informational power
reward power
coercive power
expert power
legitimate power
referent power
reactance
internalization

Chapter 7

HOSPITAL STAYS AND MEDICAL PROCEDURES

Chapter Outline

Key Questions

1. What are the psychological effects of high-tech medical procedures?
2. What is it like to be a patient in a hospital?
3. How does the experience of being a patient in a hospital differ from one department to another?
4. What are the factors affecting a person's ability to cope with a hospital stay and what roles do staff play in that coping process?
5. In what ways does a person attempt to regain a sense of control when in the hospital?

As soon as Hanna walked into the hospital, she was reminded of all the hospital dramas she had watched on television. Staff were scurrying through the halls with a sense of purpose and urgency. Families sat in waiting areas, talking quietly among themselves, some looking composed, others worried and anxious.

Today Hanna was part of the drama. Her doctor had made an appointment for her to have a mammogram. She had never had one before, and her doctor had said that it was a good screening procedure. Early detection was very important. But early detection of what? Hanna hoped that the mammogram would detect nothing.

Hanna finally found the radiology department after following a blue line on the floor that wound through the halls of the hospital. She was shown to a small changing room where she was asked to take off her upper garments and put on a gown that looked more like a discarded bed sheet. Where else would she be asked to put on something like this and then sit in a waiting room with a bunch of other people wearing discarded bed sheets? And there were so many people. The nurses and technologists were obviously used to the crowds, though. They were moving people in and out very efficiently.

When Hanna's name was called, she jumped to her feet a bit more quickly than she wanted to. She could feel the butterflies in her stomach as she went into the examination room. The procedure went smoothly, though Hanna would never have called it comfortable. Fortunately, she had a technologist who seemed to know just how to empathize with her and make her feel at ease. Before she knew it, she was in her own clothes and out in the hall, following the blue line back to the main entrance.

Most of us have been inside the confines of a hospital. However, unless you work in a hospital or have spent a considerable amount of time in one, you probably feel a bit out of place when you walk through the doors. People in unique garb might be wheeling unfamiliar machines through the halls, sometimes connected to other people! The place has its own collection of peculiar smells, and it's full of sick people, some of them dying. Indeed, a hospital is its own world. It is this world that we will be investigating in this chapter. If you have ever walked through the halls of a hospital and wondered about the psychological impact of the place, then you have thought like a health psychologist.

Hanna's example reminds us that, not only is a hospital an unfamiliar and somewhat dramatic place, we often encounter it when we are not at our best. We might be worried or anxious, or just plain unwell. In this state, we are put through procedures that can feel quite intimidating and that are designed to look for things we didn't want in the first place.

In this chapter, we will start by looking at a hospital the way an anthropologist might look at a different culture. We will move through it, from department to department, investigating the psychological impact as we go.

THE HOSPITAL AS A DISTINCT CULTURE

Imagine being asked to spend a week in a place you have never been before. In this place, most of the people dress quite differently from you. They speak your language, but they also speak another language to one another. It is a language that you cannot comprehend. They will speak this language even when you are with them and they are talking about you. In fact, these people have very different rules of social interaction. They will ask you very personal questions and expect detailed answers, even though they have just met you. They will wake you in the middle of the night. They will prevent you from getting out of your bed, even though you want to. And yet, at other times, they will make you get up when you want to stay in bed.

And there are rituals. Many visitors to this place must first provide a small amount of their blood to the inhabitants before they are allowed to stay. These people take some of their visitors and make large incisions in their bodies, often removing body parts. They may discard these body parts or keep them and study them. When it is time to leave, you may be made to exit in a chair with wheels, even though you would rather walk.

Does this sound like the sort of place you would like to visit? Does it sound rather primitive? Like the sort of place explorers would stumble upon in an Indiana Jones movie? The place we are describing is, of course, a hospital. When viewed as a distinct culture, with its own set of interaction patterns, rules, and rituals, it is easy to see why hospital stays can be quite disorienting and stressful.

The average length of a hospital stay is getting shorter as medical technology advances and budgets shrink. Nevertheless, a stay in hospital is still a very significant event in most people's lives. In Canada, the average length of a hospital stay in 1993 and 1994 was 11.1 days (Health Canada). This average includes psychiatric patients, whose stays tend to be much longer, averaging over 30 days. Stays for other problems range from 3.3 days for pregnancy complications to 24 days for diseases of the nervous system and sense organs.

While hospital stays can be difficult and lengthy, there are a number of different ways that people can experience them. Many people are like Hanna from our opening vignette. She is an **outpatient**, which means that she will not be staying overnight. Her particular procedure, a mammogram, is quite brief and fairly **non-invasive**. This means that she did not have an incision or have anything inserted into her. Nor did she have to ingest substances to aid in the radiographic procedure. Even so, as we will see in a moment, a mammogram can bring on its share of anxiety.

Other patients will be **day care patients**. This usually means they will be having a procedure that is more involved than Hanna's mammogram but still will not be staying overnight. They might be having laser surgery to remove cataracts from their eyes. Or they might be having tubes inserted in their ears to treat recurring infections. Daycare patients might be put under general anesthetic, and so they tend to be admitted early in the day and discharged by late afternoon. These patients usually need to be accompanied by someone who can be sure they get home safely and comfortably after the procedure. These patients will get one of those identification wrist bands that are so often associated with hospital stays.

Still other patients enter the hospital under emergency circumstances. They may enter by way of the emergency room and be treated and released from there in the same day. Others may be admitted through emergency and end up staying overnight or longer. Indeed, some may be unconscious when admitted and must have their circumstances explained to them when they regain consciousness in some other part of the hospital. Clearly, this is a very different experience from daycare patients or others who have had their procedure booked for a long period of time and have gone through the anticipation and waiting. Some will have gone through this waiting only to be told just before their scheduled admission day that their procedure has been postponed to accommodate more critical cases.

Each of these admission patterns can have a different effect on the patient's psychological response to being in hospital. For some, it is a sign that something traumatic and frightening is going on. For others, there is a sense of relief that the waiting is over and something constructive is going to be done. Whatever the pattern of admission, it must be emphasized that the admission procedure often constitutes a patient's first encounter with the hospital. As such, it carries all the weight we would expect of a first impression in shaping the patient's perceptions of the hospital experience.

Spencer and colleagues (1995) document the case of a 30-year-old man who suffered a spinal cord injury and had to spend 116 days rehabilitating in hospital. You can well imagine the challenges associated with learning to adapt to the disability incurred by a spinal cord injury. Interestingly, the investigators discovered through daily interviews with the patient that adaptation to his longterm hospital stay was almost as challenging. In fact, the injury and the hospital had a similar effect on the patient. Each took away some of the control he once had over his life. Adaptation to both hospital and injury meant regaining as much of that control as possible.

A study conducted in the Netherlands showed clearly that patients feel they have relinquished control to others during hospital stays (Halfens, 1995). Seventy-two people were asked to complete the Health Locus of Control Scale, which measures their sense of internal control, external control (luck, fate, and circumstance), and control by powerful others. Participants completed the scale three times: 9 days before admission, during their stay, and 7 days after being discharged from the hospital. Figure 7.1 shows the significant increase in people's scores on the powerful-other subscale during their hospital stay. Their scores on the internal and external subscales did not change over time, suggesting perhaps that, in the face of all this control by powerful others, we still try to maintain the belief that we are in as much control as we were before being admitted to hospital. Let's look more closely at the effect that loss of control has on a hospital patient.

FIGURE 7-1 Change in Powerful-Other Control Beliefs during Hospital Stays

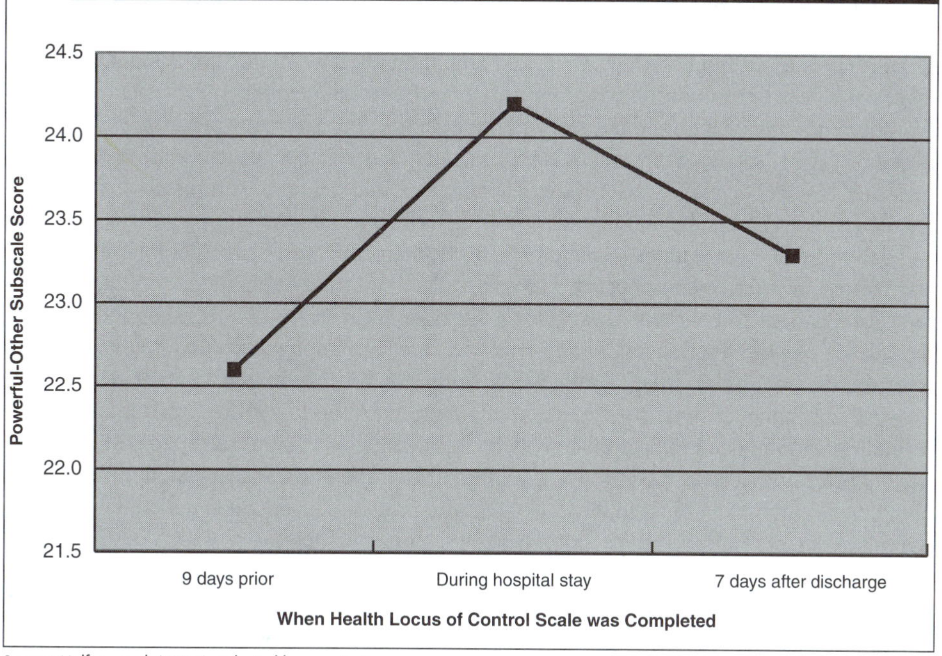

Source: Halfens et al. (1995). Adapted by permission.

A Hospital Patient's Loss of Control

People receive most of their medical care as outpatients, in a clinic, or in a doctor's office. However, there are times when a person needs to be hospitalized, either for treatment or to receive tests that, for one reason or another, cannot be performed on an outpatient basis. Upon entering the hospital, the person finds it to be what Erving Goffman (1961) describes as a **total institution**. In other words, the hospital takes control of virtually every aspect of a patient's life. Patients are expected to adapt to the hospital's schedule, to eat and sleep at specified times, to receive visitors only during designated hours, to conform to hospital procedures, and to make their bodies available for examination when requested. This lack of control is the number one complaint patients have about hospitals (Taylor, 1979).

How patients react to this loss of control in the hospital environment obviously varies from person to person. Yet, some patterns have been noted in terms of patients' reactions to the hospital environment. Judith Lorber (1975) investigated the behaviour of over 100 patients who entered a hospital for elective surgery. The patients were selected to represent people having surgeries ranging from routine to very serious. Lorber interviewed the patients when they began and ended their hospital stays. The patients were asked to indicate their degree of agreement or disagreement with a number of statements, such as, "The best thing to do in the hospital is to keep quiet and do what you're told", "I cooperate best as a patient when I know the reason for what I have to do", and, "When I'm sick, I expect to be pampered and catered to." The participants' responses to such items indicated whether they thought patients should take an *active* or *passive* role while in the hospital. Participants' agreement with the first of these items and disagreement with the second two, for example, would indicate that they believe patients should be passive, or "conforming." Lorber discovered that patients who had passive beliefs when they were admitted to the hospital were less likely than those with active beliefs to disagree with the staff and complain about minor discomforts. Obviously, these passive patients would be feeling little control in the hospital environment.

The reactions of the medical staff to the patients' behaviours were also examined in Lorber's (1975) study. After each patient was discharged, the medical staff rated the patient as a "good", "average", or "problem" patient. "Good patients" comprised 25 percent of the patient population. The good patient was described as uncomplaining, non-demanding, and generally passive. The good patients had simple medical problems, took up little of the staff's time, and had uncomplicated recoveries. The important thing to note is that, although the "good patient's" behaviour may appear ideal from the perspective of the medical staff, the patient may be experiencing helplessness and anxiety. Tagliacozzo and Mauksch (1972) point out that the "good patient", rather than being the calm, accepting, contented person the hospital staff believes him or her to be, is often torn between the desire for attention and information and the need to be well-behaved. Tagliacozzo and Mauksch state that many patients prefer not to risk appearing too demanding: "They anxiously watch a medication being late, rather than object to the delay, and they watch the specimen get cold rather than point this out to a nurse" (1972, p. 164). The result can be helplessness.

Seligman (1975) investigated the idea that constant frustration can produce **learned helplessness**. Seligman's research with animals demonstrated that some learn to do *nothing* when put into stressful situations in which no control is possible. Because these animals learned that there was no solution for their predicament, they simply gave up. They also failed to make helpful responses when put into similar situations where they could have gained some control; that is, they generalized their learned helplessness. The concept of learned helplessness has also been applied to humans in situations in which they experience or perceive loss of control (Abramson, Garber, & Seligman, 1980; Raps, Peterson, Jonas, & Seligman, 1982).

Taylor (1979) used the learned helplessness model to explain patient behaviour. When experiencing helplessness, the patient seems incapable of doing anything to improve his or her own health status. In addition, the patient fails to disclose pertinent information to the staff members. Consequently, the hospital staff cannot provide the best and most appropriate care for the patient. It is also likely that a patient who is experiencing learned helplessness will have a difficult time dealing with day-to-day responsibilities once he or she is discharged from the hospital. A person who is accustomed to having every aspect of care and treatment monitored and administered by others may have considerable difficulty assuming these roles once discharged. Consistent with this point is Coser's (1962) observation that "good patients" tend to be more reluctant to leave the hospital than "average" or "bad patients."

Half of all patients are considered "average patients" (Lorber, 1975). Average patients are very similar to good patients except that they have some minor complaints that the medical staff can usually accommodate quite easily. In contrast, "bad patients" tend to require a lot of the medical staff's time. Lorber distinguished between two types of bad patients: those who are seriously ill and complain, and those who are not seriously ill but complain anyway. While both types of bad patients require a lot of attention, the staff are more forgiving of those who complain but are seriously ill. The "complainers" who are not seriously ill usually exhibit this behaviour in an attempt to regain some control in the hospital environment. In addition to complaining, arguing, and failing to cooperate with the staff, bad patients may exhibit petty violations of hospital procedures, such as smoking or drinking, in an attempt to assert control. Many of these behaviours might simply be annoying to others, however, other behaviours may lead to more serious health consequences for the patient, such as when the patient fails to take medication or prematurely leaves the hospital.

One example of a problem patient was a 74-year-old man who had had his gallbladder removed and had postoperative psychological and medical complications. He "was labeled a problem patient by the surgeon, resident, intern, and day staff nurse. In the questionnaire, the resident said the patient's uncooperativeness made it difficult to perform routine procedures on him. The surgeon wrote that the patient was 'lachrymose, combative, and generally impossible'...the surgeon added that the patient had called him names, lied, and generally carried on" (Lorber, 1975, p. 218).

The behaviours of the "bad patient" are viewed as a form of **reactance** (Brehm, 1966). For these patients, loss of control is perceived as an unacceptable challenge to the person's freedom, which may arouse anger and must be resisted. Thus, the so-called problem patient's complaints and demands for additional attention may be angry attempts by the patient to reestablish at least a small measure of personal freedom. Patients who are younger, better educated, or accustomed to being able to control their environment are more likely to respond with reactance (Taylor, 1979).

Medical staff respond to the "bad patient" in a variety of ways. In most cases, they do so in a pleasant manner, for example by providing reassurance or explanations (Lorber, 1975). In other cases, the response is not so positive. Lorber claims that medical staff may respond with condescension, or by scolding or ignoring patients' complaints. They may respond less quickly to the patients' calls, or in the most extreme cases administer sedatives or arrange for premature discharge.

We have discussed how loss of control may cause reactance or helplessness in hospitalized patients. Neither behaviour is likely to be adaptive for the patient. Although good patients may be well liked by the hospital staff, they may be suffering from learned helplessness, which is associated with possible norepinephrine depletion, general erosion of health, and the possibility of sudden death. Patients who respond with reactance, by contrast, are likely to experience anger, heightened secretion of stress hormones, and the possible aggravation of cardiovascular problems (Taylor, 1979). Research findings germane to the patient role have prompted hospitals to provide patients with more information and give them as much control in the hospital setting as possible.

Providing information to patients has been found to reduce their anxiety before surgery, reduce the pain they experience after surgery, and reduce the number of days they spend in hospital after surgery (see Johnston & Vogele, 1993, for a review). For example, Lawrence Egbert and his colleagues (Egbert, Battit, Welch, & Bartlett, 1964) provided one group of abdominal surgery patients with information about the kind of pain they could expect to experience after their surgery, along with advice on how to minimize that pain. A control group was given routine treatment without specific information on pain. Patients in the information group, on the whole, reported less pain, requested fewer pain relievers, and spent 2.7 fewer days in the hospital than did patients in the control group.

Other studies have noted that the kind of information provided to the patient has a psychological impact on the patient. For example, Anderson (1987) documented the importance of both *informational* and *behavioural* control in a study he conducted with 60 male cardiac patients. Anderson randomly assigned the patients to three groups. The first group received the *standard* pre-surgery preparation, in which the nurse discussed two pamphlets with each of the patients that outlined the procedures related to the upcoming surgery. The second group of patients received the standard preparation plus training to increase *informational control*. The training included procedural information whereby the patients watched a videotape called "Living Proof." This video presented interviews with recovered bypass patients and followed a patient from admission through various preoperative tests and exercises, preparation for surgery, recovery, and discharge. The informational control group also received sensory information by way of an audiotape that described sensations they might experience. The third group received training in both *informational* and *behavioural control*. In addition to receiving the same training as the informational control group, this group was also provided with behavioural information such as coughing exercises they would need to do after the operation and ways to turn in bed.

Patients were assessed using a number of methods to determine the effects of the different kinds of control on patient adjustment and recovery. They completed questionnaires to measure their anxiety when they were admitted to the hospital, the day before the bypass surgery was to take place, and one week after the surgery. The patients' anxiety levels were very similar when they were first admitted to the hospital. Anxiety levels actually rose before surgery for those patients who were given the standard preparation. In contrast, both types of psychological preparation reduced the patients' anxiety both before and after surgery. Patients' use of pain medication and their length of stay in the hospital did not differ for the three groups. However, the additional psychological preparation had tremendous effects on patients' blood pressure levels in the 12 hours following surgery, when acute hypertension can become extremely dangerous. Of the patients who received the standard preparation, 75 percent developed acute hypertension and required medication as a result. In contrast, 45 percent of the patients in the informational control group and only 40 percent of the patients in the informational and behavioural control group required medication for acute hypertension.

Numerous studies have reported the benefits of providing information to patients in preparation for surgery. However, people differ as to how they respond to the information, and not all people react favourably. For example, some people, known as **monitors**, welcome information and seek it out, whereas others, called **blunters**, avoid it. A study by Suzanne Miller and Charles Mangan (1983) demonstrates how individual differences may affect responses to information about medical procedures. In this study, women about to undergo a diagnostic procedure for cervical cancer were divided into monitors and blunters based on their preference for information in a variety of naturalistic stress situations. Half the monitors and half the blunters were randomly assigned to either a high- or low-information condition. Patients in the former group were given a 20-minute verbal and visual preparatory communication detailing the procedure they were about to undergo. The other half of the monitors and blunters also spent 20 minutes with the research assistant but were given only minimal information about the upcoming procedure; the rest of the time was spent providing information on general nutrition. Measures of the patients' distress were taken in the form of pulse rates at three times: before receiving the information, after receiving the information but before the examination, and after the examination. Patients who showed the least physiological stress in response to the exam were those who were given the amount of information that fit their preferences. In other words, monitors given a large amount of information showed low physiological stress. As well, blunters given little information showed low physiological stress. However, monitors who were given little information and blunters given a large amount showed much greater stress. Other research has confirmed these findings and shown that psychological preparation for medical procedures is most effective when its content matchs the needs of the person (Carpenter, Gatchel, & Hasegawa, 1994; Litt, Nye, & Shafer, 1995; Ludwick-Rosenthal & Neufeld, 1993).

There are other ways of improving psychological control in patients. For example, researchers in Hamilton, Ontario increased patients' perceptions of control by giving patients the option of walking to the operating room rather than being transported on a stretcher (Porteous & Tyndall, 1994). During the study, 111 of 160 patients chose to walk to the operating room. Only two of these patients were not satisfied with their choice. The reasons given by the two patients included becoming uncomfortable waiting and believing that he or she "would have felt more pampered on a stretcher" (Porteous & Tyndall, 1994, p. 23). However, the majority of patients were satisfied with their decision, stating that as a result they "felt better, less like a sick person...more in control" (Porteous & Tyndall, 1994, p. 23) Thus, there are ways that hospitals can increase patients' perceptions of control and some solutions may be fairly easy to implement.

A feeling of lack of control is only one of the complaints patients have about hospitals. They also report experiencing **depersonalization** or **dehumanization**. Depersonalizing environments take away people's sense of individuality, making them feel more like objects than people (in a similar vein, perhaps you have felt this way if you have been asked for your student number rather than your name).

Depersonalization can result from many things one encounters in the hospital setting. For example, if you need to undergo even a fairly simple medical procedure it is likely that you will be required to follow a set procedure or routine and that the medical staff will also follow a routine. For instance, a pregnant woman may be required to undergo a glucose tolerance test to ensure that she has not developed gestational diabetes. Before this test begins, it will be explained to the woman that she must drink a very sweet Kool-aid like "cocktail" then remain in the hospital or lab for a number of hours so that her blood sugar can be monitored at various points. To aid the technician and ensure all pertinent information is shared with the patient, it is likely that the technician will begin a spiel (which obviously has been repeated many times) whereby he or she talks, or "runs on", for a period of time, somehow never seeming to pause for a breath, before finishing what he or she has to say. Although all the facts may have been relayed to the patient during this interaction, it is unlikely that she will be able to retain all this information. The routine of the technician has resulted in a very impersonal interaction.

Depersonalization can also result from providing little information to the patient regarding the state of his or her health or the nature of his or her treatment or by non-personal treatment by medical staff (Taylor, 1979). Phillip Zimbardo, a psychologist, has described the following example of depersonalization from his own experience as a patient:

> Recently when I was being given emergency treatment for an eye laceration, the resident surgeon abruptly terminated his conversation with me as soon as I lay down on the operating table. Although I had no sedative, or anesthesia, he acted as if I were no longer conscious, directing all his questions to a friend of mine—questions such as, "What's his name? What occupation is he in?"...As I lay there, these two men were speaking about me as if I were not there at all. The moment I got off the table and was no longer a cut to be stitched, the surgeon

resumed his conversation with me, and existence was conferred upon me again (Zimbardo, 1970, p. 298).

Depersonalization may be experienced when one is required to wear a hospital gown and even hospital-issued socks, when one is referred to by ailment rather than by name, and when one's privacy is not respected. However, hospitals are improving. Today, many hospitals encourage their patients to bring their own pyjamas and other personal effects. As well, patients are made as comfortable as possible in their environment. Have you been to a children's hospital lately? The rooms are colourful, there are play rooms filled with toys, and there are sometimes visitors, including clowns and animals; even Santa Claus has been seen on the children's ward.

How Patients Cope with the Hospital Culture

There appear to be two main ways that patients cope with this loss of control and exposure to surroundings that are so strange to them. One is by relying on other patients, the other is to adopt either a passive or active approach to the stay. Regarding patients helping each other cope, Zussman (1993), and before him Coser (1962) provide some clear analysis.

In her book, *Life on the Ward*, Coser points out that the social support patients provide each other is based on their shared submission to what we now call "powerful others" (Wallston, Wallston, & DeVellis, 1978). This support is also based on shared disability and inconvenience. Even though these might be temporary conditions, patients are brought together like motorists in a snow storm. They provide support by joking together about their conditions and generally by building solidarity. Interestingly, this probably helps patients cope with the hospital culture, but it may make it harder to adapt to life outside the hospital if the stay is a long one.

Coser's book was published in the 1960s, during a time when patients' experiences in hospitals were being studied extensively. By the 1970s, however, this study had diminished considerably. Zussman (1993) suggests that this was due, in part, to the nature of the modern hospital. In it, stays are short and technology dominates the medical landscape. To make his point, he refers to intensive care units (ICU). In these facilities, which are taking up more and more of a hospital's floor space, "technical virtuosity" (p. 176) and frequent deaths prevent patients from forming bonds with each other, and these factors discourage staff from forming therapeutic bonds with patients.

Indeed, the ICU, with its strong orientation to physiology, can create the sense of depersonalization we discussed earlier. At the same time, it must be emphasized that lives are saved in ICU. Those who work in these units may argue that there is no point in forsaking technical intervention for personal care if it means the person is more likely to die. Clearly, the ideal is a balance between technology and a human touch.

The Role of Nurses in Hospital Culture

The hospital is populated by people taking on a wide variety of roles and includes physicians, orderlies, administrators, technologists, and other staff. Arguably, though, a hospital's culture is affected most by its nurses. This is usually the largest group in the hospital, and nurses have the most person-to-person contact with patients. Indeed, nurses are called "patient advocates", in large part because they get to know the patients better than other hospital staff and they are most responsible for the day-to-day care of the patient. We will be talking about the profession of nursing in more detail in Chapter 8. For now, let's look at the ways nurses affect hospital culture and patients' ability to cope with it.

Cultures have their rituals, or shared activities that take on meaning in terms of defining those cultures. Hospitals are no exception. Not surprisingly, nursing practice has been analyzed regarding the rituals common to it. Two general types of nursing rituals have been identified—**therapeutic rituals** and **occupational rituals**. Therapeutic rituals deal mostly with patient-nurse interactions. Occupational rituals concern the socialization of nurses into the profession. As such, they focus on interactions between nurses (Wolf, 1993).

People studying hospital culture (medical anthropologists using ethnography) have identified the administration of medication and bathing patients as two important therapeutic rituals (Holland, 1993). Physicians prescribe medication patients must take, and it is the nurse's job to see that this is done. Often, patients are very cooperative and nurses reward this with a show of appreciation. Sometimes, however, patients resist their medication, and the ritual changes to one that some nurse educators have called "assertive empathy." In other words, the nurse is saying, "I know you don't like this, and I can understand why, but you are going to take it."

Patient bathing is done systematically. It connotes a level of helplessness on the part of the patient and caring on the part of the nurse. Again, some patients are more comfortable with this relationship than others. Having the process ritualized makes it easier for the nurse to complete the task, maintaining a controlled and appropriate level of intimacy and, when necessary, a firm resolve that the job must be done.

In terms of occupational rituals, Holland (1993) identifies at least four important components. First, of course, there is the uniform. Nursing uniforms vary from hospital to hospital, though they have a long history of meaning in relation to hospital culture and its association with religious institutions. Whatever the uniform may look like, the function is the same. It identifies the person as a member of the profession, subject to the codes of conduct and ethics that go with it.

The second component is the hierarchy of authority, both within the profession, with head nurses and so on, and between professions, between physicians and nurses. Ritual in this context extends to the allowable nature and direction of criticism; namely, it rarely flows *up* the hierarchy. In fact, it has been discovered that violations in hospital-infection prevention practices are less likely to be acted upon if someone lower in the hierarchy finds someone higher violating the practice (Raven, Freeman, & Haley, 1982).

The second component of occupational ritual is language. For language to define a culture, it must be unique to that culture. For example, nurses will say of a patient, "He's nil by mouth" (Holland, 1993, p. 1466). This isn't the sort of phrase you would hear anywhere else but in a hospital. Language is also used to ritualize the delicate decisions surrounding death. A decision may have been made not to resuscitate a patient if heart or respiration stops. Nurses may call this situation a "no code." Much of this language is used when nurses communicate their change-of-shift reports (Wolf, 1993). As such, this represents a clearly ritualized activity for nurses, and one in which the norms of the profession are maintained.

Whether given the description "no code", "nil by mouth", or something healthier, patients have their needs and expectations regarding the care they receive from nurses when they are in this strange world called a hospital. What are these needs and expectations and how well do the rituals of nursing meet them? In answering these questions, the two types of care nurses provide should be taken into consideration. These are **technical care** and **socioemotional care**. The former refers to the handling of prescribed medical procedures; the latter to the interpersonal skills required to help patients maintain a sense of optimism and psychological well-being.

Generally, patients aren't great judges of technical care. Most are lay people when it comes to medicine and don't have much experience with medical procedures. It would be like asking them to judge a figure skating competition when they don't know a Lutz from a triple toe loop. On the other hand, patients are good judges of socioemotional care. They know what a pleasant disposition looks like. They know what kindness and patience look like. They know when they have been treated with respect. For these reasons, patients often articulate their needs and expectations in terms of socioemotional care (Leiter, Harvie, & Frizzel, 1998).

There is an exception to this, however. Patients' satisfaction is determined by nurses' technical expertise when the patients' physical comfort and pain levels are involved. In one study, when nurses were asked what constituted the most important aspects of good nursing care, they cited listening to the patient. This answer acknowledges the value of socioemotional care. In that same study, however, when patients were asked, they said the most important aspect of good nursing care was knowing how to give shots and IVs and managing equipment (Larson & Ferketich, 1993).

Whether patients' expectations focus on the technical or socioemotional care they receive from nurses, there is little doubt that their overall satisfaction with their hospital stay is determined, in large part, by the care the nurses provide. This relationship between patient satisfaction and nursing care is highlighted in a fascinating study conducted by researchers at Acadia University in Nova Scotia (Leiter, Harvie, & Frizzel, 1998) (see Focus on Research 7.1). In this study, Leiter and colleagues correlated patient satisfaction with nurses' self-reports of professional burnout. **Burnout** is a state that results from excessive patient loads, or as Leiter and colleagues put it, nurses experience a "gap between expectations to fulfill their professional roles and the structure of the organization" (p. 1613). The most common symptoms of burnout include exhaustion, cynicism, a lack of belief in one's professional competence, and a low sense of accomplishment. Burnout is an all-too-common problem in health care that we will address further in Chapter 8.

If patients' satisfaction is determined primarily by socioemotional care, then their satisfaction should be affected by the degree of burnout existing in the hospital unit in which they are treated. The question is, does nurse burnout show itself enough to be correlated with patient satisfaction? It is this question that Leiter and colleagues addressed. Focus on Research 7.1 describes a study in which a number of strong correlations were found between elements of burnout and patients' ratings of nurses. This study provides convincing evidence that patients' ratings of nursing care are based primarily on socioemotional aspects of that care and that when nurses are overtaxed, their ability to provide that care is seriously compromised.

Patient-Centred Care: An Ideal in the Hospital

In Zussman's words, hospital patients are more than just "the human backdrop for dramatic enactments of professional socialization" (Zussman, 1993, p. 173). There is hardly a health care professional who would disagree. Regarding hospital care, however, the question remains

FOCUS ON RESEARCH 7-1 Burnout and the Capacity to Care

Title: The correspondence of patient satisfaction and nurse burnout.

Researchers: Micheal Leiter, Phyllis Harvie, and Cindy Frizzel

Purpose: To determine whether there was a relationship between nurses' self-reports of burnout and patients' ratings of nursing care.

Method: More than 700 nurses completed the Maslach Burnout Inventory. This measured the extent to which they felt exhausted, cynical, and critical of their professional ability. Burnout is related to high demands created by such things as patient overloads. Nine hundred and thirty-one patients completed the Patient Judgments of Hospital Quality Questionnaire. This is a measure of their satisfaction with various aspects of their hospital stay. Of special interest was the subscale in which patients rate nursing care. Average scores for nurses working within a hospital unit were correlated with average nursing care ratings given by patients in that unit. A wide range of hospital units was used in the analysis.

Results: Strong correlations were found between nurses' reports of various aspects of burnout and patients' ratings of nursing care.

Nurse Self-Report	Correlation with Patient Rating of Nursing Care
Exhaustion	-.73
Cynicism	-.53
Intention to quit	-.53
Work meaningfulness	.79

Conclusion: Patients' impressions of the care they receive from nurses is related to the nurses' feelings about their work as expressed in their self-reports of burnout. This is a correlational study, so we cannot draw conclusions regarding cause and effect. Having said this, it is worth exploring the very real possibility that burnout seriously affects nurses' capacity to provide socioemotional care for their patients. This study suggests that patients are sensitive to nurse burnout. This is a particularly important topic, given the vital role nurses play in helping patients cope with their hospital stays.

as to just how far we can go in dedicating resources to patients' psychosocial needs. In a San Francisco-area hospital, model units were created that featured home-like environments, art, and music. The nurses were specially trained to promote greater patient involvement in decision making, to provide more personalized care, and to increase the health education provided to patients. This was called **patient-centred care**. Not surprisingly, patients who were randomly assigned to these patient-centred units reported greater satisfaction with their stays (Martin et al., 1998). Administrators of Canadian hospitals must strike a balance between dedicating such extensive resources to patients' psychosocial needs and providing environments that address patients' fundamental biomedical needs.

THE PSYCHOLOGICAL IMPACT OF MEDICAL PROCEDURES

In our opening example, Hanna came to the hospital as an outpatient to undergo a medical procedure. Because this is the way many people experience a hospital, it is a good idea to look at the psychological impact of some of these procedures as we look closely at the ways people cope with hospital stays. In this analysis, we will make the point that there is always more to a medical procedure than what meets the practitioner's eye. Patients attach considerable meaning to the process that may go well beyond the biomedical purpose of the procedure. To illustrate this, let's return to Hanna, who is having a mammogram, and explore the psychological impact of this procedure.

The Psychology of Mammography

One valuable way to understand the potential negative psychological impact of a medical procedure is to consider its **invasiveness**. The term is self-explanatory, though it is worth noting that invasiveness has both physical and psychological components. In a physical sense, health practitioners determine the invasiveness of a procedure by the extent to which it involves piercing the skin or entering the body with instruments—physically "invading" the body. In a psychological sense, a procedure is invasive if it has the potential to cause embarrassment, shame, or discomfort. This is often the result of procedures that intrude into sexual and intimate parts of the body (Weller & Hener, 1993).

Invasiveness isn't an all-or-nothing thing. Rather, procedures can be placed on a *continuum* of invasiveness based on the definitions we have just introduced. If you have experienced a range of medical procedures in your life, you could probably rank them in terms of their invasiveness; even the different parts of a general physical examination vary in this way.

Weller and Hener (1993) conducted a study in Israel in which patient anxiety was assessed for three different procedures that varied along a continuum of invasiveness. These procedures were, in increasing order of invasiveness, abdominal ultrasound, mammogram, and hysterosalpingography (HSG). Ultrasound is a minimally invasive procedure in which the abdomen is coated with a gel and a transducer run over the area, producing a vibrating sensation as it sends out sound waves that bounce back to form an image. The gel can be a bit cold, and some procedures require a full bladder. Otherwise, there is usually little discomfort associated with the procedure. It is a different story with HSG. In this procedure, contrast material is injected through the cervix to examine the uterine cavity and fallopian tubes as part of a treatment for infertility. Women report that this procedure is very uncomfortable and difficult. Mammography falls between these two procedures on a continuum of invasiveness. There are no injections. However, the patient's breasts are pressed down during the procedure, which can be uncomfortable.

Not surprisingly, Weller and Hener found that anxiety went up with the invasiveness of the procedure. The authors don't state exactly when they measured this anxiety, however. The timing of the measurement is important. If the women completed the State Anxiety Inventory *after* the exam, then we would have a measure of how much anxiety they *experienced*. If they completed the Inventory *before* going through the procedure, then we would have a measure of how much anxiety they *anticipated*. There can be quite a difference between perceived and anticipated anxiety in this context. Often, patients feel some relief after a procedure is over and report that the experience wasn't as bad as they had anticipated.

Also, the source of the anxiety is quite different in each case. Asking patients after the procedure to report retrospectively on their anxiety has the advantage of linking anxiety to physical sensation and other real aspects of the procedure. It has the disadvantage of being distorted by relief or something idiosyncratic that may have happened during that particular test. Anticipatory anxiety is based on what the patient has heard about the procedure and on their general tendency to be anxious in situations of this kind. It may be that anticipatory anxiety can be influenced, either up or down, by the provision of information regarding the procedure.

Whether the patients were asked before or after the procedure in the Weller and Hener study, we can still be confident that mammography is, at most, moderately invasive. Nonetheless, there is considerably anxiety surrounding the procedure, not so much because of what is done but because of what might be found. Abnormal mammogram results can bring on fear, anxiety, and depression. This is also true for other screening tests, such as Pap tests for cervical cancer (Pasket & Rimer, 1995). As we will see in a moment, the real concern regarding these psychological consequences is that they decrease the likelihood that some women will return for treatment.

It could be argued that psychological distress is a necessary element of cancer treatment. As such, it is a relatively small price to pay for the lives that are saved by the early detection provided by mammography. Estimates vary considerably regarding just how many lives are saved this way, but some studies have suggested that annual mammograms for women over the age of 50 years can reduce mortality rates by as much as 30 percent (Shapiro, 1977; Tabar, Fagerberg, Duffy, & Day, 1989). Clearly, the benefits of reduced mortality outweigh the psychological costs in these cases.

When calculating this cost/benefit ratio, however, we must also take **false-positive** results into consideration. These are results that indicate abnormality when none actually exists. A perfectly reliable test has no false positives, but mammograms are not perfectly reliable. The rate of false positives for mammograms is generally considered to be quite high. In fact, it has been estimated that the results of first-round mammograms send 12 women for further investigation (often a biopsy) for every one true case of cancer (Chamberlain et al., 1984). This high rate of false positives creates a dilemma regarding mammography screening. It is a procedure that, on the one hand, saves many lives and, on the other, puts many women through unnecessary anxiety. If Hanna learns that her test has yielded abnormal results and that she is to return for follow-up testing, she will likely see herself as a cancer patient until proven otherwise. And even if follow-up tests prove negative, she may well think it is just a matter of time before the cancer appears for real (Wardle & Pope, 1992) (see Box 7.1).

In spite of these real concerns about the effects of false positives, the fact remains that most women who go through mammogram screening have negative results—they are healthy. A study that measured women's anxiety at three points in time showed that women who receive negative results are not unduly anxious, either at baseline (before being invited for screening), immediately before screening, or 9 months after the baseline measure. Women who receive false-positive results, however, do report anxiety at the 9-month mark (Sutton, Saidi, Bickler, & Hunter, 1995).

Box 7-1 False Positives in Mammography Screening

In mammography screening, a "false positive" occurs when a woman's first mammogram yields results that are sufficiently abnormal to required further testing, at which time no cancer is found. False positives are very important phenomena to study because of the psychological consequences they can have. It has been discovered that many women who are put through further tests, whether another mammography or a biopsy, suffer adverse longterm psychological effects such as depression or anxiety. These might stem from the belief that the original screen was correct, or that it is just a matter of time before they really do get cancer (Wardle & Pope, 1992).

There are a few different ways to measure false positives. In one, the number of false positives is divided by the number of true negatives plus false positives. The formula for this fraction looks like this:

$$\frac{\text{\# of false positives}}{\text{\# of true negatives + false positives}}$$

This fraction tells you the proportion of women *without* breast cancer who are called back for further testing. Six large studies of false positives were reviewed using this formula (Mushin, Kouides, & Shapiro, 1998). This review discovered false positive rates that varied from 0.9 percent to 6.5 percent, with an average of around 4 percent. In other words, for every 100 women who were actually without cancer at first screening, about four were sent for biopsies (false positives were defined in terms of negative biopsy in this review). In contrast, the same review discovered that, for every 100 women who *did* have cancer at first screening, successful identification took place between 83 and 95 percent of the time. This constitutes a high rate of early detection.

While comparison of false positives to true positives is encouraging, it must be remembered that there are many more women who don't have cancer than do, so the absolute number of false positives might be quite high compared to the number of correct detections. To investigate this, some researchers have looked at the ratio of the number of women who went for biopsy to the number who actually had cancer. Even under optimal conditions, in which mammograms are read by highly trained radiologists who do nothing else during their day and do so in undistracted surroundings, one confirmed case of cancer is found for every 10 women called back for repeat testing (Roux, Markle, & Diamond, 1998). This means that if Hanna is called back for a repeat test or biopsy, there is only a one-in-ten chance she has cancer.

We must also take into account the fact that the chances a woman will experience a false positive goes up each time she has a mammogram. Analysis of the experiences of just under 300 000 women in British Columbia revealed that, after 10 screenings, the chances that a woman between the ages of 50 and 59 years will have a false positive result is 35.1 percent. Many physicians recommend yearly mammogram screenings for this age group (Olivotto, Kan, & Coldman, 1998).

In many clinics, women are informed of these ratios and percentages when they are called back for repeat testing. However, there is some question whether this information is reassuring, or if it is akin to a judge telling a jury to disregard a piece of testimony. This turns out to be very difficult to do. It has also been argued that a retest does not constitute a false positive because no diagnosis has been made at that point (Gross, 1998). Again, health psychologists would be concerned that the patient has made a *self-diagnosis* as a result of the callback, and this can be distressing.

Regardless of how distressing a callback or negative biopsy might be, there is reassuring evidence that women who experience these false positives are not more likely to stop regular screening. In fact, they may be *more* likely to have attend regular screening appointments, because they feel more susceptible to breast cancer (Pisano, Earp, & Gallant, 1998; Pisano, Earp, Schell, Vokaty, & Denham, 1998). This is important because it has been estimated that, for women over the age of 50 years, regular screening can reduce breast cancer mortality rates by as much as 30 percent. The challenge, clearly, is to refine the screening procedure to reduce the number of false positives and thus improve the balance between early detection and unnecessary psychological distress.

It is interesting to note that, while positive and false-positive results may bring on anxiety that inhibits a person from going to follow-up appointments, a general concern regarding breast cancer prior to any screening *increases* the likelihood that a woman will take part in the screening (McCaul, Schroeder, & Reid, 1996). It seems that the screening can work to allay that concern. However, a positive or false-positive result can only worsen the concern, to the point where it is more inhibiting than motivating.

The extent to which a positive result will be inhibiting or motivating will also be influenced by other psychological factors. Lauver and her colleagues (Lauver, Nabholz, Scott, & Tak, 1997) have used something called the theory of careseeking, which focuses on **habits** and **norms**, to predict whether women will pursue mammogram screening. In terms of habit, some people are generally more likely to seek medical care when symptomatic, and these same people are more likely to engage in preventive behaviour. When this habit is combined with the belief that other people think screening is a good thing (the norm), then we should be able to predict motivation to attend screening and follow-up. This is just what Lauver and colleagues found for 178 women between the ages of 40 and 89 years.

The vast majority of mammograms are performed on women. This does not mean, however, that the anxiety accompanying positive and false-positive results is a female phenomenon. Let's look at a slightly more invasive procedure that is equally common for men and women, to develop an understanding of how the nature of the machine can affect patients' psychological response to the procedure.

The Psychology of Magnetic Resonance Imaging

Magnetic resonance imaging (MRI) has become a very popular diagnostic tool. This is because the images produced are superior to those obtained through radiography and the patient is not exposed to radiation (x-rays). The procedure is moderately invasive for at least two reasons. First, it is not uncommon for patients to require an injection of a contrast solution prior to their scan. Second, the patient must enter a confined space, in some cases for 30 minutes at a time, for tests that can last over 2 hours in total, if the patient is having a complete head and neck scan.

How confining is the space? Patients must enter a long cylinder, called a bore, that is either 55 or 70 centimeters in diameter. People with wide shoulders must pull them in to enter the bore. Once inside, the person must remain very still. To achieve this, the person's head may be held in place with Velcro straps. The temperature in the bore often reaches 27 degrees Celsius, and the magnet makes a loud banging sound during the scan.

Claustrophobia is the greatest psychological concern for those undergoing MRI procedures. This is most prevalent for people who are having scans that require them to enter the bore head first. Before their scan, these patients are asked, often repeatedly, if they have problems with enclosed spaces. The newest design of MRI scanner features an open side so the patient isn't completely enclosed, thereby reducing claustrophobic reactions. At present, though, most hospitals use closed-bore models. Let's look at what research has discovered regarding the psychological effects of going through an MRI procedure.

It is important to acknowledge that these effects can be either short-term or longterm. Short-term effects include anxiety and claustrophobia during the exam as well as something called **motion artifacts**. These are distortions to the MRI image caused by a patient's movement. In some cases, these artifacts can make diagnosis difficult; in others, they can render the scan useless and require a re-scan. It has been estimated that up to 40 percent of all scans have motion artifacts to varying degrees, impairing the quality of the diagnosis 8 to 17 percent of the time. Some motion artifacts are caused simply by the patient's breathing. Longterm psychological effects might include a newly formed apprehension of enclosed spaces that surfaces weeks or months after the MRI experience.

To assess short-term effects, researchers measured pre-exam worry in 297 patients over the age of 16 years who were about to undergo a head-first MRI. They also asked them after the exam to indicate how anxious they had been during the exam (this was measured by way of the State Anxiety Inventory.) In addition, motion artifacts were noted, to determine whether they were related to patient anxiety (Dantendorfer et al., 1997). Only 1.2 percent of the participants found the MRI "hardly bearable." On average, anxiety levels dropped from pre-exam to post-exam, and females experienced significantly more anxiety than males. The size of the bore (55 or 70 cm) had no effect on anxiety. When asked what was most unpleasant about the experience, participants cited the fact they had to stay still, the banging sound, and the narrowness of the bore. Motion artifacts occurred in 17 cases. Twelve of these cases had expressed pre-exam worry. It should be noted, however, that over 100 patients expressed pre-exam worry and the majority of these (88.5 percent) did *not* have motion artifacts.

Other studies have discovered that claustrophobic reactions are not uncommon during MRI procedures. Some researchers report such reactions in up to 20 percent of cases (Lukins, Davan, & Drummand, 1997). Others estimate that claustrophobia occurs about 5 to 10 percent of the time, though moderate to severe anxiety has been reported in 37 percent of cases (Katz, Wilson, & Fraser, 1994).

Longterm psychological effects have also been found. In one study, 10 percent of patients reported feeling nervous in enclosed spaces one month after their scan (Kilborn & Labbe, 1990). In another, it was discovered that a small percentage of people had their first claustrophobic experience *after* having their MRI (Melendez & McCrank, 1993). McIsaac and her colleagues found that 30 percent of their participants' feelings of claustrophobia had increased 1 month after their MRI, and 33 percent said they were reluctant to have another scan (McIsaac et al., 1998).

Anxiety and claustrophobia are obviously linked in MRI procedures. For this reason, studies have attempted to apply what is known about claustrophobia to better understand the aversiveness of these procedures. One widely accepted view of claustrophobia is that it is composed of two fears—**fear of suffocation** and **fear of restriction** (Rachman & Taylor, 1993). Studies have measured these fears in MRI patients to determine the extent to which they predict adverse reactions to the procedure (McIsaac et al., 1998). Of 80 participants, 11 reported that they felt panic during the exam. Not surprisingly, these people did score higher on measures of claustrophobia. In fact, McIsaac and her colleagues found a correlation of .51 between anxiety experienced during the exam and their measure of claustrophobia. More specifically, they found a .41 correlation between fear of restriction and exam anxiety, and a .57 correlation between fear of suffocation and anxiety. These researchers suggest that fewer problems would occur during the MRI exam if, prior to an exam, hospital staff administered a short version of the questionnaire that assesses these fears rather than simply asking patients if they are claustrophobic. It is interesting to note that, while other studies have found that claustrophobia worsens 1 month after an MRI, one study found that fear of restriction and suffocation improved when the MRI had been completed without anxiety (Harris, Robinson, & Menzies, 1999).

The general conclusion from this work is that most adults can get through an MRI, though many are made uncomfortable or anxious by the experience. If an MRI exam has these effects on adults, how does it affect children? One study of pediatric oncology patients (children with cancer) found that 30 percent reported moderate to extreme distress during an MRI. The worst part for them, though, was not claustrophobia; rather, it was the insertion of an intravenous line (Tyc et al., 1995). This same study found that parents' estimates of their children's distress were higher than that actually reported by the children, even though the youngest child was just 8 years old.

Just under 4 percent of the 491 children in another study were unable to complete the exam, though it should be noted that children under the age of 8 years were routinely sedated for their MRI. In that study, children said that, apart from injections, the banging sound was the worst part of the MRI experience (Marshall, Smith, & Weinberger, 1995).

Sedation is one way to help children get through an MRI exam, although it is not an ideal technique. Other interventions have been introduced that reduce the need for sedation. For example, in a hospital in which children under the age of 6 years were routinely sedated for MRI, 10 children averaging under 5 years of age were given audio tapes containing music and a story that invited the children to create mental pictures. It was discovered that only 3 of these 10 children required sedation, compared to 8 of 10 in a matched control group (Smart, 1997).

For adults, the intervention of choice is sedation. However, it is not always effective. In fact, one study found that 13 percent of patients had taken medication to reduce their anxiety (called anxiolytic medication), yet they were the very patients who reported the most pre-MRI anxiety, in spite of having taken the anxiolytic medication (Katz, Wilson, & Fraser, 1994). Of course, this doesn't mean that the medication did not reduce their anxiety levels, since we don't know what those levels were prior to their taking the sedative. Still, we do know that sedation did not bring their anxiety levels down to the average.

In an analysis of sedative usage for MRI patients, Murphy and Brunberg (1997) found that over 14 percent of 939 patients over the age of 18 years required sedation. Of these, 36 percent were male and 64 percent were female. Murphy and Brunberg also discovered that sedation was more common for patients having MRI brain scans. This means that about 14 out of every 100 MRI patients are being given medication that isn't always effective.

Non-pharmaceutical interventions are geared toward relaxation and distraction from the aversive properties of the MRI experience (Quirk & Wagner, 1995). The effect of anxiety-reducing audio tapes was assessed in a study that divided adult patients into three groups. The first acted as a control group, with no tapes. The second listened to anxiety-reducing tapes before their scans. The third listened to the tapes before and during their scans. All participants completed the State Anxiety Inventory as well as the Fear Survey Schedule (a measure of phobias) before and after their scans. Compared to the control group, anxiety decreased for both groups listening to the tape; however, there was no added benefit from listening to the tape during the scan. Interestingly, all groups reported increased MRI fears at a 1-month follow-up, regardless of which group they'd been in. This indicates that the tapes helped relieve short-term but not longterm effects.

In summary, the clear images produced by MRI scans come with certain psychological costs, especially for people who enter the bore head first. Generally, about 70 percent of all people cope with the procedure reasonably well, though some may find that their general discomfort with enclosed spaces has worsened as a result of their MRI experience. Between 10 and 20 percent of patients find that experience to be very difficult, and 3 to 5 percent cannot complete the exam. The open-sided design of new machines should make for a significant improvement in people's ability to cope with the procedure.

DAY SURGERY

The procedures we have described so far have varied in their invasiveness, but none have involved surgery. However, *day surgery*, also called *day care surgery*, is another common way in which people experience hospital settings. As the term suggests, this is surgery in which patients do not stay in the hospital overnight. They may have cataracts removed from their eyes through laser surgery, they may have urological procedures like cystocopies to investigate urinary infections or widen the urethra, or they may have surgery to implant tubes in the ears to treat recurring ear infections. In fact, there are many procedures that are now conducted such that the patient does not have to stay in the hospital overnight. When this is handled well, there are considerable advantages, both in terms of hospital costs and patient welfare.

Research conducted in England in the mid-1990s confirmed that patients' satisfaction with day surgery was generally quite high (Ghosh & Sallam, 1994). Only 2.5 percent needed to contact the hospital within 25 hours of discharge. Another 4.3 percent contacted their family doctor within 48 hours, and 1.4 percent contacted a district nurse. The most common reason for this contact was pain management.

Another British study identified the key elements to successful day surgery in pediatrics then assessed the extent to which these elements were in place (While & Wilcox, 1994). The three key elements were: (1) adequate preparation, in the form of information for parents and children; (2) timely, as opposed to premature, discharge; and (3) adequate home support. Data collected in British hospitals in 1992 indicated that there was room for improvement in these areas. Some of the information presented was inappropriate for pediatric day surgery patients, for example, "The patient must not operate heavy machinery for 24 hours." Often, there was no information given regarding post-discharge care. One of the results was that children experienced considerable emotional upset when they returned home. We can speculate on the extent to which these findings apply to modern Canadian pediatric units. Regardless, they provide a valuable template for successful pediatric day surgery experiences.

In many ways, the day surgery experience is like a compressed hospital stay. There is the admission procedure, which is probably set up well in advance of the surgery. There is the procedure itself, featuring considerable loss of personal control, from wardrobe changes to general anesthetic. There is postoperative recovery, discharge, and home care. All of these are important features of hospital stays as well. Let's look at the psychology of these stays, starting with the admission process and moving through various departments in the hospital. Then we will talk about discharge and what must be taken into account at that point.

IN THE HOSPITAL

We now shift our focus to those people who spend at least one night in hospital. In the language of health statistics, this is called a **hospital separation**. According to the 1994/95 National Population Health Survey, 2.2 million Canadians aged 15 years or older spent at least one night in a hospital in the 12 months leading up to the survey. In this case, "hospital" was broadly defined to include nursing homes and convalescent homes. However, this figure did not include people who were institutionalized on a longterm basis (Wilkins & Park, 1997).

The Emergency Department

The emergency department of a hospital deserves the attention of health psychologists for a number of reasons. First, it is a common point of entry for many patients. Second, patients often come to emergency in a state of distress or even disorientation, depending on the nature of their problem. Their treatment needs are pressing, and they are in a setting where it is likely that many other people have equally pressing treatment needs. The way hospital staff interact with these people from their first encounter in admission is very important.

In psychological terms, admission procedures are important because they constitute the patient's first impression of the hospital. Have you ever noticed that hotels spend a disproportionate amount of money on the architecture and furniture in the lobby, and that the reception staff is trained to be extremely pleasant? Clearly, hotel owners have read the literature on first impressions. But Canadian hospitals are not hotels. The admissions area associated with emergency departments can get very hectic, and the questions that need to be asked are far more personal than those asked at the reception desk of a hotel. Still, patients' impressions of the care they receive in a hospital will be affected by the demeanor and efficiency of the admissions staff. This "personal touch" might be easier to implement for patients who are coming into the hospital for a planned procedure. There is little sense of urgency and the patient might be prepared to provide the information required. However, many hospital admissions are not planned. They occur through the emergency department, which is arguably the toughest test of a hospital's admission procedures and the one that can have the greatest impact on the patient, provided he or she is conscious.

As an example of this, researchers have looked at the needs of stroke patients when they first come to the hospital (Pound, Bury, Gompertz, & Ebrahim, 1995). These patients are often frightened and disoriented. They often can't explain what has happened to them, but they know it is serious. They represent a rather extreme example of what most people feel when they enter a hospital through the emergency department with a problem that is serious enough to warrant at least an overnight stay.

Psychologically, stroke victims need three things upon being admitted to hospital. First, they need someone who is perceived to be an expert to make sense of the event. Second, they need assurance that they will survive. Once these basics have been attended to, they need to be provided with a sense of comfort and human warmth. In other words, they need to feel that the hospital staff cares about them (Pound et al., 1995).

What is required to meet needs of this type? At the very least, there must be an emergency department that has sufficient staff and organization to provide expert attention as soon as possible after the patient has entered the hospital. Then, the admission and other staff must have the interpersonal skills to communicate a sense of caring. Asking questions while fixing one's gaze on a computer screen doesn't do this. Neither does stoicism. Sometimes, all that is required is to pay some immediate attention to the patient-to-be, by indicating that someone will be with him or her as soon as possible. Patients and their families appreciate knowing if there is going to be a wait and why.

In Britain, standards of hospital care are dictated by the Patient's Charter, published by the Conservative government in 1991. The Patient's Charter serves as a good set of guidelines regarding admission procedures through the emergency department, called in Britain Accident and Emergency, or A & E. Here are a few of the stipulations of the Charter.

Patients have a right to an explanation of the proposed treatment. The explanation must be in terms that the patient can understand. It is also hoped that the patient will have some involvement in the choice of treatment. Second, the patient has a right to privacy. In an emergency department, this can be difficult to achieve because of lack of space. At the same time, patients want a balance between having their privacy and being given adequate attention by emergency staff. They don't want to be "stored" and forgotten. Third, the Charter stipulates that waiting times for treatment must be kept as short as possible. Of course, this leaves open the possibility that a wait can be hours long and still be as short as possible.

When actual A & E experiences were compared with the standards presented in the Charter, some discrepancies were discovered that may apply just as well to Canadian hospitals (Britten & Shaw, 1994). First, patients tended to feel underinformed regarding the proposed treatment. Also, there was no evidence that patients were able to exercise any choice in that treatment. The realities of A & E care may not allow for a lengthy dialogue with patients regarding treatment choices. Also, patients may be incapacitated to the extent that they are not capable of making thoughtful choices. Still, improvements could be made in this regard.

Second, most A & E departments featured a decided lack of auditory and visual privacy. Other patients, their family, and their friends could hear all the words and sounds associated with treatment. And while some beds could be cordoned off by curtains, busy times often necessitated keeping patients on beds in open areas and hallways. Finally, there is the wait time. Interestingly, this study found that patients expect a certain amount of wait time when they come to A & E. They are surprised when wait times are short. However, they are distressed when wait times are very long.

It could be argued that the realities of emergency room work clash with the expectations of the Patient's Charter, and that, in general, emergency departments are simply not the sort of places where psychological issues can be given any priority. For example, pain relief is a top priority for most people coming to emergency, yet it might not be so for hospital staff. This is because pain relief may require medication that must be authorized. Also, an accurate assessment of that pain may be essential to a proper diagnosis.

It could also be argued, however, that there are some things that can be done to improve patients' psychological experiences in emergency. This could start with the admission procedure, which we have already discussed. Indeed, it has been suggested that admission be taken away from the emergency area and be staffed by physicians and nurse practitioners who can send patients directly to the appropriate part of the hospital, perhaps radiology for x-rays, or elsewhere for emergency suturing (Mayled, 1998). In addition, clear yet brief explanations of diagnosis and treatment options are always helpful. This is a skill that we should not assume all people naturally possess; training is required to hone it (see Chapter 6 on communication in medical settings.) Patients in emergency departments also benefit from **continuity of care**. This means that one named staff person (usually a nurse) takes primary responsibility for a patient for the duration of his or her stay in emergency. The most expensive improvements may well be architectural. Crowding in emergency departments reduces privacy and increases distress. Well-designed departments can reduce crowding and provide adequate spaces for consultation with patients while at the same time minimizing staff movement between treatment stations.

Recovering From Surgery

We have looked at people who enter the hospital for just one day to have some surgical procedure performed. Of course, there are also many people whose surgical procedures are major enough to require hospital-based recovery. For a number of reasons, postoperative recovery can be a difficult time psychologically. In addition to having to cope with the unfamiliar surroundings of the hospital, postoperative patients must manage varying degrees of incapacitation, unfamiliar bodily sensations, instructions that may be painful or uncomfortable (like forced deep breathing and coughing), and the uncertainty surrounding the normality of the rate of recovery.

One way to help patients through the postoperative period is by providing good preoperative education. This is designed to make clear to the patient just what to expect in terms of sensations, recovery rates, instructions, etc. Indeed, we have known for some time that good preoperative instructions can reduce postoperative pain and length of stay (Egbert, Battet, Welch, & Partlet, (1964). A more recent meta-analysis of studies in this area confirms the benefits of what is sometimes called **psychoeducational care** (Devine, 1992). When applied to the postoperative period, psychoeducational care refers to the provision of information regarding self-care practices, further procedures, and typical patterns of recovery.

Pain Management following Surgery

One of the most important factors determining a patient's satisfaction with recovery from surgery and the length of his or her hospital stay is pain management. Pain affects mood, and mood (depression, in particular) affects length of stay for certain patients (Schubert, Burns, Paras, & Sioson, 1992; Zalewski et al., 1994). We will be discussing pain and pain management more generally in Chapter 10. At this point, we will look specifically at patients recovering from surgery. Of course, pain levels vary, though moderate to intense pain is not uncommon following some surgical procedures. In these instances, the pain is most often treated through pharmacological analgesics such as morphine, though relaxation and other non-pharmacological techniques are also used.

A number of challenges arise when providing pain medication for postoperative patients. One challenge is to ascertain correct dosage. Undermedication will discourage the patient and be ineffective. Overmedication may be harmful when strong drugs such as opioids are used. Another challenge is the psychological issue of control we discussed earlier in the chapter. Patients may not like being dependent upon other people to relieve their pain. In asking for pain medication, patients might feel that they are being weak or "whiny." Perhaps they don't want to give the impression that their recovery is not going well and thereby risk lengthening their stay in hospital (Taylor, Hall, & Salmon, 1996).

To deal with these challenges, back in the 1980s, hospitals introduced **patient-controlled analgesia (PCA)**. As the term suggests, PCA puts the control of analgesic administration in the hands of the patient. This can be done a number of ways, from intravenous administration to oral tablet. One common way is to give the patient a devise that, when pressed, releases a certain dosage of the prescribed analgesic intravenously. The devise allows practitioners to set the dosage as well as the **lock-out interval**, which is the time period between allowable dosages.

What happens when the responsibility for analgesic administration is passed to the patient? In general, studies have had encouraging outcomes. For example, colon surgery patients who were in the PCA group used less sedation and analgesia and enjoyed faster recovery times than did the group whose medication was administered by staff (Roseveare et al., 1998). Similarly, bone marrow transplant patients reported lower pain intensity and used less medication when in the PCA group (Zucker et al., 1998). A study of cardiac surgery patients found that the PCA group reported less pain postoperatively but that they used more medication than the nurse-administered group did (Boldt et al., 1998). All of these studies were prospective in design, with randomized assignment to group.

Another study included a third group of patients who were in a patient-controlled condition but received a placebo rather than an analgesic (Stainer, Grond, & Maier, 1999). A placebo is a substance that does not contain active medication but might bring about desired effects for psychological reasons, such as the patient's belief that it will work. Interestingly, patients in this "patient-controlled placebo" group administered twice the amount of medication as patients receiving opioid analgesic. Of course, the placebo group thought they were receiving a real analgesic. This study also found that 60 percent of the abdominal surgery patients responded well to PCA.

While results using PCA are generally positive, studies that have used different surgical procedures have produced varying results. For example, a study of patients undergoing gynecological surgery (laparoscopy) showed no difference between PCA and intermittent injection regarding pain, sedation, nausea and vomiting, hospitalization, or patient satisfaction with postoperative analgesia. The authors of that study do not recommend PCA for this surgery (Rosen et al., 1998). One study of children found that the PCA group used more morphine than the staff-administered group following appendectomy (Villareal, Brown, & Lawson, 1998).

It has been suggested by some that PCA will be more successful if patients receive training in the procedure before their surgery (Owen & Plummer, 1997). As a test of this, a group of patients was shown an educational videotape on PCA prior to surgery. This group had more positive attitudes toward PCA and greater pain control and satisfaction 4 and 8 hours after surgery than did the group not shown the tape (Knoerl, Faut-Callihan, Paice, & Shott, 1999). Another study placed half of the PCA patients in a preoperative tutorial group and half in a control group (Griffin, Brennan, & McShane, 1998). It turned out that both groups used the same amount of morphine and reported similar pain levels, but the tutorial group experienced less nausea between 6 and 24 hours after surgery.

The efficacy of PCA might also be affected by staff attitudes toward it. For example, nurse-patient relationships can be strained if nurses feel that they should have the responsibility for analgesic administration (Taylor, Hall, & Salmon, 1996). This may be one reason why Fulton (1996) found that nurses' attitudes toward PCA ranged from being very in favour of it to rejecting it absolutely. Nurses may very well believe that they are accountable for their patients' pain levels, and this belief may run counter to PCA. Other nurses may believe that they are being accountable by introducing PCA properly and providing good patient teaching regarding its use.

The research on PCA is generally quite positive. It restores some sense of control for the patient and results in effective pain management in the majority of cases. It is not surprising, therefore, to find that it is at present commonly used in Canadian hospitals. The research is inconsistent, however, in terms of amount of analgesic used in the PCA approach compared to staff-administered approaches. The differences between studies may be due to differences in the nature of the surgery featured in each. Also, it is possible that there are some patients who are not well suited to PCA. Certainly, education regarding its use is advised for all patients.

The Intensive-Care Unit

Nowhere in the hospital is modern technology more prominent than in the intensive-care unit (ICU). It is the unit in the hospital where life-support machinery is employed and where patients are closely monitored by a staff whose nurse-to-patient ratio is the lowest in the hospital. We made the point earlier in this chapter that the intensive-care units of hospitals are becoming more prevalent in terms of the number of beds dedicated to them. For these reasons, the ICU is an important area of study for health psychologists.

Interviews with patients after they have been in ICU have yielded some very interesting data regarding their experiences. Pallavicini-Gonzalez and colleagues (1995) discovered that patients in ICU go through three distinct stages. First, there is what the authors call the **incommunication stage**. In this stage, patients are either unconscious or barely conscious. Their memories of the experience are poor, but the memories they do have are somewhat strange. The equipment is imposing and the passage of time is unclear. The second stage is called the **readaptation stage**. At this point, the patient can sense a struggle to recover. It is during this stage that the patient recognizes his or her dependence on the machines, especially the ventilator, which helps them breath. The equipment provides some reassurance and the staff is seen as helpful. The final stage is the **reflexion stage**. In this stage, the patient tries to piece together the details of the experience, wanting to know what happened to him or her.

Of course, not all patients experience these stages, and some are moved out of ICU before they get through all three stages, which might explain why some patients have no recollection at all of their time in the unit. In fact, Russell (1999) discovered that 34 percent of the 298 patients he interviewed had no memory of being in ICU, 42 percent had some memory of it, and 24 percent reported having clear memories of their ICU experience.

Russell's interviews of patients 6 months after they had been in ICU in Melbourne, Australia represent some of the most comprehensive data currently available on the ICU experience. Some of the people interviewed said it was like being in a science fiction movie. Others likened the experience to being in a factory, and still others said it was like being in a war zone.

Consistent with the readaptive stage identified by Pallavicini-Gonzalez, Russell's participants remembered the close surveillance of technology and staff providing them with a sense of safety. Interestingly, though, they also reported that the staff provided a feeling of safety more than the machines did. In fact, 76 percent of the participants had either a vague memory of the technology or no memory of it at all. Of those who did remember it, some found it reassuring, while others were frightened by it because of a lack of knowledge regarding what the machine was for. Many of these machines monitor vital physiological processes and can be set to sound an alarm if levels drop below or rise above a set level. Not surprisingly, patients found these alarm sounds to be quite frightening when they did not know what they signalled. Much of this fear can be alleviated if nursing staff provide basic explanations of the functions of the machines.

Indeed, the data from Russell's interviews suggest strongly that *communication* is a key factor in determining a patient's psychological reaction to ICU. However, there are a number of reasons why communication is sometimes poor in ICU. For example, it has been suggested that minimizing communication with the patient also minimizes nurses' anxiety (Leathart, 1994). By not talking to patients, it is easier to *dehumanize* them. This concept, taken from social psychology, refers to the tendency to see people as objects rather than as human beings. Health practitioners may do this, not because they are uncaring, but because it is easier emotionally to think of an ICU patient as "the acute MI in bed three" rather than as Mr. Chen who has six grandchildren.

Communication is also inhibited by the fact that patients in ICU tend to be unresponsive (Turncock, 1991). Some, of course, are unconscious. If they are conscious, they may have tubes inserted in their throats. Nevertheless, communication is still important. Just because a patient can't respond does not mean he or she can't *hear*. This is illustrated most graphically by the recollection of one of Russell's interviewees:

> I remember hearing a voice saying "His blood pressure's dropping, it's 60, 57, 55." Another voice saying, "Tell me when it is 50 and we can all knock off." I still think of that sometimes (p. 789).

Overheard remarks like these carry a great deal of psychological weight for patients. Russell discovered that these remarks were remembered 6 months later and, as the quote suggests, may be remembered forever. These remarks were cited by Russell's participants as a major source of upset. Another patient recalled hearing one staff person telling another that they might as well pull the plug. It is doubtful that the staff member would have made that remark had he or she known the patient could hear.

When staff do talk to patients, they tend to focus on procedure—what is going to be done—rather than on the patient's condition and progress (Baker & Melby, 1996). Information regarding progress may be very important for patients who have entered the readaptation stage and are aware of the struggle that faces them.

Russell also asked participants if they would want to go in ICU again if they were seriously ill or injured. Eighty percent said they would, ten percent said they would leave that decision to the doctor, and ten percent said they would not want to be a patient in ICU again, even if their condition warranted it. Finally, Russell discovered that some patients need to revisit the ICU after their recovery to put the experience behind them. These revisits can be good for staff morale, too. Unfortunately, they can be difficult to schedule in a unit in which trauma is an everyday experience.

From the work of Russell and others, we can conclude that the psychological impact of ICU can be strong and lasting. Many patients credit the technology and staff with saving their lives, though recurring thoughts or dreams about the experience are not uncommon. As is the case throughout the hospital, communication is central to reducing the distress of being in ICU. Staff must assume that patients can hear them, and they must provide feedback regarding the patient's condition and progress.

This feedback must also be provided for the families of the patients, who, in the spirit of family-centred care, are very important people in the patient's treatment. They experience many stressors. They see the patient critically ill and in an unpredictable condition (a simple cough might be alarming). They see other patients who may be dying, and they hear alarms sounding on a regular basis (Gibbons, 1990). Unfortunately, communication with family and visitors is often a low priority for ICU nurses who are busy with critically ill patients (Greenwood, 1998).

Discharge

For some patients, leaving the hospital involves more than simply gathering up one's belongings and walking out the front door. It is often the case that further treatment is required, or at the very least rest and general convalescence. This means that there must be some form of support provided for patients after discharge. All of these considerations require **discharge planning**, a process in which post-hospital care is organized and risk is assessed. By risk, we are referring to such things as social problems, a lack of support, and medical conditions that result in a high degree of dependency (Evans & Hendricks, 1993).

Caring for a family member who has just returned home from the hospital can put a strain on family resources. Someone might have to take time off work. Special equipment may be required. There may be added expenses for such things as in-home nursing care.

BOX 7-2 The Neonatal Intensive-Care Unit

We have looked at what it is like for adults to be in ICU with its collection of machines, tubes, and IV drips. But can you imagine a patient who weighs less than 1 kilogram (under 2 pounds) being hooked up to all this, caught in a battle for life? These are some of the patients in the neonatal intensive care unit (NICU). Some have been born prematurely, and then taken quickly away from the delivery room to NICU. Other newborns (neonates) may be full-term births but have suffered from some prenatal (before birth, in the womb) or perinatal (during birth, a birth complication) condition that requires intensive care. It could be argued that the NICU is the most emotionally intense unit in the hospital, for both parents and staff.

This emotion is captured well by the words of Ellen Morris (1999), a nurse in NICU:

> The daily span of emotions in the NICU is long and varied: unspeakable sadness when parents have to make the soul-destroying decision to take their baby off life support—a decision that deserves respect—and the inescapable feeling of having little control over the unexpected death of an infant thought to be doing well. But balancing the sadness is the elation we all feel when a baby no longer needs to be intubated, when a mother and father hold their baby for the first time, or when an infant finally breastfeeds months after birth. My greatest satisfaction, though, comes from seeing a child born with the odds against him, discharged home at last to a loving family (p. 23).

This mother's description reminds us that parents might not know just what emotions to feel when their baby is taken to NICU:

> The delivery was bittersweet: my husband caught a glimpse of Alyssa as they whisked her away. We didn't know if we should be thrilled to be parents of a tiny girl who weighed little more than a loaf of bread or brace ourselves for the real potential for tragedy. Our friends and relatives didn't know whether to offer congratulations or condolences (Jed, 1999, p. 22).

Parents' stress levels are often high in NICU. One factor that predicts parents' stress is when and where they first see their baby (Shields-Poe & Pinelli, 1997). Even parents of full-term infants are shocked when they first see the wiring, tubing, and blinking lights, combined with the noises the machines make in NICU (Jamsa & Jamsa, 1998). With this in mind, staff and psychologists can help prepare the parents by giving them a sense of what to expect and what is common in NICU. Family-centred care is obviously very important in NICU, as is *primary care*, which means that the same nurse cares for a given baby throughout the stay (Morris, 1999). Parent involvement is encouraged. They must learn to care for their new baby and may be able to notice subtle but important changes that the busy nursing staff could miss.

In working with the parents, an approach has been advocated that goes by the acronym TEAM (Ward, 1999). In the TEAM approach, the practioner will *T*each, by preparing the parents for the NICU and explaining the equipment,

*E*mpower the parents by giving them tools to be involved in the care as soon as possible, *A*ssess the family's needs and develop a discharge plan, and *M*onitor how well the program is meeting the parents' needs and how well the parents are coping. Health psychologists can play an important role in the TEAM approach, especially given that NICU can be a hectic place for nursing staff.

In addition, there will be instructions to follow regarding such things as medication, diet, and activity levels. These can be complicated, and they can be made worse by a patient who stubbornly refuses to follow the regimen. All of these potential strains are magnified in a home where relationships are not strong to begin with. Good discharge planning tries to take as many of these factors into account as possible.

There might not be a great deal the hospital staff can do to optimize discharge arrangements in high-risk situations. After all, if the patient is physically able to be discharged, there will be another patient ready to be admitted and use the bed. Still, other professionals can help. For example, social workers and psychologists can help make the transition from hospital to home go more smoothly. This is particularly true for elderly patients who are likely to need longer-term home care that can be a full-time job in itself.

It has been estimated that the average hospital stay for people under the age of 65 in Canada is 7.7 days (Wells, 1997). Compare that to the average for people 65 years and over, which is 35.3 days. Elderly patients, then, are likely to have a more difficult time at discharge because they have grown accustomed to hospital support and routine. Problems with discharge planning for elderly patients are compounded by the fact that the planning is time consuming, and so it must be started early. This means that discharge planning is taking place before the patient's medical condition has been clearly ascertained and effectively treated. One study that analyzed the discharge-planning process for 31 elderly patients discovered that, for 27 of the patients, their planning started before their medical status was clearly determined. As a result, discharge plans had to be altered in 26 of these 27 cases (Wells, 1997). As you can imagine, patients find these changes upsetting, especially when it means lengthening the hospital stay. In fact, even the communication of early discharge decisions can be stressful because, at that point, the patient might have trouble imagining being capable of managing at home.

There are other challenges involved with discharge planning for elderly patients. They may have other functional problems secondary to the medical condition being treated but still very important to consider regarding discharge. Can they walk unaided? Can they see and hear well? Also, what are the physical capabilities of the principle caregiver? This question is especially important if the person is an elderly spouse. One way to take these functional limitations into account is to involve family members in the discharge-planning process. In the study of the 31 patients mentioned above, it was found that this involvement was sporadic (Wells, 1977), even though the staff regularly discussed discharge.

The major dilemma for elderly patients involves the balancing of adequate care with the patient's desire for autonomy. Patients may have realistic worries about "never being the same again" after their hospital stay. To cope with these worries, they may shun assistance or attempt to veto discharge plans that create an impression of dependence rather than independence. Social workers, psychologists, health care workers, and family members must help the patient make discharge plans that achieve this balance between safety and autonomy, and they must do so without being patronizing or dictatorial. The key is to involve the patient in the discharge-planning process as much as possible. This requires a sensitive understanding of the patient, the options available, and his or her health. This understanding can only be achieved if all involved adopt a team approach.

Palliative Care

For many patients, discharge from the hospital comes because their condition is improving and their prognosis is good. This does not apply to all patients, though. Some have illnesses that are called **progressive**, meaning they will continue to worsen in spite of treatment. The progressive illness of some patients is **advanced**, which means it is at a stage where death is imminent. For these patients, care shifts from an attempt to cure the illness to a regimen intended to control pain and other symptoms. A primary goal becomes the pursuit of as good a quality of life as is possible for the remaining time the patient is expected to live. Another goal is reducing distress for the patient, family, and loved ones (Hearn & Higginson, 1998). This is the goal and focus of **palliative care**.

One important decision here concerns just where the palliative care will be administered. There are three common choices: the hospital, the home, or a hospice. Hospice facilities represent a compromise between the comfort of home and the medical support of a hospital. At this point, we will focus more on palliative care as provided by hospitals. Having said this, it is important to note that hospital palliative care may also involve discharge planning and all the issues we discussed earlier in relation to that process, if the patient and family express a desire to move the site of care to the home or elsewhere. Because of this, palliative care is most successfully provided by multidisciplinary teams that include such people as physicians, nurses, social workers, chaplains, and psychologists. A review of studies assessing the effectiveness of such teams discovered that they yielded as good or better outcomes than individual planners concerning patient and family satisfaction, patients being cared for as they wished, a reduction of family anxiety, and patient pain and symptom control (Hearn & Higginson, 1998).

We have said that one of the goals of palliative care is pain management. However, in many cases pain is undertreated in palliative settings. A study of over 2 800 seriously ill patients revealed that 23 percent were living with moderately severe or extremely severe pain. No wonder that 49 percent preferred a course of treatment aimed at relieving that pain, and that 51 percent said they would rather die than permanently live with their pain. Half of the patients who are able to communicate during the last few days of their lives report moderate to severe pain (Ng & von Gunten, 1998).

It is difficult to know why pain is undertreated in palliative care. It is possible that patients, trying to appear stoic or brave, do not communicate their pain very well (Poole & Craig, 1992). It is also possible that practitioners working in palliative care see so much pain that their sense of what is normative is quite high. In other words, a patient might be in moderately severe pain but not in an *abnormal* amount of pain compared to other patients. Whatever the reason, it is clear that we have yet another problem that is best approached with clear communication. Family and friends can help give practitioners a clear sense of the patient's discomfort, and practitioners can learn to read non-verbal cues that indicate pain.

Staff working in palliative care face death on a daily basis. To cope with this, they must shed the prevailing belief in acute care that death is tantamount to failure (Payne, , & Kalus, 1998). They must adjust their goals so that they are consistent with those of palliative care. Moreover, they must come to grips with their own anxieties and fears about death. Perhaps this is why one study found that hospice nurses were less death avoidant and less concerned about their own death than emergency room nurses were (Payne, Dean, & Kalus, 1998).

While practitioners in acute care do everything they can to keep patients alive, practitioners working in palliative care must make difficult decisions that will actually result in a patient's death. Technology exists to keep patients alive virtually indefinitely—long after there is any hope that the patient will regain consciousness. Independent of debates about **euthanasia** (the deliberate ending of a patient's life to relieve suffering), palliative care practitioners must decide when it has become futile to keep a patient alive. It is a physician's responsibility to give a **do not resuscitate order**, meaning that CPR or other interventions will not be used if the patient stops breathing.

The ethics of this decision are complex. Most practitioners believe that seriously ill patients deserve the right to be involved in resuscitation decisions. However, how does the physician decide which patients are sufficiently "seriously ill" to warrant that discussion? When this decision is made, the patient moves from the world of the living to that of the dying (Teno & Coppola, 1999). In some palliative care units, these discussions are initiated with patients who are expected to live less than 6 months. At this point, palliative care units provide what has been called a **mixed management model of care**. They prepare the patient for eventual death while at the same time providing life-sustaining treatments (Teno & Coppola, 1999). We will talk in more detail about acceptance of death and stages of dying in Chapter 11. For now, try to get a sense of what this unit of the hospital would be like, with a very different focus from the rest of the hospital and many difficult decisions to be made. At the same time, nurses working in palliative care do not report higher levels of stress than do nurses working in other units. Many palliative care nurses will tell you that their patients have come to terms with their own death, and face the prospect calmly.

Focus on Research 7.2 — Children in Hospital: The Role Parents Play

We have seen in this chapter that a hospital stay and the procedures patients go through in the hospital can be difficult to cope with. But what about children who must be hospitalized? How do they fare? It has been discovered that 83 percent of children hospitalized for tonsillectomy and/or adenoidecomy displayed distress 5 to 7 days after discharge. This was according to their parents.

Perhaps one way to reduce this distress is to involve the parents as much as possible during the hospital stay. While this may seem reasonable, there is considerable debate in health care regarding the value of parental involvement in pediatric procedures. Some physicians say they are less proficient when parents are present, perhaps because the parents make them nervous. Also, parents' anxiety can become distracting or difficult. This can make the child more anxious and cause parents to get in the way physically. In fact, parents have been known to faint at these times, becoming yet another patient. Having parents present is more time consuming because the staff must explain each step of the procedure as they go along (Bauchner et al., 1996). On the positive side, parents can help reduce the child's anxiety that would have been caused by separation. They can generally help calm the child and help monitor his or her condition (Smith & Bassett, 1996).

The debate about parental presence was addressed in a study of children under the age of 3 years undergoing stressful procedures such as receiving needles for blood drawing, or urethral catheterization (Bauchner et al., 1996). The children were placed in one of three groups in which parental involvement varied. In the first group, parents were present and were given instructions regarding touching, talking, and eye contact. In the second group, parents were present but no instructions were given. In the third group, parents were not present.

Parents and clinicians were asked to rate the child's pain during the procedure. In addition, the children's crying was analyzed. The parents' assessments and the clinicians' assessments were unaffected by whether the parents were present or whether they had received instructions. There were, however, significant differences between the parents' assessments and those of the clinicians. Fifty-two percent of the parents rated their children's pain as extreme or severe; only 15 percent of the clinicians gave that rating. It is impossible to determine who is correct here, but it is probably safe to say that parents and clinicians' are using different comparison processes. For the parent, the comparison is the amount of pain their child usually experiences. For the physician, it may well be the amount of pain that is common for the procedure. Psychologists who study pain (see Chapter 10) would say that both perspectives are valuable, especially if parents are able to stay calm enough to be supportive. Some physicians may argue that many parents can't.

In the study by Bauchner and colleagues (1996), 78 percent of parents wanted to be present for these procedures. Of these parents, 80 percent said it would make them feel better, 91 percent said it would make their child feel better, and 73 percent said they thought it would help the physician. This study also found that parents are actually present for procedures such as these about 62 percent of the time.

KEY TERMS

outpatient
non-invasive procedures
day care patients
total institution
learned helplessness
reactance
monitors
blunters
depersonalization
dehumanization
therapeutic rituals
occupational rituals
technical care
socioemotional care
burnout
patient-centred care
invasiveness
false positive
habit
norm
claustrophobia
motion artifacts
fear of suffocation
fear of restriction
hospital separation
continuity of care
psychoeducational care
patient-controlled analgesia (PCA)
lock-out interval
incommunication stage
readaptation stage
reflexion stage
discharge planning
progressive illness
advanced illness
palliative care
euthanasia
do not resuscitate order
mixed management model of care

Chapter 8

THE HEALTH CARE PROVIDER

Chapter Outline

Key Questions

1. What is medical school like? What sort of practitioner does medical school produce?
2. What are the common challenges and stressors in medical practice?
3. What are the possible consequences of excessive stress for a physician?
4. What do nurses do?
5. How stressful is nursing and what are the factors affecting that stress?
6. What are the main gender-related issues in health care?
7. What are the psychological factors relevant to physical rehabilitation, and what role do physical therapists play in addressing those factors?
8. How do technologists help people cope with potentially stressful high-tech diagnostic and treatment procedures?

Jason's older sister was a doctor. He remembered how she had studied for an entire summer for her MCAT exams, a requirement for entrance to medical school. Then came the interviews and the anxious waiting to see if she had been accepted. Jason also remembered very clearly the day his sister learned that she had been accepted into medical school. She was thrilled, her parents were thrilled. Even Jason was thrilled even though he had only been 10 years old at the time.

Jason remembered all this because he was now studying for his MCAT exams. Like his sister, he had given up an entire summer to study, putting in 40 or 50 hours a week. There were times, though, when he doubted whether it was all going to be worth it. When he talked to his sister recently, she made it clear that the practice of day-to-day medicine, and the rigours of medical school, weren't always as thrilling as that day when she found out she had been accepted into medicine. The workload at medical school was staggering. And when she became a physician, she discovered that her ability to actually cure people was more limited than she had expected.

On her more discouraging days, she felt as though her job was to help people cope with conditions that either never went away or went away only to come back. Certainly, medical science was not magical in its power to heal. And there was the pager. At first, it had seemed like a symbol of her success. Now it felt more like a ball and chain. It beeped at the most inconvenient of times, and she had to answer it. Finally, Jason's sister had told him that she was proud to be a physician and that she really did feel that she was helping people in important ways, but that being a doctor wasn't as glamorous as it might appear to people outside the profession.

> Very little of my work was glamorous in the TV drama sense, but much of it was intense.
> A family physician (Coombs, 1998, p. 175).

In Chapter 1, we made the point that health psychologists receive different training from most other people working in health care. The main difference is, of course, the emphasis placed on biomedical knowledge in the training of physicians, nurses, technologists, physiotherapists, etc. These differences in background make for understandable differences in perspective when it comes to health and health care. While understandable, these differences still must be overcome if health psychologists are to make contributions regarding people's health.

It is important for health psychologists to have an appreciation for the training health care providers receive and the stresses they deal with on a daily basis. For example, it is of little use to simply tell a family physician that he or she must spend more time listening to patients and explaining things to them if we have no appreciation for the number of patients that physician must see in a given day. Similarly, a nurse may appear less compassionate than a patient would like because that nurse has a large patient load that includes some seriously ill people. In short, health psychology must often be practised within the realities of the health care system, which includes the lives of health care professionals.

In this chapter, we will look closely at what it is like to be a health care provider. Our main objective is to provide some understanding of the realities of their work. The hope is that the interventions we suggest as health psychologists will be better received and more feasible if we have this understanding.

PHYSICIANS

Few professions match medicine for responsibility and status. The ability to alleviate suffering, and the responsibility for life itself can make a career in medicine both intensely satisfying and extremely stressful. In this section, we will explore reasons why people want to become physicians, then we will look closely at the medical school experience. We will then discuss some of the realities of day-to-day practice.

Why People Choose a Career in Medicine

People are drawn to medicine for a variety of reasons. A study comparing over 2 000 male and female physicians (Neittaanmaki & Luhtala, 1993) discovered that 42 percent of women and 30 percent of men chose medicine because it was a lifelong calling. They were interested in helping people (78% of the women and 71% of the men). Fifty-eight percent of the female physicians and 47 percent of the males said success in school was an important factor. High status and high pay were also important, though men were more likely to cite these reasons than were women. Not surprisingly, physicians are more likely than the general population to have a mother or father who is a physician.

As far as the type of person who goes into medicine, research indicates that there are very few differences between medical students and others on personality characteristics. Medical students don't score higher on measures of altruism, for example. They do, however, score consistently higher on compulsivity (Krakowski, 1985). This can manifest itself as meticulous attention to detail or the repeated checking of procedures to reassure oneself that things have been done correctly. In fact, research has shown that 80 percent of physicians show marked compulsivity, and 20 percent have what the authors called compulsive personality disorder. The same study found that only 28 percent of lawyers were compulsive and that 12 percent met the criteria for the disorder (Krakowski, 1983).

It appears, then, that physicians are similar to others in terms of personality. But what about differences among specialties within medicine? Is there, for example, such a thing as a "surgeon personality?" While you may know people who can tell stories of surgeons with large egos or a flare for the dramatic, research shows that surgeons are no different from other medical specialists in terms of personality. In this research, even surgeons and anesthesiologists believed that surgeons' personalities were different from those of others in medicine (Coombs & Fawzy, 1993). However, it is common for people to believe that personality differences exist, even though data from personality tests do not indicate such differences. This may be because it is easier for us to understand our social world if we stereotype people by making mental connections between profession and personality. Rather than acknowledging the reality that there are many different types of people who perform surgery, we simplify things by creating an image of the egotistical, decisive, and aggressive surgeon and assume this image applies to all of them.

Medical School

We have stated in this chapter that health psychologists must have a clear understanding of what it is like to be a health care professional. We also made the point in Chapter 1 that the intense training a physician receives equips him or her with a biomedical view of health and illness, just as a psychologist's training equips him or her with a psychosocial view. For these reasons, it can be very helpful for people studying health psychology to have an appreciation for the nature of medical school training. From this appreciation, we may be able to understand the comments of one medical student who said of his sociology class, "I waited for a half an hour for a *fact* to write down" (Sinclair, 1997, p. 166; author's emphasis). Or another student who said of his psychology class, "Psychology's interesting when she (the lecturer) is talking about (doctor-patient) interaction, but nothing much else" (Sinclair, 1997, p. 166).

There have been a number of good books written on medical school, some for premed students who want to know how to survive medical school, others by anthropologists and other social scientists trying to understand the culture of medical school. One book that actually does both is *Surviving Medical School*, by Robert Coombs (1998). In his book, Coombs takes the reader through medical school, year by year.

The Premed Syndrome

If there is such a thing as a medical school mentality, and Coombs presents a convincing case that there is, it may well start before students even enter medical school. Premed students are often considered to be highly competitive and non-cooperative. In fact, cases have been documented of students sabotaging other students' labs to gain a competitive edge. Students exhibiting the premed syndrome are more likely to take classes solely to meet requirements and improve their GPA. They cannot afford to try a course that might expose an academic weakness. Finally, these students tend to have romanticized expectations of medical school. Of course, not all premed students fit this syndrome, but enough do to make this sense of extreme competitiveness and glorified expectations a problem for those who are accepted into medical school.

First Year

No matter how much warning an incoming student may have had, he or she is always surprised by the workload in first-year medicine. The volume of work and the time pressure are overwhelming. One student said, "It's like trying to drink from a fire hose" (Coombs, 1998, p. 19). In fact, it is virtually impossible to learn everything that is presented. This causes first-year students to wonder if they should have gone to medical school in the first place. Their self-confidence plummets. Yet, they don't complain to their peers because they would look weak, and there is a social taboo against weakness. Despite the onslaught of material, few students fail first year. Somehow, they survive.

Another very important part of first year is what is called dissection. If you have performed a dissection, it was probably on a frog or fetal pig or some other animal. First-year medical students dissect **cadavers**, bodies that have been donated to medical school. The cadaver experience is a major one for almost all first-year students. Some cover the face of their cadaver with a towel while they dissect other parts of the body. Some students report disrupted patterns of eating and sleeping, complete with nightmares (Finkelstein, 1986). Simon Sinclair, in his revealing description of a British medical school, refers to the dissection experience as a "rite of passage" (Sinclair, 1997, p. 171). For those students who keep their cadaver's face covered during most of the dissection, things become very difficult when they are required to *dissect* that face. This may come after the cadaver's skull has been removed to expose the brain. As you can imagine, some students cope by using dark humour, others by being highly professional. Most report that, during the dissection, the work becomes so interesting that they forget they are working on a body that once belonged to a living human being.

Second Year

The second year is often considered the most stressful academically. Having said that, students come to accept the fact that they can never know everything there is to know. They tell first-year students not to be upset by the fact that they can't learn everything, but first-year students don't usually listen.

For second-year students, a transformation begins to take place. They tend to become more assertive and confident. They will ask questions that show they are now focusing on what needs to be known for the patient's sake, rather than for the exam. Concurrent with this, second-year students begin to really feel the financial strain of medical school. Most don't feel they can continue to rely on their families for financial support, and costs continue to mount.

The social relationships of many second-year students begin to take on a unique quality. A differentiation emerges between those on the "inside" and those on the "outside" of medical school. Second-year students report enjoying an elevated status among those on the "outside"; yet, loneliness is common. This is due in part to the fact that many people on the "outside" don't understand medical school and are generally unsympathetic to students' complaints about it. They reason, "How hard can school be? You don't have to work for a living. And besides, you're going to be a doctor and make lots of money." It is at this point that a supportive spouse is worth his or her weight in gold.

Third Year

In most medical programs, third-year students begin to receive their clinical experience. They interact directly with patients in a hospital setting. This yields a whole new set of insecurities, for, in spite of the fact that they have learned a great deal in their first 2 years, they still do not know enough to take on the duties of a physician. They are not a physician yet but are expected to act like one. This becomes especially evident when third-year students must perform physical examinations. Students say that their lack of confidence was blatant when they were drawing blood or starting IVs, for example. Third-year students in clinical training are struck by the large gap between their textbooks and the real patients they are treating. Patients almost never lay out their symptoms as neatly as in a textbook. This leaves the student feeling uncertain and inadequate. Interestingly, Coombs reports that patients are usually quite accepting of these students. For them, the student is providing treatment, so she must be a doctor.

In these clinical settings, it is imperative that students learn as much as they can. However, the teaching in these situations can be sporadic, given the demands on the physicians of clinical work. Not surprisingly, students report that sometimes they are taught and other times they feel they are just getting in the way.

A number of challenging issues emerge for third-year students—issues that they must either come to grips with or be plagued by throughout their careers. For example, they must accept that they will make mistakes. They must strike a balance between clinical competence and unrealistic expectations of perfection. Unfortunately, mistakes are rarely discussed in medical school, so students get little help in how to deal with them.

There is also the challenge of contagion. Many of us deal with people in our jobs, but few of us worry that we will get seriously ill by doing so. The physician, however, must deal with this all the time. There are many contagious diseases physicians are exposed to, for example, AIDS. One student admitted to spending less time than he should have with a typhoid fever patient because of fear of contagion. That student is not alone. Closely related to this is susceptibility to accidents that may compromise a student's health. In a study of medical students at the University of Washington School of Medicine, almost half of one graduating class reported having had a needle-stick injury or being splashed with fluids that were infectious (Turk, 1993).

It is in the clinical training of third year that most students have their first encounter with critically ill patients. The intensive-care unit (ICU) is a good example (see Chapter 7 on hospital stays for a review of psychological issues associated with ICU). Students are taught to cope by immersing themselves in the work, using humour, and coming to realize that death is not always tantamount to failure.

In fact, dealing with death is another major challenge. Students learn to dehumanize the patient in order to cope with death. They may refer to patients in parts and pieces, talking about "the pancreas in 371." The practice of medicine can become a battle between death and medical science—a battle in which the patient becomes an object or "playing field." When personal feelings about death do arise, they are rarely discussed, again for fear of appearing weak or unsuited to the profession.

It is important to note that, while our discussion focuses on physicians, many of these challenges also apply to other health professionals. Nurses are an excellent example. In one case, a nurse was reported to have organized a service for a patient who had died after a long hospital stay. No other nurses attended the service. When asked why, one nurse said that if she started to cry for this patient, she would cry for all the patients she had seen die and would never stop crying (Coombs, 1998).

Fourth Year

By senior year, a student's socialization into the medical community is virtually complete. He or she will likely have developed a manageable level of emotional distancing from patients. This is to say that the student is not so distant as to appear uncaring, but not so close as to suffer from the exhaustion of limitless caring. Also, by this point most students have lost their sense of idealism regarding medicine, beginning to accept that there are limits to a physician's powers to heal and always be correct.

Internship and Residency

In the first year post-graduation, a physician does a year of **internship**. Rather than marking the end of the labour-intensive training period, internship, if anything, appears more demanding still. Work schedules of 90 to 120 hours per week are not uncommon in some hospitals. After internship, comes **residency**. Residents, or house officers, as they are sometimes called, are susceptible to burnout. They encounter a rather sudden increase in accountability, and a decrease in sleep. A study of residents found that the length of uninterrupted periods of sleep ranged from 40 to 86 minutes (Lurie et al., 1989). This is the case for a resident's on-call nights, when he or she is in the hospital for the entire night. To help residents cope with the demands of on-call nights, they are advised to prioritize their sickest patients, respond to their beepers quickly, and always try to prevent rather than treat (Peterkin, 1998). To make matters even more challenging, residents who work in urban hospitals, especially late at night, must be aware of danger signs signalling potentially violent patients. No wonder they are encouraged to use the support of people like the chief physician and chief resident (Peterkin, 1998).

Physicians' Emotional Involvement in Their Work

At the beginning of this chapter, we quoted a family physician who said that his work wasn't as dramatic as television but that it was still intense. It is important for health psychologists to have an appreciation of that intensity and to know how many physicians deal with it. One of the best ways to do this, of course, is to talk with physicians and get first-hand accounts. This would require a close enough relationship for the physician to feel comfortable disclosing some personal feelings and accounts, however. We must remember, also, that physicians themselves report a reluctance to discuss emotional aspects of their work. Another way to gain insights into what physicians face on an emotional level is to read sections of medical journals in which physicians write candidly about dilemmas they have faced. For example, try reading the section entitled "Heart and Soul" in the *Canadian Medical Association*

Journal, "A Piece of My Mind" in past issues of the *Journal of the American Medical Association*, or "Personal Views" in the *British Medical Journal*.

In a recent issue of the *British Medical Journal*, a physician describes clearly and concisely the dilemma presented by uncertainty in medical diagnosis:

> In a burst of honesty her doctor had the temerity to admit that variations in practice exist. Instead she wants a cut-and-dried answer because that is her expectation. Behind her are years of conditioning to believe that as medicine is a science it must produce hard facts and straightforward answers (Harrison, 1999, p. 793).

Later in this chapter, we will discuss the extent of decision-making uncertainty in medicine and explore its effects on physician stress levels.

In these sections of medical journals, you may read articles like "No Pretending Not to Know" , in which a physician recounts a case in which an ultrasound exam confirms that a woman's fetus has no skull or brain. At first, he grapples with the question of who should inform the woman who has just undergone the exam. In this case, as the radiologist, he could have let her own doctor tell her, or perhaps the resident obstetrician. However, the woman could sense something was wrong. There is no avoiding the truth, as the physician's description makes abundantly clear:

> "Did you see the baby's head?" Her question couldn't have been more to the point. My internal debate about who should tell her the results becomes academic. I pull up a chair next to her. "We've found something wrong with your baby, Mrs. J. Your baby's brain didn't develop." She is stunned, and for what seems like several minutes she says nothing. From her facial expression I can tell that she doesn't really understand. I try again to explain what is wrong with her baby. "What will happen when the baby is born?" she asks. I tell her that her baby will live a very short time and then die. She wants to know if there is any way her baby can live and even be somewhat normal: I have to tell her no (Brown, 1988, p. 2720).

Few professions feature this type of conversation. Of course, not all conversations between patients and physicians feature negative emotions. There is the elation of normal childbirth and the relief patients feel when they are informed they are not seriously ill. The point is that such extreme emotional experiences are potentially exhausting and distracting. For this reason, most physicians find that they must learn to control their emotions, avoiding the peaks and valleys their patients may encounter. To do this requires the ability to distance oneself from one's patient. It is difficult, however, to do this and still make it clear that the physician truly cares for his or her patient's well-being.

As we saw in our discussion of medical school, medical students learn to dehumanize their patients by referring to them as body parts rather than people. This is another way to maintain emotional control. Another is to use humour, which can neutralize situations that would otherwise be very sad. Thus, some physicians will use the initials **CTD** to describe a patient who is about to die; CTD stands for "circling the drain" (DiMatteo, 1991, p. 267).

Physicians and Stress

The responsibility that is an integral part of a physician's life has the potential to be very stressful. A study of over 2 000 Canadian physicians discovered that 38 percent described their practice as being very or extremely stressful (Burke & Richardsen, 1990). In addition to the basic responsibilities that come with caring for patients, there are other aspects of a physician's work that can add to the problem. For example, physicians often work under time pressure (Richardsen & Burke, 1991). If you have ever sat in your doctor's waiting room for any length of time, you will probably have noticed how often the phone rings as people try to make appointments. Many of these people want to see the doctor as soon as possible and so they are "fit in." While we appreciate this consideration as patients, it makes for a hectic day for the physician, who must try to somehow strike a balance between giving people ample time and moving patients through in a timely fashion. And all of this is thrown into chaos if an emergency occurs. It is not surprising that work overload is cited by physicians as a significant source of stress (Burke & Richardsen, 1990).

Medicine is not the only profession in which time pressure and work overload are commonplace. In medicine, however, there is always the possibility that a patient's condition may be life threatening, and this is something that doesn't enter into many other professions. Indeed, **fear of death** has been identified as a source of stress for physicians. It has been suggested that, for some physicians, it was fear of death that motivated them to go into medicine in the first place (Krakowski, 1982). They wanted to be able to stave off death for others. The problem, of course, is that some patients will die, no matter how skilled a physician may be. It is at these times that the physician runs headlong into a contradiction between the realities of everyday practice and the ideals of medicine. For many physicians (with the possible exception of those working in palliative medicine), the death of a patient is viewed as a failure. A physician must overcome this view to reduce the stress attendant upon patient of death, which is more difficult to do if the physician fears death.

Even if physicians do not fear death and have accepted the fact that, despite their best efforts, some patients will die, they still must face the stress of communicating bad news to patients and their families. This stressor is more common in some specialties than others, such as oncology. In a study of this source of stress, 38 physicians were asked to recall a time when they had given a patient bad news. The physicians were then asked some questions based on their memory of the encounter. Most physicians followed published guidelines when giving bad news, though this did not eliminate the stress they felt when doing so. They felt that they had done an effective job of reducing their patients' distress but that their own discomfort and stress had started prior to the encounter and lasted beyond the end of the encounter. The conclusion of this research was that published guidelines on the giving of bad news are helpful in reducing patient distress, but more attention has to be paid to the distress felt by the physician (Ptacek, Fries, Eberhartd, & Ptacek, 1999).

There are a number of other aspects of the job that can be stressful for physicians. As we mentioned earlier, doctors working in hospitals in residency or as house officers often suffer from sleep deprivation (Walerstein & Rosner, 1989). There is also the stress that comes from concerns over malpractice litigation (Charles & Wilbert, 1985). Not surprisingly, physicians who have been sued report more stress than those who have not.

Uncertainty as a Source of Stress

Another significant source of stress that is not always obvious to the general public is **uncertainty**. We like to think that medicine is a precise science, but it is not. In an article by Lurie and Sox (1999), the authors make two important points regarding uncertainty. First, "Clinical examinations and other diagnostic tests are imperfect" (p. 493); and second, "The consequences of medical decisions are inherently uncertain at the decisive moment" (p. 493).

This means that a given diagnosis is often accompanied by a degree of uncertainty, and **prognosis**, a prediction of how a medical condition will change in the future, is even more uncertain. Like most people trying to predict the future or analyze something that is difficult to see, physicians work with probabilities rather than absolute certainties.

Indeed, Lurie and Sox (1999) advocate the use of probability statistics varying from 0 to 1 when talking about prognosis and health outcomes, rather than imprecise language such as "possible" or "unlikely." This assumes that patients can understand the meaning of something like a .7 probability and that physicians can adjust probabilities, based not only on what research and experience tell them regarding the frequency of a given medical outcome, but also on the unique characteristics of the patient being treated.

Imagine a dialogue between a neurosurgeon and a patient who is trying to decide whether or not to have back surgery.

Patient: I don't mind going through the surgery if I know it will work. Will it take my pain away?

Physician: For people with your condition, the probability that the surgery will relieve your pain is .7.

Patient: .7? That would be great a batting average in baseball, but I'm not sure what it means for me.

Physician: It means that for every ten times I performed this operation on someone like you, I would expect it to be successful seven times.

Patient: Yeah, but you're only going to perform it once on me.

It is likely that the majority of patients don't have a good understanding of the meaning of probability statistics (Kahneman & Tversky, 1973). It is also likely that they do not have a good idea of how much uncertainty exists in medical decision-making. In a study of this, patients were asked to estimate the accuracy with which diagnosis would be made for six different conditions presented to them as written descriptions (Hamm & Smith, 1998). Interestingly, the patients' estimates did not differ across conditions. This suggests that people have a general belief about how correct medical science is and apply that belief regardless of the condition in question. The medical truth is that some conditions are considerably easier to diagnose than others and so certainty varies from one situation to the next.

Further, the patients' estimates of accuracy were quite unrealistic. In particular, they underestimated the likelihood of a false-positive diagnosis. Taken collectively, then, this means that patients believe that diagnostic certainty is greater than it really is, regardless of the condition being diagnosed. It should be noted, though, that patients who have direct experience with a given condition were slightly better at estimating the diagnostic accuracy associated with it.

This level of faith in medical science only adds to the potential stressfulness of uncertainty for the physician. A patient thinks a physician should know and does know exactly what the diagnosis is and what the treatment should be. On the other side of the consultation, the physician is very aware of the level of uncertainty that exists. The physician's response to this situation ranges from communicating that uncertainty with a probability statistic to denying the uncertainty altogether (Hamm & Smith, 1998).

All of this takes place in a context in which each party may be concerned with some possibility of which the other isn't even aware (Bergh, 1998). In addition, physicians commonly identify a treatment plan and then name the illness to fit the plan (for example, bronchitis; see Bergh, 1998). Patients are also often more interested in the physical explanation than in the treatment anyway. Taken together, you have two people who aren't really interacting in a way that makes it any easier for the physician to deal with the stress of uncertainty (Bergh, 1998).

Of course, one way for the physician to cope with uncertainty is to deny it. When a group of physicians was presented with an identical video depicting an atypical breast case, half of them diagnosed benign breast disease, one-third identified breast cancer as the most probable initial diagnosis, six percent called it normal, and nine percent gave a diagnosis unrelated to breast disease (McKinlay et al., 1998). Generally, physicians' reports of certainty were high in this study. Now, before you give up on medical decision-making altogether, remember that the decision-making simulated in this study is *preliminary* in nature. Further tests would likely be ordered to yield a more definitive diagnosis. However, diagnostic uncertainty may result in excessive testing, which is another source of stress for physicians and patients.

As we have already mentioned, medical tests don't completely eliminate uncertainty, either. Tests differ in their **sensitivity** and **specificity**. Sensitivity refers to a test's ability to pick up true positives—actual cases of the disease. Specificity refers to its ability to pick up true negatives—cases where disease is definitely *not* present (see Lurie & Sox, 1999).

A final point to make about uncertainty in medical decision-making is that it is more common in primary-care physicians than it is among specialists. **Primary-care physicians** include those in general and family practice. Differences between primary-care physicians and specialists regarding certainty are not due to differences in skill levels. They exist because physicians of all types tend to solve problems through pattern recognition. Primary-care physicians see a wider range of symptoms; therefore, they would have far too many patterns to remember and possibly too few of any particular symptom to even form a pattern in the physician's experience. Also, more problems are presented early in their history to primary-care physicians, so patterns have not yet been well defined. A physician may reasonably say to a patient, "There are three possibilities. It will either get better, worse, or stay the same. If it starts to get worse, see me right away." By contrast, the specialist sees a much narrower range of problems and symptoms, usually when they have reached a stage where the diagnosis has become more clear.

In spite of these differences between primary-care physicians and specialists, patients usually report greater satisfaction with their primary-care physician than with their specialist, because the former provides continuous, person-focused care. By contrast, the specialist tends to provide low-continuity, disease-focused care (Rosser, 1996). This means that patients are less concerned about specialized diagnostic certainty than they are about the nature of the relationship they have with the physician. This may be because patients generally believe that levels of certainty are high and similar across diagnostic settings (Hamm & Smith, 1998).

Regardless of these patient perceptions, the most important point to remember here is that physicians tend to find decision-related uncertainty to be a significant source of stress for them and that there is no easy solution to the problem. Perhaps this is why physicians sometimes cope by using rather dark humour. For example, DiMatteo (1991) describes physicians telling one another a patient has **GOK** (p. 267), which stands for "God Only Knows."

The Consequences of Stress for Physicians

Prolonged stress can have physical and psychological consequences for everyone. We outlined these in Chapter 5 in our discussion of stress and coping. In medicine, the consequences can be more severe because the care of the patient might also be compromised if a physician is not coping well with stress. Physicians are well aware of this, and this awareness can create a vicious cycle in which the physician experiences *more* stress from the guilt and pressure of not providing adequate care.

Physicians are no more likely than people in other professions to suffer from physical illness, but they are more likely to suffer from psychological problems. Affective disorders (for example, depression), suicide, and addiction are problems in medicine (Krakowski, 1982). Other research has identified exhaustion, depression, drug and alcohol dependency, and suicide as consequences of stress for physicians (Vincent, 1983).

Physician impairment

The conditions accompanying stress are doubly problematic. Not only do they compromise the physician's quality of life, they compromise the physician's ability to provide care. For these reasons, researchers looking at physician stress have coined the term **physician impairment**. It refers to a state in which stress-related symptoms interfere with the physician's ability to perform his or her job.

Writing in the *Psychiatric Journal of the University of Ottawa*, Merville Vincent (1983) discussed the difficulties experienced by some 300 physicians who had been admitted as inpatients over a 22-year period. Vincent identified physical and social consequences of stress that could lead to physician impairment, though the focus was on the symptoms rather than impairment. Vincent identified such things as overwork, exhaustion and depression, alcohol and drug dependency, marital problems, and suicide as symptoms of physician stress. Regarding marital and family problems, physicians often find themselves caught between the enormous obligations they feel toward their patients and their families. Spouses of physicians sometimes say their partners are "married to their work." This means that an important source of stress-buffering support is lost to the physician.

The physician has at his or her disposal medication that can, at least on a short-term basis, relieve the symptoms of stress. It is tempting to take these drugs to manage the symptoms but not deal with the underlying cause. Unfortunately, this can lead to dependency that only makes the situation worse. It has been estimated that 10 percent of physicians use drugs such as tranquillizers and analgesics to treat themselves (McAuliffe et al., 1986, cited in DiMatteo, 1991). A study from the 1970s estimated that drug addiction was 30 to 100 times more prevalent among physicians than in the general population (Vaillant, Sobowale, & McArthur, 1972, cited in DiMatteo, 1991). In contrast, a study in the early nineties (Flaherty & Richman, 1993) concluded that addiction to tranquillizers, alcohol, and psychedelics was no greater among members of the medical community than it was among age-matched controls. Yet another study suggests that illicit drug use is no more prevalent among physicians but that abuse of prescription drugs might be (O'Connor & Spickard, 1997).

A study published in the *Canadian Journal of Anaesthesiology*, surveying over 1 600 physicians, found that impairment rates varied from 14.4 percent in surgery to 19.9 percent in medicine (Lutsky et al., 1994). The General Medical Council in Great Britain has reported that half of the physicians who present with health difficulties serious enough to affect professional competency also had an alcohol problem (Harrison & Chick, 1994). In a 30-year retrospective study of anesthesiologists in the United States, 15.8 percent provided responses indicating a substance dependency, either drug or alcohol related (Lutsky et al., 1993). While there may be debate regarding the extent to which alcohol and drug misuse are more common among members of the medical community than in the general population, this misuse is considered a serious problem because the *consequences* can be so significant for health care providers and their patients.

GENDER ISSUES IN MEDICAL PRACTICE

No analysis of health care practitioners would be complete without a discussion of gender issues. Among physicians, men and women bring different attributes to their work, they make somewhat different career choices, and they perceive their work differently from one another. Further, there is evidence that they communicate with their patients differently, and that patients have some specific preferences for their physicians based on the patient's and physician's gender.

The "Feminization" of Medicine

In Canada in 1991, 26 percent of all physicians were female. By 1996, the figure had jumped to 30 percent (Statistics Canada). The number of female medical students in Canada went from 33 percent in 1981 to 44 percent in 1989 (Williams et al., 1990). Others have estimated that in most Canadian medical schools today, females constitute 50 percent or more of the students (Sullivan, 1990). In Finland, the percentage of female physicians has gone from 22 percent in 1960 to 45 percent in 1993 (Mattila-Lindy et al., 1998). In general, women outnumber men four to one in Canadian health care (Statistics Canada). The trend toward increased proportions of female physicians has caused some theorists to speculate on the changes this will bring to the profession. The **feminization of medicine**, as this trend has been called, may bring about changes to the balance between cure and care we talk about later in the chapter in our discussion of nursing. It may also affect the nature of interactions between patients and physicians (De Koninck, Bergeron, & Bourbonnais, 1997). To get a clearer sense of how this could happen, let's look at some specific ways in which male and female physicians differ in their practice of medicine.

Male and Female Physicians' Perceptions of Themselves, their Work, and their Careers

Male and female medical school graduates present somewhat different assessments of their personal attributes (Clack & Head, 1999). A study in Britain found that men were more likely to cite leadership potential, spirit of curiosity, and tolerance of ambiguity and uncertainty as personal attributes. Women were more likely to identify their ability to inspire confidence in others and their ability to listen as well as their caring and compassionate nature (Clack & Head, 1999). As we will see, these differences in the way medical graduates see themselves play themselves out as differences in the way men and women go about the business of medicine as well. In the Clack and Head study, men and women were equally likely to make reference to their excitement with the subject of medicine, their perseverance, and their open-mindedness.

A study in Finland assessed physicians' self-reported values. These were defined as desirable goals that serve to guide the physicians through their lives (Neittaanmäki et al., 1999). It was found that female physicians were more likely to value close friends and what the authors called "universalism", which referred to world peace and an unpolluted environment. Women were also more likely to say they valued doing a good job and gaining the respect of others. Again, these values are manifest in some of the differences in the career choices and interaction styles of male and female physicians. This also applies to a study conducted in North America in which male medical students said the quality they most valued in their own physician was competence, whereas for female medical students this quality was compassion (McFarland & Rhoades, 1998).

Regarding career choices, a study by researchers at Université Laval in Québec City discovered that female physicians place more importance on their private lives when making professional life decisions than do their male counterparts (De Koninck, Bergeron & Bourbonnais, 1997). Interviews with female physicians yielded some clear statements about the way values affected their career choices:

> What is important for women is not the size of their practice, the income, or publications, but the type of practice, personal satisfaction, fulfilling needs…" (a female physician interviewed, De Koninck, Bergeron, & Bourbonnais, 1997). Another woman put it this way: "I didn't want to be just a doctor...I wanted a family, children...I wanted a life that I would call normal...I said to myself, if I go into neurosurgery, I'll never be able to" (a female physician interviewed, De Koninck, Bergeron, & Bourbonnais, 1997).

In a study of medical students at the University of Toronto, 27 percent of the men said they would choose surgery compared to only 10 percent of the women (Baxter, Cohen, & McLeod, 1996). These differences were based, in part, on perceptions regarding the lifestyle demands of the work and the amount of interaction (or lack thereof) surgeons have with patients. Other research with medical students has found that men say they wanted to work longer hours than women did and that women are more likely to want to spend leisure time with their family and friends (McFarland & Rhoades, 1998). Consistent with this, only four percent of orthopedic surgeons in the United States are women (Rowley, Baldwin, & McGuire, 1991).

Once they have made their career choice, female and male physicians have different perceptions of their work. Females are more likely to feel what is called **role strain**. This means that they feel torn by the demands of multiple roles, never being able to handle either to their satisfaction. These roles may include physician, mother, and wife, to name a few. This is compounded by the fact that women report feeling a greater sense of responsibility to others (Gross, 1998).

Given that medicine has historically been male dominated, it is not surprising that women physicians are more likely to perceive discrimination than men are (vanIneveld et al., 1996). A study of internal medicine housestaff in Canada found that 70 percent of female residents said they had experienced discrimination by attending physicians, whereas only 23 percent of male residents reported such discrimination. Similarly, 88 percent of female residents reported discrimination from patients (38% of male residents reported this) and 71 percent of female physicians reported discrimination from nurses, compared to 35 percent for male residents (vanIneveld et al., 1996). Female physicians were also much more likely to state that they had experienced sexual harassment from attending physicians, peers and patients than male residents were. In a study of over 450 female physicians in Ontario, 76 percent said that they had experienced sexual harassment from patients (Phillips, 1996). Perhaps one of the most upsetting findings from the vanIneveld study was that 40 percent of all residents reported having experienced physical assault.

You might think that all this would add up to more stress for female physicians compared to their male colleagues. Research investigating sex differences in stress levels among physicians has yielded mixed results, some showing females to experience more stress and others showing no differences. Gross (1998) analyzed these inconsistent findings, discovering that the studies showing no difference tended to use close-ended scale items to measure stress (e.g., Richardsen & Burke, 1991), whereas the studies finding sex differences used open-ended measures.

Joyce Tinsley (1998) makes the point that discrimination can work both ways. Tinsley presents examples of males in an otherwise all-female medical team who report that their opinions are devalued and that they are excluded from the group's conversations.

Gender Differences in the Provision of Patient Care

Clear differences emerge when the communication styles of male and female physicians are studied. For example, females tend to be more in favour of collaboration with their patients in treatment, they spend more time with their patients, and they are more likely to discuss psychosocial issues and deal with patients' emotions (Roter & Hall, 1998). Women have been found to be more egalitarian than authoritarian in their use of language with patients, preferring words like, "Let's" (West, 1993).

Concerning medical decisions, some research suggests that female and male physicians differ while other research does not. For example, a study in Finland (Mattila-Lindy et al., 1998) looking at medical decisions regarding women's reproductive health found very few differences between male and female physicians. This includes such areas as obstetric practices and hormone therapy during and after menopause. In contrast, a study of physicians across Canada found that female doctors were more liberal regarding their patients' access to amniocentesis than male physicians were. Female physicians also favoured broader access to prenatal diagnoses such as ultrasound (Bouchard & Renaud, 1997). In the United States, it was found that women were more likely to get mammograms if they had a female physician (Lurie et al., 1993). Consistent with this, a study in Washington State showed that female patients of male physicians were twice as likely not to have had a mammogram in the last 2 years (Anderson & Urban, 1997). The interesting thing about the Washington State study is that it controlled for patient characteristics. For example, women with female physicians tended to be younger than those with male physicians.

Still, the differences among these studies could be attributed to differences in physicians' attitudes toward women's health issues in the countries involved. The differences may also be due to differences in the treatment being studied—obstetrics and pre-natal diagnosis versus mammogram.

It is also possible that differences between men and women regarding their clinical decision-making could be explained by differences in their training. Consistent with this, an analysis of over 70 000 patients seen at the Queen's University Family Medical Centre over a 5-year period between 1988 and 1993 found that female residents in family medicine saw 68.4 percent of the female patients. This means that, in the final stages of their training, female physicians see significantly more female patients than male physicians do, at least in family medicine (Sabir, Godwin, & Birtwistle, 1997).

Given these differences, what do we know about patients' preferences for female or male physicians? You might hypothesize that patients generally favour a physician whose gender is the same as their own. Indeed, a study in the 1960s found that urban women preferred female physicians, even at a time when there were significantly fewer of them than there are today (Hopkins et al., 1967). However, more recent research indicates that this preference exists in some cases but it is not a universal law. A study in the Netherlands found that patients had virtually no preference regarding physician gender when the treatment was **instrumental** in nature (this includes such things as surgery and anesthesiology). On the other hand, for physicians with whom they expect a closer relationship, such as general practitioners and obstetricians, patients prefer physicians of the same gender as themselves (Kerssens, Bensing, & Andela, 1997). For example, 88 percent of men and 82 percent of women expressed no preference regarding a surgeon. However, only 72 percent of men had no preference regarding a GP and 53 percent of women had no preference regarding a gynecologist. In that study, 16 percent of men expressed a preference for a male GP and 42 percent of women wanted a female gynecologist. (Five percent of women wanted a male gynecologist.) Similar results have been obtained in Britain (Nichols, 1987). Another interesting finding in the Kerssen and colleagues study is that, of those who expressed a preference regarding a *hospital nurse*, those choosing a female outnumbered those choosing a male 11 to 1.

It is important to note that these preferences are not simply related to the sex-role stereotype that men are supposedly more technically competent and women more humane. In the Netherlands study, men said they thought their male physician was more humane than a female physician would be. The most common reason patients give for a same-sex preference is that they feel they can talk more easily to someone who is the same gender as themselves.

It might also stand to reason that patients' preferences regarding the gender of the physician would depend on the nature of the examination being conducted, given that some exams are more personally intrusive than others. With this in mind, researchers looked at patients' perceptions of male and female physicians giving anal and vaginal exams (Van Elderen, Maes, Rouneau, & Seegers, 1998). Both male and female patients rated female physicians higher than males on a curing dimension for giving anal examinations. For vaginal exams, which were of course rated only by female patients, females were rated more highly on the curing dimension, the caring dimension, and a consulting dimension (see "Nursing" section below for more on curing and caring). So you can see that patient preferences can be more complex than simply having men wanting male physicians and women wanting female ones.

NURSING

Modern nursing in Canada is a profession facing many challenges. The changes in medical science demand that nurses stay current in their knowledge level. The roles that nurses play in modern hospitals are expanding to include many advanced areas such as transplant specialization and cardiac care. In fact, the area of advanced practice nursing is a rapidly expanding one in Canada. Let's take a closer look at advanced practice in nursing to develop a better understanding of what the profession entails today.

The Nature of Modern Nursing

When most lay people think of nurses, they think of people who are involved in **caring** for patients in hospital. This is distinct from the role of the physician, which focuses on the **curing** of people (Watson, 1988). In providing care, nurses make sure that medication is properly administered, that hygienic and dietary needs of the patients are taken care of, and that the emotional needs of the patient are considered as well. In general, they are patient advocates in the hospital setting. Of course, nurses work in settings other than hospitals. They also work in community settings, as public health nurses, as home care nurses, and so on. All of these roles that we commonly associate with nursing have been in place for many years.

There are those who believe that the caring side of health care is being eroded somewhat as modern medicine becomes more technical and specialized (Krebs et al., 1996). This change shifts health care to a cure orientation. Of course, there is nothing wrong with cure. However, when the cure-care balance is disrupted, two problems can arise. First, a two-tier system is created in health care whereby cure is given higher status. This can result in a devaluing of the nurse's role, which is a problem because the reality in health care is that care is more prevalent than cure. Second, cure isn't preventative.

There are two ways that nurses are attempting to make the importance of their role clear. First, they remind us of the importance of a care orientation. Second, they engage in training and job re-definition such that they become more actively involved in cure-related practice.

This advanced training and re-definition of roles in modern nursing has given rise to **advanced practice nursing**. The Canadian Nurses Association (CNA) defines advanced practice as "the role of a nurse working within a specialty area where superior clinical skills and judgement are acquired through a combination of experience and education" (CNA, 1997a, p. 2). In advanced practice, nurses' roles expand to include teaching, consultation, and research.

There are a number of general categories of advanced nursing practice. One is the **clinical nurse specialist**. Nurses with this specialty will hold a master's or doctoral degree in nursing and will have extensive experience in a given clinical specialty. Another category is the **nurse practitioner**. The nurse practitioner often works in rural, remote settings. In these settings, where physicians are often in short supply, the nurse practitioner performs functions that might otherwise be performed by a physician. Thus, the Canadian Nurses Association points out that, for the nurse practitioner, "caring and curing overlap" (CNA, 1997a, p. 4). This category is formally recognized in Ontario, where university-level programs exist for the training of nurse practitioners, and health legislation is now reflecting this expanded role for nurses in provinces such as Alberta and Ontario. As is often the case when roles change and expand, there is debate in health care regarding the most appropriate scope and boundaries of positions such as the nurse practitioner.

Nursing, then, is a profession in which ongoing education has become essential to keep up with advances in technology and nursing research. Many people entering the profession come in with a 4-year bachelor's degree in nursing rather than a registered nursing degree that may take 2 to 3 years to attain. It is clearly a field with exciting challenges. At the same time, nursing can be a stressful profession, as we will see later in this section. Funding cutbacks in health care affect nursing significantly, and so we have a profession in which the demands are high and the resources can at times be inadequate.

Add to this the prediction by the Canadian Nurses Association that, according to an independent study, we will have a shortage of nurses in the order of 59 000 to 113 000 by the year 2001, and there is cause for concern (CNA, 1997b). This projected shortage will result from an aging workforce in nursing and a lack of young people entering the profession. In addition, the population in general is aging, putting increasing demands on the health care system. The Canadian Nurses Association predicts that the demand for registered nurses will climb by 46 percent between 1993 and 2001 (CNA, 1997b).

Why should all this matter to health psychologists? There are a number of reasons. First, increased demands combined with a shortage of resources is a recipe for stress. As we will see in this section, stress is a problem in nursing, for both nurses and patients. You may remember from our discussion of hospital stays in Chapter 7 that we cited Canadian research indicating patient satisfaction was correlated with nurses' self-reports of burnout (Leiter, Harvie, & Frizzel, 1998) (see Focus on Research 7.1). Burnout and stress are closely related. Second, people in health care are not immune to lifestyle-related illnesses—illnesses they spend so much time treating. Third, a considerable amount of hospital research in health psychology involves nurses. Nurses may be asked to administer research protocols in addition to their regular duties. When conducting this research, it is essential to have some understanding of the demands such involvement places on the nurses' already hectic schedules and the implications that our conclusions and recommendations will have for nurses' work.

Stereotypes in Nursing

We referred to stereotypes when we talked about people's impressions of surgeons and how those impressions are often inaccurate. In nursing, stereotypes are even more prevalent. They are propagated by everything from the way nurses are portrayed in get-well cards to the limited knowledge the general public has about the wide range of skills and tasks involved in modern nursing. Dahl (1992) points out that the lay public correctly sees nurses as "professionals who provide care and compassion." The stereotype this engenders is the nurse as handmaiden to the physician, as some people have called it.

Other researchers (Kalisch & Kalisch, 1987) have identified three common stereotypes in nursing. They are based on the erroneous generalization that almost all nurses are young, Caucasian females. These stereotypes, which are exploited in some get-well cards, are the **innocent angel**, the **sex symbol**, and the **frustrated battleaxe**. None of these helps to present nursing as a credible medical profession.

Stereotypes associated with nursing are, of course, gender based. We discussed gender issues in more detail earlier in the chapter. Regarding nursing, consider the following list of traits that one group of participants said were more common in nurses than in doctors:

Extroverted	Follower	Warm
Other-concerned	Generous	Honest
Emotional	Feminine	Emotional

These judgments were derived by presenting people with polar-opposite word pairs and asking them to say which was more like a nurse and which was more like a doctor. For example, nurses were seen as being more "emotional" and doctors more "logical." Nurses were considered more "other-concerned" and doctors more self-concerned (Kaler, Levy, & Schall, 1989). One of the main problems with these stereotypes is that, when nurses accept them, they become more susceptible to stress-related problems such as burnout (Krebs et al., 1996).

Because of the prevalence of stereotypes in nursing, feminists tend to be divided in their opinion of the profession (Reverby, 1993). There are those who believe the profession should be valued because it is important work that women do well. Others, adopting a feminist perspective, criticize the profession for propagating stereotypes of nurturance and subservience. This division of opinion puts female nurses in a no-win situation, which can also be stressful.

Stress in Nursing

Nursing ranks near the top among service occupations in terms of stress (Cooper & Baglioni, 1988). This is not surprising, given the nature of the work nurses do. Indeed, to truly understand what nurses deal with on a daily basis one must have an appreciation for the stressors they face. In 1993, the absenteeism rate at one New Brunswick regional hospital averaged 10.3 days per annum per nurse (Larocque, 1996), and this was related to job dissatisfaction.

People who work in professions in which suffering is common are susceptible to something called **compassion fatigue** (Schwan, 1998). Even for the most caring of people, there are limits to the amount of energy one can dedicate to other people's welfare. When those limits are exceeded, the person with compassion fatigue must either become less compassionate or reduce the number of patients he or she treats. For nurses who work in trauma-related settings, the symptoms of compassion fatigue mimic those of post-traumatic stress disorder, including such things as anxiety, exhaustion, and sleep disruption.

Closely related to compassion fatigue is **burnout**. In a landmark article, Christina Maslach (1979) identified the symptoms of burnout. They are physical exhaustion, depersonalization of patients, and feelings of discouragement and low accomplishment. People suffering from burnout seem to be experiencing an internal conflict between the jaded feelings accompanying the syndrome and the guilt that comes from not caring as much about their patients and their jobs as they believe a professional should.

As we have mentioned, the consequences of stress and its related conditions, compassion fatigue and burnout, are significant. One study found a significant relationship between patient incidents over a 3-month period, such as falling and medication errors, and nurses' scores on a stress index (Dugan et al., 1996). Not only do patients notice burnout when being cared for (Leiter, Harvie, & Frizzel, 1998), nurses with burnout miss more shifts, so patients may miss the nurses entirely (Parker & Kulik, 1995). Worse still, nurses who suffer prolonged burnout tend to leave the profession altogether (Parker & Kulik).

The causes of stress are clear and numerous and begin as soon as someone enters nursing from training. In fact, the transition from student nurse to practitioner can be the first major source of stress. This has been called **reality shock** (Kramer, 1974) and is defined as the reaction to the discrepancy between a training environment and an actual work environment. Newly hired nurses will report that they thought they had been adequately trained but have quickly realized that they still have much to learn, and that it must be learned quickly (Charnley, 1999). The sudden role shift from student to practising nurse can be frightening, since nurses now feel that they should know everything. They find it hard to cope with the volume of work and feel guilty when things don't get done in a timely way. New nurses sense a gap between the high standards they were taught and the lower standards that are the reality of nursing due to heavy demands and limited resources. One conflict many nurses must resolve is the one that exists between the humanistic, nurturing nature of nursing on one hand, and the high-tech, high-traffic demands of modern medicine on the other. Finally, there is the stress of "learning the system", which entails finding out where things are kept and what the norms are and developing relationships with colleagues (Charnley).

For experienced nurses, the sources of stress appear to take on two common forms: understaffing and relationships with managers (Taylor, White, & Muncer, 1999). Regarding the latter, a study of 270 nurses in Australia reported that their main source of distress was abuse from colleagues. This took the form of abusive language, rudeness, and humiliation (Farrell, 1999). Also, multitasking is common in modern nursing and a source of increased stress. At any given moment, a nurse may be required to take numerous tests, manage supplies, complete paperwork, administer medications, and reassure worried family members (Flakus, 1998).

It would stand to reason that some nursing specialties are more stressful than others. For example, oncology (pediatric oncology, in particular) features higher degrees of turnover than some other specialty areas (Hinds et al., 1998). Booth (1998) has studied the intense stress that accompanies unexpected patient death during surgery. This is particularly stressful because the surgical staff may feel that the death was caused by the intervention (and they may be correct). Even if the surgery was the only hope for the patient, staff are often left with the feeling that unexpected death during surgery was due to human error, whether it was or not. Few other professions feature such confrontations with mortality and one's own sense of competence.

While it would be reasonable to expect that some nursing specialties are particularly prone to stress, it would be ill-advised to assume that everyone working in those areas suffers from stress. For example, the main sources of stress for psychiatric nurses come from working with violent or difficult patients. In addition, psychiatric nurses often feel they do not receive the same level of recognition that other nursing specialties enjoy regarding the importance of their work. Given this, one would expect a higher rate of stress among psychiatric nurses, yet one study found that general hospital nurses working in acute care experienced significantly more stress than psychiatric hospital nurses did (Muscroft & Hicks, 1998).

Stress is a significant problem in nursing but is not an insurmountable one. There are ways in which nurses can cope effectively with the stressors of their job, and there are ways institutions can improve the work environment to reduce those stressors. For the nurses themselves, coping depends on personal factors and social factors (Boey, 1999). **Personal factors** include personality characteristics and coping strategies. For example, nurses with high self-esteem and a clear sense of control are less prone to stress. In terms of coping strategies, those who are more stress resistant tend to avoid negative emotion-focused coping. Instead, they use problem-focused coping, trying to find ways to make their job more manageable rather than dwelling upon the frustration and anxiety they may have felt. **Social factors**, as the term implies, refer to those elements of the nurse's social network, such as family, friends, and coworkers.

One of the grand ironies of work in the helping professions is that many people working in them spend most of their energy looking after other people and considerably less looking after themselves. After all, most people who are drawn to professions like nursing want to help others. The problem, of course, is that if nurses don't look after themselves they become less effective at helping others. They become more vulnerable to stress and burnout.

In this vein, we are reminded of what airline flight attendants say to passengers before takeoff. It goes something like this: "In the unlikely event of cabin depressurization, a yellow mask will drop from the overhead compartment. Place the mask over your nose and mouth and begin breathing normally. *If you are travelling with young children or others who need assistance, put your mask on first, before assisting others*."

At the heart of this advice is the common sense notion that we can't help others if we pass out ourselves. This works as an excellent metaphor when talking with nurses about their own health. It is particularly relevant in light of research that has shown nurses to be more overweight than the general population (Pratt, Overfield, & Hilton, 1994) and that student nurses smoked more than those in other professions, had irregular eating habits, and reported some binge drinking (Diltmar, Haughey, O'Shea, & Brasure, 1989). On the optimistic side, research in Ireland has shown that practicing nurses engage in more health-related behaviours than student nurses do (Hope, Kelleher, & O'Connor, 1998).

It is important to note that the feeling of control that can be so helpful in reducing stress is also influenced by hospital management. According to the **Job Strain Model**, a job with high strain is one that features both high demands and low control (Karasek, 1979). This would suggest that policies intended to enhance nurses' sense of control should reduce stress and burnout. Such policies include group meetings, better communication up and down the hierarchy, more say in job design, etc. (Felton, 1998). When these are in place, it is also likely that nurses will feel more committed to their institutions, which is another antidote to burnout (Hinds et al., 1998).

BOX 8-1 Problem-Based Learning: Training Students to Think Like Practitioners

Problem solving is, perhaps, the most important and common mental task for physicians. A patient presents one or more symptoms and it becomes the physician's job to ask the right questions to determine the cause of the symptoms and what to do about them. What brings the symptoms on? What relieves them? What further information is needed? What tests need to be done? When these questions have been answered, a diagnosis must be made and a course of action determined.

Expert physicians and novices don't tend to think the same way (Thomas, 1997). Experts begin rapidly generating hypotheses from the beginning of a consultation with a patient. They are able to test a number of these hypotheses simultaneously as the consultation progresses. In general, they generate better hypotheses because they have a better knowledge base.

Other health care professionals must also be problem solvers, though they may focus more on becoming skilled at carrying out certain procedures. Incoming students have little or no experience with this form of problem-solving or the procedures involved in health care. How can they best be trained, in a relatively short period of time, to be practitioners?

One of the most popular approaches to this training challenge is called **problem-based learning (PBL)**. The curricula employed in PBL use actual cases in an attempt to simulate practice settings (Doucet, Purdy, Kaufman, & Langille, 1998). Students are given a case and must work in groups to solve the problems presented in it. With PBL, students spend more time working autonomously, using resources such as the library to learn what they need to know to solve the problems presented in the case. It is believed that, in doing so, they will retain the knowledge longer and develop better clinical skills (Antepohl & Herzig, 1999). Three hallmarks of PBL are the stimulation of prior knowledge (what do I already know that will help me with this case?), learning in context to improve retention, and the elaboration of knowledge through discussion with other group members (Saarinen-Rahiika & Binkley, 1998).

Problem-based learning was first developed in Canada. It was introduced into the curriculum at McMaster University in Hamilton, Ontario in 1965 (Saarinen-Rahiika & Binkley, 1998). Since then, it has been adopted at a number of Canadian universities and at institutions around the world, including Harvard. In some schools, the entire curriculum is taught this way; in others, PBL is introduced after 1 or 2 years of lecture-based presentation. In still others, individual courses are taught using PBL.

Some of the most extensive research on the effectiveness of PBL has been conducted by David Kaufman and his colleagues at Dalhousie University in Halifax, Nova Scotia. Problem-based learning was implemented at Dalhousie in their Faculty of Medicine in 1992. The first PBL graduating class in 1996 was compared to previous lecture-based classes in their performance on Canadian national licensing exams. It was discovered that the PBL class performed better than previous classes on the psychiatric, preventative medicine, and community health components of the exam. There were no differences between the PBL class and other classes on clinical reasoning scores (Kaufman & Mann, 1998). Problem-based learning has also been used in **continuing medical education (CME)** and has been shown to be superior to lecture-based approaches (Doucet, Purdy, Kaufman, & Langille, 1998). This might be expected, given that CME is intended for practitioners who are returning for further education and have a greater wealth of experience to draw on when working with PBL cases.

Problem-based learning may well alter the way students think during their training, but it doesn't necessarily affect *what* they think about. Susan Philips (1997) from Queen's University in Kingston, Ontario has analyzed the content of a number of cases used in PBL curricula. She concluded that the biomedical, body-as-machine focus of medical training is not altered or augmented in these cases. Phillips also contends that gender bias continues to be present in the way patients are represented in cases.

FOCUS ON RESEARCH 8-1

Hospital Cleaners: Invisible Yet Vital Members of a Hospital's Staff

In this chapter, our discussion of health practitioners has focused on physicians and nurses. This is because these are the most prevalent people in health care. However, they are certainly not the only people who play important roles in health care and, in particular, in the hospital. There are dieticians and people who prepare meals, orderlies, administrators, psychologists, and lab technologists, to name a few.

One group that is essential to the provision of health care in a hospital is the hospital cleaners. However, they are often placed at the bottom of the hospital's hierarchy, which has negative consequences associated with it. In an in-depth study of cleaners in Québec hospitals, Messing (1998) explored both the reasons for this problem and its consequences.

In Messing's study, hospital cleaners told her that there was a common misconception that their job was easy. In fact, this was reflected in their pay scales, which were divided such that "heavy" cleaners were paid more than "light" cleaners. The irony was that "heavy" cleaners used machines to do their work and "light" cleaners did their work by hand, often on their knees. Also, like so many jobs, the cleaners were only noticed when there was a problem. No one seemed to notice the pride they took in their work; to make things shine and improve the cleanliness of the sections they were responsible for, many cleaners found ways to combine their cleaning agents to improve their effectiveness.

Others brought some of their own supplies to do the work.

There are also broader, sociologically based reasons for the devaluing of cleaners. The majority are women, who historically have been expected to clean things up without getting recognition for the importance of the job. The cleaners' work becomes associated with housework, which has been labelled "unproductive" by a society that values the money-making capability of a job. Also, many of the cleaners are members of cultural minorities and are of lower socioeconomic status than other hospital workers, and so a lack of respect for their work carries overtones of cultural, racial, and social prejudice.

You may ask why this should matter to those running hospitals or, in fact, to health psychologists. There are a number of reasons. First, cleaners actually interact with the patients quite a bit while doing their work, yet, because the cleaners are an "invisible" component of the system, they rarely receive any training on how to do so. For example, cleaners must regularly decide whether or not to disturb a patient without having any clear sense of the patient's current condition.

In other cases, patients ask cleaners to do things for them that might be contraindicated, but the cleaner doesn't know this. In Messing's study, she was told of a cleaner who got in trouble for getting a glass of water for a preoperative patient who was to have no fluids. Better communication between cleaners and other staff would have avoided that problem. Further, cleaners worry about contagion. One cleaner reported that, after cleaning a patient's room for a number of days, she arrived to find a quarantine sign on the door. Understandably, she wondered just how serious the problem was and how long it had been a problem. No one had told her. Finally, because there is so little communication with hospital cleaners, spaces are sometimes poorly designed and equipment poorly placed so that it is hard to clean. This can result in absenteeism as cleaners deal with musculoskeletal and cardiovascular problems, which are common to their job.

Hygiene is clearly essential to the effective running of a hospital. However, for reasons relevant to psychology, namely communication problems and stereotyping, this vital aspect might be compromised.

OTHER HEALTH CARE PROFESSIONALS

Focus on Research 8.1 serves as a reminder that physicians and nurses are not the only health care professionals worthy of a health psychologist's attention. In this section, we will look at two other professions in which psychology can play a central role. Certainly, our list of professions discussed in this chapter is far from exhaustive. You are invited to think of ways in which psychology can make constructive contributions to the work of others providing health care.

CASE 8-1 The Long Road Back

One of the most disturbing things for May was that she has no memory whatsoever for the event that has left her feeling so debilitated. One minute she felt fine, and the next she woke up in a hospital, having no idea how she got there. She did know, however, that something terrible had happened. This was because she could feel nothing in her right arm or right leg and she couldn't talk.

May, who was 61 years old, had suffered a stroke, or cerebrovascular accident (CVA), as it is known medically. During the stroke, the blood supply to the left side of her brain had been cut off due to a blockage in the artery. May's family had been told that no one could say for sure just how profound her disability would be. It would depend on biology, medicine, some luck, and May's will to go through rehabilitation.

Over the first few days in the hospital, May did show some improvement. Some of her speaking ability returned, much to the relief of her family, but she still found verbal communication enormously frustrating. And then there was the difficulty she was experiencing with movement. Getting up to go to the bathroom was a major undertaking. She wondered how she and her husband would ever manage outside the hospital; maybe she would never leave. All of these thoughts were very discouraging for May, so much so that there were times when she wished the stroke had just killed her and put an end to everything.

That cloud began to lift, however, when May met Joyce. Joyce was the physical therapist who was assigned to help May on her long road to rehabilitation. Joyce's skill and encouragement became vital to May, who found herself working harder than she had at any time in her life. Soon, May started to feel like a professional athlete, training for the biggest game of her career.

Physical Rehabilitation and Physiotherapists

In Case Study 8.1, you met May, a 61-year-old woman who suffered a stroke that affected every aspect of her life. In reading that case study, can you imagine the challenges faced by May and her physical therapist as they work on May's rehabilitation? Of course, many of those challenges are psychological in nature. In addition to knowing what May is capable of and what exercises to give her each day, Joyce must be sensitive to issues of motivation, adherence, mood, and social support.

Somewhat surprisingly, there is not a large literature investigating many of these issues in physical rehabilitation. Rather, most attention has been paid to psychological issues surrounding drug and alcohol rehab. While this is a vital area in its own right, much can be learned by studying the way physical therapists work with their patients. In addition, health psychology can contribute to the effectiveness of that work. Let's look at some of these psychological issues in more detail.

Goal Setting

It is clear that physiotherapists must enter into a partnership with their patients if they hope to be successful. In other words, the relationship cannot be one in which the patient is passive and dependent upon the therapist. Nowhere is this more evident than in the area of goal setting (Taylor & Taylor, 1997). We know from sport psychology that people are much more likely to work toward a goal if they have had a say in *choosing* that goal. This is not usually done by the athlete alone, nor should it be done by the patient alone. This is because the athlete and patient cannot be entirely objective regarding what is possible. In some cases, patients might let discouragement get the better of them, and so they set goals that are not ambitious enough. In other cases, they may become impatient and set goals that cannot be reached in the short-term, setting themselves up for frustration.

An interesting observational study looked at the goal-setting behaviour of male stroke patients when they had physical therapy in the hospital versus receiving it in their own homes (von Koch, Wottrich, & Holmqvist, 1998). It was observed that the patients seemed to take on different roles when at home. They were more likely to express their goals and take initiative when working with their therapist. Remember, this study looked at the same patients in both settings.

Adherence

Closely related to goal setting is adherence (Sluijs, Kerssens, van der Zee, & Myers, 1998). The physiotherapist cannot oversee all the work a patient must do. For improvement to occur, a patient such as May must work diligently on rehabilitation on her own. She must adhere to the rehab regimen that she and the physiotherapist have agreed upon. All the factors we will be discussing in this section on physical rehabilitation are interrelated. For example, if May feels that she was part of the goal-setting process, then she will feel more committed to achieving these goals. For this reason, she is more likely to adhere to the regimen. You will see that education, cognitive interventions, and behavioural interventions also affect adherence.

Behavioural Interventions

Most rehabilitation patients need some form of **external reinforcement**. That is to say, the physiotherapist, friends, family, and other practitioners must encourage and praise the patient's successes. For May, improvement will not be measured on a minute-to-minute basis. She will need to be reminded of what she can do today that she could not do during the early weeks of her rehabilitation. Also, May will need to find ways to **self-reinforce**. She must pat herself on the back and maybe even give herself tangible rewards, like a new dress or a best-selling book, for achieving certain goals. One of the best things about physical rehabilitation is that at least some of the success can be *measured objectively*. May can measure how much further she has walked, and how much more clearly she can speak as she progresses through the regimen. Objective criteria for success are the bread and butter of behavioural interventions. They allow for reinforcement to be directly contingent upon desired behaviour and allow the patient and physiotherapist to *shape* the program by gradually increasing observable standards.

Cognitive Interventions

The power of effective behavioural interventions is clear in physical therapy. However, May's program cannot rely solely on behavioural strategies. It must also focus on her thinking, and that is the stuff of cognitive interventions. There are at least two areas in which this is crucial. First, May must believe that she can reach an identified goal. You may remember from Chapter 1 that we call these *efficacy beliefs*. These beliefs can be tricky to instill. It isn't usually enough to simply *tell* someone that he or she is capable of doing something. Those messages must be based on some *evidence* that the patient will accept as being reasonable. Efficacy beliefs, then, are often built on past successes. A classic example is an attained goal that the patient initially thought was unattainable. Also, it is possible that experienced physical therapists alter their patients' efficacy beliefs simply by the way they interact with them. In other words, they assume that the patient is capable, and the patient lives up to that assumption. More research needs to be done on the efficacy-enhancing strategies employed by physical therapists, however, to confirm this.

The second crucial target for cognitive interventions is the patient's **attributions**. These are the explanations a person gives for his or her successes and failures. In May's case, as with all patients, it will be essential that she attribute her success *internally* (Wiegmann & Berven, 1998). In other words, she must take credit for her improvement, citing things like her hard work and fighting spirit. If she tries to attribute her success to Joyce, her physiotherapist, Joyce must politely deflect that back to May. So, if May says, "You're a saint, Joyce. I could never do this without you", this may feel great for Joyce, but she must reply with something like, "Thanks for the compliment, May, but you're the one who's the great worker here."

Positive efficacy beliefs and internal attributions of success greatly increase the likelihood that May will adhere to her regimen when Joyce is not around. Most of all, these ways of thinking move May toward *independence*, which is an important goal of physical rehabilitation.

Pain Management

In our discussion of physical rehabilitation, we must address the issue of pain management, since pain is a common problem for many patients in rehabilitation. Chapter 10 addresses pain in detail, so we will not repeat the concepts presented there. At this point, it is important to remember the obvious—pain makes rehabilitation harder. This means that all of the pain management strategies discussed in Chapter 10, such as relaxation, distraction, and interpretation of pain, are major topics for people working in physical therapy. Also, pain is very informative regarding the patient's progress.

In our discussion of physical rehabilitation, we have not included a separate section for motivation. This is because motivation is involved in each of the sections we did include. Partnerships improve motivation, as do reinforcers and effective cognitive interventions. In fact, motivation is such a pervasive issue that we are often drawn to athletic metaphors to help us understand the psychology of physical rehabilitation. This makes sense, because there is considerable overlap between health psychology and sport psychology in the area of rehabilitation. You will note this overlap again when you read about recovery from athletic injuries in Chapter 12 on exercise and sport.

The literature that does exist in the area of motivation and rehabilitation makes clear reference to sport contexts when it introduces topics such as goal setting, relaxation, mental imagery, and positive thinking (Taylor & Taylor, 1997). Having said this, it is important to acknowledge that May does not have to be an ex-professional athlete to do well in her rehabilitation (though she reports feeling like one at times). This point is made very well in a discussion of motivation factors associated with the physical rehabilitation of five women between the ages of 80 and 94 (Resnick, 1996). In this discussion, Resnick makes reference to goal setting, the use of humour, communicating a sense of caring, and engaging in a partnership with the patient that acknowledges the power of each partner to effect successful rehabilitation.

Technologists

Much of the high-tech equipment found in hospitals and clinics is operated by technologists who go through 2 or more years of training. They learn how to operate the equipment and about the biomedical assessments the equipment performs. Technologists, then, combine a desire to help others with an interest in technology. They often represent the human side of what has become a highly mechanized world of diagnostic and treatment procedures.

In diagnosis, experienced technologists can often tell a normal test result from an abnormal one, yet they are not allowed to pass these impressions on to the patient. This can be particularly difficult, because the patient might desperately want to know the technologist's opinion. Since many patients know that the technologist cannot make a diagnosis, the patients will subtly probe the technologist with phrases like, "Well, what do you think?" or "How does it look?" The technologist, in reply, must say something like, "The radiologist will go over your test results with you", or, "We'll be sending the results to your doctor." The patient may interpret this as an attempt on the technologist's part to avoid giving bad news, which makes the patient anxious.

CASE 8-2 Can High-Tech Be Human?

Chen consulted his doctor about a recurring pain on the right side of his abdomen. His apprehension level went up measurably when he heard the words "barium enema." He had never had one before, so he wasn't exactly sure what it was. All the same, it sounded embarrassing and awful. To make matters worse, the enema was only part of the examination he was to go through to discover the source of the pain. A machine was going to be pushed into his abdomen like it was some sort of balloon. And what was this pain anyway? The very imposing machinery and embarrassing procedures made him feel as though he had something seriously wrong with him.

Thankfully, Chen met an experienced technologist who had a pretty good idea of what he was feeling. She told him just what the enema would involve. It didn't sound too pleasant, but at least he knew how long it would take and what it would feel like. She explained just what she was doing each step of the way. Just as important, she talked with Chen about things that had nothing to do with the test, giving him the sense that he was, indeed, a normal person going through a common experience.

As Case Study 8.2 portrays, experienced technologists are very good at helping patients through procedures that may be physically or psychologically difficult. These include everything from nuclear medicine tests to radiation therapy for cancer. When helping patients, technologists tend to engage in three different topics. They may present **procedure-based information**, which addresses *what* will be done and why. They may present **sensation-based information**, concerning what a procedure will feel or sound like and how long it will last. Or they might engage in **interpersonal small talk**, which has nothing to do with the procedure but passes the time by distracting the patient onto topics like the weather or parking around the hospital (Poole & Kallhood, 1996).

A FINAL WORD

In this chapter, we have presented a series of profiles of health practitioners and the work they do. Of course, since we are not physicians, nurses, physiotherapists, or technologists (or other practitioners), we had to rely on published research and first-hand interaction with practitioners to create these profiles. Given the consistency with which such phenomena as stress, training, and other issues are discussed, it is clear that there these profiles apply widely across the professions we have discussed. By the same token, we must never lose sight of the fact that there is considerable variation among practitioners. Some never experience stress or gender-related discrimination. Some find medical school to be quite straightforward and manageable. Others have been virtually paralyzed by these things. Finally, we urge you to talk to people who work in health care to get first-hand accounts of their work. Certainly, the main objective in this chapter has been to convince you that it is vital for people in health psychology to make the effort to get to know what it is really like to work in health-related professions.

KEY TERMS

cadavers
internship
residency
CTD
fear of death
uncertainty
prognosis
sensitivity
specificity
primary-care physicians
GOK
physician impairment
feminization of medicine
role strain
instrumental treatment
caring
curing
advanced practice nursing
clinical nurse specialist
nurse practitioner
innocent angel
sex symbol
frustrated battleaxe
compassion fatigue
burnout
reality shock
personal factors in stress
social factors in stress
job strain model
problem-based learning (PBL)
continuing medical education (CME)
external reinforcement
self-reinforcement
efficacy beliefs
attributions
procedure-based information
sensation-based information
interpersonal small talk

Chapter 9

HEALTH ACROSS THE LIFESPAN

Chapter Outline

Child Health
- Child Poverty
- Prenatal Influences
- Unintentional Injuries
- Immunization
- Chronic Illness in Childhood

Adolescent Health
- Eating Disorders
- Smoking
- Alcohol Use
- Illicit Drug Use
- Unsafe Sexual Behaviours

Geriatric Health
- Personal Autonomy and Physical Decline
- Dementia
- Unintentional Injuries
- Death among the Elderly

Key Questions

1. What is the most common cause of unintentional injury in children?
2. What factors prompt adolescents to begin smoking?
3. How can we help people addicted to smoking, alcohol, or illicit drugs quit these habits?
4. Why do people engage in unsafe sexual behaviours?
5. What are the most common causes of unintentional injury in the elderly?
6. What factors are responsible for loss of autonomy in the elderly?
7. Why is the death of an older person seen as less tragic than the death of a younger person?

Jennifer began to smoke in high school. She was a bright girl who enjoyed the academic side of school but didn't always find the social side of school easy. When she began junior high school, also known as middle school, she noticed a radical shift in how her friends spent their time. Instead of playing sports and watching movies, her friends were now more interested in partying and meeting guys. For a time, Jennifer resisted her friends' suggestions that she not be so uptight, that she learn to relax and start socializing at parties. However, Jennifer found that she was spending more and more time by herself and grew lonely. It seemed to her that the easiest way to fit in and regain friendships was to begin smoking. So she did and continued to smoke even after graduating from high school.

After high school, Jennifer went in search of a job. She wanted to work as a journalist or perhaps behind the scenes at a radio or television station. She was told that the best experience she could gain would be at a small-town radio or television station, where she would be expected to complete all the tasks of producing a story by herself: find a story, write the story, take pictures, and deliver the story on air. So Jennifer followed this advice. She found a job in a small town working for a local television station. In this new environment, Jennifer was able to give up smoking. Very few of the other people who worked at the television station smoked and, of course, she no longer saw her high school friends, at least not on a regular basis. Jennifer was lucky. Unlike so many people who have a difficult time quitting, Jennifer was able to quit smoking on her own relatively easily.

Many years later, when Jennifer was going through the turmoil of a "messy" divorce, she began to smoke again. She was surprised one day when after a lengthy meeting with her lawyer she found herself craving a cigarette. After a couple of days she gave in to this craving and bought a package of cigarettes. She smoked a single cigarette and found that this did alleviate some of her stress—she welcomed the relief. Yet, she knew smoking was unhealthy. She didn't want her children to model her behaviour and didn't want their health endangered as a result of her behaviour, so she never smoked indoors or let her children see her smoke. Fortunately, once the divorce was settled and she had obtained custody of her children, she was again able to "kick" the habit.

In this chapter, we will focus on specific health conditions, health behaviours, and related psychological issues for three distinct age groups: children, adolescents, and the elderly. The research presented in the other chapters in this text generally focuses on the adult population, with little attention given to other age populations. This chapter will focus on important health-related issues for each of the three age groups. For example, we'll examine the leading cause of death in children, the behaviour that begins in adolescence and is the number one preventable cause of death in Canadians, and barriers to seniors' autonomy. The scenario of Jennifer reminds us that some behaviours, such as smoking, affect people in more than one age group. For example, a developing child (fetus) is affected when parents smoke; adolescents are affected by seeing their peers smoke, because they often succumb to peer pressure and join the ranks of smokers; and adults and seniors often die prematurely as a result of smoking behaviours.

CHILD HEALTH

On November 11, 1999, the United Nations commemorated the tenth anniversary of the Convention on the Rights of the Child. This Convention was adopted in 1989 and ratified in Canada in 1991. In addition, in 1998, the United Nations General Assembly proclaimed that 2001 to 2010 would be the International Decade for a Culture of Peace and Non-Violence for the Children of the World. Non-discrimination against children is to be guaranteed and the best interests of the child "must guide all actions" (UN press release, 1999, www.un.org/News/Press/docs/1999). It has been determined that the largest barrier to children's rights is poverty, therefore the emphasis is on implementing measures that ensure and maximize survival and development. The United Nations has ranked Canada first in the world in terms of human development but only tenth in the world when a poverty index is included.

Child Poverty

In 1996, 730 000 children under the age of 18 years lived in two-parent families whose income was below the poverty line. Another 673 000 impoverished children resided in a household led by their mother only. As many as 200 000 Canadians live in substandard housing or are homeless, and a growing proportion of these individuals are women and children. Six percent of households in the general population in 1996 (approximately 1.5 million people) reported that they did not have enough money to buy food. Consequently, nearly one-half million individuals relied on donations from a food bank or similar charitable organization. Unfortunately, as the income of a family decreases, rates of poor health, hyperactivity, and delayed cognitive development will increase in the children present in that family (Ross, 1998). Moreover, children from impoverished homes are less likely to participate in organized athletic and sporting activities, which, in turn, affects physical health. Poverty has an overarching effect on health. Let us now turn our attention to more specific issues. We begin by talking about factors that negatively affect a child's health before the child is born.

Prenatal Influences

The psychological and physical development of the child is determined, in part, by the physical and socioemotional health of the mother. Maternal age and nutrition influence child development. In addition, embryonic and fetal development can be affected by many viruses (e.g., herpes virus), chemicals (e.g., environmental pollutants such as carbon monoxide and lead), or drugs (e.g., tobacco and alcohol). Any agent that causes a birth defect is called a **teratogen**. The effect of these agents depends on the type of agent and the genetic characteristics of the fetus. The time at which the fetus is exposed is also important, because some teratogens are more likely to produce birth defects if they are encountered at certain times, or critical periods, during the pregnancy. The period when the organ is developing most rapidly is the period of greatest vulnerability, referred to as the **critical period** (Moore & Persaud, 1993). The **germinal stage** is the earliest stage of prenatal development, lasting from conception to about 2 weeks. During this stage, the developing child or blastocyst is not susceptible to teratogens. During the **embryonic stage**, which occurs from about 2 to 8 weeks after conception, the organism is most vulnerable to teratogens. This is the time when the most extreme growth occurs. The central nervous system, heart, limbs, eyes, ears, teeth, and palate are extremely susceptible during this stage. The **fetal stage** of prenatal development begins at approximately 8 weeks and continues until birth. The brain and central nervous system as well as external genitalia are at the greatest risk from teratogens during this stage.

Maternal Substance Abuse

Drinking during pregnancy increases the risk of **fetal alcohol syndrome (FAS)** and **fetal alcohol effects (FAE)**. Fetal alcohol syndrome commonly causes mental retardation, central nervous system disorders, cardiac abnormalities, growth deficiencies, and facial abnormalities. Behavioural concerns often involve inattentiveness, poor concentration, memory deficits, impulsivity, and hyperactivity. "Fetal alcohol effects" is the term used to describe children who have some of the characteristics of FAS (when prenatal alcohol use is a possible cause). Although there is no national surveillance of FAS, conservative estimates suggest that 0.33 cases of FAS occur in every 1 000 births in western countries (Health Canada, 1999). The incidence of FAE is approximately three times higher than that of FAS. Although some case studies suggest that FAS is more common among Canadian aboriginal children than non-aboriginal children, there currently is no empirical evidence to support this conclusion. Health care costs for the residential care of children with FAS are approximately 11 percent of the costs for care of all children with a mental handicap (Harris, 1995). This figure elucidates the seriousness of this disorder. Not surprisingly, abstinence from alcohol is recommended for women who are pregnant or who are planning to become pregnant. How many women drink when pregnant? According to the 1996/97 National Population Health

Survey, seven percent of Canadian women report drinking at any time throughout their pregnancy. Interestingly, women who drink during pregnancy tend to be older and of higher socioeconomic status than those who do not.

Infants born to women who have smoked throughout pregnancy often have a low birth weight (less than 2 500 grams or 5.5 pounds) and experience perinatal distress. Low birth weight can result in mental and physical disabilities and sometimes death. In 1996, 36 percent of new mothers reported that they had smoked during their pregnancy (146 000 women) (Health Canada, 1999). The prevalence of smoking in mothers has been linked to education level. Over 60 percent of pregnant women who had not graduated from high school smoked during their pregnancy, whereas only 14 percent of those with a university education smoked. (Sudden infant death syndrome [SIDS] is also linked to smoking behaviour of the mother and the presence of environmental tobacco smoke.)

The thalidomide tragedy in the 1960s prompted researchers to investigate the effects of other drugs (e.g., cocaine) on the fetus. Chasnoff, Landress, and Barrett (1990) found that 11 to 14 percent of women tested positive with urinary screening for cocaine, marijuana, or heroin use during pregnancy. Researchers testing for the presence of drugs in the neonate's meconium indicate that the rate may be closer to 45 percent (Ostrea, Romero, & Yee, 1993). Keep in mind that this doesn't necessarily mean that these newborns will have symptoms suggestive of a toxicology. The symptoms most often noted as a result of maternal drug use include poor muscle tone and motor movement, irritability, and poor self-quieting (Schuler & Nair, 1999).

Maternal Age

Maternal age is also a factor in the fetus' developmental outcome. Adolescent mothers are at risk for delivering their babies prematurely and with low birth weights. Babies born to adolescent mothers also have an increased incidence of neurological disorders. Over 40 percent of teenage mothers who are pregnant smoke. In addition, teenage childbearing is related to a number of other risk factors, including poorer social and economic outcomes. In 1995, there were 38 502 reported teenage pregnancies in Canada (including live births, abortions, and stillbirths) (Health Canada, 1999).

There may also be negative health consequences to infants born to mothers over the age of 40 years. For instance, genetic disorders such as Down syndrome, phenylketonuria, and Tay-Sachs disease are more prevalent in babies born to older mothers. There is also a greater risk of developmental delay in babies born to mothers over 40 years of age than in babies born to younger mothers.

Unintentional Injuries

Once a baby is born, there are innumerable factors that may affect the infant and result in tragic health consequences or even death. Unintentional injuries are the leading cause of death in children and youth (and the third-leading cause of death in the population as a whole). Death rates resulting from injuries are much higher among aboriginal children. For example, when First Nations children are compared with the total Canadian population of children, the rate of death from injuries is almost four times greater for infants and five times greater for preschoolers (Health Canada, 1999).

Most fatal unintentional injuries result from motor vehicle accidents. A large majority of these injuries result from an adult's failure to properly restrain an infant or toddler in the back seat of a car (Saldana & Peterson, 1997). Unfortunately, several infants and young children have been killed or seriously injured in the front seat of a car by the deployment of passenger-side air bags. Nearly all of these injuries could have been avoided if the child was properly restrained in the back seat (National Highway Traffic Safety Administration, 1993–96).

A large proportion of deaths among children result from drowning. Not all drownings occur at pools or beaches, although for older children, swimming pools are the most common place for drowning. For children under the age of 5 years, bathtubs and large buckets filled with water are potentially deadly receptacles (Saldana & Peterson, 1997). Many children are also killed or injured by burns, most of which result from house fires. Children under 5 years of age have an increased risk of death from house fires; the younger the child, the greater the risk (Saldana & Peterson, 1997). Many residential fires are due to adults' smoking. Unfortunately, children are often the victims (Miller, 1993).

There are many other causes of unintentional childhood injury, including falls, poisonings, and bicycle mishaps. A cross-national survey of school-aged children found that the largest group of injuries for 11-year-old Canadian children occurred during sporting activities and play. The second largest group were those that involved the child falling off or tripping over something. In general, falls are the most important cause of injury (rather than death) in children and youth under the age of 20 years (Health Canada, 1999). Sadly, children under the age of 4 years can be badly injured or killed from falling relatively short distances, such as from a bunk bed, the top of a slide, or through an open window. Poisoning deaths have decreased for young children in recent years, but they are the next-most frequent cause of injury-related admission to hospitals (Health Canada, 1999). This decrease in poisonings is mainly due to increased use of child-resistant containers. Thousands of children become ill each year from exposure to dangerous chemicals. It has been estimated that for each poisoning death of a child under the age of six years, there are 20 000 calls to poison control centres (Saldana & Peterson, 1997). Finally, bicycle mishaps are responsible for many deaths and injuries. Many bicycle fatalities could have been prevented by the proper use of bicycle helmets. Bicycle injuries are related to both age and gender; the number of deaths and injuries increases up to early adolescence, with boys between the ages of 10 and 14 years having the highest rates (Saldana & Peterson, 1997).

There are pronounced gender differences for unintentional injuries in children. Specifically, boys have a greater incidence of injuries at all ages and stages and suffer more severe injuries than girls do. The reasons for these differences—which may include boys engaging in more risk-taking behaviour than girls, the different nature of childhood activities for boys and girls, and inborn differences in impulsivity and activity level—are still a matter of debate (Bradbury, Janicke, Riley, & Finney, 1999; Health Canada, 1999).

Psychologists have played an increasingly important role in developing and implementing strategies for reducing unintentional injuries over the last couple of decades. Death rates from unintentional injuries have been decreasing, and much of this decline has resulted from interventions aimed at (1) changing individual behaviours, (2) changing the environment, or (3) changing the law. The most effective interventions to reduce children's injuries have been those directed at parents. Peterson and Schick (1993) discovered that most injuries experienced by second-grade children in their homes could have been avoided if children had followed some basic rules (e.g., "Don't walk backwards", "Don't run with anything in your mouth", or "Don't touch, taste, or smell medicines or cleaners"). If parents are willing to implement these general rules, it is likely that there will be a reduction in injuries. The environment can be changed by building safer cars and roads, manufacturing better bicycle and motorcycle helmets, and making the home safer (e.g., by installing smoke detectors or putting toxic medicines and cleaners out of reach of children). However, the most effective strategies in preventing unintentional injuries are legal interventions. For example, the use of infant car seats is mandatory in all provinces, and the use of bicycle helmets is mandatory in many provinces (Zador & Ciccone, 1993).

As there are interventions available to reduce morbidity and mortality rates from unintentional injuries, so there are interventions available to reduce the incidence of disease. In the next section, we'll look at one of these interventions.

Immunization

Since vaccines were first introduced, Canada has seen a 95 percent reduction in vaccine-preventable diseases. Polio has been eliminated and it is expected that measles will be eradicated by the year 2005. In contrast, the reported incidence of pertussis, commonly referred to as whooping cough, was higher in 1994/95 then it had been in the preceding 10 years (Health Canada, 1999).

The success of immunization programs has recently been challenged. Generations of children have grown up in the absence of diseases that previously wreaked havoc on the population. As a result, it seems that parents are becoming complacent and less likely to have their children immunized. In addition, parental confidence in some vaccines has been eroded by "exaggerated and often erroneous reports of serious adverse reactions" (Health Canada, 1999, p. 80). It has also been noted that life is becoming more hectic for parents and that in the ever-increasing dual-working-parent families and single-parent homes, children are less likely to be vaccinated because of time constraints ("The Homestretch", CBC Radio, January 3, 2000). Unfortunately, children from these homes are the children who are more likely to have interactions with larger numbers of other children in daycare situations and be exposed to more germs than those children who are at home full-time. Vigilance in attaining and maintaining a national commitment to immunization programs remains a public health priority (ACPH, 1999).

The changing face of disease within our country due, in part, to immunization, has presented new challenges for researchers. Approximately 10 to 15 percent of Canadian children have chronic illnesses. Researchers are now exploring how children and their families manage and cope with chronic illness as well as continuing to search for cures for childhood diseases.

Chronic Illness in Childhood

There is no single, agreed-upon definition of chronic illness in childhood. Commonly, definitions of chronic illness include a longevity of the disease or illness for extended periods of time, often for life. A chronic illness is usually treatable but not curable. This means the disease must be "managed" (e.g., pain reduced or a reduction in attacks or seizures) in some way for long periods of time, usually until the patient's death (Bradford, 1997; Eiser, 1990;

Hobbs & Perrin, 1995). Most researchers, health care providers, and psychologists agree that the nature of chronic illnesses includes "emotional, behavioural, and perceptual processes and disease- or treatment-related symptoms [that] occur on multiple levels" (McQuaid & Nassau, 1999, p. 305).

A child's perception of illness is, not surprisingly, related to cognitive maturation (Brewster, 1982). Brewster (1982) examined fifty chronically ill children (i.e., children with diabetes, asthma, sickle-cell anemia, and multiple congenital anomalies) between the ages of 5 and 13 years to determine how they conceptualized their illness. The young children viewed illness as the direct result of human behaviour and viewed treatments or medical procedures as punishments for wrongdoing. Older children believed that physical causes (e.g., germs) rather than personal behaviours were responsible for illness. The older children also understood that medical treatments were designed to be curative and not punishing. The oldest children in Brewster's study were able to recognize that there are multiple causes of an illness, some intrinsic and some extrinsic. However, even among the most cognitively advanced children there was still evidence of attributions of self-blame and egocentric thinking. For example, a 12-year-old leukemic patient remarked, "I know that my doctor told me that my illness is caused by too many white cells, but I still wonder if it was caused by something that I did" (Brewster, 1982, p. 361). Brewster speculates that chronically ill patients may retain illogical beliefs in their own responsibility for illness, not out of an inability to think logically but more out of an attempt to maintain a sense of personal control to thwart feelings of helplessness.

Often children with chronic illnesses may not feel in control of their illness. Frequently, children must involve parents and family members to help with their medical management. Parents often must assume responsibility for the child's treatment, and the family as a whole must adapt to the demands of the child's illness (Bradford, 1997). The process of adaptation is best viewed by both patient and family as a process that changes over time, because the disease itself may change in time or the child may become capable of taking on more responsibility with age (Reiss, Steinglass, & Howe, 1993).

How a child with a chronic illness adjusts to or copes with the illness can be influenced by the disease itself, individual characteristics of the child, and environmental factors within the child's life (Johnson, 1985). Each illness places different limitations on the patient's functioning. Treatment requirements differ in difficulty, complexity, frequency, discomfort, and resultant side effects. Further, some diseases are linked with other disorders or "complications" that place additional demands on the patient and family. Finally, each disease has its own special characteristics, and the illness itself can change over time, becoming more or less severe with resultant changes in treatment, prognosis, and the patient's functional capabilities. For example, a diabetic child must lead a life of daily injections, urine tests, and dietary constraints. A youngster with leukemia must endure painful spinal taps, hair loss, and the imminence of death. A child who has been severely burned must initially endure great pain and then cope with the effects of disfigurement.

Most children coping with chronic disease do so fairly well. Researchers have not found individual characteristics that help or hinder coping with chronic illness in general. One notable exception is patient age. As discussed previously, a child's age or cognitive developmental level is an important contributor to what he or she is capable of understanding about the disease and treatment. The child's cognitive developmental level will also affect how well he or she communicates concerns to parents or health care providers.

Children with chronic illness may experience numerous hospitalizations and resultant separation from their families (Johnson, 1985). Similarly, frequent illness episodes require school absences and separation from peers. These factors can lead a child to feel jealous of others who are healthy and who can lead a less constricted existence. Feelings of being different from peers and siblings may lead to a sense of isolation and loneliness. The greatest environmental factor affecting the child is the child's family. Caring for a chronically ill child may cause considerable personal strain and distress for one or both parents. Siblings of the ill child may receive less parental attention; and a financial burden may be placed on the family. It is also possible, however, that the illness may have a positive effect on the family's functioning. There may be increased sharing, support, and heightened self-esteem gained by the family's efforts to cope with and master the stress of the illness.

ADOLESCENT HEALTH

Many health habits are formed in adolescence and continue into adulthood and sometimes even for the rest of a person's life. In our opening example, Jennifer began smoking while in junior high school. She continued smoking for a number of years then quit shortly after high school. Later, however, when Jennifer was going through a period of stress in her life she reverted to her former strategy of dealing with stress by resuming smoking. In our discussion of health-compromising behaviours that begin in adolescence, you'll notice that many of the behaviours become habitual and are difficult to terminate.

CASE 9-1 Bulimia Nervosa in Teenagers

Julia is an attractive girl of normal weight who has always been concerned with her appearance. If you ever want to know what clothes are trendy, take a peek at what Julia is wearing. She can even tell you what colour of lipstick and fingernail polish are "in" this month. How does she know this? She reads the magazines *Elle* and *Cosmopolitan* religiously. Her friends are also very "up to date", and in junior high school they jointly began to engage in a behaviour they felt was "fashionable." As a group, the girls would go into the washroom and throw up. Julia says she was not all that concerned with losing weight but she didn't want to gain any either. In fact, the purging began more because it seemed to be a "cool" thing to do rather than resulting from concerns Julia might have had about her own weight. Unfortunately, the purging changed from a "group activity" to something she did frequently on her own. It became a habit for Julia to vomit after eating, a very unhealthy habit.

Eating Disorders

Julia's behaviour is indicative of an eating disorder known as **bulimia nervosa**. Bulimia involves recurrent episodes of binge eating followed by purging. The purging strategies used most frequently are vomiting and laxative use. This disorder can result in numerous medical problems, such as anemia, inflammation of the digestive tract, heart arrhythmias resulting from electrolyte imbalances (which may cause sudden death), and irreversible erosion of dental enamel (British Columbia Eating Disorder Association [BCDEA], 1998). Although some bulimics are overweight like Julia, most are of normal weight. Bulimics are aware that their behaviour is not normal, and they are ashamed of it. Because of this, they usually try to hide their behaviour from others. The binge portion of the bulimic episode is often impulsive, and bulimics are likely to engage in other impulsive and reckless behaviours as well. For example, kleptomania is more common among bulimics than among the general population. Although the items stolen would usually be associated with the bulimic's binging and purging, such as food or laxatives, it wouldn't be uncommon for a bulimic to steal clothing, cosmetics, alcohol, or other unneeded items. Bulimics are also more likely than the general population to engage in spending sprees or sexual promiscuity because of their impulsive nature.

The number of patients being diagnosed with eating disorders is increasing (BCEDA, 1998; Rosen & Neumark-Sztainer, 1997). A 1992 survey of adolescents across British Columbia found that in the 7 days preceding the survey, unhealthy weight control practices (e.g., purging after meals or using diet pills) were acknowledged by 6 percent of the male students and 7 percent of the female students (McCreary Centre Society, 1993). Although eating disorders are most common among adolescents and adults, even children suffer from eating disorders. Seventy percent of children with eating disorders are female. In the adolescent and adult eating disorder population, 90 to 95 percent of those with eating disorders are female. How prevalent are eating disorders? Although there are no Canadian statistics available, in the U.S. bulimia has been found to occur in 1 to 20 percent of individuals, depending on the population under study (BCEDA, 1998).The University of Toronto Programme for Eating Disorders (Kruger, McVey, & Kennedy, 1998) has noticed an increasing proportion of patients who suffer from bulimia nervosa compared to those who suffer from anorexia nervosa.

Anorexia nervosa is an eating disorder that is characterized by a dramatic reduction in food intake and extreme weight loss. Anorexics are very fearful of gaining weight and consequently will refuse food and may engage in excessive exercise. Yet, anorexics are very preoccupied with food and may spend a lot of their time cooking for others or engaging in other pursuits that revolve around food. The self-starvation in anorexia will lead to low blood pressure, heart damage or cardiac arrhythmias, and eventually death. When one has reached a state of near starvation, the person will lose the hair on his or her head and fine hair growth (lanugo) will appear on one's face and body. Anorexics are also at increased risk of osteoporosis (BCEDA, 1998).

Anorexia is less prevalent in the general population than bulimia (ranging from 0.5% to 4%). Anorexia occurs most often in Caucasian adolescent females from the upper social classes and those who practise ballet, model, or are competitive in sports (Steinhausen et al., 1997; Garner & Garfinkel, 1980; Thompson & Sherman, 1993). Yet, anorexia is increasingly being seen in patients who are very young, male, less affluent, and people of colour (Gard & Freeman, 1996; Story et al., 1995; Thompson & Sherman, 1993). There is some indication that gay men are slightly over-represented among anorexics (Carlat, Camargo, & Herzog, 1997). However, researchers state that both male and female anorexics are more likely than the general population to identify themselves as asexual.

Biological, Cultural, and Psychological Contributors to Eating Disorders

Biological, cultural, and psychological factors may all be possible contributors to eating disorders. Twin studies have documented that both twins are more likely to suffer from eating disorders if the twins are identical rather than fraternal twins (Kendler et al., 1991; Walters & Kendler, 1995). Other researchers have also reported an increased risk of eating disorders among relatives (Cooper, 1995). Hypothalmic abnormalities have been noted in anorexics, and an association has also been noted between anorexia and Turner's syndrome (a disorder among females who lack a second X chromosome) (Gold et al., 1986).

In North American society, there is pressure on individuals to be thin and stay youthful. This expectation is learned at a very young age. Then, when children reach puberty and naturally gain weight many become distressed. Often adolescents will try to control their weight by dieting. Unfortunately, this strategy is sometimes carried too far, and this is when many eating disorders begin. In fact, dieting is the most important predictor of new eating disorders (Patton et al., 1999). Eating disorders are more likely to occur in individuals from families in which eating disorders, psychopathology, alcoholism, or sexual abuse exist or have taken place (BCEDA, 1998; Wonderlich et al., 1997). The media is also partly to blame for this pressure. Researchers (e.g., Stice, 1994) have documented that females who have greater exposure to media containing a high concentration of body images show more characteristics of eating disorders than do females with less exposure to this media.

Psychological factors associated with eating disorders include issues of control, low self-esteem, extreme sensitivity to other's feelings, perfectionism, maturity fears, and distorted body image (BCEDA, 1998). Hilde Bruch (1973, 1978, 1982), who spent more than 40 years studying eating disorders, reported that anorexics typically are troubled female adolescents who feel incapable of changing their lives. These young women are from families that do not encourage autonomy and are perceived by the adolescent as overdemanding. To exert some control in their lives, they exert control over the thing closest to them, their bodies. Many individuals who suffer from eating disorders do not perceive their bodies accurately. Research has shown that women, in general, see themselves as one-fourth larger than they really are (Thompson, 1986). Men may also see themselves as larger than they really are but they do so to a lesser degree and, unlike women, many of these men may want to be larger (Geist et al., 1999). Both anorexics and bulimics tend to overestimate their body size to a greater extent than does the general population.

Treatment for Eating Disorders

Successful treatment for eating disorders is literally a matter of life or death. This is particularly true for anorexics, because nearly six percent of all anorexics die from their disorder (Neumarker, 1997). Not surprisingly, anorexics are very difficult to treat because they believe that the one aspect of their environment they can control is their own body. As long as they refuse to eat they maintain control. As starvation continues, anorexics eventually reach the point of exhaustion and possible physical collapse. At this point, treatment is usually forced on them. The first goal of treatment is to medically stabilize the patient and increase his or her weight (Goldner & Brimingham, 1994). Weight restoration is a step in the treatment process but is not a cure. Anorexics need to change both their body image *and* their eating habits. Cognitive behaviour therapy attempts to eradicate the irrational beliefs of patients while maintaining a warm and accepting attitude. For example, anorexics are taught to avoid absolutist thoughts like, "If I put on one pound, I'll go on to gain one hundred." Similarly, they are educated about nutritional facts. Superstitious beliefs like, "Laxatives prevent the absorption of calories" are dispelled. Patients are also encouraged to recognize that others do not have the same high standards for their behaviour that they do (Thompson & Sherman, 1993). Family therapy is often included in the treatment process. It has been found that family participation positively influences the results of therapy (Eisler et al., 1999).

Bulimia is much easier to treat than anorexia, because bulimics are aware that their eating habits are not normal. As a result, they are motivated to change these behaviours. Treatment for bulimia usually includes cognitive-behavioural therapy. This is often combined with drug therapy. Typically therapy begins by patients being instructed to monitor their eating habits. An individualized treatment program is then developed to help break down patterns of behaviour that maintain disordered eating and will include such things as reinforcement, relaxation training, and cognitive restructuring (Thackwray, Smith, Bodfish, & Meyers, 1993). Specific techniques might include increasing the regularity of meals, eating a greater variety of foods, delaying the impulse to purge as long as possible, and eating foods in new settings not previously associated with binges (Agras et al., 1989; Kirkley, Schneider, Agras, & Bachman, 1985). The cognitive-behavioural techniques implemented should address the pathological concerns bulimics have about their weight and eating in addition to increasing perceptions of self-esteem. Drugs, especially antidepressants, are used in managing bulimia. It has been determined that they decrease the frequency of binges (Mitchell & de Zwaan, 1993). However, drugs do not treat the cause of the problem and as such, they should only be used to treat bulimia in conjunction with other forms of therapy (Compas et al., 1998).

Unfortunately, as many as half of previously treated eating-disorder sufferers will continue to have eating problems. The difficulty in treating eating disorders effectively, coupled with their increasing prevalence, suggests that researchers should focus more on ways to prevent eating disorders rather than focusing almost exclusively on treating them after they have developed (Battle & Brownell, 1996; Mann et al., 1997). In the next section, we discuss a health-compromising behaviour that, like eating disorders, often begins in adolescence. This behaviour contributes to a large number of deaths among Canadians.

Smoking

Age and Gender Differences in Smoking

There are few habits as potentially deadly as smoking cigarettes. Smoking is the number one preventable cause of death and disease in Canada. In 1996, smoking accounted for approximately 45 000 deaths. It has been estimated that at least one-quarter of all deaths among persons aged 35 to 84 years in Canada are attributable to tobacco use (Ellison, Morrison, de Groh, & Villeneuve, 1999). The National Population Health Survey (1996/97) documents that more than 25 percent of Canadians 12 years of age and older smoke. Rates of use were highest among those aged 20 to 24 years (35.1%) and lowest among those aged 75 years or older (11.2%). Traditionally, more males than females have smoked cigarettes. However, more and more females are smoking. This trend will likely continue, as we note that more and more adolescent girls are smoking. It is also worth mentioning that although more adolescent girls than boys smoke, adolescent boys smoke more than do adolescent girls.

Sociocultural Differences in Smoking

Rates of smoking vary substantially by socioeconomic status (National Population Health Survey, 1996/97). The percentage of people who smoke tends to decline with increases in income as well as education and job prestige. Those in the lowest income bracket report the highest rates of smoking (40% of men and 36% of women). Smoking rates decrease with an increase in income, to lows of 16 and 13 percent among men and women, respectively, in the highest income bracket. The highest rates of smoking in Canada occur among aboriginal people, about double the overall rate in the Canadian population as a whole (Reading, 1997). In 1997, adult smoking rates within the aboriginal population were highest in the youngest age groups surveyed, those between the ages of 20 and 24 years (72%) and 25 to 29 years (71%). There is a steady decline in smoking with increasing age—those 75 years of age and older report the lowest rate of smoking, at 23 percent. Prevalence of smoking has also been documented by immigrant status (Chen, Ng, & Wilkins, 1996). Recent non-European immigrants are significantly less likely than the Canadian-born population to smoke. In fact, for all immigrants, the number who smoke generally increased with the length of time in Canada. This leads us to conclude that there is something about our Canadian culture that promotes smoking. Unlike for the Canadian-born population, there is no clear relationship between smoking and income status for immigrants.

Why Do People Smoke?

Considering that most people are aware that smoking is bad for them, that is, that smoking is linked to a wide variety of health consequences, it is puzzling that so many people smoke. This behaviour becomes even more puzzling when we realize that the first few times people smoke, they likely cough, find the taste unpleasant, and may even experience dizziness and nausea. Why would someone voluntarily engage in this behaviour? Why after their first experience would they want to smoke again? Strangely enough, they do. Let's take a look at why people begin to smoke and why they continue to smoke.

Beginning to Smoke

Smoking often begins during adolescence, when peer influence is strong. Numerous studies have found that adolescents are more likely to smoke if their friends smoke (Biglan, Duncan, Ary, & Smolkowski, 1995; Conrad, Flay, & Hill, 1992; Jansen et al., 1987; Mittelmark et al., 1987; Stanton, Mahalski, McGee, & Silva, 1993). When adolescents first try smoking, they usually do so in the company of their peers and with their peers' encouragement (Leventhal, Prochaska, & Hirschman, 1985). Once adolescents begin to smoke, this behaviour is reinforced by their peers. Consider the fact that adolescents who smoke receive 26 times more offers of cigarettes than do adolescents who are non-smokers (Ary & Biglan, 1988). Also, girls are repeatedly offered cigarettes more than are boys (Charlton, Minagawa, & While, 1999). Further, researchers estimate that more than 70 percent of all cigarettes smoked by adolescents are done so in the presence of a peer (Biglan et al., 1984).

Do you remember Jennifer who we introduced you to at the beginning of this chapter? Jennifer was greatly influenced by peer pressure in her decision to begin smoking. Both her parents and many of her friends smoked. In a sense, the cards were stacked against Jennifer, as there were many situational factors present that are associated with smoking. Researchers have documented that adolescents are more likely to smoke if they have parents or older siblings who also smoke (e.g., Biglan et al., 1995). These findings suggest that both modelling and peer pressure are likely important causative factors of smoking.

BOX 9-1 Canadian Tobacco Advertising

Tobacco companies spend a lot of money each year to persuade people to buy cigarettes and other tobacco products. Obviously, these companies would have a difficult time selling tobacco if their advertising campaign focused on the qualities of the product itself—a product that shortens one's life and causes pain and suffering is not one that most people want to spend their hard earned money on (particularly if the product is for themselves rather than for their worst enemy). Therefore, tobacco companies usually highlight the product's positive image.

Parliament has been trying to curtail tobacco advertising for decades. In 1972, tobacco companies voluntarily withdrew from television and radio advertising. In 1988, the tobacco industry spent an unprecedented $33 million on advertising in Canada. The same year, the Tobacco Products Control Act banning tobacco advertising was passed. However, a loophole was discovered by the tobacco industry that would allow them to sponsor events such as car races, fireworks competitions and jazz festivals. In 1997, Parliament reintroduced restrictions on cigarette promotions in the 1997 Tobacco Act to eliminate tobacco sponsorships. However, Federal Health Minister Allan Rock delayed implementation of restrictions on tobacco sponsorships to honour a promise to car racing organizations. In the year 2000, tobacco advertising will be restricted to the sites of the events that they are promoting. By the year 2003, tobacco advertising will be banned everywhere.

It is interesting to note that in 1998, after Parliament reintroduced restrictions on cigarette promotions advertising, expenditures were as high as they were before any legal restrictions were imposed. Sponsorship promotions in 1998 were 380 percent higher than they were 5 years previously. And, if you remember, tobacco promotion supposedly disappeared from television screens in Canada in 1972. Yet, sponsored events (and advertisements for the events) have kept tobacco brands alive on Canadian television networks. In fact, it has been reported that tobacco logos were on air longer than all other commercials combined during these sports broadcasts (see web site, www.smoke-free.ca). For example, the 1997 du Maurier Open Mens Tennis Tournament that aired on CTV consisted of 1 hour and 45 minutes of programming time. For 46 minutes of that programming time, the tobacco logo was in view. In contrast, paid advertising time made up only 24 minutes of total measured air-time.

The image of the smoker also seems to be important. One study (Stanton et al., 1993) showed that "image" was a major reason for smoking among 11-year-olds. Other studies have found that boys and girls between the ages of 11 and 15 years often associate smoking with being attractive to the opposite sex, being "glamorous" and "exciting." The image of the smoker is also that he or she is rebellious, tough, and mature (Barton, Chassin, Presson, & Sherman, 1982; Dinh, Sarason, Peterson, & Onstad, 1995). The media certainly plays a role in formulating an image associated with smoking. Youngsters dealing with the insecurities of adolescence may find that cigarettes enable them to communicate the image they would like to convey (Aloise-Young, Hennigan, & Graham, 1996). Researchers estimate that advertising is responsible for 34 percent of experimentation with cigarettes (Pierce et al., 1998). The extent of tobacco advertising in Canada is described in Box 9.1.

Although situational factors (e.g., peer pressure) are thought to be the most important determinants in the initiation of smoking, personal characteristics also seem to be related to smoking behaviour. For example, characteristics such as low self-esteem, dependency, powerlessness, and social isolation all increase the tendency to imitate others' behaviour (Ennett & Bauman, 1993). It follows that low-achieving students, students with an external locus of control, and students with a low sense of self-efficacy are more likely to smoke than are students with high self-esteem, an internal locus of control, and a high sense of self-efficacy (Clark, MacPherson, & Holmes, 1982; Stacy et al., 1992). People who are rebellious and engage in risk-taking behaviours such as having multiple sex partners, using marijuana, and binge drinking are more likely to smoke than are people who do not engage in such behaviours (Emmons, Wechsler, Dowdall, & Abraham, 1998; Lipkus, Barefoot, Williams, & Siegler, 1994). To summarize, adolescents tend to begin smoking because of four factors: parental modelling, peer influence, cigarette advertising, and personal characteristics. But what factors are responsible for people becoming regular smokers?

Becoming a Regular Smoker

Although the majority of people try smoking at least once in their lives, most people do not become regular smokers. Researchers have not discovered why some people become regular smokers and others do not. There does not seem to be a single reason why people smoke. Rather, it appears that different people smoke for different reasons.

Much of the research investigating this topic has stemmed from the theoretical position of Silvan Tomkins (1966, 1968). Tomkins put forth four explanations as to why people who begin to smoke continue to smoke on a regular basis. Some people smoke to achieve a positive affect. In other words, a **positive-affect smoker** smokes to increase stimulation, to relax, or to gratify sensorimotor needs. In contrast, **negative-affect smokers** are people who smoke to reduce negative affect such as anxiety, distress, fear, or guilt. You may recall that Jennifer from our opening vignette first began to smoke to reduce loneliness. Later, she began to smoke again to deal with the stress in her life resulting from divorce proceedings; Jennifer would be considered a negative-affect smoker. Other people smoke simply out of habit. **Habitual smokers** probably initiated smoking to achieve a positive affect or reduce a negative affect but continue to smoke without awareness that they are doing so. These people do not derive any benefits from smoking. Finally, **addictive smokers**, those who develop a psychological dependence on smoking, are keenly aware of when they are not smoking. Addictive smokers can tell you exactly how long it has been since their last cigarette and how long it will likely be before their next one. These people have cigarettes with them at all times and usually keep at least one extra package on hand for "emergencies."

Because different people have different reasons for smoking, strategies to quit smoking vary in their effectiveness. For example, one study found that people who smoke for pleasure show a sharp drop in the number of cigarettes they smoke when their cigarettes have been dipped in vinegar, whereas those who smoke for other reasons (e.g., addiction) do not. In contrast, people who smoke primarily from habit show a marked reduction in the amount they smoke when asked to keep a record of cigarettes smoked, whereas this is not the case for those who smoke for pleasure (Ikard & Tomkins, 1973; Leventhal & Cleary, 1980).

We have discussed psychological reasons why people continue to smoke, but heredity may also play a role. Researchers have not definitively determined the link between heredity and smoking, but three possible explanations have been put forth. First, genetic factors may underlie certain personality traits associated with smoking (e.g., rebelliousness). Second, heredity may determine the extent to which people find tobacco pleasant or unpleasant. Third, genetically based differences in reaction to nicotine influence the degree to which people exposed to nicotine become dependent on it (Pomerleau, Collins, Shiffman, & Pomerleau, 1993).

Once people begin smoking regularly, they become physiologically dependent on the nicotine in cigarettes. However, before discussing the theories that attempt to explain the addictive quality of nicotine, we should first describe how nicotine initially affects us. When a person inhales smoke from a cigarette, nicotine passes through cell membranes in the mouth and nose on route to the lungs, where alveoli absorb it and carry it to the blood (e.g., Henningfield, Cohen, & Pickworth, 1993). In a very short, time the blood has carried the nicotine to the brain. In the brain, nicotine triggers the release of various chemicals that activate both the central and sympathetic nervous systems, resulting in increases in heart rate and blood pressure. This entire process takes approximately 7 seconds. Now, let's return to our discussion of nicotine addiction.

The exact nature of nicotine addiction is not clear. However, a number of theories have been put forth in an attempt to explain it. The **nicotine fixed-effect model** maintains that nicotine produces addiction by stimulating specific reward centres in the central nervous system (Hall, Rappaport, Hopkins, & Griffin, 1973). According to this model, nicotine has the paradoxical capacity to produce feelings of mental alertness and relaxation simultaneously. In contrast, the **nicotine regulation model** proposes that smokers develop an optimal level of nicotine in their bodies and then smoke in order to maintain this level and avoid withdrawal symptoms (Jarvik, 1973). These models both have limitations and have also been criticized because they focus entirely on the physiological aspects of addiction (e.g., Shiffman et al., 1995).

The **multiple regulation model** of smoking is a more comprehensive model of smoking than either the nicotine fixed-effect model or the nicotine regulation model (Leventhal & Cleary, 1980). The multiple regulation model maintains that the physiological effects of nicotine interact with the psychological functions of smoking to produce addiction. According to this model, emotional regulation is central to smoking, with nicotine levels being regulated because they have become conditioned to various emotional states. Let's demonstrate this by way of example. Consider Kelly, who is a 15-year-old shy, socially anxious teenager. To reduce her social anxiety, Kelly tends to smoke at parties and in other social situations. Once Kelly finishes a cigarette, however, the anxiety reappears and the level of nicotine in her blood begins to drop. As this is repeated over time, an increase in anxiety becomes conditioned to the decline in nicotine levels. This reinforces smoking by way of increasing nicotine level and also avoiding anxiety. Although this model seems to account for the addictive nature of smoking better than theories that focus exclusively on either psychological or physiological aspects, it too does not account for all that is known about smoking.

The **biobehavioural model** developed by Pomerleau and Pomerleau (1989) maintains that people use and come to depend on the effects of nicotine to regulate cognitive performance and emotional affect. More specifically, when nicotine reaches the brain it triggers the release of such chemicals as acetylcholine, norepinephrine, dopamine, endogenous opiods, and vasopressin. These chemicals improve memory, enhance pleasure, and facilitate task performance. Further, these chemicals decrease symptoms of nicotine withdrawal and feelings of anxiety, tension, and pain (McGehee et al., 1995). According to the biobehavioural model, regular smokers have trouble quitting because when they decrease their nicotine level they notice a reduction in concentration, attention, and memory performance, and an increase in anxiety, irritability, and moodiness.

Health Consequences of Smoking

As previously mentioned, smoking is the number one preventable cause of death and disease in Canada. Research conclusively documents that smoking reduces life expectancy by several years. Ellison and his colleagues (1999) at Health Canada determined that the rate of premature deaths (before age 70) was twice that among lifelong smokers compared to never-smokers for both males and females. Smoking also increases the risk of many illnesses, including cancer and cardiovascular disease (Thun et al., 1995). In fact, the more you smoke, the worse your odds become. The good news is that if you do quit smoking, your odds steadily improve. After 15 or 20 years as a non-smoker, your odds are similar to those of people who have never smoked (LaCroix et al., 1991; Ockene, Kuller, Svendsen, & Meilahn, 1990).

Smoking and Cardiovascular and Cerebrovascular Disease. Together, cardiovascular and cerebrovascular diseases were responsible for 73 000 deaths (34.7%) in Canada in 1995 (Statistics Canada, 1999). In general, the risk of dying of cardiovascular disease is about twice as high for smokers as for non-smokers (CDC, 1993). The risk is slightly higher for men than for women (Colditz et al., 1988).

Smoking is thought to contribute to cardiovascular disease in a number of ways. There is some evidence that cigarette smoking increases the level of serum cholesterol and the size of plaque within the arteries. Amazingly, the progression of atherosclerosis is estimated to increase by as much as 50 percent during a 3-year period (Tell et al., 1994; Howard et al., 1998). Nicotine itself may also contribute to heart disease. Nicotine has a stimulant effect on the nervous system, resulting in increases in heart rate, blood pressure, and cardiac output, combined with constriction of blood vessels. Fortunately, the risk of heart attack and stroke, like that of cancer, decline when people quit smoking (Kawachi et al., 1993; Negri et al., 1994).

Smoking and Cancer. Cancer is one of the leading causes of death in Canada. In 1995, 27.4 percent of deaths in Canada were attributed to various forms of cancer (Statistics

Canada, 1999). Although almost 80 percent of smoking-related deaths in Canada result from lung cancer, smoking is also responsible for deaths from cancer of the lip, oral cavity, pharynx, esophagus, pancreas, larynx, urinary bladder, and kidney (Ellison et al., 1999). Researchers in the United States have documented the correspondence between the rise in lung cancer deaths and the prevalence of smoking since the 1930s. These researchers (e.g., McGinnis, Shopland, & Brown, 1987; Shopland & Burns, 1993) state that the rate of mortality from lung cancer began to rise approximately 15 to 20 years after the rate of smoking started to rise. Not surprisingly, these rates have paralleled each other since that time.

Numerous retrospective and prospective studies have consistently demonstrated the link between tobacco use and cancer in humans (e.g., Lam et al., 1997). Experimental studies on laboratory animals have gone a step further and identified the tar in tobacco as a likely carcinogen. The research findings overwhelmingly demonstrate that tobacco tars and likely other by-products of tobacco smoke cause cancer (e.g., Denissenko, Pao, Tang, & Pfeifer, 1996).

Smoking and Chronic Obstructive Pulmonary Diseases. Chronic obstructive pulmonary diseases (COPD) include a number of respiratory and lung diseases, such as chronic bronchitis and emphysema. They accounted for 9 185 deaths (4.4%) in Canada in 1995 (Statistics Canada, 1999). Virtually all COPD are experienced by smokers. In other words, these conditions are relatively rare in non-smokers (Whitemore, Perlin, & DiCiccio, 1995). In general terms, smoking irritates and damages respiratory organs. This damage leads to reduced airflow when breathing and is particularly noticeable when the person tries to exhale with force.

Environmental Tobacco Smoke

We have looked at what happens to the health of people who smoke. What we have not considered is the number of people who are affected by **environmental tobacco smoke (ETS)**, also known as secondhand smoke. Most Canadians spend more time indoors than outdoors, and tobacco smoke is a key contaminant in indoor air quality. Breathing ETS is called **passive smoking**. Health Canada estimates that more than 300 Canadian non-smokers die each year from lung cancer caused by exposure to ETS (Health Canada, 1999). The number of non-smokers who die from cardiovascular disease as a result of ETS is likely much higher, given that researchers have estimated that at least 10 times the number of non-smokers die from ETS-related cardiovascular disease than do from ETS-related lung cancer. Pregnant women, fetuses, and young children are especially susceptible to the effects of ETS. Resulting health consequences include complications of pregnancy and low birthweight, increased risk of sudden infant death syndrome and ear infections, reduced lung development, and increased severity of asthma and other respiratory illnesses. In an effort to protect people many municipalities now have restrictions on smoking in public settings. Municipal bylaw coverage has continued to increase since 1991 (Health Canada, 1999).

Quitting Smoking

As previously mentioned, smoking is an **addiction**. That is, once people begin to smoke regularly most become physically or psychologically dependent on it. Therefore, if someone wanted to quit smoking he or she would have to go through a period of **withdrawal**. Withdrawal refers to the unpleasant symptoms that people experience when they stop using a substance they have become dependent on. As previously mentioned, when one reduces or eliminates nicotine intake he or she will experience a reduction in concentration, attention, and memory performance as well as an increase in anxiety, irritability, and moodiness.

Quitting on One's Own. The vast majority of individuals who quit smoking will quit on their own, without any professional help (Schacter, 1982; Cunningham, 1999). Though heavy smokers report finding it more difficult to quit and experience more unpleasant effects from quitting than do light smokers, there is no difference in success rates between the two groups. However, there are age differences in success rates. Younger light smokers are more likely than heavy smokers to give up smoking. In contrast, among older smokers, heavy smokers were more successful at quitting. This age difference may result from older smokers having experienced health problems due to their smoking habits that necessitate they quit smoking (Cohen et al., 1989; Coambs, Li, & Kozlowski, 1992). We should point out that most people can stop smoking on their own but that most do not succeed in their first attempt (Rose, Chassin, Presson, & Sherman, 1996).

Quitting with Therapy. If people cannot quit smoking on their own, they often seek help from others. Most therapies include nicotine-replacement therapy, psychological interventions, or both. Therapies that combine both nicotine replacement therapy and psychological interventions, known as multidimensional approaches, are considered most effective (Cinciripini et al., 1996; Laforge, Wiley, Prochaska, & Levesque, 1995).

Nicotine-replacement therapy provides some form of nicotine replacement for the nicotine former smokers previously obtained through smoking. Typically, nicotine gum or the nicotine patch are used. **Nicotine gum** provides small amounts of nicotine to the person when chewed. The **nicotine patch**, on the other hand, resembles a large bandage and releases a small continuous dose of nicotine into the body's system. Patches with smaller and smaller doses of nicotine are worn until the person is no longer addicted to the nicotine. A 17 to 18 percent cessation rate is achieved by people who use nicotine gum versus 9 percent for placebo gum, whereas a 22 percent cessation rate is achieved by those who use the nicotine patch compared to about 9 percent for a placebo patch (Tsoh et al., 1997). Recently, it has been discovered that if the drug bupropion is combined with the patch, a 35 percent cessation rate is obtained (Jorenby et al., 1999). No matter what form of nicotine replacement is used, it will be more effective if various psychological approaches to treatment are used as well (Cinciripini et al., 1996; Laforge et al., 1995).

The psychological approaches to smoking cessation generally take one of two different forms: aversion therapies or self-management strategies. **Aversion therapies** involve pairing the behaviour to be eliminated, in this case smoking, with some unpleasant stimulus so that smoking will elicit negative sensations. The three most common forms of aversion therapies are electric shock, imagined aversive scenes, and rapid smoking. *Electric shock* can be paired with smoking situations so that when a person smokes they are shocked and made uncomfortable. When *aversive scenes* are employed, people are directed to think of an aversive scene that includes the smoking behaviour when they are about to begin smoking and then something disgusting (e.g., you take the cigarette out of the pack and are about to light it when you suddenly vomit all over your cigarette, your hands, and the lighter. The smell is so foul you can hardly stand it. You drop the cigarette and the lighter and as you turn away and head toward the bathroom to clean yourself up you begin to feel much less nauseous). The third technique, *rapid smoking*, is very seldom used. Rapid smoking involves placing the smoker in a small, enclosed room where he or she is to inhale from a cigarette rapidly every few seconds while concentrating on the smoke, the stinging burn in the throat, and other unpleasant elements. Aversion strategies may help in the initial stages of quitting smoking but the effects are seldom longterm.

Self-management strategies are designed to help people overcome the environmental conditions that perpetuate smoking. *Self-monitoring* requires that people record each cigarette smoked, the time of day, where they were, who they were with, and their mood. Self-monitoring in itself reduces smoking, but the information obtained also aids in formulating other approaches to smoking cessation. *Stimulus control* strategies focus on removing the cues that lead a person to smoke. For example, if a person always smokes during their coffee break when they are sitting in the staff room, that person may want to go for a walk or have their coffee break in a different location. *Behavioural contracting* involves establishing a contract so that a person will be rewarded if they fulfill the contract or punished if they do not. These contracts often involve the person depositing a large sum of money that they will lose if they do not adhere to the contract.

These are only a few of the strategies that can be used to help people quit smoking. Focus on Research 9.1 outlines a large-scale attempt to encourage people to quit smoking.

FOCUS ON RESEARCH 9-1

COMMIT: The Community Intervention Trial for Smoking Cessation

The National Cancer Institute's Community Intervention Trial for Smoking Cessation (COMMIT) was a 7-year, multicentre, cooperative research project involving 11 pairs of matched communities (10 in the U.S. and 1 in Canada). It is the most extensive tobacco-control study ever undertaken in North America. Branftord, Ontario served as the intervention community in Canada and Peterborough, Ontario as its comparison. The goal of COMMIT was to increase the priority of smoking cessation as a public health issue and to increase social norms and values supporting non-smoking. Initially, surveys were conducted at each site to determine both the prevalence of smoking and attitudes towards smoking (c.f., Taylor, Goldsmith, & Best, 1996). Anti-smoking intervention strategies were then implemented and the effects of these interventions measured.

Researchers worked with each intervention community to determine and implement the most suitable intervention strategies for their population. Some of the intervention strategies used in Brantford were: smoking policy workshops and consultations at the worksite; between-worksite challenges and competitions; publicizing smoking-control activities and awareness campaigns through the media; development and maintenance of a cessation resources guide; and preparation and distribution of a semiannual newsletter. In addition, heavy smokers were recruited and became part of the "Smokers' Network." These individuals were provided with "survival kits" (both humourous and useful contents for stopping smoking) and were encouraged to participate in a Quit and Win contest. Contest participants were asked to commit to remaining smoke-free for 30 days in exchange for the chance to win a substantial prize. This strategy proved quite popular and was repeated numerous times. There were between 50 and 200 participants each time. A final strategy worth mentioning is the "Sting" operations. These involved young people under legal age attempting to purchase cigarettes. The results of these attempts were then made public to inform the community about the ease of access to tobacco for underage smokers. The smoking cessation interventions took place for 4 years, from 1989 to 1993 (Lindsay et al., 1996).

Results of these interventions were somewhat disappointing. For example, the number of heavy smokers in the intervention communities who quit smoking was not significantly different from the number who quit in the comparison communities. However, light-to-moderate smokers in the intervention communities were more likely to quit than those in the comparison communities (COMMIT Research Group, 1995a, 1995b). There were also substantial changes in favour of stronger anti-smoking attitudes over the course of the trial. However, this attitude change occurred in both intervention and comparison communities and was consistent with findings across North America (Taylor et al., 1998). It may be that global attitude changes need more time to develop in response to the intervention. Certainly, a change in public attitude was witnessed in response to the sting operations in Brantford from one year to the next (Lindsay et al., 1996). As well, change resulted when a representative from Alcoholics Anonymous spontaneously initiated the establishment of a non-smoking chapter of AA (Zanna et al., 1996).

Alcohol Use

Alcohol Consumption

About 53 percent of Canadians (63% of men and 43% of women) drink alcohol at least once per month (Health Canada, 1999). Women are more likely than men to be non-drinkers. Men are more likely than women to report being "heavy" or "binge" drinkers, that is, to have consumed five or more drinks on at least one occasion in the past year. The proportion of men and women who drink at least one drink per month rises steadily with increases in income. This is a trend that is in direct contrast to smoking. You may remember that smoking rates decrease steadily with income level. If we look at episodes of binge drinking, we see that 24 percent of men in the two lowest income levels who were drinkers reported at least one episode of binge drinking, compared to 43 percent of men in the highest income bracket. A "J" shape is produced when the rate of binge drinking among women according to income level is plotted. The rate of binge drinking among women drinkers in the lowest income level was 13 percent in the Health Canada study. This dropped to 10 percent at the next income level then slowly climbed to 19 percent at the highest income level.

Age is another factor associated with drinking. Although rates of drinking for adults have been decreasing over the last couple of decades, there are disturbing indications that the proportion of adolescents who drink is increasing (Canadian Centre on Substance Abuse, 1999). For example, the Nova Scotia Student Drug Use Survey reported that 57 percent of students drank alcohol in 1998, an increase of 12 percent from 1991. Similar rates of drinking are reported by students in the other Atlantic provinces (Prince Edward Island, 53%; New Brunswick, 56%; Newfoundland, 58%) and in Ontario (60%) (cited in Health Canada, 1999). Not surprisingly, the percentage of adolescents who have tried alcohol increases with age. In British Columbia, 47 percent of boys and 41 percent of girls have tried alcohol by age 13 (McCreary Centre Society, 1999). This figure increases to 80 percent for both males and females aged 17 years. Other provinces have also noted an increase in drinking with age (Health Canada, 1999). In Nova Scotia, 21 percent of Grade 7 students and 58 percent of Grade 9 students reported drinking alcohol in the previous year. The rates are similar in Newfoundland and Labrador (20% of Grade 7 students and 59% of Grade 9 students) and in Ontario (32% of Grade 7 students and 56% of Grade 9 students). Previously, we discussed the prevalence of binge drinking in adults. Unfortunately, this rate seems to be even higher in adolescents. In British Columbia, more than 40 percent of the 12 to 18-year-olds who reported ever having a drink had engaged in a binge at least once during the past month! This figure had increased seven percent from 1992 to 1998 for both males and females (McCreary Centre Society, 1999). And, aboriginal Canadian adolescents are reported as having a risk that is as much as six times greater than other Canadians for developing alcohol problems (Canadian Centre on Substance Abuse, 1999).

American studies indicate that the use of alcohol is lowest among older adults (U.S. Department of Health and Human Services, 1998). However, this may be due more to heavy drinkers dying younger than to older people modifying their drinking habits as they age. Prospective studies have found only a small decline in alcohol use as people become older (National Institute on Alcohol Abuse and Alcoholism, 1988).

The Effects of Alcohol

The alcohol used in beverages is called **ethanol** or **ethyl alcohol**. This alcohol is a depressant drug and, like other depressant drugs (e.g., tranquillizers and painkillers), it slows down the nervous system, which may cause drowsiness, induce sleep, or relieve pain. Even the initial apparent stimulant effect actually results from depression of centres in the brain that inhibit our actions and control our behaviour. After one drink, the majority of people report feeling more relaxed. With more than one drink, a person may feel more outgoing and self-confident, but some people will become aggressive, depressed, or withdrawn. At higher doses—even below a blood-alcohol concentration of 0.08, the legal limit for driving a car in Canada—thinking, judgment, and ability to estimate distance can be impaired and reaction times increased (Alberta Alcohol and Drug Abuse Commission, 1999).

Excessive use of alcohol can have adverse effects on almost every system of the body. For example, chronic alcohol abuse causes liver disease and damage to the stomach, pancreas, and intestines. Moreover, chronic drinking causes high blood pressure, depression of the immune system, and is associated with coronary artery disease, cancer of the throat, larynx, mouth, esophagus, and liver (Alberta Alcohol and Drug Abuse Commission, 1999). Other consequences of drinking include blackouts, hangovers, and even death. Blackouts are periods of memory loss that occur while a person is drinking heavily. Hangovers, on the other hand, occur after drinking has stopped. Hangovers are caused by mild alcohol withdrawal and may be experienced 8 to 12 hours after a bout of heavy drinking. The symptoms of a hangover include fatigue, headache, nausea, and sometimes vomiting and shakiness. Death may occur following moderate doses of alcohol taken together with other depressant drugs, such as sleeping pills and tranquillizers, or from an overdose of alcohol as a result of excessive consumption. This kind of consumption has been associated with events such as college fraternity initiations. For example, some college students have been known to participate in the dangerous behaviour of "funneling", putting a funnel in someone's mouth and pouring liquor into the funnel. This method of drinking can be lethal because it easily provides too much alcohol to the person.

Although, as noted above, there are many dire negative consequences to excessive drinking, there are, in fact, health benefits for light to moderate drinkers. Numerous studies (Berkman, Breslow, & Wingard, 1983; Friedman & Kimball, 1986; Cullen, Knuimon, & Ward, 1993; Kitamura et al., 1998) have reported that moderate drinking has survival advantages for men. Specifically, this research has shown that light to moderate drinkers are at less risk of developing coronary heart disease and possibly stroke (Maclure, 1993; Sacco et al., 1999). Although the relationship between drinking and survival is less clear for women, one study found that women who drank from three to eighteen drinks per week had a reduced risk of death, particularly from cardiovascular disease (Fuchs et al., 1995). However, women who drank more than 18 drinks per week had an increased risk of death from other causes (e.g., breast cancer and cirrhosis). We should point out that early studies indicated that red wine was the kind of alcohol that resulted in survival advantages. More recent research has found no particular advantage of one kind of alcohol over another. Wine, beer, and liquor are all thought to produce the same advantages (Parker et al., 1996; Rehm et al., 1997). Researchers believe that consuming alcohol increases levels of high-density lipoprotein (HDL), which is responsible for a decreased risk of heart attacks (Gaziano et al., 1993; Linn et al., 1993).

Explaining Drinking Behaviour

It has been suggested that drinking is well accepted and therefore commonplace in North America. One wonders if, in fact, drinking is so commonplace that it is well accepted. Regardless, drunkenness or problem drinking is not acceptable, and it is therefore important to explain why this behaviour occurs (McMurran, 1994). The **disease model** of problem drinking maintains that alcoholism is a disease brought about by the physical properties of alcohol (Jellinek, 1960). The **alcohol dependency syndrome model** states that at certain times and for a variety of reasons people do not exercise control over their drinking and this leads to problem drinking (Edwards & Gross, 1976). A number of elements are said to be essential for alcohol dependency syndrome to develop, including a salience of drink-seeking behaviour (meaning that drinking begins to take priority over all other aspects of life) and an increased tolerance for alcohol. Someone with an increased tolerance for alcohol may gradually become accustomed to going about their daily routine "at blood alcohol levels that would incapacitate the non-tolerant drinker" (Edwards & Gross, 1976, p. 1059). Although this model remains popular in certain circles it has been criticized because of its emphasis on the physical properties of alcohol and its neglect of the cognitive and social learning aspects of drinking (McMurran, 1994)

Cognitive-physiological models propose that people drink because alcohol influences cognitive functioning, allowing people to escape tension and negative self-evaluations. One of these models, the **tension reduction hypothesis**, maintains that people drink alcohol because of its tension-reducing properties (Conger, 1956). Although there is little empirical support for this theory, some research suggests that alcohol may lead people to avoid tension-producing behaviours or situations (Sher & Levenson, 1982). The **self-awareness model** suggests that drinking inhibits the use of normal, complex information-processing strategies such as memory and information acquisition, making people less self-aware (Hull, 1981, 1987; Hull & Bond, 1986). Decreased self-awareness leads to decreased monitoring of behaviour, resulting in the disinhibition and decrease in self-criticism that often occurs when people are drinking. Simply stated, some people may consume alcohol to avoid self-awareness. A third cognitive-physiological theory developed to explain drinking behaviour is called **alcohol myopia** (Steele & Josephs, 1990). Alcohol myopia refers to a drinker's decreased ability to process information outside a narrow range (myopia). This effect also helps to lower inhibition of impulsive responses. Alcohol myopia is characterized by people behaving more excessively (i.e., more friendly, more aggressive, etc.), having a tendency to inflate self-evaluations, and experiencing *drunken relief* or a tendency to worry less and pay less attention to their worries.

The **social learning model** proposes that people drink because they experience positive reinforcement for doing so (e.g., the taste or the effects of alcohol are pleasant) or because they observe others drinking and model this behaviour. For example, you may try drinking because your friends drink and you may continue to drink in the company of your friends. Or, once you have tried drinking you may like the taste of the beverage or you may notice a change in your behaviour that you find appealing (e.g., you feel less shy after having a drink). Social learning theory can explain why people begin to drink, why they continue to drink in moderation, and why some people drink to excess. Excessive drinking may occur because of modelling (your friends are also drinking to excess) or because once you stop drinking you experience negative reinforcement in the form of a hangover or withdrawal symptoms. According to the social learning model, drinking behaviour is learned and can therefore also be unlearned. A number of treatment techniques to help people overcome excessive drinking habits rely on social learning principles.

Preventing and Treating Alcohol Abuse

Attempts to prevent alcohol abuse have taken a number of forms. Public policy and legal approaches include implementing age restrictions for individuals buying or consuming alcohol. Health promotion and education strategies incorporating social influence approaches are found to be useful in helping adolescents avoid drinking heavily. These may include discussions and films regarding how peers, family members, and the media influence drinking, or modelling and role-playing of specific refusal skills (e.g., "No thank you, I don't drink") and how to deal with high-risk situations (Donaldson, Graham, Piccinin, & Hansen, 1995; Kivlahen et al., 1990; Klepp, Kelder, & Perry, 1995).

Like quitting smoking, the majority of people stop drinking without treatment (Cunningham, 1999). Authorities in the field of problem drinking prefer to use the term *unassisted change* (McMurran, 1994). This term may be somewhat misleading, because support is likely provided to the individual by many people in an informal manner (Sobel, Sobel, Toneatto, & Leo, 1993). However, many individuals who cannot quit drinking on their own seek formal treatment. All formal treatments strive to achieve immediate abstinence. Some programs may permit light drinking to resume at a later point in time. Twelve-step programs such as Alcoholics Anonymous (AA) have become increasingly popular. Yet, this kind of program doesn't seem to be more effective than other formal treatments. One controlled study (Brandsma, Maultsby, & Walsh, 1980) found that participants who were seeking treatment through AA had a higher dropout rate (68%) than those in any of the other treatment groups in the study (57%). Psychotherapy, drug therapy (e.g., disulfiram, commonly known as Antabuse) and aversion therapy (e.g., electric shock or with the drug emetine) have all been used with limited success (Miller & Hester, 1980; Schuckit, 1996). Relapse is a persistent problem with all alcohol treatment approaches. Most often, a relapse will occur within 3 months after the end of treatment. After a year, only about one-third of those who complete the program are still abstinent (Baker, Cooney, & Pomerleau, 1987).

Drinking and Driving

We mentioned previously that drinking influences our thought processes. Unfortunately, alcohol causes people to think less negatively about drinking and driving (MacDonald, Zanna, & Fong, 1995, 1998). The result is disastrous—people drink and drive and are often involved in motor vehicle accidents. According to the 1996/97 National Population Health Survey, 10 percent of Canadians who have a driver's licence and consume alcohol admitted to driving after consuming "too much" alcohol. Men (13%) are more likely than women (5%) to report drinking and driving, and young drivers aged 18 and 19 years report drinking and driving more than do other age groups (Health Canada, 1999). Because judgment and decision making are impaired it is not surprising that intoxicated individuals are often involved in traffic accidents. Fortunately, there has been a significant decline in the number of fatal injures resulting from drinking and driving over the last 20 years. The rate of alcohol involvement in traffic deaths, however, remains unacceptably high. According to Transport Canada, there were 3 082 motor vehicle traffic deaths in 1996 (cited in Health Canada, 1999). Among fatally injured drivers, 35 percent were legally impaired. Statistics are not available for the number of innocent victims injured or killed.

Illicit Drug Use

Compared with the effects of smoking cigarettes and drinking alcohol, relatively few people die from the effects of illegal drugs. For example, cocaine, the most lethal of the illicit drugs, kills only one person for every 1 000 killed by tobacco products (Rouse, 1998). Of course, even one death from illicit drugs is too many. Illicit drugs present certain risks not found with legal drugs, regardless of pharmacological effects. A person purchasing illicit drugs may be told he's buying one drug and then receive another; illegally manufactured drugs may be contaminated with other very toxic chemicals; and users never really know what drug or how much of a particular drug they are taking.

How prevalent is the use of illicit drugs? The most commonly used illicit drug in North America is marijuana. Seven percent of Canadians reported using marijuana in the 1994/95 National Public Health Survey. However, the rate of young people using marijuana (young people are the most frequent users of illicit drugs) has been increasing. In 1998, 40 percent of students in British Columbia reported using marijuana, up from 25 percent in 1992 (McCreary Centre Society, 1999). Similar increases have been found in Nova Scotia (from 17% in 1991 to 38% in 1998) and in Ontario (from 12% in 1991 to 25% in 1997) (Health Canada, 1999). About half of those who have used marijuana report having done so in the past month.

Adolescents are also most likely to use other illicit drugs. Surveys of the general population indicate that fewer than one percent of Canadians use crack cocaine, LSD, or speed. However, eleven percent of adolescents in British Columbia report using hallucinogens (e.g., LSD and ecstasy) seven percent report using cocaine, and two percent report using heroin. Studies conducted in other provinces have shown significant increases in the use of a number of drugs by students. For example, LSD, non-prescription and prescription stimulants, mescaline, cocaine or crack, PCP, heroin, and inhalants have all been reported as being used more in 1998 than in 1991 (Health Canada, 1999). Let's turn our attention to some of the health problems associated with some of the more common illicit drugs.

Marijuana

Marijuana is composed of the leaves, flowers, and small branches of *Cannabis sativa*, a plant that grows in almost every climate. Delta-9-tetrahydrocannabinol (THC) is the intoxicating ingredient of marijuana. Is smoking marijuana a potential health hazard? Marijuana leads to disturbances in short-term memory, judgment, and time perception (Ferraro, 1980). When large doses are consumed, heart rate is increased. A rapid heart rate may lead to health hazards for people who have coronary problems. However, few authorities regard marijuana as a major health risk. One study (Sidney et al., 1997) found no increase in mortality rates of marijuana users, with the exception of men who died of AIDS. This study does not determine cause and effect. However, we can probably assume that marijuana did not cause death from AIDS. Instead, we might assume that men who received a diagnosis of AIDS subsequently increased their use of marijuana. Marijuana has been used in medical situations because of its effects. It has been used as an appetite stimulant for AIDS patients and has been used medically to treat glaucoma and prevent the vomiting and nausea associated with chemotherapy (Grinspoon & Bakalar, 1995). Although marijuana is used as a medical treatment, it remains illegal even for this purpose.

Why do people use marijuana in spite of the aforementioned side effects? They do so to experience euphoria, a sense of well-being, feelings of relaxation, and heightened sexual responsiveness. The desired psychological effects of marijuana seem to depend, in part, on setting and personal expectation. It's not surprising that those who attain these psychological effects are usually experienced marijuana smokers who expect to attain them. Marijuana use does not lead to physiological dependence and withdrawal symptoms do not occur with cessation of marijuana use.

LSD, PCP, and MDMA

LSD (lysergic acid diethylamide, commonly referred to as "acid"), PCP (phycyclidine, commonly referred to as "angel dust"), and MDMA (3,4-methylenedioxymethylamphetamine, most often referred to as "ecstacy") are drugs that are classified as **hallucinogens**. These drugs dramatically affect perception, emotions, and mental processes. As their name suggests, they can cause hallucinations. Hallucinations can elicit feelings of euphoria but can also cause one to feel threatened; because of fear, anxiety, or panic, the user can behave quite violently. More often, however, users report a sense of well-being and heightened tactile sensations and emotions. The effects of MDMA usually last up to 8 hours and those of LSD up to 12 hours, while the effects of PCP usually disappear within a few hours or days when taking a single dose. However, the effects of high doses of PCP have lasted from 10 days to 2 weeks (Alberta Alcohol and Drug Abuse Commission, 1999).

Short-term physiological reactions to hallucinogens include increased blood pressure, heart rate, and temperature; dilated pupils; impaired motor skills and coordination; dizziness; and nausea. Larger doses can cause convulsions, coma, and death. Persistent speech problems, memory loss, severe depression and anxiety, and social withdrawal have also been noted following prolonged use.

Cocaine

Cocaine is a **stimulant** drug, extracted from the coca plant indigenous to the Andes Mountains in South America. Cocaine is most often snorted through the nasal passages but is also smoked and "freebased", that is, injected intravenously. Cocaine provides a strong sense of well-being, heightened attention, and a powerful euphoria. This effect lasts approximately 15 to 30 minutes. When the effects wear off, the user is often left with a feeling of fatigue, sluggishness, and a strong desire to "use" again. Increased doses do not make the euphoria last longer and can endanger the cardiovascular system.

One study of lifetime cocaine use among young adults found no relationship between heavy use of cocaine and various cardiovascular risk factors (Braun, Murray, & Signey, 1997). However, other research has shown that cocaine does have negative effects on the cardiovascular system (Rowbotham & Lowenstein, 1990). Using cocaine causes the person's blood vessels to constrict, their heart rate to increase, and their blood pressure to speed up suddenly. It can also trigger cardiac arrhythmia. These factors may cause a stroke or myocardial infarction. Physiological withdrawal symptoms do not accompany cessation of cocaine use but psychological dependence does seem to occur.

Preventing and Treating Illicit Drug Use

Programs aimed at preventing teenage drug abuse are similar to those aimed at preventing smoking. Children and adolescents can be educated through the schools and mass media about the deleterious effects of drug abuse. These educational programs are based on social influence and life skills training methods that teach children and adolescents how to resist starting to use drugs (Botvin et al., 1990; Botvin & Willis, 1985). A second preventative technique is common in all Western countries: the use of laws to limit the legal access to drugs. Unfortunately, this approach may produce other social problems (e.g., a large criminal enterprise) (Robins, 1995). Finally, encouraging parental monitoring of their children was found to reduce the likelihood that children will try drugs (Chilcoat, Dishion, & Anthony, 1995).

Treatment programs for drug abuse are similar to those for alcohol abuse. In fact, it's not uncommon for formal treatment centres to treat both forms of abuse. The most promising treatment approaches include both behavioural and cognitive methods, such as self-management techniques (Tims, Fletcher, & Hubard, 1991). Unfortunately, as with the treatment of alcohol and smoking, there is a high rate of relapse, and the first 6 months after treatment are critical. Many drug treatment programs now include follow-up or "booster" sessions to help people remain abstinent.

The use of drugs and alcohol directly results in numerous health consequences. Their use also leads to indirect health consequences. For instance, individuals who are intoxicated are more likely to engage in risky behaviours such as unsafe sexual practices (MacDonald, MacDonald, Zanna, & Fong, in press; MacDonald, Zanna, & Fong, 1996, 1998). Let's explore the practice of unsafe sexual behaviours further.

Unsafe Sexual Behaviours

The effects of unsafe sexual behaviours are both numerous and negative. In addition to unplanned pregnancies, unsafe sexual behaviours can lead to serious health consequences, such as sexually transmitted diseases (STDs), infertility, and HIV infection. Results from the 1994/95 National Public Health Survey indicated that 51 percent of female and 29 percent of male sexually active 15- to 19-year-olds (excluding those with a single sex partner and who were married, in a common-law relationship, divorced, or widowed) had had sex without a condom in the past year. Among youth aged 20 to 24 years, 53 percent of sexually active females and 44 percent of sexually active males reported having had sex without a condom during the previous year.

Few studies have investigated the sexual behaviour of Canadian aboriginal populations (Calzavara et al., 1999). However, Canadian aboriginals have rates of sexually transmitted disease as much as four times higher than the rate in the general population. This may indicate that aboriginals may be more likely than the general population to engage in unsafe sexual behaviours (Jolly, Orr, Hammond, & Young, 1995). A recent survey (Calzavara et al.) of 11 reserve communities in Ontario found that only 9 percent of those who engaged in vaginal intercourse in the previous year reported always using condoms. Moreover, only 11.2 percent of those who engaged in anal intercourse reported always using condoms. These statistics were derived from a sample of individuals who were 15 years old or older and single (32%), married or common-law (45%), and separated, divorced, or widowed (29.4%).

Why do people not use condoms when engaging in intercourse? Researchers (MacDonald et al., 1990) attempted to gain insight into this question by conducting a national survey of 5 500 first-year Canadian college and university students between the ages of 16 and 24 years. The students reported not using condoms because they were embarrassed about purchasing them, they had difficulty discussing condom use with their partner, they believed that condoms interfered with sexual pleasure, and because they already used oral contraceptives. Another factor associated with not using condoms was insufficient knowledge of HIV/STDs. Amazingly, in the study with aboriginals mentioned previously, nine percent of those who reported being sexually active over the previous year had not heard of AIDS (Calzavara et al., 1999). A number of factors were not significant in influencing condom use among the students surveyed, including grade point average, fear of acquiring an STD or AIDS, history of STDs, and trust in partner's information about previous experiences. While almost half of the students believed that carrying a condom makes others think that an individual is willing to have sex, this belief was not related to condom use. The reasons provided by the general population for participating in unsafe sexual behaviours are similar to those provided by the students surveyed in the study by MacDonald et al. (e.g., Boroditsky, Fisher, & Sand, 1995).

A variety of theoretical approaches have been used in an attempt to determine sexual and reproductive health behaviours (see Fisher & Fisher, 1998, for a review of these theories). Some of these theories have been developed outside the domain of sexual and reproductive health and applied within it, for example, the health belief model (Rosenstock, Stretcher, & Becker, 1994), the theory of reasoned action (Fishbein & Ajzen, 1975), the theory of planned behavior (Ajzen, 1991), and the stages of change model (Prochaska & Velicer, 1997). You may remember reading about these theories in Chapter 1. Other theories have been developed and applied specifically within the area of sexuality and reproductive health, including the sexual behavior sequence (Byrne, 1977), the AIDS risk reduction model (Catania, Kegeles, & Coates, 1990) and the information–motivation–behavioural skills model (Fisher & Fisher, 1992, 1999). Let's take a closer look at one of these models.

The **information–motivation–behavioural skills model** (Fisher & Fisher, 1992; Fisher & Fisher, 1999) maintains there are a number of steps one must go through to successfully achieve safe sex practices. First, a person must recognize and accept that he or she is sexually active. Second, the person must create a "sexual and reproductive health agenda." In other words, the individual must be motivated to engage in safe sex practices to prevent pregnancy and infection. Third, the individual must be capable of engaging in behaviours that fulfill this agenda. For example, he or she must be able to negotiate cooperation in contraceptive and condom use with a partner. If cooperation is not forthcoming, the individual must be able to exit the situation. This model also acknowledges that it is frequently necessary to engage in public sexual and reproductive health behaviour acts (e.g., condom purchasing, HIV testing). To maintain safe sexual practices over time, an individual must be able to reinforce this behaviour (this could be done by such behaviours as acknowledging one's relief or gratitude). Finally, the individual must be able to adjust sexual and reproductive health behaviour scripts appropriately as his or her needs change over time. For example, it may be appropriate to shift from condom use to monogamy after a window period, mutual STD and HIV antibody testing, and discussion of how to continue mutual monogamy and how violations of this agreement will be handled. Of course, this change in practice can only take place if both the relationship and the individuals in the relationship are mature enough to entertain the responsibilities and risks associated with this agreement. We cannot emphasize enough that it is inappropriate to shift from condom use to monogamy as a strategy for safe sex behaviour after a brief period of "getting to know" one's partner or for younger couples, whose relationships tend to be less stable and long lasting (Misovich, Fisher, & Fisher, 1996).

GERIATRIC HEALTH

Twelve percent of the Canadian population is over the age of 65 years and there has been a 31 percent increase in the number of elderly over the age of 85 years in the past 5 years

(National Advisory Council on Aging, 1997). These demographics point to the importance of examining issues and concerns regarding healthy aging.

Personal Autonomy and Physical Decline

Personal autonomy is very important to our sense of well-being. When an individual has independence, they have control over their lives. When independence is taken away, control is taken away. This results in a feeling of helplessness. People who feel in control are happier, are less likely to experience stress, and even recover from surgery faster than patients who do not experience control (this finding is discussed in more detail in Chapter 7).

Sensory Changes

A number of physical changes occur when one ages. Some of these changes become barriers to older people's autonomy. For instance, changes in vision occur as a result of the normal aging process. By the age of 50 years, many people have become aware of vision changes. Typically, older adults will experience a gradual decline in the ability to read small print or to focus on objects. This is called **presbyopia**. With increasing age there is a decrease in the sharpness of vision, double-vision or "haloes" around bright lights might appear, and more light may be needed for certain activities like reading or driving. Serious visual problems, such as cataracts, glaucoma, and macular degeneration will lead to vision loss or blindness if not treated. Visual impairments affect one senior in eleven. There is no question that a loss in vision would hamper one's autonomy. People with limited vision are unlikely to be able to drive, their recreational pursuits would be limited (playing cards would be difficult if you could not read the number on the corner of the card, and you'd never find your ball on the golf course), and daily household chores would be difficult.

Impaired hearing might also limit one's autonomy. The rate of impaired hearing is less than 1 percent for those under age the age of 25 years but increases to 47.5 percent for those 85 years old and older. Most hearing loss is sensorineural. **Sensorineural hearing loss** is caused by problems of the nervous system in the inner ear. This loss can result from changes that come with age, with exposure to environmental noise, or from using some medications (e.g., aspirin). People with sensorineural hearing loss generally do not suffer from total deafness. Rather, they may have problems comprehending what people are saying, and they are very sensitive to loud sounds. The person may hear clicking, ringing, or hissing noises. The hearing loss occurs bilaterally and symmetrically. Although people with hearing losses will not be as limited as those with visual problems, some difficulty in driving may ensue. The siren of an ambulance coming up behind you or the honking horn of someone who is trying to get your attention may be inaudible.

Smell and taste disorders are also more common in old age. Although smell and taste disorders may not have an effect on one's autonomy, they may lead to health consequences. A person suffering from a smell or taste disorder is deprived of an early warning system that we often take for granted. Decreased smells will delay the detection of fires, poisonous fumes, and leaking gas, and decreased smell combined with decreased taste will limit the detection of spoiled food and beverages.

Longterm Activity Limitations

To this point, we have discussed physical changes that commonly occur as people age and that are associated with a loss of independence. Longterm activity limitations or disabilities also result in a loss of personal autonomy. In 1996/97, 28 percent of Canadians aged 65 to 74 years and 44 percent of those aged 75 years and over reported a longterm activity limitation or disability resulting from a health problem. Men aged 65 to 74 years were more likely than women to report an activity limitation; after the age of 75 years, rates of longterm activity limitations were slightly higher for women than for men (44% for men and 45% for women).

The primary condition responsible for activity limitations varies considerably depending on age and gender. Arthritis is the primary cause of activity limitations for all women over the age of 55 years (24% of those aged 55 to 64 years; 32% of those aged 65 to 74 years; and 21% of those over the age of 75 years). In contrast, the major causes of activity limitations for men vary in each age category. Men aged 55 to 64 years reported that back problems (23%) were primarily responsible for their activity limitations, whereas men aged 65 to 74 years reported that heart problems (20%) led to activity limitations. Finally, men over the age of 75 years stated that heart problems (16%) and nervous system problems (15%) were the major causes of their activity limitations (Health Canada, 1999).

Sensory declines and activity limitations both take away from an individual's independence. Declines in cognitive abilities are also responsible for a lack of personal autonomy. The probability of suffering from dementia, a condition which results in decline of mental functions, increases with age. In the next section, we'll take a closer look at dementia.

Dementia

Dementia refers to a group of diseases characterized by a progressive and usually irreversible decline of mental functions. The symptoms of dementia are memory loss, disorientation, cognitive decline, and inappropriate social behaviour. Tom is an example of someone who has lived with dementia (see Case 9-1). If someone you know appears confused and has trouble making decisions, forgets the names of people and places, does or says things repeatedly, has problems with physical ambulation and difficulty completing household tasks, you should recognize that these signs may indicate dementia. In later stages, loss of motor and physical functioning occur. The patient becomes dependent on others to manage even the simplest physical functions (Biegel, Sales, & Schulz, 1991).

Among the elderly, there are two major forms of dementia: **senile dementia**, which is officially referred to as "diseases of the Alzheimer's type" and **multi-infarct dementia**, also called cerebrovascular disease (Tatemichi, Sacktor, & Mayeux, 1994). Multi-infarct dementia is an indirect result of a hardening or a narrowing of the arteries supplying blood to the brain. In what is essentially a series of small strokes, several small areas of the brain are destroyed, or "infarcted." These multiple infarcts (many small areas of tissue death) are the direct cause of the dementia. Rather than a complete loss of intellectual abilities, symptoms are usually "spotty" and variable.

Senile dementia is characterized by brain atrophy, hard plaques, and neurofibrillary tangles on autopsy. Although the exact causes of dementia are not known, researchers speculate that genetic defects, infectious disease, abnormal protein functioning, toxic substances (e.g., aluminum), decreased cortical blood flow, and reduced acetylcholine levels may be

CASE 9-2 A Former Writer

Tom had been a successful writer for most of his life, celebrated for his ability to remember the intricate details of a complex and fascinating story without using notes. At the age of 68 years, soon after his retirement, Tom began to experience difficulty in finding the right words to express himself and often lost his train of thought. Within months, he couldn't remember his schedule for the day. Within a few years, he couldn't remember if he had just eaten.

Tom began to wander around the house at night. He sometimes became irritable and even violent. Eventually, he moved to a nursing home where he continued to decline until he was unable to perform even the simplest functions for himself. He forgot names and eventually could not recognize those who were close to him (Fischman, 1984).

responsible. Multi-infarct dementia, like all heart and arterial diseases, has been attributed to various factors, including poor diet (too much fat), lack of exercise, smoking, and genetic predisposition. Hence, much of its incidence could be reduced by the lifestyle changed advocated for vascular disease in general.

Between the ages of 65 and 85 years, the prevalence of all dementia doubles approximately every 5 years (National Advisory Council on Aging, 1996). In 1991, 2.4 percent of those aged 65 to 74 years, 11.1 percent of those 75 to 84 years of age, and 34.5 percent of those 85 years of age or older suffered from dementia. In Canada, 10 000 deaths per year can be attributed directly to dementia. Alzheimer's disease is the fourth most common cause of death among Canada's elderly after cancer, heart disease, and stroke. Once a person displays symptoms of Alzheimer's disease, they have a life expectancy of 8 years. Persons diagnosed with multi-infarct dementia, overall, have fewer years of life remaining after diagnoses compared to those diagnosed with Alzheimer's disease.

Patients diagnosed with dementia, dementia of the Alzheimer's type in particular, respond to this diagnosis with a variety of strong emotions, including shock, anger, fear, despair, and disbelief; some deny or refuse to acknowledge their condition altogether. Most want to talk about their condition. Yet they are sad and fearful because they know that as the dementia progresses, they will no longer be able to relate to their family with dignity and respect. Perhaps the most distressing aspect of dementia is the awareness of having profound cognitive deficits that will only get worse. Observing the unravelling of a self-identity that one has spent a lifetime creating is virtually impossible to bear with equanimity (Biegel, Sales, & Schulz, 1991; Cohen & Eisdorfer, 1986).

Unintentional Injuries

Older adults have mortality rates from unintentional injuries more than twice that found in any other age group. It may seem strange, but older people die from many of the same unintentional injuries as children, for example, falls, fires, and motor vehicle accidents. Falls are the leading cause of accidental death for both men and women 65 years of age and older. Studies conducted in British Columbia and Ontario document that falls are also the number one reason for hospitalized injury of older adults (Gallagher & Scott, 1997; Pickett, Hartling, & Brison, 1997). For persons aged 65 years and over in British Columbia, 84 percent of days spent in hospitals are attributed to falls. Injuries sustained from motor vehicle accidents and "other" unintentional injuries contribute to only 16 percent of days seniors spend in hospitals (Gallagher & Scott, 1997). Mortality and morbidity from falls among the elderly are due to fractures in the neck or femur (hip) (Millar & Hill, 1994). While more older women than men are hospitalized for fall-related injuries, more men than women die from these injuries (Scott & Gallagher, 1999). Deaths due to femoral fractures have declined consistently since the 1970s. However, researchers have not yet determined whether this downward trend has resulted from changes in surgical treatments or from a drop in incidence (given observed hospital admission rates) (Millar & Hill, 1994).

Research indicates that falls occur most frequently on sidewalks and crosswalks (Gallagher & Scott, 1997). Not surprisingly, research conducted in Montreal indicates that most falls occur on days with inclement weather (Levy, Bensimon, May, & Leighton, 1998). Days with lower temperatures, snow, and freezing rain had higher rates of hip fracture. Oddly, occurrence of hip fractures peaked in mid-December for women but not until the first week of January for men.

Older people are at an increased risk from residential fires. There are two possible explanations for this—infirmity, which can make escape more difficult, and diminished cognitive functioning, which can lead to cooking devices left unattended or being improperly used (Center for Disease Control, 1998). Although children under the age of 5 years have an increased risk of death from residential fires, older people have an even greater risk. Past the age of 65 years, the death rate from residential fires rises sharply as people age.

Older people also have fairly high rates of motor vehicle deaths. Some research has suggested that older drivers diagnosed with dementia are involved in more motor vehicle deaths than healthy older drivers and are therefore viewed as "high-risk" drivers (Parasuraman & Nestor, 1993). However, other research has refuted these claims (Tuokko et al., 1995). The inconsistency of these findings suggests that the diagnosis of dementia is not an adequate predictor of driving function (Odenheimer, 1993). To maximize the autonomy of older people, a diagnosis of dementia in a senior should not automatically lead to revocation of their driver's licence. Rather, renewal of a license should be based on criteria related to driving competence. Parasuraman and Nestor (1993) suggest that testing attentional abilities important for safe driving would be a better determinant of license issuance.

Throughout this chapter we have focused on both intentional behaviours (e.g., smoking) and unintentional behaviours (e.g., falls) that will lead to premature death. Elimination of health-compromising behaviours will help us live longer but we must all die eventually. Next, we will discuss how death of older persons is perceived by society.

Death among the Elderly

In our society, the death of older people is perceived as less tragic than the death of a person in any other age group. A number of explanations may account for this belief (Feifel, 1977). First, it has been suggested that when older people die fewer role substitutions must be made than when younger people die. For example, older adults are not usually the primary caregiver or primary breadwinner in a household. Therefore, these roles will not need

BOX 9-2 How Can You Be Healthier, Happier, and Cheaper to Care For?

What personal health practices should you engage in to increase your chances of maintaining health, mobility and independence in old age? The National Advisory Council on Aging (1994) and Health Canada (1999) has the following recommendations:

1. Maintain an adequate income throughout life:

   As one's income increases, the incidence of emotional disorders, heart trouble, and arthritis/ rheumatism decreases.

2. Obtain an education:

   People with low levels of education tend to have more disabilities and chronic illnesses, regardless of age. A low level of education is a significant predictor of dementia.

3. Maintain relationships with family and friends:

   People who have social support are healthier and live longerthan those who do not.

4. Obtain information about maintaining health and treating symptoms of common ailments yourself:

   These behaviours have been shown to reduce visits to physicians by 50 percent in cases of cold and flu.

5. Before using medication, consult a health professional, get written information, and use memory aids:

   These strategies increase knowledge of medications and reduce errors in medication use.

6. Become more physically active:

   A year of physical endurance training improves heart function in men and women in their 60s by 25 to 30 percent. Regular physical activity can reduce risk for the two major causes of disability in older men, back problems and heart disease. Physical activity also has an important role in the management of arthritis, the number one cause of disability in older women. Adults (aged 45 to 64 years) who are physically active are less likely than sedentary adults to report heart trouble, diabetes, bronchitis, arthritis, and high blood cholesterol. Remaining physically active helps maintain intellectual functioning, reduces stress, and improves sleep. Seniors who are active are less likely to be depressed.

replacement when the older person dies. Second, the elderly are viewed to have had the life they are entitled to so they will not be cheated of anything if they die. Third, contact with the elderly by all other age groups diminishes. Therefore, there are few interactions for other age groups to miss out on when an elderly person dies compared to when a person of a younger age group dies. Fourth, many elderly people experience such a marked physical, social, or psychological deterioration that they are no longer perceived as living a valuable or gratifying life. Fifth, death is a normal aging process and therefore is expected. Finally, the elderly have a significantly larger number of friends and family members who have died and, therefore, they are prepared to die.

We have presented a very brief view here of what death in the elderly means to society as a whole. A more thorough discussion of death in the general population, the process of dying, and how people cope with the death of others will follow in Chapter 11 which discusses chronic and life-threatening illness.

KEY TERMS

teratogen
critical period
germinal stage
embryonic stage
fetal stage
fetal alcohol syndrome (FAS)
fetal alcohol effects (FAE)
bulimia nervosa
anorexia nervosa
positive-affect smoker
negative-affect smokers
habitual smokers
addictive smokers
nicotine fixed-effect model
nicotine regulation model
multiple regulation model
biobehavioural model
environmental tobacco smoke
passive smoking
addiction
withdrawal
nicotine-replacement therapy
nicotine gum
nicotine patch
aversion therapies
self-management strategies
ethanol
ethyl alcohol
disease model
alcohol dependency syndrome model
tension reduction hypothesis
self-awareness model
alcohol myopia
social learning model
hallucinogens
stimulant
information–motivation–behavioural skills model
presbyopia
sensorineural hearing loss
dementia
senile dementia
multi-infarct dementia

Chapte

10

PAIN

Chapter Outline

Key Questions

1. What are the benefits to experiencing pain?
2. How do early theories of pain differ from more contemporary theories?
3. How does acute pain differ from chronic pain?
4. How does the culture people belong to influence their experience of and response to pain?
5. What are the different methods used to measure pain?
6. How does pain measurement differ in children versus adults?
7. What are some of the pain control techniques available to the pain sufferer?
8. Why are multidisciplinary pain management programs so successful?

At 22 years of age, Jake was a happy-go-lucky, athletic, apprentice chef in an exclusive restaurant. He loved his job and took it very seriously. One day, when the master chef was away, two boxes of chickens were delivered. Jake cut up the chickens and packaged them for the freezer. Not long after, he became very ill. Jake was finally diagnosed as having been infected with Salmonella, resulting from a bacteria that is usually present on raw chicken meat. Jake was quarantined in the hospital where he spent 10 days and lost 30 pounds.

Upon his discharge from the hospital, Jake rapidly resumed his old activities—he went back to work and immediately returned to playing soccer. However, 6 weeks later, a host of new symptoms appeared: joint pain, urethritis (inflammation of the urethra), and conjunctivitis (inflammation of the eye). This triad of symptoms is indicative of Reiter's syndrome. Reiter's syndrome occurs in 2 to 3 percent of patients exposed to bacteria known to promote Reiter's (such as that which produces *Salmonella*). In North America, 30 in every 100 000 individuals will experience this syndrome at some point in their lives. The incidence rate is five times higher for males than for females. Although most people recover from this illness in 6 months, some have it "grumble on" for 12 or more months, and a small minority develop unremitting and potentially disabling arthritis. Unfortunately, Jake was one of the unlucky ones. His physician told him his pain would increase over time and that he would eventually lose mobility—not an easy prognosis for anyone to accept and especially not for an active person at such a young age.

With his eternal optimism, Jake continued to embrace life. He made a career change and found a job where he would be interacting with others all day—he became a bus driver. This job was the perfect fit for Jake, because he loved people and almost everyone with whom he came in contact with became an instant friend. Rarely did Jake exhibit any pain. He married and had two children. As the years passed, his pain increased and, as a result, he took more and more pain killers. It got to the point where the pain became excruciating and he was consuming 14 Tylenol Threes in a day (far exceeding the recommended dosage). Then, 13 years after the initial diagnosis, he just couldn't keep it "together" any longer.

Jake became extremely depressed and began to experience anxiety attacks. He was off work for a few months but he then returned to his jovial self. Once back at work, he drove a bus for only 3 weeks before he had to go on leave again. Emotionally, he was sinking deeper than he had ever been. He became suicidal and began abusing his medication, taking far more than the physician had prescribed. Secretly, he also began abusing alcohol. Jake was checked into a hospital where he would receive psychiatric help. After a number of weeks in the hospital, Jake was discharged and seemed to be in better spirits. Unfortunately, Jake will have to live with physical pain for the rest of his life. He has tried, in his words, "every pain management technique available." In addition to pharmacological treatment, he has tried acupuncture, guided imagery, meditation, physical exercises, and massage therapy. He recently returned from a 10-day stay at a pain clinic. Jake said that the pain management techniques at the clinic ranged from group hugs to a few very painful procedures where he screamed louder than he had ever screamed before. Jake states that the most beneficial aspect of this visit was that he learned that he really wasn't "so bad off." Many of the other patients were currently experiencing more pain than he was, and the ordeals that they had gone through were heart-wrenching. Currently, Jake continues to be in good spirits, he participates in aqua therapy, and visits a massage therapist.

He knows that he will be taking medication for the rest of his life, and very recently his physician has stated he may have to give up the idea of ever driving a bus again.

Jake's pain is considered chronic or longterm. The pain that Jake has experienced as a result of Reiter's syndrome has affected him in many ways. It has affected him emotionally. Jake can no longer work in the job he loves. In fact, he is currently living on disability payments. Both of these factors are hard on his self-esteem. It is not surprising that depression and anxiety are often experienced by people with chronic pain. His social life has changed considerably and for more than a year he didn't want to see even his closest friends. Obviously, the pain has affected him physically as well. Jake can no longer play soccer with his teammates. He only hopes that he will still be able to kick the soccer ball around with his children when they are old enough. It is true that pain of any kind usually leads people to change their activity level. As this chapter explains, such pain behaviours are an important component of the pain experience.

THE SIGNIFICANCE OF PAIN

After reading about Jake, a life without pain sounds appealing. You would feel no pain when falling down, when stubbing your toe, or when slamming your finger in the car door. Headaches would not exist. You would feel no pain while exercising, and giving birth might even be considered a pleasant experience. Doesn't that sound appealing? Before you conclude that life would be wonderful with no pain, consider the case of Miss C., a young Canadian girl who was a student at McGill University (Melzack & Wall, 1996). Miss C.'s father, a physician in Canada, suggested to his colleagues in Montreal that they should examine her. Miss C. was highly intelligent and seemed normal in every way except that she had never felt pain. As a child, she had bitten off the tip of her tongue while chewing food and had suffered third-degree burns on her legs after kneeling on a hot radiator to look out a window. In fact, Miss C. could not remember ever sneezing or coughing, and she had neither the gag reflex nor the corneal reflex that protects the eyes.

The physicians who examined Miss C. subjected her to tests that would have been considered forms of torture in a normal person. They administered electric shocks to different parts of her body and immersed her limbs in hot water at temperatures that usually produce reports of burning pain. They immersed her limbs in cold water for prolonged periods and pinched tendons. She felt no pain. In addition, her heart rate, blood pressure, and respiration remained normal throughout the tests.

As a result of her inability to experience pain, Miss C. had severe medical problems, including pathological changes in her knees, hip, and spine. Melzack and Wall (1996) explain that insensitivity to pain can lead people to remain in one position too long, causing inflammation of the joints. Even worse, the failure to feel pain leads one to neglect injuries. As a result, healing is obstructed. Injured tissue can easily become infected. These infections are very difficult to treat, particularly if they extend to the bone.

Miss C. died when she was only 29 years old of massive infections that could not be brought under control. During the last month of her life, Miss C. complained of discomfort, tenderness, and pain in her left hip. This pain was relieved by aspirin. Although she felt practically no pain during her life, her insensitivity to pain directly contributed to the infections that killed her.

Thus, there are benefits to experiencing pain. Pain is known to serve at least three functions. First, the pain that occurs before serious injury, such as when we step on or pick up hot, sharp, or otherwise potentially damaging objects, has real survival value. It produces immediate withdrawal or some other action that prevents further injury. Second, the pains that prevent further injury serve as the basis of learning to avoid injurious objects or situations that may occur at a later time. Third, pains due to damaged joints, abdominal infections, diseases, or serious injuries set limits on activity and enforce inactivity and rest, which are often essential for the body's natural recuperative and disease-fighting mechanisms to ensure recovery and survival.

PAIN PERCEPTION

When a person comes in contact with injurious stimuli, signals of tissue damage follow a particular route from **afferent (sensory) neurons** of the peripheral nervous system to the spinal cord and then to the brain. The afferent nerve endings that respond to pain stimuli are called **nociceptors**. When activated, these nerve endings generate impulses that travel to the central nervous system. The afferent peripheral fibres that transmit pain impulses are **A-delta fibres** and **C-fibres**. A-delta fibres are associated with sharp, distinct pain. The A-delta fibres are small, myelinated fibres that transmit impulses very quickly. In contrast, C-fibres transmit impulses more slowly because they are unmyelinated. The C-fibres, which comprise over 60 percent of all sensory afferents, are involved when pain is diffuse, dull, or aching (Chapman, 1984; Melzack & Wall, 1996). The afferent fibres group together after leaving the periphery, and this grouping forms a nerve. The nerves then enter the dorsal horns of the spinal cord; these contain several layers, or laminae, each of which receives incoming messages from afferent neurons. The cells in the first two layers form the substantia gelatinosa, and it is here where sensory input information is thought to be modulated (Melzack & Wall, 1965). Sensory aspects of pain are strongly influenced by activity in A-delta fibres, which send messages through the thalamus on their way to the brain's cerebral cortex. Here the A-delta fibres signal sharp pain. The motivational and affective elements of pain appear to be more heavily determined by the C-fibres, which send pain messages to the brain stem and lower portions of the forebrain.

THEORIES OF PAIN

Early Theories of Pain

In the early 1900s, the dominant theories of pain took a very mechanistic view of pain perception. Von Frey argued for a **specificity theory** of pain, suggesting that pain was an independent sensation like heat, cold, or touch. He proposed that there were different kinds of receptors in the skin and that each kind of receptor responded to a particular kind of stimulus. These different receptors were thought to be structurally different in ways that made them sensitive to different kinds of stimulation (e.g., pain, heat, cold, or touch). In addition, specific routes of transmission in the central nervous system were proposed, as were special centres in the brain, that registered and interpreted only one kind of stimulus. Current evidence contradicts this theory. We now know that pain is not an experience separate from other sensory experiences. Rather, pain can result from excessive heat, cold, or pressure. Further, pain sensations do not seem to follow dedicated nervous pathways.

Around the same time that the specificity theory was proposed, Goldschneider proposed another theory of pain. His **pattern theory** posits that there is no separate system for perceiving pain and that the receptors for pain are shared with other senses, such as the sense of touch. According to the pattern theory, pain results from the patterning and quality of stimulation from peripheral nerve endings. So, for example, mild stimulation, perhaps resulting from a caress, might result in the sensation of touch; whereas intense stimulation, such as when one is hit, would result in the sensation of pain. The pattern theory also holds that sensations can summate. In other words, nerve impulses are conducted to the spinal column and, only after reaching a certain threshold, are conducted to the brain. This summation can account for the short delay experienced between the onset of tissue damage (as in a cut or burn) and the actual experience of pain.

Current research suggests that components of both specificity theory and pattern theory may be correct. Although there are specialized nerve fibres that conduct pain, there are others that can give rise to pain when they are stimulated beyond a certain threshold. Further, as the pattern theory predicts, receptors do respond to patterned information, but there is no direct connection between the pain receptors in the peripheral nervous system and the brain centre where pain would be perceived. These theories identified the role of the brain as a passive receiver of messages. We now know the brain plays a much larger role in the experience of pain (Melzack, 1993).

Gate Control Theory

In 1965, Melzack and Wall proposed the **gate control theory** of pain. In their view, pain is not a sensation that is transmitted directly from the peripheral nerve endings to the brain. Instead, the theory emphasizes that sensations are modified as they are conducted to the brain by way of the spinal cord. They are also influenced by downward pathways from the brain that interpret the experience. Melzack and Wall propose that there is a structure in the dorsal horns of the spinal column, a gatelike mechanism, which is able to control the flow of pain stimulation to the brain.

According to the gate control theory, information enters the dorsal horns of the spinal cord by way of primary afferent neurons. This information passes through the substantia gelatinosa, where the information is modulated by stimulation from the periphery as well as feedback from the fibres descending from the brain. This then affects the activity of the transmission cells, causing them to either conduct (excitatory influence) or not conduct (inhibitory influence) pain sensations to the brain.

Melzack and Wall (1965) proposed that the experience of pain is affected by the balance of activity in the small and large nerve fibres. This activity determines the patterning and intensity of stimulation. Activity in the small A-delta and C-fibres causes prolonged activity in the spinal cord. This type of activity promotes sensitivity and opens the gate, which produces pain. In contrast, activity in the large A-beta fibres tends to close the gate.

The gate may be closed by activity in the spinal cord and also by messages descending from the brain. A specialized system of large-diameter, rapidly conducting fibres, called **the central control trigger**, activates selective cognitive processes that then influence, by way of descending fibres, the opening and closing of the gate. That is, the experience of pain is influenced by past experience, attention, and other cognitive activities through the central control trigger. Consequently, affective reactions such as anxiety, depression, fear, or focusing on an injury can exacerbate the experience of pain by affecting the central control trigger, thus opening the gate. Intense involvement in other activities, or relaxation, or positive experiences can mute the pain experience by causing the gate to close.

Consider observations made by Beecher (1959) during World War II. An injury or wound sustained by a civilian produces pain (the gate is open). However, a soldier with the equivalent injury does not experience the same amount of pain, because the soldier is distracted by the environment (the gate is closed). Evidence in support of this observation can be seen in the amount of analgesic requested by patients from each group. A civilian patient will ask for significantly more analgesic than will a soldier who sustained the same injury.

This theory also explains how injuries can go virtually unnoticed. If sensory input is sent into a heavily activated nervous system, the stimulation may not be perceived as pain. A hockey player may fracture a rib during a game but not notice the acute pain because of excitement and concentration on the game. It isn't until after the game is over that the player notices the pain. At this time, the nervous system would be functioning at a different level of activation, and the gate is more easily opened.

The gate control theory is arguably the leading theory of pain. Melzack (1993) states that the gate theory's most important contribution to biological and medical science was that it "highlighted the central nervous system as an essential component in pain processes" (p. 619). The brain and the dorsal horns are no longer viewed merely as passive transmission stations. In addition, psychological factors, previously dismissed as "reactions to pain", are now seen as an integral part of pain processing. Finally, new avenues for pain treatment resulted. Cutting nerves and pathways is no longer the treatment method of choice. The gate control theory remains basically intact after more than 25 years, despite a subsequent massive amount of research. Further, it continues to spur research and generate interest in the psychological and perceptual factors involved in pain. However, the gate control theory is not able to explain several chronic pain problems, such as phantom limb pain (see Box 10.1).

BOX 10-1 Phantom Limb Pain

In 1866, the first account of phantom limbs was published. It appeared not in a scientific journal as one might expect but in the *Atlantic Monthly*, as an anonymously written short story. In "The Case of George Dedlow", the main character loses an arm to amputation during the Civil War. At one point, he awakens in the hospital after, unbeknownst to him, both his legs have also been amputated.

> [I was] suddenly aware of a sharp cramp in my left leg. I tried to get at it...with my single arm, but, finding myself too weak, hailed an attendant. "Just rub my left calf...if you please."
>
> "Calf?...You ain't got non, pardner. It's took off" (cited in Melzack, 1992, p. 120).

The author happened to be Wier Mitchell, the foremost American neurologist at the time. Historians have proposed that Mitchell chose to publish this account in the *Atlantic Monthly* anonymously because he was unsure how his colleagues would respond to the concept of phantom limb pain. He feared that they would not believe amputated arms and legs could be felt by their previous owners.

In fact, the phenomenon of phantom limbs is common to those who have undergone amputation. The limb is very vivid to the amputee, who can usually tell you the precise location of the phantom. A phantom limb behaves very much like a normal limb. Usually, a phantom arm hangs straight down at the side when the person sits or stands but moves in perfect coordination with other limbs during walking. Similarly, a phantom leg bends like a normal leg would when its owner sits; it stretches out when the individual lies down; and it becomes upright during standing (Melzack, 1992).

Occasionally, the amputee is sure the limb is stuck in an unusual position. Melzack (1992) noted that one man believed his phantom arm extended straight out from the shoulder, at a right angle to the body. Consequently, whenever the man walked through a doorway he would turn sideways so that his arm would not hit the wall. Another man slept only on his front or side because his phantom arm was bent behind him and got in the way when he tried to rest on his back.

Particularly initially, the phantom limb may seem so real to the amputee that the amputee might try standing up on a phantom foot or answering a phone with a phantom hand. The most extraordinary feature of phantom limbs is their reality to the amputee. A phantom limb can experience many sensations including warmth, cold, and pressure. A phantom limb can feel wet (as when an artificial arm is seen entering into the lake during a swan dive). It can also feel itchy, which can be very annoying. Fortunately, scratching the apparent site of discomfort can actually relieve the distress sometimes. It may sometimes seem that the phantom limb is sweaty, prickly, or even being tickled (Melzack, 1992).

Of course, the sensation in phantom limbs that causes the most distress to the sufferer is pain. Researchers (Jensen, Krebs, Nielsen, & Rasmussen, 1985; Krebs et al., 1984) have found that 72 percent of amputees had phantom limb pain 1 week after amputation, and that 60 percent had pain 6 months to 7 years later. Although the pain usually starts soon after amputation, sometimes it does not appear for weeks, months, or even years. The pain is often characterized as burning, cramping, or shooting and can vary from being occasional and mild to continuous and severe (Melzack, 1992).

Originally, it was believed that one must first possess and then lose a limb and the corresponding nerves to experience phantom pain. However, there is now considerable evidence of phantoms in people born without limbs and in those who experienced limb amputation in very early childhood (e.g., Melzack, Israel, Lacroix, & Schultz, 1997; Ramachandran, 1993).

Melzack (1993, 1998) has proposed an extension to the gate control theory entitled the **neuromatrix theory**. This theory places a greater emphasis on the brain's role in pain perception. According to this theory, a neuromatrix or network of brain neurons, "distributed throughout many areas of the brain, comprises a widespread network of neurons which generates patterns, processes information that flows through it, and ultimately produces the pattern that is felt as a whole body" (Melzack, 1993, p. 623). The neuromatrix-generated patterns are called *neurosignature patterns*. These patterns may be generated from sensory inputs, however they may also be innately produced, such as in the case of phantom limb pain. The neurosignature patterns are responsible for producing a multidimensional experience of pain. Like the gate control theory, the neuromatrix theory maintains that pain perception is part of a complex process that is affected by sensory input, activity of the nervous system, and past experiences and expectations.

NEUROCHEMICAL BASIS OF PAIN AND PAIN INHIBITION

The gate control theory of pain asserts that the brain can control the amount of pain an individual experiences by transmitting messages down the spinal cord to block the transmission of pain signals (Melzack & Wall, 1965, 1996). There is evidence that supports this view. David Reynolds (1969) conducted a study in which he implanted an electrode in the midbrain portion of a number of rats' brain stems. The exact location of the electrode varied from one rat to the next. Then, he made sure that each rat could feel pain by applying a clamp to their tails. Not surprisingly, each rat responded by demonstrating pain. Several days later, Reynolds tested whether stimulation through the electrode would block pain. At the same time as the rats were electrically stimulated he again applied the clamp. Those rats with electrodes in the area of the midbrain known as the **periaqueductal gray area** did not exhibit pain. Those rats that did not experience pain in response to having their tails clamped later had abdominal surgery performed on them while the periaqueductal gray area of their brains was being electrically stimulated. Again, the rats did not feel any pain. This phenomenon has been termed **stimulation-produced analgesia (SPA)**. Reynolds' findings encouraged researchers to look for the neurochemical basis of pain. Subsequently, **endogenous opioids** were identified.

Endogenous opioids are opiate-like substances produced within the body that regulate pain. They are naturally occurring substances in the brain, spinal cord, and glands. They appear to act as an internal pain relief system by slowing or blocking the transmission of nerve impulses, in much the same way as do exogenous opioids such as the drugs heroin and morphine. Researchers have identified three main groups of these endogenous opioids: beta-endorphin, proenkephalin, and prodynorphin (Akil et al., 1984).

The system of endogenous opioids and their function in the body is very complex. Researchers do not have a full understanding of the mechanisms by which they work. However, it is apparent that having internal pain-relieving chemicals serves an adaptive function. It may be that because pain and emotions are closely linked, studies have found that psychological stress can trigger endogenous opioid activity (Bloom, Lazerson, & Hofstadter, 1985; Winters, 1985). There is also evidence that intense physical exercise can trigger the release of beta-endorphin, resulting in natural, short-term pain suppression and subjective feelings of physical well-being (Akil et al., 1984). The release of endogenous opioids may help

CASE STUDY 10-1 Acute versus Chronic Pain

Riley is 28 years old and is just finishing his residency in anesthesiology. Medical school was not easy for Riley. He had to study harder than most of the other students, but he was determined to do well and he graduated close to the top of his class. Today, Riley received an invitation in the mail to his high school reunion. Riley had enjoyed high school and been quite popular. This popularity probably arose, at least in part, from his participation in school sports. He played volleyball and basketball, but the sport he enjoyed most was football. He decided that returning to his home town for his high school reunion would be just the break he needed from life at the hospital.

The first night of the reunion weekend was a wine and cheese reception in the old gymnasium. Riley met up with many of his former buddies and they reminisced about their football success. It really was remarkable how they could collectively recall every play and detail of each game they played in their senior year. They really had been one of the greatest teams in the high school's history. In fact, six of the team members had gone on to play football in university, and four others had turned professional. The guys decided that they had to get together for a scrimmage before the weekend was out.

On Sunday morning, 16 members of the former team gathered for a scrimmage. The guys played hard and even the spectators were impressed with the quick moves the players exhibited. After the game, the guys vowed to get together every year on the last weekend of August for a scrimmage.

Riley flew home on Sunday night. When he tried to rise from his seat at the conclusion of the flight, he experienced a sharp pain in his back. Slowly and carefully, he eased himself into a standing position. He had obviously overdone it at the scrimmage earlier that day. Riley knew he was going to be extremely stiff the next day. He decided that a walk before bed and maybe even a soak in the apartment's hot tub might help ward off some of the stiffness.

Compare Riley's experience of pain to that experienced by Michelle.

Michelle has been a professional pairs figure skater for almost 20 years. She and her partner have decided they will call it quits at the end of the current season. One factor that played a part in this decision is Michelle's pain. For the last few years, Michelle has found it increasingly difficult to land the jumps and throws that she and her partner practise over and over on a daily basis. After landing each throw and after landing each jump, Michelle experiences a sharp searing pain in her knees. After each practise session, Michelle must ice her knees to help alleviate the pain, swelling, and tenderness. Not only does Michelle have a hard time landing her jumps, she has also noticed that she is having some difficulty simply walking. It is likely that Michelle will be diagnosed with osteoarthritis. Although Michelle is going to miss skating, she hopes that a less physically demanding schedule will ease some of the pain she has been experiencing.

to explain how injured athletes in competition and soldiers on the battlefield continue to function with little or no perception of pain.

ACUTE VERSUS CHRONIC PAIN

Medical professionals make an important distinction between two main kinds of clinical pain: acute and chronic. Case Study 10.1 presents these two different types of pain in the examples of Riley and Michelle's individual experiences. Riley is suffering from **acute pain**. Acute pain seems to serve to warn of impending tissue damage or the need for convalescent rest. A toothache, the discomforts of childbirth, a broken limb, and postoperative pain are all forms of acute pain. Acute pain is by definition temporary and lasts less than 6 months (Turk, Meichenbaum, & Genest, 1983). The physiological responses to acute pain seem partly proportional to the stimulus intensity. However, it can cause considerable anxiety and distress. Fortunately, painkillers can often ease the discomfort, and as the injury begins to heal, the anxiety subsides.

But sometimes the pain lingers on. When it lasts longer than 6 months, pain is considered **chronic**. Any condition that is expected to bring only acute pain but continues for 6 months without resolution is considered to be chronic pain. Michelle, like Jake at the beginning of this chapter, is experiencing chronic pain. Chronic pain can be intermittent or constant, mild, or severe. It varies a great deal depending upon its type (Turk et al., 1983). **Chronic recurrent pain** does not become progressively worse. It is characterized by intense episodes of acute pain followed by relief. For example, a person who suffers from migraine headaches may have excruciating headaches lasting from hours to days, but then may have several pain-free weeks or months. By comparison, the person who has **chronic intractable benign pain** has pain all the time, with varying intensity. People who suffer from lower back pain generally experience their pain continually and find that they can do little to reduce it. Finally, **chronic progressive pain** involves continuous discomfort that gradually intensifies as the condition worsens. It is typically associated with malignancies or degenerative disorders such as cancer and advancing arthritis.

In many types of chronic pain, the disease process is primarily responsible for the pain experienced. However, psychosocial factors may also play a role. At times, tissue damage may result in the initial acute pain that the person experiences. Subsequently, psychosocial factors may play a more prominent role. To clarify this process, we must distinguish between respondent and operant pain (Fordyce, 1976, 1978). **Respondent pain** refers to pain that occurs in response to noxious stimulation or tissue damage. In contrast, **operant pain** is pain that is reinforced by the person's environment. Typically, people in pain will alter their behaviour in an attempt to reduce the pain. For example, a person may limp, guard a painful arm, avoid exercise, or even stay in bed to avoid pain. When such **pain behaviours** either reduce the pain or prevent it from getting worse, the tendency to continue the behaviour is reinforced. As the pain behaviours appear successful at preventing or reducing the pain, the person will want to continue to engage in these behaviours for fear that the pain will return if they are discontinued. Consequently, these behaviours are particularly resistant to change, as they are specifically aimed at avoidance. Because the person fears the recurrence of pain, they no longer engage in normal behaviours.

The verbal and behavioural expressions of pain also have a powerful effect on other people. When an individual complains of pain, displays pain on his or her face, or exhibits an abnormal gait or posture, he or she may receive attention, concern, and even assistance from those witnessing these behaviours—this can further reinforce pain behaviour (von Baeyer, Johnson, & McMillan, 1984). Researchers have discovered that chronic pain sufferers who report higher levels of satisfaction with social support also exhibit higher levels of pain-related behaviours (Gil, Keefe, Crisson, & Van Dalfsen, 1987). Positive attention provided by supportive spouses in response to the expression of pain may inadvertently maintain or increase an individual's expression of pain and the experience of disability (Turk, Kerns, & Rosenberg, 1992). In one study, the best predictor of a person's pain and activity level was the individual's perception of their spouse's solicitousness in response to the expression of pain. Chronic pain sufferers whose spouses showed higher levels of concern reported greater levels of pain and lower activity levels compared to those whose spouses exhibited less concern (Flor, Kerns, & Turk, 1987).

One of the most common complaints described by those with chronic pain is the resulting sleep disturbance (American Pain Society, 1999). A large majority (79%) of those experiencing moderate or severe chronic pain complain about the difficulties they have in falling to sleep. As well, these individuals frequently are awakened as a result of the pain. In the morning, they wake up exhausted. They are tired and drained of energy, not merely from lack of sleep but also because the continuous pain wears them down (Sternbach, 1986). It is not surprising that these chronic pain sufferers also find themselves irritated by little things and trivial comments of those around them. These people recognize that they are snapping at their friends and family for insufficient reasons, yet they cannot seem to stop. This often leads those with chronic pain to withdraw from their families and friends.

The chronic pain sufferer who withdraws from family and friends experiences little social or recreational life. In addition, 59 percent of those with moderate or severe chronic pain have had to leave their jobs (American Pain Society, 1999). As a result, people's standard of living is reduced and an added strain is put on the family. Ironically, if compensation is received for the pain experience because it resulted from an injury on the job or perhaps in an automobile accident, this may exacerbate the perceived severity of pain and distress (Turk & Okifuji, 1996). In addition, both personal and career goals may be set aside because the sufferer's life is beginning to revolve around pain (Karoly & Ruehlman, 1996).

All of the previously mentioned behaviours resulting from the experience of pain have an impact on one's emotional state. As formerly stated, many chronic pain sufferers are irritable. In addition, chronic pain sufferers report being listless, unable to cope, and depressed (American Pain Society, 1999). Chronic pain and depression sufferers share many of the same characteristics (Sternbach, 1974). Merskey (1986) reports that almost all published studies of psychiatric and psychological test findings of chronic pain patients report mild but significant depression. Further, approximately 50 percent of hospitalized depressed patients report pain as a major symptom. These are daunting statistics, especially when one considers that depression is known to exacerbate pain and pain-related behaviours (Kessler, Kronstorfer, & Traue, 1996; Kroner-Herwig et al., 1996). Fortunately, once pain is controlled there is a significant improvement in individuals' abilities and moods. For example, a national study in the U.S. found that 84 percent of chronic pain sufferers whose pain is now under control feel happy and upbeat, compared to 41 percent who provided this response before their pain was controlled (American Pain Society, 1999).

BOX 10-2 Chronic Pain On Trial

In a recent article entitled "Chronic pain on trial: The influence of litigation and compensation on chronic pain syndromes", Thomas Hadjistavropoulos (1999), from the University of Regina, describes a current controversy surrounding chronic pain. According to Hadjistavropoulos, many argue that the litigious nature of North American society influences the symptoms reported by patients.

Crosscultural research suggests there may be some truth to this argument. For example, Bella (1982) contrasted the proportion of patients in Australia who reported "late-whiplash syndrome" resulting from car accidents with patients in Singapore. In contrast to its frequency in Australia, the late-whiplash syndrome was extremely rare in Singapore, and when it occurred it often involved patients of European background. Another study contrasted American patients to patients from New Zealand (Carron, DeGood, & Tait, 1985). New Zealand's nonadversarial system compensates all victims regardless of fault and without the need to prove injury at work. The results of this study determined that 49 percent of the American sample received pain-related compensation compared to 17 percent of the New Zealand sample. Further, the American patients reported greater emotional and behavioural disruption as a result of chronic low back pain. This occurred even though the two samples of patients initially described experiencing similar degrees of pain. Carron et al. concluded that the absence of an adversarial system in New Zealand contributed to the crosscultural difference.

The results of this crosscultural research may have lead, in part, to the conclusions drawn in a report by the *Task Force on Pain in the Workplace* of the International Association for the Study of Pain (IASP) (Fordyce, 1995). The task force implied in their report that extended pain and disability following certain kinds of low back pain are primarily the result of operant and societal factors. Specifically, assigning an individual disability status was said to expose that individual to "potentially debilitating circumstances that include excessive rest, well-intentioned but harmful treatments, and overprotection by family members" (Hadjistavropoulos, 1999, p. 62). The report outlines that disability claims resulting from low back pain have shown enormous increases. Yet, there is no evidence that back injuries are becoming more frequent or severe. The report characterized individuals with non-specific low back pain as "activity intolerant" and suggested that wage replacement benefits should not exceed 6 weeks unless there was evidence to indicate a disabling condition other than non-specific low back pain.

The IASP report has led to considerable controversy (e.g., Block, 1997; Craig, 1996; Fordyce, 1996; Loeser, 1996; Merskey, 1996a, 1996b). The Canadian chapter of IASP, for example, characterized the report as incomplete and as representing the opinion of a limited number of individuals. Hadjistavropoulos (1999) states that despite good intentions, if followed the report could have disastrous consequences for some injured persons. In an attempt to remedy this situation, Hadjistavropoulos has developed a number of strategies that may reduce compensation costs for chronic pain while also reducing patient suffering:

1. Health care practitioners can do more to encourage patients to return to work. Rather than prescribe rest for musculoskeletal pain patients, these patients should be encouraged to return to work. Catchclove and Cohen (1982) show that this encouragement has a significant impact on the number of individuals that will return to work.
2. Employers should attempt to reduce job dissatisfaction in the workplace. Studies have shown that improvements in work conditions and the work environment facilitate the recovery of many injured workers (see Turk, 1997).
3. Enhance diagnostic accuracy. Research suggests that pain patients are frequently inaccurately or incompletely diagnosed. For example, Hendler and Kozikowski (1993) found that 66.7 percent of patients referred to a pain diagnostic centre had been misdiagnosed.
4. Continue research on malingering. Health care practitioners need to be able to determine when someone is pretending to be in pain or exaggerating the severity of their symptoms. At present, there is not a method to confidently assess when someone is malingering (Main & Spanswick, 1995).
5. Identify types of patients who may be particularly susceptible to the effects of compensation and litigation.
6. Modify the adversarial nature of the North American litigation/compensation system. Countries (e.g., New Zealand) that have removed the adversarial relationship between employer, claimant, and the insurer allow income compensation for accidental injury without the need to prove the injury at work and by allowing rapid rehabilitation intervention (Walsh & Dumitru, 1988).

PSYCHOSOCIAL FACTORS AND PAIN

Gender Differences

Clinical research has documented that women are more likely than men to experience a variety of recurrent pain. Recurrent pain can result from many ailments, including migraine and other headaches as well as musculoskeletal, back, and abdominal pain (e.g., Pryse-Phillips et al., 1992; Lee, Helewa, Smythe, Bombardier, & Goldsmith, 1985; Lester, Lefebvre, & Keefe, 1994; Magni, Rossi, Rigatti-Luchini, & Merskey, 1992). In most studies, women report more severe levels of pain, more frequent pain, and pain of longer duration than men (Unruh, 1996; Unruh, Ritchie, & Merskey, 1999).

Researchers agree that there are also gender differences in the perception and response to pain (see Unruh, 1996 or Vallerand, 1995 for reviews). The extent of these differences is under debate. Unruh (1996) has identified three key issues surrounding gender differences and pain: (1) the manner in which women and men perceive and respond to pain; (2) the psychosocial and biological factors that may influence gender variations in pain experience; and (3) the response of the health care system to the pain presented by women and men.

Laboratory research has documented how men and women differ in their pain responses (Riley et al., 1998; Koltyn & Vaughn, 1999). For example, Vallerand (1995) reported that women have a lower pain threshold and lower pain tolerance than men have. To determine a participant's pain threshold, researchers will inflict pain on the participant by one of a number of methods. A commonly used method is known as a "cold-pressor task." This entails participants submerging their hand in cold water until they experience pain. They indicate to the researcher, usually by pushing a button, when this point is reached. At this time participants are said to have reached their **pain threshold**.

Researchers are sometimes interested in identifying participants' **pain tolerance** levels rather than their pain threshold. The pain tolerance level is either the duration of time a person is willing to endure a stimulus beyond the point where it began to hurt or the stimulus a person will endure beyond that point (Sternbach, 1968). When the participants "can't stand it" any longer, they have reached their level of pain tolerance. Once the participants have indicated that they have reached their limit, they can remove their hand from the noxious stimuli. Laboratory studies investigating gender differences in pain threshold and pain tolerance have not yielded consistent results (e.g., Kuhl et al., 1999). Some researchers argue (e.g., Berkley, 1997; Lautenbacher & Rollman, 1993) that these inconsistent results are due to the variety of noxious stimuli used by investigators to determine pain threshold and pain tolerance. In a recent study, Koltyn and Vaughn (1999) documented that men and women differed in heat and pressure pain ratings but not in cold pain ratings or pain thresholds.

Other critics argue that gender differences in response to pain are actually due to differences in reporting pain. Robinson (Azar, 1999), a pain researcher, states, "It's my belief that women in the lab give a more unbiased report of their pain" (p. 7). He goes on to say that men feel there is a social cost to admitting publicly that something hurts. Men are taught to "tough out" pain and so in the lab they endure more discomfort. In contrast, women feel little pressure to endure unnecessary pain and therefore have no trouble admitting when something hurts. Robinson has presented research that may provide some support for his claims (Robinson et al., 1999). Robinson's study investigated gender-related stereotypes about pain. This study, based on the responses of almost 400 university students, discovered that men are perceived to be less willing to report pain than women and that women are perceived to be more sensitive and less enduring of pain. Other researchers (e.g., Jones & Rollman, 1999) are now exploring how these gender-role stereotypes influence the different responses men and women have to pain. One study has documented that individuals who obtain high masculinity scores on Bem's Sex Role Inventory (Bem, 1974) demonstrate an increased pain threshold in laboratory pain research (Otto & Dougher, 1985).

It is plausible that societal beliefs about gender differences in response to pain are a product of different societal gender-role expectations. A pain event may have different risks of interference on roles and responsibilities for men and women. Unruh (1996) points out that when we experience pain, we engage in a process of cognitive appraisal. That is, we determine what this experience means to us. To determine the meaning of an event we ask ourselves the following questions: "What does it mean?" "In what way does it affect me?" "Should I be concerned?" and "Is any action required on my part?" (Kreitler & Kreitler,

1976). The meaning given to an event is an important consideration in determining one's response to the event. Women with multiple roles and responsibilities resulting from childcare, care for elderly parents, household management, and paid employment have more than one reason to appraise pain as threatening. They may therefore attend to pain sooner in an effort to minimize its intrusiveness (Johnson, 1991; Crook, 1993).

Although psychosocial factors may influence pain perception, underlying biological differences in pain mechanisms may also predispose women to have more pain. Unruh (1996) comments on the lack of research addressing gender differences in terms of biological mechanisms that may influence the pain experience. However, she postulates that known gender differences in brain chemistry, metabolism, physical structures, and hormonal variations may influence the biological mechanisms of pain transmission, pain sensitivity, and pain perception. Polleri (1992) and Berkley (1997) also argue that there are sufficient biological factors to predict gender differences in pain.

Both biological and psychosocial factors related to the experience and reporting of pain by men and women may lead to differences in the way men and women are treated by the health care system. For example, psychosocial factors may be responsible for women describing their pain in more detail and with more expressive and social language than do men (Crook, 1982). As a result of these descriptions, women are more likely to receive a psychogenic interpretation of their pain by their physicians, particularly when the pain is not directly related to tissue damage (Wall, 1984). Unruh (1996) claims that these interpretations may "cause women to receive more attention for psychological aspects of pain but inadequate pain relief" (p. 159).

Women are also perceived by physicians and nurses to dramatize or exaggerate their pain. As a result, they are provided less analgesia than are men. For instance, in a matched-pairs design investigation of patients following coronary artery bypass graft, Calderone (1990) found that men were significantly more likely to receive pain medication and at more frequent intervals than women. In fact, the group of women who were 62 years of age or older were the least likely to receive pain medications. Another study (McDonald, 1994) reported that women received significantly less pain medication than men following appendectomies with no postoperative complications. The trend to undermedicate women is further complicated by the gender of the physician prescribing the analgesic. Weisse, Sanders, Syat, & Sorum (1999) report that male physicians prescribe higher doses of analgesic for male patients than for female patients whereas female physicians prescribe higher doses for female patients.

While women are thought to exaggerate their reports of pain, men are thought to minimize their pain and its consequences. This attitude may lead men to seek medical attention only when the pain characteristics have become more extreme, which may result in the pain being more difficult to treat. Perhaps this is why men are twice as likely as women to undergo pain-related surgery (Lack, 1982; Burns et al., 1996). It is also true that men seem to implement fewer coping strategies than women in response to pain. Unruh, Ritchie, and Merskey (1999) documented that men have less social support and are less likely to engage in problem-solving and palliative behaviours to deal with their pain than women. Until there is conclusive evidence to explain pain-related gender differences, health professionals should be attentive to possible biases in expectations about pain response and pain behaviour in men and women.

Cultural Differences

Pain is something that people all around the world experience. However, cultural background and social context will affect each person's experience, expression, and treatment of pain (Gureje, Von Korff, Simon, & Gater, 1996; Wise et al., 1999; Zatzick & Dimsdale, 1990). These differences result from the meaning each culture attaches to pain and from stereotypes associated with various cultural experiences.

Since the 1940s (e.g., Chapman, 1944), researchers have compared pain expression for people from various cultural backgrounds. Although many of these early studies report cultural differences in the expression of pain, they have been criticized for their inclusion of stereotypical biases (Streltzer, 1997). For instance, Italians are stereotyped as being very demonstrative. Italians have cultural approval for public expression of pain. Because of this, they are not inhibited in their expression of pain and their public suffering is designed to bring family and professional support and sympathy. Consistent with this stereotype, research indicates that Italians express a desire for immediate pain relief (Zborowski, 1958). In contrast, "Old Americans" (Caucasions of northern European origin) who have more stoic, matter-of-fact attitudes toward pain are reported to react to pain as calmly as possible, withdraw when in strong pain, and cry or moan only when alone (Zborowski, 1952). These differences in pain behaviours may reflect how people in different cultures learned to respond to pain. Alternatively, the perceived cultural differences might result from the researchers' expectations and the subjective measures used in these early studies.

More recent studies have used more objective measurements of pain behaviours. Many of these studies have also documented cultural differences in the experience of pain (Wise et al., 1999). For example, Europeans and North Americans consider pain to be a common experience for cancer patients. Pain experts in those countries state that pain is undertreated (Calvillo & Flaskerud, 1991; Streltzer, 1997). In contrast, experts from Asian countries do not consider cancer pain to be as much of a problem. These different attitudes lead to differences in treatment: approximately 70 percent of patients in Europe receive opiates for cancer pain. In contrast, only about 4 percent of Asian cancer patients receive this medication. It is possible that these variations may be due more to physicians' beliefs than to patients' pain. Support for this idea is provided by an American study that reported that the culture of the nurse influenced the interpretation of patients' pain (Calvillo & Flaskerud, 1991).

Ethnicity does influence the amount of pain medication patients receive. In particular, minorities are frequently prescribed less pain medication. One study reported that African-American and Hispanic-American patients received significantly less postoperative medication than Causcasian-Americans (Ng, Dimsdale, Shragg, & Deutsch, 1996). It is unclear whether this difference is due to the health professional's perceptions of need or to the patients' pain behaviours. To further complicate the issue, it appears that there is a difference in pain medication dosages depending on the gender of the prescribing physician. A study of Causcasian-American physicians found that male physicians prescribed significantly lower doses of analgesic to African-American patients than to Causcasian-American patients, while the female physicians did the reverse. (Weisse, Sanders, Syat, & Sorum, 1999). Further research is required to adequately explain the discrepancies in cultural research related to pain.

THE MEASUREMENT OF PAIN

Pain is a challenge to assess because people have difficulty describing pain objectively. If you have cut your arm, you can point to the wound. Or, if you are concerned that you might have broken a bone, this can be determined by radiography. Pain lacks these objective referents. Yet, assessing pain is very important in determining treatment for patients and evaluating the effectiveness of different pain-reducing methods. As a result, clinicians and researchers have developed many techniques for measuring the pain felt by an individual. These generally fall into three major categories: (1) psychophysiological measures; (2) behavioural assessment; and (3) self-reports. Each technique has certain advantages and certain limitations.

Psychophysiological Measures

Pain has both sensory and emotional components that can produce changes in the autonomic nervous system as well as other physiological conditions. Psychophysiological measures assess pain as it is reflected in changes produced in an individual's physiological activity (Lykken, 1987).

One psychophysiological measure researchers use for assessing pain is an **electromyograph**, or EMG, which measures the electrical activity in muscles. This electrical activity reflects the level of muscle tension. Because muscle tension is associated with certain pain states, such as headaches and low back pain, we would expect that EMG recordings would be different between people experiencing pain and those not experiencing it. However, the findings have been mixed. Blanchard and Andrasik (1985) conducted a study with headache patients and found that these patients demonstrate different EMG patterns when they are having headaches compared to when they are not. However, other studies have found no consistent results to support the idea that the level of muscle tension is an accurate predictor of headache pain or low back pain (Andrasik et al., 1982; Wolf, Nacht, & Kelly, 1982). More research is needed to verify that EMG measurements provide a reliable and valid index of pain.

Researchers have also attempted to assess pain with measures of **autonomic activity**, such as heart rate, respiration rate, blood pressure, hand surface temperature, and skin conductance. These measures assess generalized arousal that may be the result of reactions to the pain or to other stimuli. There has been only limited success in adopting these methods to measure pain. The use of **thermography** to measure skin temperature is one exception to these generally negative results (LeRoy & Filasky, 1990). Thermographic instruments measure subtle changes in skin temperature and provide an estimate of autonomic nervous system functioning. Thermography has shown some success in measuring some types of pain, however, pain is only one of many factors contributing to changes in skin temperature (Nigl, 1984). In general, measures of autonomic activity are believed to be most useful in simply assessing the emotional components of pain (Chapman et al., 1985).

Another instrument that measures pain is the **electroencephalograph**, or EEG. The EEG measures electrical activity in the brain. When a person's sensory system detects a stimulus, such as a clicking sound, the signal to the brain produces a change in EEG voltage. Electrical responses produced by stimuli are called **evoked potentials**, which the EEG records as sharp surges or peaks on the graph. Responses increase with the intensity of stimuli and decrease when people take analgesics. The EEG responses also correlate with subjective reports of pain (Chapman et al., 1985).

Even though psychophysiological measures objectively assess bodily changes that occur in response to pain, these bodily changes may also occur in response to other factors (e.g., attention, diet, and stress). Therefore, whenever possible, psychophysiological measures should be used in conjunction with other approaches in assessing pain.

Behavioural Assessment

Other measures of pain have focused on **pain behaviours**. Pain behaviours are behaviours exhibited when a person is in discomfort. They include non-verbal expressions (e.g., facial and vocal cues), distortions in movement and posture, irritability, and restrictions or avoidance of activity (Turk, Wack, & Kerns, 1985). Analyses of pain behaviours provide a basis for assessing how pain has disrupted the life of patients. Procedures have been developed for assessing specific pain behaviours in both daily activities and structured clinical settings.

Assessment of Pain Behaviour in Day-to-Day Activities

In assessing day-to-day activities, researchers and clinicians might be interested in the amount of time the person spends in bed, for example, or how many complaints he or she expresses. Does the person bend over very carefully or not at all? Does the person seek help in moving, walking, or climbing stairs? Does the person walk with a limp? Family members or significant others in the patient's life are often the best people to make these assessments. If these people are willing to help, they can be trained to make careful observations and keep accurate records. A procedure documented by William Fordyce (1976) recommends that the assessor compile a list of from five to ten behaviours that generally signal when the patient is in pain. This list might include such behaviours as requesting medication, moaning, or verbalizing pain. The assessor is then trained to watch for these behaviours in the patient and to keep track of the frequency and/or amount of time the patient exhibits them. The assessor is also trained to monitor how people, including the assessor, react to the client's pain behaviour. This procedure is useful for assessing the patient's pain experiences and also the impact they have on the patient's life and the social context that may maintain these behaviours.

This system has been modified and refined by other researchers (Turk, Meichenbaum, & Genest 1983). These refinements include the addition of a spouse diary and a significant-other pain questionnaire. The supplemental spouse diary requires the spouse to record the time, date, and location (e.g., in the car or at home in bed) of severe pain episodes. The spouse records his or her own actions and feelings in response to these pain episodes. In addition, the spouse estimates the effectiveness of such actions along a six-point scale from "did not help at all" to "seemed to stop the pain completely." The second supplement, the significant-other pain questionnaire, is made up of 30 items inquiring about the patient's severity of pain and its effect on work, recreation, and family relations. A number of the questions pertain to the significant other's feeling and responses toward the patient and the pain situation. These supplemental assessment devices can be compared with the patient's own diary and pain questionnaire over the same period.

Assessment of Pain Behaviour in Clinical Settings

In clinical settings, procedures are available for health care practitioners to assess the pain behaviour of patients. For example, in hospitals nurses may use the UAB Pain Behavior Scale (Richards, Nepomuceno, Riles, & Suer, 1982) during routine care of patients. The nurse has the patient perform several activities and rates ten pain behaviours (e.g., mobility, medication use) on a three-point scale: "none", "occasional", and "frequent." These ratings are assigned numerical values and summed for a total score.

A number of studies have focused on assessing discomfort in patients suffering from low back pain (Follick, Ahern, & Aberger, 1985; Keefe & Block, 1982; Kleinke & Spangler, 1988; Ohlund et al., 1994). In each study, patients performed a standard set of activities. For example, Chris Kleinke and Arthur Spangler (1988) asked patients to walk, pick up an object on the floor, remove their shoes while sitting, and perform several exercises such as trunk rotations, toe touching, and situps. In each study, the patients were videotaped, and trained assessors rated their performance for several pain behaviours, including sighing, grimacing, rubbing, bracing, and engaging in guarded movement. Patients are also asked to rate the intensity of their pain, thus allowing a validity check of the observers' ratings. For each behaviour except grimacing, the observers' and patients' ratings were highly correlated. These studies suggest that behavioural assessments of pain can be made relatively easily and reliably.

Self-Reports of Pain

The third and most obvious approach to pain measurement is to ask people to describe their pain, either in their own words or by filling out a rating scale or questionnaire. These are the most common types of pain assessment. In treating a patient's pain, health care practitioners ask where the pain is, what it feels like, how strong it is, and when it tends to occur.

Interviews

Interviews about pain can provide valuable information. In addition to a description of pain, such interviews can determine the history of the pain problem. The history would include when the pain was first experienced, how it developed, and the techniques used for controlling it. Factors seeming to trigger or exacerbate the pain can be discussed. The patient's emotional adjustment and whether or how the patient's lifestyle has been altered can also be explored. The information obtained in these interviews can be supplemented with information provided by significant others in the patient's life.

Rating Scales

Rating scales are one of the simplest and most direct measures of pain. Therefore, it is not surprising that rating scales are the most frequently used measures of pain (Reading, 1989). These scales are usually used to measure pain intensity. Sometimes, patients are asked to simply verbally respond to the statement, "On a scale from 1 to 10, with 10 being the most excruciating pain possible, and 1 being the lowest level of pain detectable, how much pain are you currently experiencing?" Or, the health care practitioner may choose to ask the patient to respond to this statement by providing a scale of 1 to 100. In either of these statements, the basic question is really the same. However, the form of the scale can vary (see Figure 10.1).

FIGURE 10-1 Rating Scales for Pain Measurement

Visual Analog Scale:

Mark a point on the line to show how strong your pain is

no pain — worst pain imaginable

Box Scale:

Rate the level of your pain by circling one number on the scale, where 0 means "no pain" and 10 means "worst pain imaginable"

1	2	3	4	5	6	7	8	9	10

Verbal Rating Scale:

Circle the phrase that best describes your pain

Not Painful   Slightly Painful   Moderately Painful   Very Painful   Extremely Painful

The **visual analog scale** (VAS) is simply a line anchored on the left by the phrase "no pain" and on the right by a phrase like "worst pain imaginable." People rate their pain by marking a point on the line. The **box scale** is similar to the VAS in that the scale is labelled at the ends with the phrases "no pain" and "worst pain imaginable." However, rather than simply marking a point on a line, patients are provided a series of numbers in boxes and must choose the number which best indicates the degree of pain they are experiencing. A third rating scale is the **verbal rating scale** (VRS). People are asked to describe their pain by choosing the phrase that most closely resembles the pain they are experiencing.

Researchers have studied the degree to which the rating scale format (visual, verbal, or numerical) influences the responses of the patients. For example, Ohnhaus & Adler (1975) conducted a study of drug potency in which participants were asked to supply verbal ratings of pain and ratings on the VAS. The authors concluded that the VAS reflected more precisely what a patient actually feels. However, other studies have compared the three kinds of rating scales and found no reliable differences in the reported intensity of pain. Yet, patients state a preference for the adjectival or verbal scales (Joyce et al., 1975; Kremer & Atkinson, 1990; Reading, 1989).

Rating scales are quick and easy to use, allowing people to rate their pain frequently. Averaging these ratings across time gives a more accurate picture of the amount of pain a person generally experiences compared to a single rating (Jensen & McFarland, 1993). Turk, Meichenbaum, and Genest (1983) describe how this method can be used to identify patterns of pain in chronic pain patients. Multiple ratings provide a record to determine if the patient's pain is generally improving or getting worse. In addition, patterns in the timing of severe pain may be recognized. For example, it may be that severe pain occurs most often first thing in the morning or later in the day. Or, it may be that on certain days the patient's pain is more severe. If these patterns can be identified, the patient may be able to alter his or her schedule or even the environment to accommodate or eradicate at a minimum the most severe pain.

Pain Questionnaires

Pain questionnaires were developed in response to the realization that pain is not unidimensional. That is, the experience of pain is much more than a feeling of discomfort that can be described in terms of its intensity. Melzack asserts that describing pain on a single dimension is like "specifying the visual world only in terms of light flux without regard to pattern, color, texture, and the many other dimensions of visual experience" (1975, p. 278). In an effort to measure the multidimensional nature of pain, Melzack (1975) developed the McGill Pain Questionnaire (MPQ).

The McGill Pain Questionnaire (Figure 10.2) offers patients the opportunity to describe their pain on three broad dimensions: sensory, affective, and evaluative. *Sensory* qualities of pain include its temporal, spatial, pressure, and thermal properties; *affective* qualities include fear, tension, and autonomic properties; *evaluative* qualities are the subjective overall intensity of the pain experience.

The MPQ has four parts. Part 1 consists of front and back drawings of the human body. Patients are asked to indicate on these drawings the areas where they feel pain. Part 2 consists of a list of 78 descriptive words, separated into a total of 20 subclasses. Patients are instructed to select a word from each subclass that most accurately characterizes their pain. The words are ordered in increasing intensity (e.g., hot, burning, scalding, and searing). Each word in each class has an assigned value based on the degree of pain it represents. In the previous example, "searing" would contribute the largest number of points and "hot" would contribute the lowest number. These points are summed across the 20 subclasses and the total score is called the "pain-rating index." This index is the most commonly used part of the questionnaire. Part 3 of the MPQ asks how patients' pain has changed with time. Part 4 contains a series of verbal rating scales. One of these scales inquires about the amount of pain the patient is experiencing at the present time. This scale provides a separate score called the Present Pain Intensity (PPI) score.

There are many advantages of the MPQ over previous instruments for measuring pain. The MPQ's largest contribution is its measurement of more than one dimension of pain. Researchers have provided evidence in support of this notion by confirming that pain is experienced on between two and four dimensions (e.g., Brennan, Barrett, & Garretson, 1987). Further, patients suffering from similar pain syndromes often identify the same patterns of words from the MPQ to characterize their pain. In addition, patients with different pain syndromes (e.g., cancer, arthritis, headaches, or phantom limb pain) identify different words to characterize their pain (Melzack & Wall, 1996). There are drawbacks to the MPQ. For instance, a fairly strong vocabulary is required to complete the questionnaire. Consequently, the MPQ is not useful for assessing pain in young children or with people who do not have a strong grasp of the English language (Chapman et al., 1985; Karoly, 1985).

FIGURE 10-2 The McGill Pain Questionnaire

Part 1 Where Is Your Pain?

Please mark on the drawing below, the areas where you feel pain. Put E if external, or I if internal, near the areas which you mark. Put EI if both external and internal.

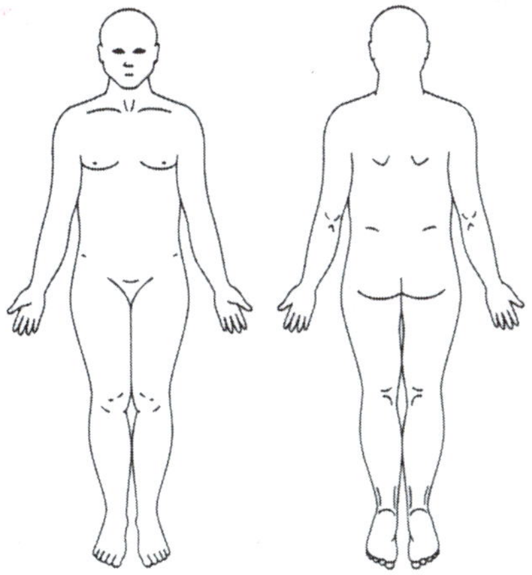

Part 2 What Does Your Pain Feel Like?

1	2	3	4
Flickering Quivering Pulsing Throbbing Beating Pounding	Jumping Flashing Shooting	Pricking Boring Drilling Stabbing Lancinating	Sharp Cutting Lacerating
5	**6**	**7**	**8**
Pinching Pressing Gnawing Camping Crushing	Tugging Pulling Wrenching	Hot Burning Scalding Searing	Tingling Itchy Smarting Stinging
9	**10**	**11**	**12**
Dull Sore Hurting Aching Heavy	Tender Taut Rasping Splitting	Tiring Exhausting	Sickening Suffocating
13	**14**	**15**	**16**
Fearful Frightful Terrifying	Punishing Grueling Cruel Vicious Killing	Wretched Blinding	Annoying Troublesome Miserable Intense Unbearable
17	**18**	**19**	**20**
Spreading Radiating Penetrating Piercing	Tight Numb Drawing Squeezing Tearing	Cool Cold Freezing	Nagging Nauseating Agonizing Dreadful Torturing

Part 3 How Does Your Pain Change With Time?

1. Which word or words would you use to describe the pattern of your pain?

1	2	3
Continuous Steady Constant	Rhythmic Periodic Intermittent	Brief Momentary Transient

2. What kind of things relieve your pain?

3. What kind of things increase your pain?

Part 4 How Strong Is Your Pain?

People agree that the following 5 words represent pain of increasing intensity. They are:

1	2	3	4	5
Mild	Discomforting	Distressing	Horrible	Excruciating

To answer each question below, write the number of the most appropriate word in the space beside the question.

1. Which word describes your pain right now? _____
2. Which word describes it at its worst? _____
3. Which word describes it when it is least? _____
4. Which word describes the worst toothache you ever had? _____
5. Which word describes the worst headache you ever had? _____
6. Which word describes the worst stomach-ache you ever had? _____

Source: Melzack, R. (1975). Reprinted with permission.

The MPQ is the most commonly used pain questionnaire (Piotrowski, 1998). It has been used to assess chronic pain in both clinical populations (e.g., patients with cancer pain and headache pain) and in laboratory research (e.g., Chapman & Syrjala, 1990; Dudgeon, Raubertas, & Rosenthal, 1993; Hunter & Phillips, 1981). A short form of the MPQ is now available (Melzack, 1987). The short form also includes multidimensional assessment and correlates highly with scores on the standard MPQ. However, the MPQ is not the only pain questionnaire available.

The West Haven-Yale Multidimensional Pain Inventory (MPI) assesses many aspects of psychological and physical functioning and could provide a comprehensive assessment of the lives of pain patients (Kerns, Turk, & Rudy, 1985). The MPI is comprised of 52 items divided into three sections. The first section measures: (1) pain severity; (2) pain's interference with patients' lives; (3) patients' dissatisfaction with their present functioning; (4) patients' view of the support they receive from others; (5) patients' perceived life control; and (6) patients' negative mood states. The second section measures patients' perceptions of the responses of significant others. The final section identifies how frequently patients engage in each of 30 different daily activities.

Many pain questionnaires have been developed for both general and specific uses, for example, the Pain Anxiety Symptoms Scale (McCracken, Zayfert, & Gross, 1993). Some of these questionnaires have been developed for use with specific populations. For instance, both the Varni Thomson Pediatric Pain Questionnaire (Varni, Thompson, & Hanson, 1987) and the Dalhousie Everyday Pain Scale (von Baeyer, Baskerville, & McGrath, 1998) were developed for use with children; the Parents' Postoperative Pain Measure was designed to assist parents in the at-home assessment of their children's pain (Finley, Chambers, McGrath, & Walsh, 1999). Other questionnaires have been developed for use with specific pain syndromes, for example, the Chronic Pain Coping Inventory (Jensen, Turner, Romano, & Strom, 1995). However, the McGill Pain Questionnaire is by far the most common instrument used by clinical practitioners and researchers (Piotrowski, 1998). In fact, it has even been adapted for use in other cultures. For example, the JMPQ is a Japanese form of the McGill Pain Questionnaire (Hasegawa et al., 1996).

Assessing Pain in Infants and Children

Assessing pain in infants and children is potentially more challenging than assessing pain in adults. Obviously, infants can not complete self-report questionnaires. Similarly, young children have difficulty expressing their experience of pain because of their limited language abilities. Therefore, pain assessments conducted on these populations cannot follow the standard questionnaire format used with adults.

At one time, it was believed that very young infants were insensitive to pain (Fletcher, 1988; Merskey, 1970; Sheridan, 1992). Currently, it is widely believed that infants feel pain with the same intensity as adults do (McCain & Morwessel, 1995). If we can not ask a newborn whether they are in pain, or how much pain they are in, what should we do? A sample of 72 neonatal intensive care unit (NICU) nurses were asked which indicators they used to interpret the experience of pain in the infants entrusted to their care (Howard & Thurber, 1998). The 10 pain indicators used by the NICU nurses, listed in decreasing order of frequency, were: fussiness, restlessness, grimacing, crying, increasing heart rate, increasing respirations, wiggling, rapid state changes, wrinkling of forehead, and clenching of fist.

Canadian researchers (e.g., Hadjistavropoulos, Craig, Grunau, & Johnston, 1994; Hadjistavropoulos, Craig, Grunau, & Whitfield, 1997) have documented the relative importance of each of the cues available when judging infant pain. They have discovered that while cry characteristics seem to command attention, cues provided through infant facial activity are weighted more heavily in adults' judgments of newborn pain. These facial characteristics include a brow bulge, eyes squeezed shut, a taut tongue and a deepened nasolabial furrow (the line or wrinkle that runs down from either side of your nose to the outer corners of your mouth). Facial characteristics also appear to convey more information to judges than does the infant's bodily activity.

Measurement of facial characteristics has been incorporated in the Neonatal Facial Coding System (NFCS). The NFCS was developed by Grunau and Craig (1987) to provide a detailed, anatomically based, and objective description of newborns' reactions to potentially painful stimuli. This instrument was developed primarily for use by researchers. It requires the researcher to assign a value of "1" or "0" to each facial action (brow bulge, eye squeeze, nasolabial furrow, open lips, vertical stretch mouth, horizontal stretch mouth, lip purse, taut tongue, and chin quiver). The scoring is completed by microanalyzing videotaped recordings of the infant.

As children get older, more instruments are available to assess their pain (Beyer & Wells, 1989). Children's behaviour can be observed and their pain rated by using scales such as the Dalhousie Everyday Pain Scale (von Baeyer, Baskerville, & McGrath, 1998). Self-report measures may also be used with children. However, these measures provide considerably less detail to the health professional than do measures used with adults. Preschool children may be asked to indicate the degree of their "hurt" by choosing a photograph from a scale of facial expressions. The Oucher scale displays six photographs of a child's face, showing increasing levels of discomfort. Colour scales, ladder scales or line drawings of faces are measures available for health professionals to use when assessing young children's pain. One visual analogue scale developed for children includes a straight, horizontal line with a happy, smiling face at one end and a sad, crying face at the other. Pain questionnaires have been developed for use with children. Examples of pain questionnaires for children include the Pediatric Pain Questionnaire (Varni, Thompson, & Hanson, 1987) and the Children's Comprehensive Pain Questionnaire (McGrath, 1987).

PAIN CONTROL TECHNIQUES

Pharmacological Control of Pain

The traditional and most common method of controlling pain is through pain-relieving medications. **Peripherally acting analgesics**, also known as non-narcotic analgesics, are probably the most frequently used analgesics (Melzack & Wall, 1996; Sunshine & Olson, 1989). Included in this group are such common pain relievers as aspirin, acetaminophen (e.g., Tylenol), and ibuprofen (e.g., Advil, Nuprin). These drugs work by reducing inflammation at the site of tissue damage and inhibiting the synthesis of neurochemicals in the peripheral nervous system that facilitate the transmission of pain impulses. Peripherally acting analgesics provide substantial pain relief for a wide variety of pain conditions, especially arthritis and other conditions involving inflammation (Anderson et al., 1985; Kanner, 1986). Although peripherally acting analgesics are generally available over the counter, they do have side effects and may interact with other drugs. Used in recommended amounts, however, they are generally safe and are effective when dealing with mild to moderate pain.

Centrally acting analgesics are pain-killing medications called narcotics. Narcotics work by binding to opiate receptors in the central nervous system (Aronoff, Wagner, & Spangler, 1986; Twycross & McQuay, 1989). These drugs are either derived directly from the opium poppy, as are codeine and morphine, or they are synthetically reproduced but based on opium molecules, as are heroin, methadone, and the brand-name drugs Percodan and Demerol. These drugs operate on the central nervous system by imitating the effects of the body's endogenous pain relief system. Specifically, the molecules in these drugs bind to receptors for endorphins and enkephalins in the brain and spinal cord, blocking the transmission of pain signals. They are considered the most potent pain relievers available. They are frequently used to alleviate labour pain, postoperative pain, and chronic progressive pain experienced by some terminal cancer patients.

Although narcotics are extremely useful for relieving pain, they also have disadvantages. For example, narcotics are known to be psychoactive, they depress respiration, they have tremendous potential to produce tolerance so that the person needs higher and higher doses to achieve the same effect, and they can be addictive (Aronoff et al., 1986).

There is considerable controversy about the likelihood of a patient becoming addicted to narcotics. Some researchers argue that this is a very real possibility (Aronoff et al., 1986) whereas others believe that this issue has been blown out of proportion (Melzack & Wall, 1996). Studies of both acute and chronic pain patients have found that few patients actually become addicted (e.g., Twycross & McQuay, 1989). Research suggests that when allowed to self-administer narcotics, patients recovering from surgery use less medication than would have been given by hospital staff. For further discussion of this topic, refer to the section on patient controlled analgesia in Chapter 7.

Local anesthetics, such as novocaine and lidocaine, make up a third category of chemicals for relieving pain (Winters, 1985). These medications can be applied topically but are much more effective when injected at the site where the pain originates. You would likely have received a local anesthetic from your dentist before he or she began drilling or pulling a tooth. Likewise, you may have received a local anesthetic before receiving sutures. Local anesthetics work by blocking nerve cells from generating pain impulses (Winters, 1985). Although they work well to block impulses in pain fibres, they also block impulses in motor neurons. Consequently, you will have little or no control over your mouth, tongue, lips, and cheeks for several hours after a dental procedure if you received a local anesthetic prior to it.

Other drugs affect pain indirectly. For example, **sedatives**, such as barbiturates, and **tranquillizers**, such as diazepam (Valium), are depressants; that is, they depress bodily functions by decreasing the transmission of impulses throughout the central nervous system (Aronoff et al., 1986). These drugs probably do not directly affect pain but, rather, reduce patient anxiety and help the patient to sleep (thereby escaping the pain for a while and resting so as to better tolerate the pain when awake). Antidepressants also help patients who are in pain by reducing the depression that may accompany pain. In addition, it is believed that they affect pain-related neurotransmitters.

There has been a dramatic increase recently in research on drug combinations that enhance pain reduction (Dalal & Melzack, 1998). This research involves: (1) drugs that have not traditionally been viewed as analgesics, such as antidepressants and sedatives; (2) drugs that have been viewed as effective analgesics in their own right, such as opioids and some antiinflammatory drugs; and (3) combinations of both types, such as opioids and antidepressants. Combining drugs in the treatment of pain increases analgesia resulting from their interaction or due to additive effects. For instance, opioid analgesia is enhanced when combined with the administration of amphetamines. Further, a combination of drugs may reduce the side effects of the drugs because the amount of each drug administered is reduced. Alternately, the side effects of some drugs can be reduced when another drug is administered and the two drugs interact. For example, the general cognitive decline and drowsiness experienced from the administration of opioids can be counteracted by introducing amphetamines.

Surgical Control of Pain

The surgical treatment of pain is the most extreme form of treatment available to pain patients. Surgery is considered only as a last resort, after all other treatment options have been exhausted. Although this treatment is radical, not all patients experience relief from their pain following surgery. In addition, surgery has its own dangers and possibilities for complications.

While some surgical techniques attempt to disrupt the transmission of pain from the periphery to the spinal cord, others are designed to interrupt the flow of pain sensations from the spinal cord upward to the brain (Carson, 1987). The least drastic surgery involves destroying the peripheral nerves close to the site of the pain. However, even this type of surgery will result in a complete loss of sensation to the area—a side effect that some patients describe as worse than the experience of pain. One must also consider that, in most cases, the peripheral nerves include both sensory and motor fibres. Thus, surgery will cause not only loss of sensation but also loss of movement.

A potentially more dangerous surgery involves severing the dorsal root ganglion, outside the spinal cord (Melzack & Wall, 1996). Just before entering the spinal cord, the nerves split into dorsal and ventral branches. The dorsal branch is entirely sensory, therefore severing it will produce only sensory loss and leave motor functioning unaffected. Like surgery of the peripheral nerves, surgery on the dorsal root ganglion will result in some patients experiencing distress because of the complete loss of sensation.

Surgery may also be performed on the spinal cord and the brain itself. Surgery to the spinal cord initially produces a complete loss of sensation below the area "damaged", thereby eliminating the experience of pain. Brain surgery as a form of pain treatment is extremely rare. Obviously, this kind of surgery is very serious, because lesions to the brain can produce many effects in addition to pain relief. One type of brain surgery, a prefrontal lobotomy, has successfully aided patients' ability to cope with pain. This type of surgery results in patients simply "not caring", and consequently they do not report pain.

Although these treatments may relieve pain for a time, usually the surgical intervention will have only short-term effectiveness. Peripheral nerves may regenerate and pain impulses will eventually find another route to the brain if neural pathways are blocked. If the surgical procedure is successful, the patient will likely experience numbness and possibly paralysis in the region affected by the nerves. The patient who chooses surgery as a treatment option may find that they must undergo numerous procedures to keep the pain "at bay."

Consider the case of a patient we'll call Tony. The metal sides of a railroad car collapsed on Tony. As a result, he was left with total and permanent motor and sensory loss below the tenth thoracic level (T10-11). Seven years after the accident, Tony underwent surgery (a high thoracic cordotomy) and was pain free for 6 months. Two years after that, he again underwent surgery (a thoracolumbar laminectomy and a spinal cordectomy), which gave him complete pain relief for 11.5 years. Again the pain returned, and once it returned every day became extremely painful. Tony reported that he was experiencing shooting pains lasting 3 to 4 seconds and, at its worst, occurring 50 to 60 times an hour (Melzack & Loeser, 1978).

Acupuncture

Acupuncture is an ancient Chinese pain control technique that has been in continuous practice for at least 2 000 years (Melzack, 1989). Basically, the procedure involves the insertion of fine needles (made of steel, gold, or other metals) through specific points in the skin then twirling or electrically charging them to create stimulation to the peripheral nerves. The effects of acupuncture are not immediate and the needles must be stimulated for approximately 20 minutes to produce analgesia. In addition, the stimulation must be fairly intense and continuous. However, the analgesia can last for hours after the stimulation has ended.

The practice of acupuncture is part of a complex theory of medicine in which all diseases and pains are believed to be due to disharmony between *yin* (spirit) and *yang* (blood). In China, where this philosophy is more widely accepted, five to ten percent of surgical operations are conducted with the use of acupuncture as the only form of analgesia. The patients must volunteer for the procedure and the surgeries using acupuncture analgesia are relatively straightforward, with little likelihood of complications. In Western countries, acupuncture is rarely used for surgery; it is seen instead as a treatment for less intense pain.

Laboratory studies have shown that acupuncture produces only mild analgesia in most people. Further, the degree of pain relief experienced is now known to be dependent on the intensity of the stimulation, rather than the exact point of stimulation. Traditionally, it was believed that exact points on the body, outlined on acupuncture charts, must be stimulated to have the desired effect. For example, certain points on the nose and ear were associated with the small intestine, whereas other points were associated with the kidneys, heart, or abdomen. Interestingly, individuals who derive the most benefits from acupuncture are the same individuals who benefit most from hypnotism.

Acupuncture is becoming more widely practised in North America, and this practice may continue to grow. A survey of health care professionals at two Cancer Care Ontario centres revealed that acupuncture was the nonpharmacolgic strategy for the management of cancer pain that participants were most interested in learning more about (Sellick & Zaza, 1998). The National Institute of Health (NIH) acknowledges that acupuncture has been somewhat successful for pain conditions involving tissue damage or tenderness, such as that experienced in postoperative dental pain. In addition, the NIH asserts that there are many situations in which acupuncture may be useful as an adjunct treatment or possibly an acceptable alternative to traditional treatments (e.g., headache, myofascial pain, osteoarthritis, low back pain, carpal tunnel syndrome, and tennis elbow) (Carlsson & Sjölund, 1994; Chapman, 1984; JAMA, 1998; Takeda & Wessel 1994).

Physical Therapy

Physical therapy involves a variety of treatment approaches to help patients who suffer from both acute and chronic pain. Patients usually work with a physical therapist to prepare an individualized treatment program. It should include daily or weekly goals that promote very gradual but steady progress. The program should progress fast enough so that the patient experiences a feeling of accomplishment but slow enough to prevent overexertion or re-injury. For example, after injury or surgery, patients perform exercises to increase muscular strength and tissue flexibility to restore their range of motion. Exercise also benefits arthritis patients because it helps maintain joint flexibility and prevents joints from deteriorating (Minor & Sanford, 1993; Wickersham, 1984). In addition, exercise is extremely beneficial for back-pain patients who need to maintain flexibility and develop strength in key muscles to provide support for their spines (Alaranta et al., 1994). As part of an exercise program, patients are typically also taught body mechanics and proper posture to prevent further injuries.

Transcutaneous Electrical Nerve Stimulation

Transcutaneous electrical nerve stimulation (TENS) involves placing an electrode on the surface of the skin, close to where the patient feels pain, and applying electrical stimulation. This stimulation affects all nerves within approximately 4 centimeters of the skin's surface. Although stimulation is usually applied for approximately 20 minutes, the duration of pain relief usually lasts several hours, and occasionally lasts for days or weeks. There is considerable individual variation in the amount of pain relief experienced. Generally, the more frequent the stimulation the longer the pain relief persists. For example, daily stimulation may provide gradually increasing relief over periods of weeks or months (Melzack, 1989).

The advantage of TENS, compared to acupuncture, is that TENS is non-invasive and does not need to be performed by a licenced practitioner. Once the appropriate points are located, the treatment can be self-administered by the patient under the physician's supervision. The electronic units which supply the electrical stimulation are often portable and can be equipped with rechargeable batteries making it relatively easy to administer TENS at home (Melzack, 1989).

The effectiveness of TENS in reducing acute muscular and postoperative pain in the majority of patients is well documented (Chapman, 1984; Hare & Milano, 1985). In a moving example, Chapman (1984) describes a 9-year-old boy who began receiving TENS while still unconscious after kidney surgery. After he regained consciousness, the hospital staff asked repeatedly if he felt pain in his belly. The boy continually replied, "No, it doesn't hurt." What is completely astonishing is that the boy did not realize he had already undergone surgery. When the surgeon left the room the boy spoke casually with the others in the room. When asked whether there was anything he feared, he began to cry and confessed his terror of the expected operation that would remove his kidney. His surprised nurse tried to reassure him that the surgery had already been done, and that there was nothing to worry about. He refused to believe her. "But don't you remember?" she contended, "that's why they put you to sleep this morning—so they could do the operation." The little boy looked very threatened. "It's not true!" he shouted, "It's not true!" When asked why it couldn't be true, he asserted confidently, "Because I haven't got any bandages." He was asked to feel his belly, since his hands were outside of the bedclothes. When he did, an expression of astonishment came over his face. At that moment, he declared he felt pain, and he began to cry. (Chapman, 1984, p. 1265).

Although TENS is useful in treating acute pain, its effectiveness in treating chronic pain is less clear (Finsen et al., 1988). Patients with arthritis have achieved substantial and long-lasting relief from pain using TENS (Bradley, 1983; Hare & Milano, 1985). In addition, studies that have compared the effectiveness of TENS to acupuncture in treating low back pain report that the two techniques are equal in terms of reducing pain (Andersson & Holmgren, 1975, Fox & Melzack, 1976; Laitininen, 1976). However, TENS produces short-lived relief to patients experiencing other chronic conditions including phantom limb pain (Johnson, 1984; Minor & Sanford, 1993).

Massage

Several years ago, a massage was considered a luxury. Today, massage therapy is one of the pain management techniques that Canadian physicians are keen to learn more about (Sellick & Zaza, 1998). Massage therapy is used to ease muscle pain and other pains, including that resulting from cancer pain. The procedure consists of systematic stroking and kneading of the body. The two main types of massage therapy are Swedish massage and Shiatsu massage. **Swedish massage** is a set routine of basic strokes to work the body and includes slow, gentle stroking movements, known as *effleurage*, to warm and relax tissue and to stimulate blood circulation. A deeper massage is also conducted with movements such as friction, percussion, and *pettrisage* (massage in which the muscles are kneaded and pressed). **Shiatsu massage** is based on the belief that there is a flow of energy through the body and that at times energy blockages develop. Consistent with this belief, energy blockages are released through the strong and sustained pressure of the massage at specific points on the body.

Research conducted with 32 hospital staff at a large teaching hospital investigated the usefulness of Swedish massage (Katz, Wowk, Culp, & Wakeling, 1999). Participants received either a series of eight 15-minute, on-site massage treatments or eight sessions of seated rest. Those in the massage group experienced significant reductions in pain and tensions levels compared to the control group that received seated rest. This pain and tension relief persisted for up to a day or longer following the massage. An added benefit experienced by those who received the massage treatments was an increase in overall mood.

Relaxation

Relaxation training has shown some evidence of being an effective treatment for both acute and chronic pain. It is often used in conjunction with other pain management strategies and is thought to be an essential part of both biofeedback and hypnotic treatment. The rationale for relaxation training is straightforward: continual muscle contraction has been considered both a cause and an effect of pain (Dolce & Raczynski, 1985). Researchers have found that muscle tension results in lactic acid build-up in muscles and also decreases blood flow to muscles. Both these factors result in significant increases in people's experience of pain.

As discussed in Chapter 5, relaxation can be accomplished with many different techniques, including progressive muscle relaxation and meditation. Psychologists have developed various methods of **progressive muscle relaxation** that concentrate on either one or several specific muscle groups (Jacobson, 1938). For example, in a quiet environment the patient is asked to close his or her eyes and concentrate on breathing in and out, taking deep slow breaths. The patient might then be asked to squeeze his or her fingers into a fist as tightly as possible. Then the individual is asked to slowly relax the hand. This demonstrates to the patient the difference between tense and relaxed muscles. Without the comparison of a contracted muscle, most people have difficulty imagining what a relaxed muscle feels like. The psychologist will guide the patient through this contraction-relaxation exercise with other muscle groups such as the arms, shoulders, neck, back, toes, feet, calves, thighs, and buttocks. Periodically, the patient will be reminded to continue to breathe deeply. In addition, the patient might be told to empty his or her mind of all thoughts and/or to focus on an image that is pleasing to them (such as waves washing over the sand at the seashore). Focusing on a pleasant, relaxing image directs attention away from sources of anxiety, pain, and stress.

Patients are encouraged to practise this technique on their own between sessions with the psychologist. If they have difficulties achieving the desired state, the patient may turn to one of many prerecorded audio- and videotapes available that aid patients in their quest for relaxation. Some of the tapes offer a soothing voice that guides one through the progressive relaxation technique, while other tapes simply provide sounds of nature (e.g., the sea, a babbling brook, or songbirds) or peaceful music. After approximately 10 sessions with a psychologist guiding the patient, the patient is usually able to enter a state of deep relaxation very easily on his or her own. This was the case with Jake, whom we introduced to you at the beginning of the chapter. Now, Jake can concentrate on achieving a relaxed state almost anytime, resulting in a peaceful and calm state. This was something that initially he wasn't able to do on his own.

How successful has progressive relaxation been in the management of pain? In a meta-analysis of studies, Carlson and Hoyle (1993) reported that progressive muscle relaxation was generally helpful in coping with stress-related disorders such as migraine and tension headache, depression, hypertension, and low back pain. However, the actual effect size varied substantially from study to study, in part because of variation in the experimental procedures. Relaxation training was most effective when patients had participated in a sufficient number of training sessions, when they had been trained individually rather than in a group, when the patients used audiotapes to supplement their training, and when the patients had enough time to master the technique.

A question may arise as to the durability of the effects of relaxation treatment for pain. Edward Blanchard and colleagues have addressed this issue by conducting a 5-year follow-up investigation of chronic headache patients (Blanchard, Andrasik et al., 1987; Blanchard, Appelbaum et al., 1987). These patients had all experienced an average of 18 years of headache resulting either from muscle-contraction (tension-type) or "vascular" headache, the latter of which includes both migraine and combined (migraine plus tension-type) headache. These patients completed training for progressive muscle relaxation in ten sessions over eight weeks. Those patients whose headache pain had not improved by at least 60 percent were offered additional treatment in the form of biofeedback. The treatment effects endured over time. That is, 5 years after the initial treatment patients reported headache pain at levels similar to those reported immediately after taking part in the treatment. The headache pain did not return to pretreatment levels. Other research has supported this conclusion, with patients experiencing durable relief from both relaxation and biofeedback for at least 2 years (Blanchard, 1987).

Meditation is another form of relaxation. *Meditative relaxation*, developed by Herbert Benson and colleagues (e.g., Benson, Beary, & Carol, 1974) is derived from various religious meditative practices but has no religious connotations. With Bensonian relaxation, the patient attempts to focus attention fully on a single thought or image. Often a very simple syllable such as "ohm" or "one" is repeated slowly over and over again with each breath. This process usually takes place in a quiet environment where the participant sits with eyes closed and muscles relaxed for a period of approximately 20 minutes.

Mindfulness meditation is a related strategy for achieving relaxation. This type of meditation has its roots in Buddhist practice. Participants engaged in mindfulness meditation do not try to ignore unpleasant thoughts or sensations. Instead, they are instructed to focus on any thought or sensation as it occurs but to view these thoughts in a non-judgmental manner. As Kabat-Zinn (1993) explains, "Observing without judging, moment by moment, helps you see what is on your mind without editing or censoring it, without intellectualizing it or getting lost in your own incessant thinking" (p. 263).

There are very few controlled studies evaluating the effectiveness of meditation. Those studies that have been published report mixed results. Some studies suggest that meditation is not successful as a pain control technique (Holmes, 1981), whereas others report that meditation is more effective than relaxation, biofeedback, or cognitive-behavioural strategies (Murphy, 1996). More studies are required to accurately determine whether meditation is a useful technique for managing pain.

Guided imagery can be considered a form of relaxation and also can be classified as a technique that relies on distraction. With guided imagery, the participant is told to imagine a calm, peaceful, and pleasant image. The image should be relatively unchanging, and the participant is told to focus all of his or her attention on the image.

Guided imagery is a technique suggested to pregnant mothers for use in childbirth. Women in labour are told to choose a focal point, either real or imagined, that they can concentrate on when giving birth. This may be a lovely country road surrounded by trees with the leaves changing colours in the fall. Alternately, the woman may choose to focus on a picture of her pet that she has brought with her to the hospital for this very purpose or a light on the ceiling of her room.

Children are also encouraged to use guided imagery when undergoing cancer treatment. One child described skiing down a mountain as fast as he could. He commented on the warmth of the sunshine but insisted that focusing on the speed with which he skied in and out of the gates was how he became most "absorbed" in his image.

The effectiveness of guided imagery has not been established. When used to manage pain, guided imagery is most often used in conjunction with other pain control techniques. Thus, the unique contribution of guided imagery is difficult to establish. Studies conducted on guided imagery suggest it is superior to biofeedback in treating headaches (Ilacqua, 1994), aids burn victims in coping with pain (Achterberg, Kenner, & Lawlis, 1988), and reduces post-operative pain in child surgical patients as well as the length of their hospital stays (Lambert, 1996).

Distraction

As with guided imagery, **distraction** involves focusing one's attention on something other than the sensation of pain. As we mentioned earlier, athletes, soldiers, and others who are "caught up" in what they are doing may not immediately notice when they have injured themselves. Certainly, the pain in these situations does not seem as extreme as it might in others. Although we sometimes engage in distraction unknowingly, it is also possible to consciously apply the technique of distraction to help control the experience of pain. We can distract ourselves by focusing on a completely different activity, such as listening to music, singing a song, playing a video game, doing arithmetic problems, or reading a book. The staff at Vancouver Children's Hospital has found that pop-up books are very good for distracting children. These are made available to children while they are undergoing cancer treatment.

Alternately, distraction can involve reinterpreting the event that is resulting in pain. Bandura (1991) provides a description from an 8-year-old boy who is re-interpreting a painful event: "As soon as I get in the dentist's chair, I pretend he's the enemy and I'm a secret agent, and he's torturing me to get secrets, and if I make one sound, I'm telling him secret information, so I never do." The boy goes on to say that this is good practice because he is going to be a secret agent when he grows up. There may be times when this technique works too well. On one occasion, the boy got quite absorbed in his role; when the dentist asked the boy to rinse his mouth, the boy snarled and said "I won't tell you a damned thing." This stunned the dentist and apparently even the boy was surprised with this outburst.

Distraction techniques are particularly useful for reducing acute pain, such as that experienced during some medical and dental procedures. Although those suffering from chronic pain may be able to divert their attention for a short time, it is unlikely that they can distract themselves indefinitely. Therefore, a patient who experiences chronic pain is likely to use distraction only when he or she anticipates a sharp rise in their pain. For example, distraction would be particularly useful when a person suffering from chronic lower back pain must endure a bumpy car ride to the physician's office or when an arthritic patient needs to climb a flight of stairs.

Biofeedback

Biofeedback is a procedure used to teach patients to exert voluntary control over a bodily process that they are usually unaware of, such as heart rate. This technique relies on the principles of *operant conditioning*. Initially, a target bodily process is identified. This bodily process is then tracked by an electronic device that presents a sensory signal (usually visual or auditory) to the patient. The sensory signal enables the patient to monitor the bodily process; with this information, the patient can attempt to modify it. For example, a person trying to lower his or her heart rate can attempt various methods to achieve this result. The feedback from the machine might provide a signal in the form of a tone that will let the patient know which methods actually alter his or her heart rate and which do not. It may be that focusing on one's breathing and ignoring everything else might lower the patient's heart rate. Or, humming a slow song or visualizing a peaceful scene might lower the patient's heart rate. The biofeedback machine will tell the patient which method is most effective. Training sessions last about 20 to 30 minutes but once patients know which strategies work best for them, they can usually implement the bodily changes on their own, without use of the machine.

There are many forms of biofeedback. Biofeedback that measures muscle tension is called **electromyographic (EMG) biofeedback**. This form of biofeedback is particularly useful for patients who experience tension headaches resulting from chronically tensed muscles in the head, neck, and jaw. It can help teach the patients how to consciously reduce the tension in their muscles. **Thermal biofeedback** measures temperature and blood flow. This is a very effective treatment for migraine headache sufferers, who can learn to bring blood to their hands, a strategy known as **handwarming**, which reduces cranial blood flow and the pain caused by dilated cranial blood vessels. Biofeedback has also been applied to the treatment of temporomandibular joint pain, arthritis, low back pain, pain associated with cerebral palsy, and Reynaud's syndrome (a condition in which the blood supply to the extremities is interrupted, resulting in pain, numbness, and tingling) (Engel, Jensen, Schwartz, & White, 1999; Turk, Zacki, & Rudy, 1993).

Although biofeedback may be used in a very specific way to deal with a specific pain problem, the power of biofeedback can be quite general as well. People have been taught to activate their parasympathetic nervous system to produce a relaxed state. This is particularly useful at times when a person may be experiencing fear or anxiety.

Hypnosis

Hypnosis is one of the oldest techniques used to control pain (Hilgard & Hilgard, 1975). In the early nineteenth century, sensational tales appeared of physicians performing major surgery on patients who had been hypnotized. In 1829, it was reported that a French surgeon, Dr. Cloquet, removed a malignant tumour and several enlarged glands from a 64-year old woman. In order to accomplish this feat, an incision was made from the woman's armpit to the inner side of her breast, in other words, the incision went half way across her chest. Yet the woman, who had not received any drugs, conversed with the physician and showed no signs of experiencing pain (Kroger, 1957; cited in Chaves & Barber, 1976).

Hypnosis is often considered an altered state of consciousness that involves several components. First, a state of *relaxation* is necessary so that a hypnotic trance can be induced. Second, *distraction* or diversion of attention from the pain experience is engendered (this step is also referred to as "narrowing of attention"). Next, the practitioner *suggests* to the patient that the pain is diminishing. In this step, the practitioner may suggest that the pain is being replaced by a more pleasant sensation, such as warmth (Barber, 1986; Orne & Dinges, 1989).

The hypnotic procedure can take one of a number of forms. Consider Dylan, a 26-year-old who is currently experiencing extreme pain in his left arm resulting from a fall he experienced while snowboarding.

> Scenario One:
> Dylan's practitioner first induces hypnosis and then suggests, "The arm is going to begin to feel numb, with a pins-and-needles sensation as though it has received novocaine, and it will go entirely to sleep." After a period of giving such suggestions, the practitioner adds, "This numbness is now so complete that there will be no pain sensation whatsoever, though you just might be able barely to feel my touch."

These suggestions rely upon Dylan imagining sensations he has had in the past: numbness, pins and needles, the feeling that novocaine has been injected and that the arm has gone to sleep. If Dylan can imagine these sensations well enough that he is actually experiencing them, he will also gain control over the pain sensation in that arm.

> Scenario Two:
> Dylan's practitioner first induces hypnosis and then suggests, "Your arm will begin to float up, bending at the elbow." After this is repeated a few times, the practitioner grasps Dylan's arm and adds, "You now see your arm floating down, slowly, and gently your arm is cradled in your lap."

This procedure, first described by Erickson (1967), is an indirect way of suggesting away pain. Dylan's actual arm no longer seems to belong to him. Consequently, he no longer feels pain in his arm.

Scenario Three:
Dylan's practitioner first induces hypnosis and then suggests, "Collect your pain in your left hand. As you do so slowly make a fist. Squeeze your fist tighter as you continue to capture the pain." After a number of these suggestions, the practitioner adds, "You have gathered all of the pain in your hand, now throw it away."

This technique relies on the experience of focusing on the left hand and providing the sensation of muscular tension and pressure to facilitate the response to suggestion. The practitioner might also have Dylan relive an experience he had before experiencing pain in his arm, thereby indirectly eliminating the pain.

Unfortunately, hypnosis does not work for everyone. For people who are highly responsive to suggestion, hypnosis can be very helpful in pain relief. However, researchers are not entirely sure whether hypnosis actually blocks pain or simply interferes with the reporting of it. Under hypnotic suggestion, people tend not to show behavioural signs of pain, such as grimacing or tensing their muscles. As well, hypnotized people report verbally that they feel no discomfort (Hilgard & Hilgard, 1975). They may recognize that they are in pain, but they indicate that the pain is not affecting them or does not matter to them. However, under hypnosis, people still show the classic physiological reactions of pain, such as changes in respiration and increased heart rate and blood pressure (Orne, 1989).

Researchers have yet to achieve a complete understanding of the mechanism responsible for the success of hypnosis. Consequently, modern physicians have been reluctant to adopt it in their clinical practice. However, there is now considerable documentation demonstrating the effectiveness of hypnosis for patients undergoing surgery, childbirth, and dental procedures as well as for those receiving treatment of burns, low back pain, cancer pain, and headaches (Barber, 1986; Iserson, 1999; Linden, 1994; Orne & Dinges, 1989; Sellick, & Zaza, 1998). For example, in a controlled clinical trial Spiegel and Bloom (1983) randomly assigned 54 women with metastatic breast cancer to three groups. Group one members met weekly for 90 minutes and comprised a support group. During the session, the women underwent hypnosis for approximately 5 to 10 minutes. The women assigned to group two also had a 90-minute weekly support group meeting but did not undergo hypnosis. The third group received only the usual medical treatment. One year later, the women in groups one and two reported significantly less pain compared to group three, with group one reporting the least pain. In fact, group three, the control group, actually reported an increase in pain and suffering a year after the experiment commenced. Many studies have reported an added benefit of using hypnosis in the treatment of pain. Patients who receive hypnosis report less anxiety than do patients who receive other forms of pain treatment (Liossi & Hatira, 1999; Mauer et al., 1999).

Multidisciplinary Pain Management Programs

Pain clinics and pain management programs have been developed to aid the chronic pain patient. The above review of existing pain treatments illustrates that no single method of treatment is completely effective. Further, the success of each method of treatment varies considerably from one patient to the next. Therefore, a treatment approach that combines several treatment methods is likely to succeed for the largest percentage of patients and provide the greatest pain relief for each individual.

The concept of having special institutions to provide a multidisciplinary treatment for pain originated with John Bonica. He founded the first pain clinic at the University of Washington Medical School in 1960. There are now thousands of pain clinics across North America. The structure, methods, and quality of pain clinics vary widely. Many pain clinics are private institutions, whereas others are affiliated with medical schools, universities, or hospitals. Some clinics provide inpatient care, while others provide treatment on an outpatient basis. Often the program will include the interdisciplinary efforts of physicians, psychologists or psychiatrists, physical therapists, and occupational therapists (Rains, Penzien, & Jamison, 1992). However, there are countless experts who can be included or consulted in any particular program (e.g., neurologists, rheumatologists, orthopedic surgeons, acupuncturists, massage therapists, etc.).

Initially, patients are assessed to determine the qualitative nature of their pain. This assessment typically involves documenting the location, sensory qualities, severity, and duration of the patient's pain as well as its onset and history. Determining the patient's current emotional and mental state, the degree to which family and work lives have been interrupted, and how the patient has coped with the pain in the past is also part of the initial assessment. This assessment allows for the program to be customized to match the needs of the patient (Chapman, 1991; Rains et al., 1992; Turk & Stacey, in press). Goals for each patient are established, and the program is constructed to help the patient attain those goals.

The goals and objectives of different pain management programs may vary. However, they typically include: reducing the patient's experience of pain, improving physical and lifestyle functioning, improving social support and family life, decreasing reliance on medications, and reducing the patient's need to use health care services (Follick, Ahern, Attansio, & Riley, 1985; Rains et al., 1992). The programs generally include specific treatment components for attaining each goal. For example, most programs include patient education to provide patients with a more complete understanding of the nature of their condition. Patients may take part in discussions of nutrition; medications; depression resulting from pain; how to combat sleep disturbances; and assertiveness or social skills. Usually patients are also educated about various methods of pain control. For instance, relaxation training and exercise are regular components of pain clinic programs. Guided imagery, acupuncture, massage, and other pain-reducing strategies may also be included. Familial and vocational counselling are also incorporated in many pain management programs.

How effective are multidisciplinary pain management programs? Numerous studies have documented that chronic pain sufferers who receive treatment at multidisciplinary pain centres report much less subsequent pain and are far more likely to return to work than individuals who receive standard pain treatment (Cutler et al., 1994; Flor, Fydrich, & Turk, 1992). Consider the evaluation of the pain management program at the Miller-Dwan Hospital Pain Control Center in Minnesota (Cinciripini & Floreen, 1982). Participants taking part in the program at the time of evaluation were men and women who had suffered intractable pain from known injuries or diseases (e.g., arthritis) for at least 1 year. At the time, all of the participants were unable to work because of the disabling pain they were experiencing. The participants took part in the program on an inpatient basis for 4 weeks, with weekends off. In this program, patients participate as part of a group. All patients took part in the full program, which comprised a medication-reduction procedure, physical therapy, relaxation and biofeedback training, self-monitoring, behavioural contracting, cognitive-behavioural group therapy, and family involvement and training. The patients' behaviour and functioning was assessed at the start of the program, at the end of the program, and follow-up assessments at 6 and 12 months following program completion, which the majority of the participants took part in. Upon completing the program, patients' activity levels had increased and their pain experiences, pain behaviours, and medication use had sharply decreased. Amazingly, 90 percent of the patients were no longer taking analgesic medication. Follow-up assessments revealed that participants continued to be physically active and that approximately one-half were employed. The participants' pain continued to decrease. The average pain rating reported by participants before treatment was 4.6 on a 10-point scale, at the time of program completion it was 2.2, and after 1 year it was 1.2. This program can certainly be regarded as successful.

Which components of a multidisciplinary pain management program make it so effective? Many would argue that it is the combination of pain treatments that make a multidisciplinary program effective. However, a recent study has documented how helpful patients believe each component of a multidisciplinary program has been for them. Perna, Durgin, and Geller (1999) randomly selected 16 female and 9 male chronic pain patients' files. All of the patients had completed a comprehensive multidisciplinary 20-day pain management program. At the conclusion of the program, each patient completed a form that asked to rate on a scale from 1 to 10 "the helpfulness" of each of the treatment modalities they had participated in; a score of "1" indicated not at all helpful whereas a score of "10" indicated the most help possible. Mean scores and the order of patient-rated helpfulness for each modality were as follows: group therapy (8.64), individual therapy (8.29), mind-body (7.95), physical therapy (7.75), biofeedback (7.68), medical office visits (6.80), occupational therapy (6.56), aqua therapy (6.33), vocational therapy (6.00), osteopathic manipulation (4.40), and trigger point injection (2.40). It is interesting that interventions aimed at mental activity were chosen as most helpful, particularly when, as the authors point out, all the patients in the study were on workers' compensation and likely stood to benefit from de-emphasizing psychological issues.

Not all chronic pain patients benefit from the treatment provided at a pain clinic, but most do. You may recall that Jake, who we introduced you to at the beginning of this chapter, had recently returned from a 10-day stay at a pain clinic. Jake was a prime candidate for this kind of treatment because his pain had not been relieved even after trying "every pain management technique available." Jake was skeptical about the benefits he might receive at the clinic and certainly some of the pain management techniques worked better for him than some of the others. For example, he felt that the acupuncturist caused more pain than he relieved. Fortunately, not all of the treatments were perceived in this way. Jake thought that many of the exercises he learned from the physiotherapist were quite helpful. Jake derived other benefits from his stay as well. He now possesses more coping skills and social support than he did when he entered the program. In addition, over the course of his stay he dramatically reduced the amount of medication he was taking.

Multidisciplinary pain management programs represent a truly biopsychosocial approach to pain management. They can provide medical, psychosocial, physical, and occupational therapy. They can also improve chronic pain sufferers' psychosocial and physical functioning and reduce their pain, pain behaviour, and drug use.

KEY TERMS

afferent (sensory) neurons
nociceptors
A-delta fibres
C-fibres
specificity theory
pattern theory
gate control theory
central control trigger
neuromatrix theory
pariaqueductal gray area
stimulation-produced analgesia (SPA)
endogenous opioids
acute pain
chronic pain
chronic recurrent pain
chronic intractable benign pain
chronic progressive pain
respondent pain
operant pain
pain behaviours
pain threshold
pain tolerance
electromyograph (EMG)
autonomic activity
thermography
electroencephalograph (EEG)
evoked potentials
visual analog scale (VAS)
box scale
verbal rating scale (VRS)
peripherally acting analgesics
centrally acting analgesics
narcotics
local anesthetics
sedatives
tranquillizers
acupuncture
physical therapy
transcutaneous electrical nerve stimulation (TENS)
swedish massage
shiatsu massage
progressive muscle relaxation
meditation
guided imagery
distraction
electromyographic (EMG) biofeedback
thermal biofeedback
handwarming
hypnosis
multidisciplinary pain management programs
phantom limb pain

Chapter 11

CHRONIC AND LIFE-THREATENING ILLNESS

Chapter Outline

Key Questions

1. How is a chronic or life-threatening illness different from other illnesses?
2. What are the most common examples of chronic and life-threatening illnesses?
3. What are the physical challenges posed by common chronic and life-threatening illnesses?
4. What are the psychological issues and sources of distress for people with chronic and life-threatening illnesses?
5. How can health psychologists and others help people cope with various chronic and life-threatening illnesses?
6. What do we mean by quality of life in this context and why is it important when treating people with chronic and life-threatening illnesses?
7. What psychological reactions are common to people who face the real possibility of premature death?
8. How can we help people cope with the possibility of premature death, and how can we help family and friends when they lose a loved one to serious illness?

At first, Mario attributed his fatigue to a lack of sleep. However, his fatigue persisted, even on days when he had slept well the night before. And then there was the light-headedness, especially when he hadn't eaten for a while. Once, it got so bad that Mario actually felt disoriented.

After a trip to his doctor and some blood tests, Mario found out that he had Type II diabetes. He was discouraged by the diagnosis. It sounded so serious. He had heard of people dying or going blind from diabetes. Just as discouraging was the fact that he was going to have to make significant changes to his life—changes that would be permanent. This was because diabetes is a **chronic** condition. It doesn't go away or get better. Instead, people with chronic conditions must learn to cope with them on a daily basis.

Mario was going to have to change his diet and closely monitor it. He was going to have to lose weight, too. These major changes were going to be even more difficult for Mario because, for the first time in his life, he was feeling very depressed and fearful. Fortunately, his wife and friends were supportive, and there were some excellent information sessions put on by the hospital, so Mario did not have to feel alone in facing the daily challenges brought on by diabetes.

In this chapter, we will look at the psychology of chronic conditions that people live with for life, and serious conditions, which are life threatening and often accompanied by severe symptoms. For most of us, illness is **acute**, which means it is episodic in nature. This means that it has a defined beginning and end. Chronically ill people might not view their illness in **episodic** terms, however, and this can make their condition hard to cope with (Nerenz & Leventhal, 1983). It is not surprising that health psychology has dedicated a great deal of research effort to understanding these conditions, which are often accompanied by emotional distress. Mario's reaction to his diagnosis of diabetes is not uncommon. Many people feel anger, depression, and fear when they learn they must cope with serious or chronic illnesses. However, in most cases these emotional reactions are not conducive to successful coping. Table 11.1 presents four different ways in which symptoms are experienced by the chronically ill. A chronically ill person may well experience each symptom pattern, which in turn produces its own set of psychological responses.

TABLE 11-1 The Range of Symptom-Related Experience for People with Chronic Illness

Symptoms That Are:	Produce:
constant	discouragement and fear
lessened or in remission	hope
unpredictably erratic	anger and frustration
relentlessly progressive	exhaustion and a sense of being overwhelmed

Source: Goodheart & Lansing, 1997. Adapted by persmission.

A person's reaction to a chronic condition is influenced by his or her cognitive representation of that condition. For example, people with cardiovascular disease can see themselves as being *chronically ill* or *at risk* (Nerenz & Leventhal, 1983). While it may be medically accurate to think of oneself as being chronically ill, it is probably more adaptive to represent oneself as being at risk. This is because the former results in a self-label that can be depressing, discouraging, and permanent. The latter promotes active involvement in problem solving in the form of risk reduction.

We'll look closely at a number of conditions that are either chronic, serious, or both. We'll also look at the factors affecting people's ability to cope with these conditions and how people can be helped to cope better. You may remember that in Chapter 1, we made the point that major causes of death have changed since the beginning of the twentieth century. While it was viruses and bacteria that were the main killers in 1900, diseases of lifestyle and environment—cancer and cardiovascular diseases—are now the main culprits. In this chapter, we are going to look closely at what it is like to have these and other diseases.

CANCER

In 1997, 181 people out of every 100 000 in Canada died from cancer (Statistics Canada, 1999). This number, which has remained relatively stable since 1980, represents 28 percent of all deaths in 1997. Consistent with this, in 1998 Statistics Canada estimated that people living in Canada had about a one-in-four chance of dying from cancer, and a 41 percent chance of getting cancer some time in their lives. Remember that these are **lifetime** statistics, describing a person's chance of ever getting cancer in their lives. As such, they are influenced considerably by the fact that a much higher percentage of older people will contract cancer. The probability that people in their thirties will get cancer is only 0.7 percent, whereas for people in their eighties, the probability is 34 percent (National Cancer Institute of Canada, 1998). The point is that, in our lifetime, we will all either know people who have cancer or we will have to cope with it ourselves.

CASE 11-1 An Unwelcome Diagnosis

Maria's life changed the day her physician discovered a lump in her breast during a routine examination. Then came the mammogram, the biopsy, and the result she had feared. She had a malignant tumour in her breast. One day, she had been most concerned about her workload, her children's over-enthusiastic soccer coach, and her husband's reluctance to paint the kitchen. Suddenly, all of that seemed to pale in comparison to the questions that now had to be answered. Had the cancer spread? Could all the cancer be removed with a lumpectomy or would she require a mastectomy? How could she cope with that? What would her husband think? There would be more tests and more procedures. She remembered a colleague at work who had died from breast cancer. Was Maria going to die? She could not answer any of these questions. All she knew for sure was that she had never been so afraid in her life.

Cancer is not one disease, but many. The experience of a patient with one form of cancer can differ radically from that of another patient with a different form. The study of and treatment of cancer is called **oncology**. Oncologists often specialized in a particular *site* where cancer occurs in the body. This specialization is further indication of the differences between types of cancers, or **sites of cancer**, as oncologists would refer to them. For example, one group of oncologists might specialize in cancers of the genitourinary system. These oncologists would treat prostate cancer. Others may focus on the central nervous system. Many factors will influence a person's psychological reactions to a diagnosis of cancer. One of these factors is the site of the disease and the symptoms associated with it.

What all forms of cancer share is the uncontrolled growth of abnormal cells. General cell growth is, of course, common throughout the body. This growth is controlled as cells wear out and are replaced. Cancer cells are different, though. They grow in an uncontrolled manner and destroy normal cells in the process. When these abnormal cells form a mass, it is called a tumour. This tumour may be localized, or cells may spread to other parts of the body. When this happens, the cancer is said to have **metastasized**, or spread. Metastasized cancer is considerably harder to treat, since the treatment must be much less localized. Early detection of tumours reduces the likelihood that the cancer will have metastasized and thus increases chances of survival. In Case Study 11.1, Maria hoped that her physician had detected the lump early, so that the cancer had not had time to spread. The Canadian Cancer Society has an informative web site for those seeking more information on cancer. It can be found at www.cancer.ca.

Whatever the site of the tumour, a diagnosis of cancer can have a profound effect on a person. Some will view it as a death sentence, others as the ultimate challenge of their lives. Many will go through strong denial in the early stages in an attempt to cope with trauma that is unprecedented in their lives. Even after receiving her diagnosis, Maria may deny that she has cancer. Interestingly, it has been found that denial can actually help as a short-term response in the early stages of the cancer experience (Meyerowitz, Heinrich, & Schag, 1983).

Patients must cope with aggressive treatments that bring on side effects that are worse than the symptoms of many other diseases. They must face the real possibility that their lives will be shortened, and they must also face the possible stigma associated with serious illness. Friends and colleagues aren't always adept at providing support for the cancer patient. Their own fear and lack of familiarity with cancer can get in the way. There is evidence, though, that the stigma of cancer is diminishing and that people are becoming more adept at lending support to friends and family members with the disease (Bloom & Kessler, 1994).

The nature of cancer patients' suffering has been categorized into three general areas: physical, psychological, and social (Kuuppeloäki & Lauri, 1998). According to research in which cancer patients were asked to complete questionnaires investigating their suffering, approximately 60 percent of cancer suffering is related to physical factors (Kuuppeloäki & Lauri, 1998). These break down further into two subcategories: illness-caused and treatment-caused. The most common complaints in this regard are fatigue, pain, and side effects of chemotherapy, which we will discuss in a moment. About 44 percent of suffering relates to psychological factors. The two most prevalent forms are depression and fear. For the patients in Kuuppeloäki and Lauri's (1998) study, the worst times for depression were at the initial diagnosis, when or if the cancer metastasized, and when the patients were in poor physical condition. About 13 percent of suffering relates to the patients' social lives. The primary problem here is withdrawal. While the stigma of having cancer appears to be lifting, as we have seen (Bloom & Kessler, 1994), it is still the case that many patients experience significant disruptions in their social lives.

Adolescents with cancer report cancer-related hassles as long as 2 years after they have been treated. These include such things as being unable to play contact sports or, for a person who had suffered a brain tumour 14 years earlier, still experiencing fear every time he had a headache.

Physical Problems

Fatigue and pain have been identified as two of the most common physical problems faced by cancer patients (Kuuppeloäki & Lauri, 1998). Pain management, then, is a major challenge for patients and for those providing treatment. One source of frustration in this regard is the fact that cancer pain tends to be undertreated. It has been estimated that more than 90 percent of cancer pain can be controlled by current treatments; however, these treatments are underused (Paice, Toy, & Shott, 1998). Why is this? It is not because practitioners are not inclined to do everything they can to reduce patients' suffering. Rather, the patients' attitudes and behaviour explain why more people are in pain than need be.

For example, patients' fears about building up a tolerance to analgesic medication and, to a lesser extent, an addiction to it, keep them from seeking adequate pain-relieving treatment (Paice, Toy, & Shott, 1998). Yet most of these fears are unfounded. Thomason and colleagues (1998) identified patient-related barriers to taking analgesics for their cancer pain. The first was forgetfulness, followed by the belief that the pain should be tolerated. Patients also reported concerns regarding side effects. For these and a host of other reasons, patients may be unwilling to report mild or moderate pain, making it difficult for practitioners to prescribe adequate medication (Thomason et al., 1998).

Psychological Distress

As you can well imagine, there are many different psychological reactions involved in the cancer experience. Two of the most common and that tend to cause the most problems for patients and their families are fear and depression. Breast cancer patients scheduled for mastectomy report that their psychological distress is greatest in the period between their diagnosis and their surgery (Jamison, Wellish, & Pasnau (1978). Maria's family and friends from Case Study 11.1 must be especially helpful during this time.

For some patients, fear and depression become chronic, even if cancer treatment is proceeding successfully. They may fear recurrence or that the cancer will metastasize. They may fear the side effects of the treatment and the changes to their self-image (Steginga, Occhipinti, Wilson & Dunn, 1998). For example, breast cancer patients have said that they fear feeling less feminine as a result of mastectomy, and that people will notice that their chest is different, or that friends will withdraw and be unable to discuss cancer with them (Steginga et al., 1998).

Depression is a common form of psychological distress for cancer patients (e.g., Payne et al, 1999; Thompson & Shear, 1998), although it is more prevalent in some forms of cancer than others. For example, depression is diagnosed at a higher rate for pancreatic cancer, a disease that tends to have a poor prognosis (Alter, 1996). A study of 52 consecutive patients undergoing radiation therapy for various forms of cancer found that 16 of them (31%) were depressed (Jenkins, Carmody, & Rush, 1998). Depression results in poorer quality of life, less compliance with medical treatment, longer hospital stays, and higher mortality rates (Newport & Nemeroff, 1998). Depressed patients also report greater pain intensity (Sist et al., 1998). To compound the problem, a patient's depression is positively correlated with family caregivers' depression (Kurtz, Kurtz, Given, & Given, 1995).

Analysis of cancer-related depression has shown that it is linked to **intrusive memories**. These are unwanted thoughts, often visual in nature, that are related to memories the patient has about cancer. They usually involve illness and death, often that of a friend, relative, or someone in a movie. These intrusive memories result in poor coping because they produce an anxious preoccupation with cancer, as well as a sense of helplessness and hopelessness (Brewin et al., 1998). Maria must try not to dwell on her colleague who died from breast cancer.

Brewin and colleagues studied 65 cancer patients who were either severely or mildly depressed, comparing them to a group of 65 non-depressed cancer patients. The participants had a mean time since diagnosis of 46.5 months. Thirty-two percent of mildly depressed patients and 43 percent of severely depressed patients reported intrusive memories. Only 11 percent of the non-depressed patients reported such memories. Also, the number of intrusive memories was greater for the depressed patients (Brewin et al., 1998).

The extent to which a person with cancer experiences depression and anxiety may be related to the person's coping style. For example, the person may cope by focusing on ways to reduce the emotional impact of the disease. This is called **emotion-focused coping**. Alternatively, the person might engage in **problem-focused coping**. In this case, the person might seek information about the disease, closely follow treatment recommendations, and actively address the stressors associated with cancer and its treatment. In emotion-focused coping, the tendency is to avoid thinking about possible stressors because to address them would be upsetting. Patients who had been diagnosed 10 weeks prior to taking part in a study of coping styles showed less depression and anxiety if they adopted a problem-focused approach. This was particularly true of participants who believed they could control the progression of their cancer (Osowiecki & Compas, 1998). However, coping style *did not* predict depression and anxiety 4 months later. Interestingly, the same study found that people using emotion-focused coping did not experience significantly less emotional distress, suggesting that the approach wasn't serving its purpose.

It has been estimated that 17 percent of children with cancer suffer from depression (Kashani & Hakimi, 1982). It is possible that this depression stems, in part, from the way children think about their cancer. For example, children who blame themselves for their cancer were rated by nurses as being more poorly adjusted than were children who attributed their cancer to external causes (Bearison, Sadow, Granowetter, & Winkel, 1993). Also, for girls with cancer depression is related to the extent to which they see their situation as being threatening (Burgess & Haaga, 1998).

Taken collectively, the research on depression and cancer suggests that the best mental approach for a patient is to believe that progression can be controlled, face the factors that are potentially stressful by treating them as problems to be solved, and avoid dwelling on memories or images associated with the disease and with death. This is easier said than done. For many patients, psychologists can help by providing interventions such as cognitive behaviour therapy (Bottomley et al., 1996).

Cancer Treatment

Cancer is most often treated through surgery, radiation therapy, chemotherapy, or hormone therapy, or some combination of these. Hormone therapy is used for cancers such as prostate and some breast cancers when tumour growth is stimulated by the presence of certain hormones. The therapy is designed to reduce the existence of these tumour-stimulating hormones. Maria will probably have surgery to remove her tumour and, possibly, part or all of her breast. She may also have radiation therapy before surgery to shrink the tumour and chemotherapy after surgery to treat any cancer that may have spread.

Some cancer patients fear the treatment more than the disease itself. For example, prostate cancer patients on hormone therapy usually experience persistent fatigue. Moreover, their sex drive is severely diminished and they may start developing female secondary sex characteristics such as breast enlargement. The other forms of treatment also come with common side effects that can make coping difficult.

We have already talked about recovery from surgery in Chapter 7 on hospital stays and medical procedures. In that chapter, we made the point that pain management was an important component of the recovery process. This is particularly true for cancer patients recovering from their surgery. Other psychological issues exist for cancer patients who undergo surgery. One is the anxiety associated with the outcome of the surgery. Were all the cancerous cells removed? Was there evidence that the cancer had metastasized? How much normal tissue had to be removed? Will this affect normal functioning when I recover from the surgery?

Another very important issue in cancer surgery is **disfigurement**. Cancer surgery that requires the removal of a considerable amount of normal tissue is called **radical**. Radical surgery has the potential to change not only a person's normal functioning but their look as well. Cancers of the head and neck may require surgery that changes facial shape. Throat cancer surgery may require the removal of the larynx that is responsible for making speech sounds. As a result of this surgery, patients would require the use of a prosthetic speech device that dramatically changes the sound of their voice. Colorectal cancer is one of the four most common cancers in Canada, afflicting 19 people per 100 000 in 1997 (Statistics Canada, 1999). If surgery is required to remove part of the colon, a patient may require a prosthetic replacement of the lower colon. This requires that the patient wear a colostomy bag to collect waste materials; the person may also lose control of the bowel.

One of the better-known surgical procedures for breast cancer patients is mastectomy, which Maria may well have to face. Patients can experience depression and disruptions in sexual activity as a result of radical mastectomy, in which part or all of a breast is removed. Not surprisingly, patients tend to cope better with much less radical lumpectomy surgery (Moyer, 1997). Surgery, then, comes with considerable psychological and physical costs. Opting against surgery, however, runs the real risk of having the tumour grow and spread. For young patients, decisions regarding surgery are usually easier to make than for elderly patients, who may end up suffering more from the surgery than they would from cancer that would not take as many years off their lives as it would off a younger person's.

Radiation therapy is used to shrink tumours. It can be used prior to or following surgery or may be used on its own. Radiation therapy is usually administered on an outpatient basis, though patients' experiences with radiation therapy will differ significantly depending on the site of their cancer. A person may have just a few treatments or as many as 30 or more over the course of several weeks, as is the case with many prostate cancer patients.

Patients with head and neck tumours may have to undergo preliminary dental work before their radiation treatments can begin. They must be fitted with a mask that will hold their heads in precisely the same position each time they come in for a treatment. Other patients with tumours in abdominal regions may be fitted with a body mold that they are placed in before treatments to ensure accuracy. They may also be "tattooed" with small cross-hair target marks to help the radiation technologists line up the beams that position the treatment. These radiation tattoos are reminders of their radiation experience and their cancer. Some patients will display them proudly; others will do their best to ignore them. Side effects from radiation therapy depend on the extent to which the radiation hits neighbouring cells and organs.

Surgery and radiation therapy are treatments intended to deal with specific sites as precisely as possible. In cases in which it is suspected that the cancer has metastasized, or to help prevent it from doing so, **chemotherapy** is used in addition to surgery and/or radiation therapy. It is called an **adjuvant therapy** when used in conjunction with other therapies in this way. Rather than attacking specific sites, the powerful drugs used in chemotherapy are distributed throughout the body, with the exception of the brain in some circumstances.

As is the case with radiation therapy, the side effects of chemotherapy are caused by unavoidable harm being done to healthy cells. They include fatigue, nausea, hair loss, erosion of oral and gastrointestinal mucosa that can result in pain and diarrhea, and increased susceptibility to infection (Stuber, 1995). The number of side effects and their intensity vary depending upon drug and dosage. Fatigue is reported in up to 70 percent of chemotherapy and radiation patients (Dimeo et al., 1999). In some cases, fatigue is severe enough that the dosages have to be limited. It has been found, however, that exercise in the form of pedalling a stationary bike while lying in bed can significantly reduce fatigue in high-dose chemotherapy treatment (Dimeo et al., 1999).

Interestingly, of all the side effects associated with chemotherapy, 35 of 60 breast cancer patients identified hair loss as being the most difficult to deal with (Tierney, Taylor, & Closs, 1992). There are a number of understandable psychological reasons for this, many of which relate to one's sense of identity. We look very different without our hair. It is a distinctive, defining characteristic for us. When Phil Zimbardo wanted to simulate a loss of identity for "prisoners" in his famous prison simulation study, he had them wear nylon stockings on their heads to simulate baldness (Haney, Banks, & Zimbardo, 1973). He did this because people look remarkably similar without their hair. Maria, then, would lose some of her former identity, albeit temporarily. At the same time, her hair loss signals a new identity—that of a cancer patient. People will differ in how comfortable they are with this new identity. Maria may find distinctive hats, scarves, and wigs to help her reestablish a sense of uniqueness and normality. One of our students who had gone through chemotherapy chose not to cut his hair for years after it grew back.

The nausea and vomiting many patients experience as a side effect of chemotherapy have received considerable study. Most chemotherapy treatments are administered in clinics on an outpatient basis or in physicians' offices. The patient then returns home to cope with the side effects. It is not uncommon for patients to begin feeling nauseated *before* they receive their treatment. This is called **anticipatory nausea**, and it is explained in terms of classical conditioning (Jacobson et al., 1995). The setting in which the treatment is administered, the medical staff involved, and the smells of the room all become potential conditioned stimuli that bring on nausea in anticipation of the treatment. In addition to making the nausea worse, it is possible that immune suppression may be another conditioned response that accompanies anticipatory nausea.

Nausea and vomiting add to the discouragement and depression cancer patients experience (Cull, 1990; Forester, Kornfeld, Fleiss, & Thompson, 1993; Kurtz, Kurtz, Given, & Given, 1995). In turn, depression may increase the risk of dying from the disease (Herrmann et al., 1998; Shekelle et al., 1981).

If Maria were to be given chemotherapy, she might also be given medication intended to reduce nausea and vomiting, called **antiemetic medication**. This can be administered before and after chemotherapy and radiation treatments. Studies have shown it to be effective for some patients (e.g., Abbott et al., 1999; Barbounis et al., 1999; Sohara et al., 1999). Whether antiemetic medication is used may depend on the nature of the cancer and whether or not it could interfere with the effectiveness of the treatment (Muustedt et al., 1999).

Helping People Cope with Cancer

Social Support

It is clear that cancer provides many challenges to a person's capacity to cope. It is important to realize also that for virtually every cancer patient there is a family and a collection of close friends who are also affected by the disease. With this in mind, comprehensive cancer care adopts a **family orientation**. In essence, the family becomes the patient. The lives of spouses and children can be changed dramatically when a family member is diagnosed with cancer. At the same time, family and friends will be called upon to provide much needed support for that person. The strain on the family can be overwhelming (Baider, Cooper, & Kaplan De Nour, 1996). The family's ability to cope with cancer will be directly related to the extent to which they have learned in the past to be flexible in stressful situations (Goodheart & Lansing, 1997). A family that has never communicated well in stressful situations will have to learn to do so if a family member gets cancer.

Modern medicine has sophisticated treatments for malignancies. It can even provide medication for depression and anxiety. However, when it comes to coping with cancer on a longterm basis, Maria will likely find that there is no substitute for a strong **social support** network (e.g., Hoskins et al., 1996).

We discussed social support in Chapter 4 on health promotion. We return to it here because of its importance as a mechanism for helping cancer patients and their families cope with serious illness. We know that social support is beneficial, but just how does it work? Those attempting to answer this question have taken a close look at the *social* nature of social support. What is it about some interactions that are so helpful and supportive?

We all know that sometimes it is enough to just "be there" as a sounding board for the person's concerns or to alleviate loneliness, which can be a serious problem for cancer patients. Also, support can be provided by helping with practical problems, like providing a ride to an appointment, doing some cooking, or taking out the garbage. Some forms of support, especially some forms of emotional support, require that people *communicate* with one another. This has been called **help-intended communication** (Goodman & Dooley, 1976) and is defined as communication that attempts to alleviate emotional distress. The interesting thing about help-intended communication is that, despite its good intentions, it doesn't always work. In fact, sometimes it can be perceived by the person with cancer as being *un*helpful (Dunkel-Schetter, 1984).

To identify some of the differences between helpful and unhelpful communication, Pistrang, Barker, and Rutter (1997) analyzed conversations between recently diagnosed breast cancer patients and their husbands. They audiotaped conversations and then played them back for the participants to get their impressions of what had been helpful and what had been unhelpful. It was discovered that a husband's attempts to lighten the conversation could be seen as unhelpful because they may make his wife feel misunderstood. In other words, Maria might not want to make light of something or change the mood until she has assurance that her husband can empathize with what she is going through. Similarly, her husband's attempts to "look on the bright side" may be seen as unhelpful because they fail to acknowledge her fears and concerns.

While microanalyses such as these can provide valuable insights into the interactive aspects of social support, they can also be somewhat daunting for those trying to provide this support. When we become preoccupied with "saying the right thing", we may become paralyzed and thus entirely unhelpful. The general conclusion to draw from work like that of Pistrang and colleagues is that support providers should acknowledge the person's concerns and fears as being legitimate while trying to help the person find effective ways of dealing with them. We can do this without dwelling on the intricacies of every word we say.

The fact that Maria's husband might think he is being helpful while she thinks he is being unhelpful indicates that perceptions are very important when it comes to social support. In fact, it may well be that our beliefs about the *availability* of our support are as important as the actual support we receive (Komproe et al., 1997). The reassurance we get from knowing that support is out there if we need it has been shown to reduce depression and encourage cancer patients to actually seek support. This, in turn, reduces feelings of helplessness. This is reminiscent of what Vancouver residents say when asked how they can appreciate the city's mountains that are so often obscured by cloud. They say, "It's important just knowing that they are there." When it comes to our social support networks, just knowing that they are there is also very important.

Empathy is an important element of support. Family and friends can provide some, but to truly empathize, two people must have experienced the same situation. For cancer patients, this means interacting with other patients in more formally organized support groups or being paired with volunteers who have had similar cancer experiences. Research has shown that a well-timed visit from a volunteer can help breast cancer patients feel less isolated and more optimistic about the future (Dunn, Steginga, Occhipinti, & Wilson, 1999).

Community agencies and cancer centres coordinate such groups. In addition to providing empathy, they can be good sources of information as new patients meet with others who have learned through experience how to best cope with various aspects of the disease. Studies have shown that support groups are of considerable benefit for prostate cancer patients. They help men feel more informed about the illness and involved in the treatment (Gregoire, Kalogeropoulos & Corcos, 1997; Kaps, 1994), and they provide opportunities to talk with other patients about difficult issues (Gray, Fitch, Davis, & Phillips, 1997). In short, support groups provide good opportunities for problem-focused coping.

Having said this, it isn't necessarily true that support groups are good for all patients. Support groups often emphasize education, and so they suit people who cope best by being informed. You may remember from Chapter 7 on hospital stays and medical procedures that these people are called **monitors**. Remember also that some patients cope best by blocking out information. These people are called **blunters** (Miller, 1980). It is very possible that blunters would have to change their coping style to benefit from support groups.

Kate White, a student from our research group at Simon Fraser University, has introduced the possibility that social comparison processes may help explain why some people benefit from support groups while others do not. When we engage in **social comparison**, we look to the opinions and experiences of others to determine what is right and wrong, normal or abnormal. We use this information to help guide us in our decision making (Festinger, 1954). This process is akin to the subjective norm component of the theory of reasoned action (Fishbein & Ajzen, 1975), which we discussed in Chapter 1. When we engage in social comparison, we can compare *upward*, by looking at people who are better off than us, or we can compare *downward*, by looking at people who are worse off.

In support groups, upward comparisons are made with group members who are seen to be coping better than the person doing the comparing, and downward comparisons are made with those seen to be doing worse. Patients who view upward comparisons as evidence that they can get better or downward comparisons as reminders that they should be thankful because they could be worse off, would be more likely to attend a support group. On the other hand, people who find upward comparisons discouraging because they feel worse off by comparison and downward comparisons depressing because they see themselves eventually declining to that state, would not be likely to attend. For example, a person recently diagnosed with a brain tumour may attend a support group and meet people whose cancer has advanced to the point where they are terminally ill. The person could be thankful that her disease isn't that bad, or she could be frightened by the prospect that her disease will progress the same way. For Maria, then, a support group would be as beneficial as her thinking and coping styles would allow it to be.

Medication and Psychotherapy

For many cancer patients, the depression and fear they experience can be adequately managed with the help of social support, whether from family, friends, or a support group. Support networks may be readily available for the patient or may be created with the help of the hospital, community, or social worker. For some patients, however, more intensive intervention is needed. These people may need to work with a clinical psychologist, counselling psychologist, or psychiatrist.

Psychiatrists might prescribe antidepressant medication such as fluoxetine (Prozac), which has been shown to be effective in treating depression in women with cancer (Holland et al., 1998). It is possible that complications may arise from taking antidepressant medication in conjunction with other cancer-related treatments, and so drug interactions have to be taken into consideration when antidepressants are prescribed (Franco-Bronson, 1996). There has also been some debate concerning the possibility that some antidepressants may stimulate tumour growth, since this outcome was reported in a study using rodents. A recent study of humans, however, found no evidence of increased risk of recurrence or further tumour growth in patients taking antidepressants or antihistamines (Weiss, McFarland, Burkhart, & Ho, 1998).

Because of the concerns associated with the use of medication, and because psychotherapy has been shown to be quite effective as a means of helping cancer patients, psychotherapeutic interventions are not uncommon. One goal of psychotherapy might be to help patients adopt a problem-focused approach to their cancer (Greer & Moorey, 1997; Nezu et al., 1998). Goodheart and Lansing (1997) have outlined a series of steps to follow when developing a psychotherapeutic treatment strategy for working with people who are chronically ill. These steps apply very well to cancer patients and their families.

The first step is to *obtain sufficient medical information*. Some of this can be obtained from the patient. This may be difficult or burdensome for the patient, however, so the therapist must communicate well with medical staff. Second, the therapist must *assess the person's psychological status and response to the illness*. In so doing, the therapist must weigh the demands of the illness against the coping resources of the patient. Also, the therapist must develop a sense of the person's psychological state before the illness. Third, the therapist must *integrate a theoretical orientation*. To probe the person's feelings and unstated anxieties, the therapies might adopt a psychodynamic orientation. To address functional quality-of-life issues, a behavioural orientation might be adopted. The key is to *offer a range of interventions* and then to *match the intervention with the patient's most pressing needs*.

Clinical psychologists, psychiatrists, and counsellors often work with people in groups. These therapeutic groups differ from support groups in that they are guided by a professional trained in psychotherapy, with the emphasis shifting somewhat from the provision of information to ways in which depression and anxiety can be alleviated. Therapy of this nature has been shown to reduce the physical and emotional distress associated with radiation therapy (Forester et al., 1993). Indeed, research reviews on the outcomes of group psychotherapy for cancer patients have identified considerable evidence that such therapy is effective (Fawzy & Fawzy, 1998; Rieger, Touyz, & Wain, 1998).

In earlier chapters, we mentioned the research of David Spiegel and colleagues (1989), in which women with metastasized breast cancer who were randomly assigned to a support group lived almost twice as long as those in the control condition. What is the content of these sessions that appear to be so effective? Spiegel and colleagues identify a number of aspects. First, the members are encouraged to express emotions and confront their concerns about death. Second, a sense of group cohesion is built, increasing the sense of social support. Third, participants are taught to improve their communication skills, given that talking about one's cancer can be quite difficult. Fourth, they are given relaxation training.

There is considerable research indicating that groups of this type (and even unstructured groups for a varied population of cancer patients) are quite effective in helping people cope with their cancer and improve their emotional outlook (for a review, see Lescz & Goodwin, 1998).

Consistent with the notion of family oriented care, psychotherapy is also often provided for families of the person with cancer. It has been estimated that 29 percent of family caregivers experience psychological distress severe enough to warrant clinical intervention (Rodrigue & Hoffmann, 1994). The roles of family members change when one of them is diagnosed with cancer. Household responsibilities must be shared as one or more members become a principle caregiver. There can also be financial difficulties if the person with cancer must take an extended leave from work. Family members may need help managing the psychological burdens associated with taking on various caregiving roles and, in some cases, being a "midwife to death" (Brown & Stetz, 1999). In these cases, grief counselling may also focus on the entire family. Whatever the outcome for Maria, it may be that her family would benefit from psychotherapeutic interventions.

Psychological interventions are also used to help patients cope with cancer-related pain. For example, hypnotherapy has shown promising results (Sachs, 1992), as has visual imagery and relaxation training with children (Kuttner, 1997). For example, Dr. Leora Kuttner works with children undergoing painful procedures at the British Columbia Children's Hospital. She has children focus their attention on bubble blowing as a form of distraction. She has also used hypnosis as well as relaxation through biofeedback. Using the latter technique, Dr. Kuttner helps children relax by giving them cues as to how relaxed they are.

Given the prevalence of cancer and the myriad of coping challenges associated with the disease, it is clear that health psychologists can make significant contributions to the quality of life of cancer patients like Maria and to the coping abilities of the patients' families.

DIABETES

Diabetes is the seventh leading cause of death in Canada. Unlike some other illnesses, such as heart diseases, the incidence of diabetes is steadily increasing. In Canada in 1996, 17 people per 100 000 died from diabetes. However, it is often the case that people with diabetes die from complications such as heart disease rather than from diabetes itself, so this death rate understates the severity of the disease. In fact, it has been estimated that deaths from diabetes-related complications are five times more common than deaths from diabetes itself (Laboratory Centre for Disease Control, 1998). Diabetes is more common in men than it is in women. Twenty men per 100 000 died from diabetes in Canada in 1996, compared to 14 women per 100 000 (Laboratory Centre for Disease Control, 1998).

Diabetes occurs when the pancreas produces too little insulin, which is needed to help the body use sugar for energy. People with Type I diabetes produce very little or no insulin. As a result, they are called **insulin dependent**. According to Health Canada, about 10 percent of all diabetics are Type I. People with **Type II diabetes** do produce insulin, but they either don't produce enough or they can't use their insulin effectively. About 90 percent of all diabetics are Type II. There is a third type, called **gestational diabetes**, which is a temporary condition affecting two to four percent of all pregnant women.

Type I diabetes is more prevalent among people of aboriginal, African, and Latin-American decent, and among people who have a history of diabetes in their family (Health Canada web site). Type II diabetes is more common among people over the age of 45 years, especially if they are obese. In fact, nearly 50 percent of Type II patients are over the age of 60 years (Morley, 1998). For people with Type I diabetes, symptoms usually come on quite quickly and are severe. They include such things as frequent urination, unusual thirst, extreme hunger, unusual weight loss, and extreme fatigue. People with Type II diabetes might also experience frequent infections, and cuts and bruises take a long time to heal.

People with Type I diabetes must monitor their blood sugar levels very carefully and take insulin, usually by self-administered injection, on a daily basis. While the vast majority of Type I patients monitor their blood glucose levels, a large study in Germany found that only 41 percent do so as often as they should (Haupt et al., 1996). People with Type II diabetes do not have to take insulin; however, they must also monitor their blood sugar and maintain a well-controlled diet. It is not uncommon for people diagnosed with Type II diabetes to become depressed and discouraged. These psychological states can have a serious effect on their willingness to follow the regimens necessary to control their disease.

Diabetes and Psychological Distress

As is the case with most chronic illnesses, fear and depression are two of the most common psychological problems for people with diabetes. Let's take a close look at each.

Fear and Diabetes

Diabetic patients' fears tend to focus on the possible longterm consequences of the disease. These include amputation, cardiovascular disease, kidney failure (nephropathy), neurological problems, going blind (retinopathy), and stroke (Hendricks & Hendricks, 1998). These fears cause problems because they tend to get in the way of disease management for the patient (Straus, 1996). Consistent with the health belief model, diabetic patients who become fearful may doubt the efficacy of the management program in the face of these potentially terrible consequences.

Another common fear for diabetics, especially Type I, concerns the times when their blood sugar levels get out of balance. This condition, called **hypoglycemia**, brings on aversive physical symptoms such as fatigue. It can also be accompanied by disorientation, confusion, and negative mood. In extreme cases, hypoglycemia can lead to seizure or loss of consciousness. The disorientation and negative mood state can have upsetting consequences socially. For example, it is very possible that one's spouse, partner, or friend will notice that a person is becoming hypoglycemic before the person notices it themselves. When the other person points this out, the suggestion might be met with anger and confusion (Ritholz & Jacobson, 1998). After the person gets his or her blood sugar stabilized, there is the guilt and discouragement of realizing that he or she can't always take quick action to remedy his or her condition, and that someone else who was only trying to help had to bear the brunt of the person's angry outburst.

BOX 11-1 Diabetes Among the Haida

Type II diabetes is becoming more prevalent in aboriginal communities than in the non-aboriginal population. For this reason, Grams and colleagues (1996) held focus-group sessions with the Haida Gwaii in the Queen Charlotte Islands, where 17 percent of the adults in one village suffered from diabetes. Through these discussions, it was discovered that the Haida found diabetes to be a very upsetting condition. They feared death and suffered grief from the loss of the things they loved to do and the things they loved to eat. They had a strong desire to regain personal control. The researchers concluded that attempts to help the Haida manage diabetes must not be dictatorial or prescriptive in nature. Rather, they must respect the way the Haida's feelings about the disease are manifest and work to give them a sense of control over their symptoms and the valued aspects of their lives that suffer because of diabetes.

Type I diabetes often occurs in childhood. When it does, parents become very involved in disease management. Because of this, the parents' fears are just as relevant as those of the child. These include longterm complications, early death, and severe insulin reactions (Drozda et al., 1997). For example, parents of children who have had a diabetes-related seizure or loss of consciousness are significantly more afraid of hypoglycemia than parents of diabetic children who have not suffered in this way (Marrero, Guare, Vandagriff, & Finebert, 1997). Parents must also find ways to help their children cope with daily routines that are usually much more structured than those of other children. These structures, and the symptoms of diabetes, can make diabetic children feel different from their healthy peers (Drozda et al., 1997).

Depression and Diabetes

Depression and discouragement are problematic, though understandable, psychological consequences of diabetes. It has been estimated that depression is found in 15 to 20 percent of Types I and II patients (Lustman, Freedland, Griffith, & Clouse, 1998). Diabetics often have trouble talking to others about hypoglycemia and the emotions associated with it. As a result, they may feel isolated or unsupported. Moreover, as we have already mentioned, they may have a difficult time accepting help when it comes during a hypoglycemic episode. It is not surprising, then, that depression is significantly related to a diabetic's quality of life (Kohen, Burgess, Catalán, & Lant, 1998).

To complicate matters, depression and blood sugar are linked bidirectionally. Low blood sugar worsens depression and, in turn, depression reduces the likelihood that people with diabetes will monitor their blood glucose levels regularly. Not surprisingly, depression is also worse for people who suffer diabetes-related complications such as cardiovascular problems. Conversely, depression increases the risk for such complications (Lustman et al., 1998; Lloyd, Mathews, Wing, & Orchard, 1992). For these reasons, it is very important to treat depression to break the cycle of depression and worsening symptomology.

Helping People Cope with Diabetes

There are at least two major goals of programs designed to help diabetics. The first is to ensure compliance with the disease-management regimen. The second is to treat psychological distress. As you can probably tell, these two goals are closely related. We have already seen that psychological distress decreases compliance with the disease-management regimen. Also, poor management results in worse symptoms and complications, which in turn bring on more distress.

One way to break this cycle is cognitive behaviour therapy (CBT). It is important to explore this option, since antidepressant medication can have unwanted side effects for diabetics. Fortunately, research indicates that CBT can be just as effective as medication (Jacobson & Weinger, 1998). Lustman and colleagues randomly assigned diabetic patients to either a CBT group or a control condition. They discovered that 85 percent of the CBT group showed relief from depression compared to only 27 percent of the control patients. It was also encouraging to note that at follow-up, 70 percent were still not depressed, compared to 34 percent of the controls.

Educational and support groups are also provided for people with diabetes. These are usually offered as part of a hospital education program that patients attend on a regular basis to learn more about the disease and its management. They will also have their blood glucose and other indicators measured. At these sessions, patients can learn more than nutrition and exercise facts. They also meet other patients, many of whom are coping well with their diabetes. This provides them with important information regarding efficacy—that diabetes can be controlled. They also get "inside information" on disease control and emotional coping that can only come from other patients.

Family and friends of people with diabetics can help by being aware of the emotional side of the disease. The fears regarding longterm consequences are real, not trivial. And when the person is experiencing hypoglycemia, it is important to note that mood changes and disorientation might make the person appear unreceptive to help. This does not mean that help shouldn't be offered.

DISEASES OF THE CARDIOVASCULAR SYSTEM

Diseases of the heart and cardiovascular system are quite common. In 1997, 526 people per 100 000 in Canada died from cardiovascular diseases, heart diseases, heart attack, or cerebrovascular diseases (most commonly, stroke) (Statistics Canada, 1999). This translates to just under 175 000 people in 1 year alone. At that, deaths due to heart disease have declined considerably. Between 1980 and 1994, there was a 34 percent decrease in deaths due to diseases of the heart. Men are still more likely than women to die from heart disease. Over each of the past 20 years, men have accounted for approximately 65 percent of heart disease deaths (Statistics Canada, 1999).

When health psychologists work with and study people with heart and cardiovascular disease, they typically focus on three types of conditions. There are people who have suffered a heart attack, or **mycardial infarction (MI)**, as it is known medically. Of particular interest are people who have had their *first* MI. The medical and psychological challenge for these people is to reduce the likelihood that they will have a second MI, which far fewer people survive. A second group consists of people who have had a **coronary artery bypass graft (CABG)**. This is commonly called bypass surgery, a procedure in which healthy arteries from other parts of the body, often the legs, are grafted into the coronary artery system to, as the term implies, bypass blocked arteries. The third group consists of people who have had **angioplasty**. In this procedure, a bubble-like device is inserted into the artery at the point of the blockage, thus expanding the artery and allowing for better blood flow. In a similar procedure, a cylindrical metal stent is inserted to support the walls of the vessel. There are other, less tested methods now in use to clear arteries, including the use of laser technology. Bypass surgery and angioplasty are used to treat a condition called **myocardial ischemia**, in which there is a lack of blood flow to the heart muscle.

Psychological Distress in Cardiovascular Disease

Patients with heart and/or cardiovascular disease often suffer accompanying psychological distress. Not only does this affect their quality of life, it puts them at greater risk for further morbidity (more disease or complications) and mortality. Lorne's reaction to being hospitalized in CCU, which we describe in Case Study 11.2, is a common one. When reality sets

CASE 11-2 Short-Term Reactions to First Myocardial Infarction

One day when Lorne was mowing his lawn, he felt a strong pain in his chest that radiated to his shoulder and down his left arm. He began to sweat profusely, feel nauseated and, had he not knelt down on the grass, would surely have fainted. It was in this position that his wife found him as she came out to do some gardening. She quickly got him to the car and to the hospital, where he was diagnosed as having had a heart attack.

When Lorne was settled in the cardiac care unit (CCU) of the hospital, he began to feel better. It struck him as ridiculous that he had actually had a heart attack and he told the nurses so. Surely they had made a mistake. He told them that he should not be made to stay in the hospital, especially hooked up to a heart monitor. He was a busy man. He had a big meeting the next day and there were things he had to prepare. In fact, Lorne became a bit obnoxious as he lay in the hospital bed. The nursing staff did their best to calm him and tell him that he really needed to be right where he was.

in and he comes to accept that he really has had a heart attack, Lorne's protests will subside (Krantz & Deckel, 1983). The question is: what will follow?

One common form of psychological distress accompanying cardiovascular disease is anxiety. Trait anxiety results in poorer quality of life for cardiac patients (Engebretson et al., 1999). A heart attack can be a frightening experience, so it is not surprising to find that some patients live in fear of having another one. As a result, these patients become cripples of their cardiac history. This means that they curtail their activity levels far more than their disease status requires. This has been called **cardiac invalidism** (Krantz & Deckel, 1983). This creates two major problems for the patient. First, the patient stops doing some of the things that defined his or her quality of life, such as tennis, golf, or sexual activity. Second, the patient lapses into a sedentary lifestyle that is not conducive to good cardiovascular health.

Anxiety is particularly strong for people who experience **cardiac arrest**, in which their heart actually stops beating and they must be resuscitated. In the first few weeks after cardiac arrest, phobic anxiety and panic symptoms are not uncommon (Dlin, 1980). One of the problems with these reactions is that panic symptoms often mimic heart problems or heart attack. This, in turn, fuels the sense of panic, and a vicious cycle is started that compromises the person's cardiac health. Fortunately, this anxiety stabilizes for most patients in time, though many experience intrusive thoughts about the event and try to avoid anything that might remind them of their resuscitation (Ladwig et al., 1999).

Perhaps the most common form of psychological distress associated with cardiovascular and heart disease is depression. Major depression is diagnosed in just under 20 percent of people who recently suffered a myocardial infarction (Frasure-Smith, Lesperance, & Talajic, 1993), and minor depression is found in over 25 percent of these patients (Schleifer et al., 1989). In fact, the incidence of major depression is three times greater for coronary artery disease patients than it is for the general population (Rozanski, Blumenthal, & Kaplan, 1999). There is also evidence to suggest that this depression could be more problematic for women, especially those who are older. It has been estimated that women are twice as likely to suffer post-MI depression than are men (Frasure-Smith et al., 1993). One study found that 23 percent of female cardiac patients, including those with problems other than heart attack, were depressed. Yet, women generally are not as emphatically encouraged to attend rehabilitation programs that would help with this depression as men are (Lavie, Milani, Cassidy, & Gilliland, 1999).

In addition to reducing quality of life, depression can have significant effects on the patient's cardiovascular health. Depressed patients are more than four times as likely to die of cardiac-related problems within 6 months of diagnosis (Frasure-Smith et al., 1993) and more than six times as likely to die within 18 months (Frasure-Smith, Lesperance, & Talajic, 1995). In fact, depression is a risk factor for first MI. It has been estimated that depressed people are four-and-a-half times more likely to suffer a heart attack than are non-depressed people (Pratt et al., 1996). Depression also yields increased reports of **angina**, or chest pain (Ladwig, Röll, Breithardt, & Borggrefe, 1999), although the nature of cause and effect in this regard has been questioned (Sheps, Sheffield, & Carney, 1999). In other words, does depression cause chest pain, or does it cause greater reporting of that pain?

Depression is particularly problematic for older cardiac patients. Patients over the age of 65 who are depressed are more than twice as likely to report difficulties with activities of daily living (ADL) (Steffens et al., 1999). Also, the consequences of depression appear to be somewhat more severe for women. In a study that monitored women for 1 year after their heart attack, 8.3 percent of depressed women died of cardiac causes compared to 2.4 percent of non-depressed women (Frasure-Smith et al., 1999).

The physiological mechanisms by which depression increases risk of mortality for cardiac patients are not entirely clear. However, it is known that depressed coronary heart disease patients have higher heart rates than do non-depressed patients (Carney et al., 1999) and that depressed patients do not adjust their heart rate in response to blood pressure changes well (Watkins & Grossman, 1999). Given the finding that people with depression are at greater risk for heart attack, it appears that there is a bidirectional relationship between depression and cardiovascular disease. It becomes imperative, therefore, to treat the depression and break this dangerous cycle.

Helping People Cope with Cardiovascular Disease

In addition to the support of family and friends, cardiac patients can benefit from rehabilitation programs and, where appropriate, psychotherapy. Modern rehabilitation programs for people recovering from heart attack, bypass surgery, or angioplasty are **holistic** in nature. That is to say, they address all aspects of the participant's life, from diet to exercise to psychological well-being. Rehabilitation programs for people who have had one myocardial infarction have been shown to reduce mortality by 20 to 25 percent and improve psychological status in terms of reduced negative affect and state anxiety (Engebretson et al., 1999) (Case 12.2 presents an autobiographical account of a person who has benefited considerably from his rehabilitation program).

Rehabilitation programs may differ somewhat from location to location, but most share certain elements in common. Participants have their physical condition monitored. They are provided with education regarding their medication and the reduction of risk factors. They are also put on programs intended to reduce those risk factors, focusing on diet, exercise, and stress reduction. One such program, which featured three 75-minute sessions a week over 12 weeks, reduced levels of anxiety, depression, and confusion while increasing the participants' sense of vigour. This was particularly true for participants with high trait anxiety, which is a risk factor for further morbidity and poor quality of life (Engebretson et al., 1999). Another program tailored specifically for women yielded lower depression, anxiety and hostility and increased exercise capacity and quality of life for the participants (Lavie, Milani, Cassidy, & Gilliland, 1999).

Another important psychological factor to address in therapy with cardiac patients is anger. Anger is a risk factor for coronary heart disease (CHD), especially when expressed as hostility. Moreover, one episode of intensely expressed anger can trigger a fatal heart attack for people with severe CHD. Therapy intended to reduce anger features a number of components. Participants are taught to monitor their emotions so they can identify times when anger is a problem (Mayne & Ambrose, 1999). They are also taught relaxation skills. In terms of their thinking, participants go through what is called **cognitive reappraisal and restructuring.** In this, they learn to think differently about the things that tend to make them angry. For example, they may have been blaming other drivers for traffic jams or may mistakenly assume that people who frustrate them do so intentionally. Also, there is time spent on behavioural change, in which they learn to control their voice tone, breathing, etc.

With all these proven benefits, you might think that cardiac rehabilitation programs are well attended, but they are not. In the United States, only 15 to 30 percent of MI, CABG, and angioplasty patients complete a rehabilitation program, and dropout rates are quite high (King & Teo, 1998). Researchers at the University of Alberta have suggested that psychological factors affect these attendance rates. Such factors as self-efficacy, motivation, and social support may all be predictive of program completion (King & Teo, 1998). Again, this suggestion is consistent with the health belief model and theory of reasoned action discussed in Chapter 1. These theories predict that attendance would be higher for people who thought the program would work and who had other people in their lives who had either attended successfully or encouraged them to do so.

For some patients, rehabilitation programs are not enough to help them overcome depression. The problem is made more complex by the fact that some antidepressant medication has adverse side effects that compromise cardiovascular functioning (Evans et al., 1999). Newer antidepressant agents, such as fluoxetine (Prozac), may be more promising, although they are not yet well tested. While results with this type of antidepressant (called selective seratonin reuptake inhibitors, or SSRI) are encouraging, there may still be problems created by interactions with other medication patients take for their heart condition (Evans et al., 1999).

Because of the uncertainty of outcomes associated with medication, psychotherapy is often the intervention of choice for cardiac patients with depression. Evidence shows that this therapy, which may be provided in groups or individually, is quite effective when presented in conjunction with a rehabilitation program (Mendes-de-Leon, Powell, & Kaplan, 1991). In addition to targeting depression, these interventions address other psychological responses, such as hostility, which are known to put people at risk for cardiovascular disease. A general rule of thumb, then, is that rehabilitation programs do an effective job of addressing medical risk factors, while psychotherapy helps address psychological ones (Evans et al., 1999).

HIV AND AIDS

Acquired immune deficiency syndrome (AIDS) was first reported in Canada in 1979. By 1995, there were an estimated 18 014 cases in the country (Health Canada, 1996). In the late 1990s, the death toll from AIDS dropped significantly in Canada. In 1995, there were 1 764 AIDS-attributed deaths. In 1997, that number had dropped to 525 (Health Canada, 1997). While the death toll from AIDS is dropping, the number of people with HIV infection continues to rise. Health Canada (1997) estimates that by 1997, there were 54 000 people in Canada who were HIV positive. These statistics are drawn from the country as a whole. As we will see when we take a closer look at AIDS later in the chapter, there are some groups that are at greater risk than others for contracting AIDS; most notably, our aboriginal population (Health Canada, 1997) (see Box 11.2.)

BOX 11-2 AIDS and Canada's Aboriginal Population

Statistics describing the incidence of HIV infection and AIDS among Canada's aboriginal peoples indicate some differences that have raised the concern of Health Canada's Medical Services Branch and members of the aboriginal community. In the fall of 1997, there were 249 reported cases of AIDS among aboriginal people in Canada (Laboratory Centre for Disease Control, 1997). Given that ethnic origin is listed in just over half of the cases reported to the Laboratory Centre for Disease Control, it is likely that this number of reported aboriginal cases is an underestimate. It is known that AIDS is more prevalent in the under-30 age group for aboriginal than for non-aboriginal people (30 percent versus 19 percent), and that the proportion of adult females with AIDS is also greater in the aboriginal population (15 percent versus 7 percent) (Laboratory Centre for Disease Control, 1997). The spread of HIV/AIDS is worsened when a population is more mobile. For the aboriginal population, this takes the form of greater mobility between inner city and rural/reserve settings. From the late 1980s to 1998, programs designed to improve prevention and education regarding AIDS among Canada's aboriginal population were not very effective. A more recent program features an increase in the involvement of aboriginal peoples to improve its relevancy, which, it is hoped, will help reduce the incidence of HIV and AIDS in this segment of our population (Laboratory Centre for Disease Control, 1997).

The symptoms of HIV (which stands for human immunodeficiency virus) include: persistent fever; swelling of the lymph glands on the neck and under the arms; frequent fatigue; diarrhea; sweating during sleep; and yeast infections in the vagina, ears, and tongue (AIDS Foundation of Canada web site, www.aidsfoundation.ca). Since these symptoms aren't unique to HIV, a person with concerns should see his or her physician.

Human immunodeficiency virus gradually breaks down the body's immune system, making it susceptible to a host of other infections, including neoplasms such as non-Hodgkins' lymphoma and Kaposi's sarcoma. Prolonged HIV infection results in AIDS (**acquired immune deficiency syndrome**). Human immunodeficiency virus can be transmitted through unprotected vaginal or anal sex, the sharing of needles, or during pregnancy or childbirth, when a mother might transmit HIV to her child (AIDS Foundation of Canada web site). To learn more about HIV and AIDS, consult the AIDS Foundation of Canada web site.

Psychological Distress and HIV/AIDS

HIV and AIDS are different from most other chronic and serious illnesses in a number of ways. First, though advances in medication have made encouraging strides in prolonging the lives of persons living with AIDS, there is still no cure for the disease, and the person living with it knows it will eventually be fatal. In addition to a set of symptoms that can be very difficult to endure, there is the fact that people living with AIDS often suffer from social isolation and stigmatization. Unlike many other serious illnesses, AIDS has the problem of contagion and the related problem of myths about contagion. Compared to other serious illnesses, AIDS patients tend to be younger, on average. Also, rightly or wrongly, AIDS patients may feel personal responsibility or guilt regarding their illness, because sexual behaviour or drug use may have been involved. Finally, many people with AIDS have lost people from their social network to the very disease they are trying to cope with. For all these reasons, people with HIV and AIDS must deal with a host of psychological challenges (Kelly, 1998).

For example, anxiety is a virtually universal problem for persons living with AIDS (PLWA) (Phillips & Morrow, 1998). This anxiety stems from uncertainty about the future, the losses that are experienced, the social stigma, the prejudice that a PLWA's offspring endure, and the disease process itself (Phillips & Morrow, 1998). An HIV-positive diagnosis can be traumatic enough to elicit symptoms of post-traumatic stress disorder (PTSD). One study discovered that 30 percent of HIV-positive gay and bisexual men showed symptoms of PTSD, and one-third of those showing such symptoms had onset that came six months or more after their HIV-positive diagnosis (Kelly et al., 1998). PTSD symptoms were more prevalent for men who had a history of PTSD prior to their HIV diagnosis. Also, PTSD was related to major depression.

The nature and development of depression among persons with HIV and AIDS appears open for debate. Some researchers have reported a dramatic increase in depression as AIDS develops (Lyketsos et al., 1996). Others have reported that depression is experienced by 22 to 61 percent of people who are HIV-positive (Rosenberger et al., 1993). Some research indicates that HIV status alone does not lead to psychological distress unless other factors are present. These factors include age, employment status, social support, coping style, and a person's sense of mastery (Dickey, Dew, Becker, & Kingsley, 1999).

On the other hand, there are those who have questioned whether depression actually increases after diagnosis, or if it is more commonly a preexisting condition that is made more salient by the diagnosis. It is known that depression is more prevalent among gay men regardless of their HIV status (Perkins et al., 1994). Also yet to be resolved is the extent to which depression affects disease progression (Evans et al., 1999).

A study in Italy discovered that people who were HIV-positive and depressed had a higher prevalence of bipolar disorder than depressed HIV-negative people did (Perretta et al., 1998). This is to say that their depression was combined with manic episodes. In fact, 78 percent of HIV-positive depressed people reported having had a bipolar episode. The interesting observation here is that bipolar symptoms tended to appear before the person was HIV-positive, leading to the conclusion that bipolar symptoms are actually a *risk-factor* for HIV.

Helping People Cope with HIV and AIDS

Providing psychotherapeutic interventions for people with HIV and AIDS can be challenging, not only for the reasons that make the illnesses themselves difficult to cope with, but because psychotropic medication may actually make other symptoms worse. For example, selective **serotonin reuptake inhibitors** (SSRIs) can increase sleep disturbances, weight loss, sexual dysfunction, and fatigue. Other medication may have fewer of these effects but still cause headache or dizziness and interact poorly with other medication the person may need to take (Elliott et al., 1999). It has also been suggested that the beneficial effects of medication may be only short-term (Evans et al., 1999).

When providing psychotherapy for people who are HIV-positive or who have AIDS, a number of clinical issues must be considered (Kelly, 1998). Unlike other diseases, it can be difficult for HIV/AIDS patients to disclose their disease status to others. Telling someone you have a blocked artery just isn't the same as telling that person you are HIV-positive. To compound things, persons living with AIDS have higher rates of bereavement and may have been caregivers themselves, especially if they are gay men or intravenous drug users (IDU). For these reasons, persons living with AIDS must often reestablish their social support systems. Regarding their behaviour, they must make and maintain major changes in terms of risk-related behaviour and adhere to medical regimens that can be complex and extensive.

Psychotherapy issues for persons living with AIDS have changed somewhat over the past few years due to advances in medicine that prolong life expectancies. **Antiretroviral medications** such as AZT and **protease inhibitor** drug combinations are significantly prolonging the lives of persons living with AIDS. The psychotherapeutic issues are changing accordingly. Not surprisingly, psychological status is often related to disease-related milestones such as the first notification of seropositive status, first symptoms, and first sign of AIDS-defining illness (Kelly, 1998). Therapy for people dealing with these and other factors is often conducted in groups. The therapist must take into account the makeup of the group, given that AIDS affects many different types of people. For example, a group consisting exclusively of gay men is quite different from one in which there are gay men, intravenous drug users, and heterosexual women.

Groups may adopt a cognitive focus when they help participants stop being plagued by intrusive thoughts, or when they address irrational beliefs that lead to depression and anxiety. Groups with this focus have been proven effective (Emmott, 1991). In addition, the groups can take on a behavioural focus, looking at ways to cope with problems at home and at work, strategies for regaining social support, and ways to relax and manage stress. In general, it has been found that psychological interventions for persons living with AIDS are effective in improving psychological status but do not affect medical status (Lamping et al., 1993).

It is also important to note that those providing care to people living with AIDS are in need of considerable support. When the person living with AIDS is from the gay community, it is not uncommon for their caregivers to be from that same community. They may well have seen many of their friends and loved ones die. They may fear HIV infection themselves or know that they are, in fact, seropositive.

Finally, we must hearken back to Chapter 4 on health promotion to remind ourselves that *prevention* is a very large issue when it comes to HIV and AIDS. All the psychological principles discussed in Chapter 4 apply well here. We cannot rely too heavily on fear appeals. Rather we must convince people of the efficacy of safe sex and careful needle use while at the same time making salient the potential threat of AIDS.

OTHER CHRONIC CONDITIONS

Cancer, cardiovascular disease, diabetes, and AIDS are four of the most commonly discussed chronic conditions in health psychology. There are, of course, quite a few other chronic conditions that are equally as pressing for patients experiencing them. Included in this list would be Parkinson's disease and arthritis. More generally, there are many people who live with physical and mental disabilities. Each of these conditions carries its own set of coping challenges.

For example, major depression occurs in 40 to 50 percent of all people with Parkinson's disease (Gotham, Brown, & Marsden, 1986, cited in Evans, 1999). This causes further problems in terms of memory, language, and motor performance. Not surprisingly, depression can also be a problem for people coping with the chronic pain of arthritis, a disease that affects about one percent of the population and between five and seven percent of those over the age of 65 years (Walsh, Blanchard, Kremer, & Blanchard, 1999). One study found that 36 percent of patients with arthritis (average age = 57 years) had scores indicative of clinical depression, which is above the norm for the general population (Walsh et al., 1999). As is the case with depression and most chronic conditions, the depression and symptoms tend to worsen together. Also, depression is related to feelings of isolation and self-blame and is worse for people who feel a lack of control over their illness (Murphy, Dickens, Creed, & Bernstein, 1999).

In a more general sense, there are many people who cope with permanent physical disabilities that may impair their movement or sensory capacities. One of the main obstacles for people with disabilities is presented by the attitudes of people without disabilities. These attitudes, which may range from pity to understanding to impatience, are often formed in childhood. They are often based on stereotypes rather than first-hand experience (Bracegirdle, 1995; Harper, 1999), and they affect the extent to which non-disabled children interact with their peers who do have disabilities (Roberts & Smith, 1999). Interestingly, elementary school children in the third to sixth grade rated their own willingness to participate in activities with children in wheelchairs higher than their perceptions of other classmates' willingness to do so (Morgan, Bieberich, Walker, & Schwerdtfeger, 1998).

The quality of life of people living with disabilities depends on their occupation or their belief that they are engaged in meaningful activities. Another important factor is their sense of social integration, which is, of course, related to the extent to which they are accepted by others (Viemeroe & Krause, 1998). When trying to understand the psychological factors associated with coping with a disability, it is important to consider when the person became disabled. People who have recently become disabled may still be struggling with changes in their sense of self and a reevaluation of their values (Iwai, 1996; Mpofu & Houston, 1998).

Psychotherapy for people with physical disabilities has yielded encouraging results, although many psychotherapists do not see clients from this population nor do they specialize in the unique needs of people with physical disabilities (Hurley, Tomasulo, & Pfadt, 1998). These unique needs include such things as an accurate assessment of the person's physical capabilities and an understanding of the person's beliefs regarding his or her disability. Also, as is the case with many chronic conditions, there are the caregivers to consider, who may be very burdened by their responsibilities (Dumont, St. Onge, Fougeyrollas, & Renaud, 1998).

QUALITY OF LIFE

In this chapter on chronic and serious illness, we have made repeated reference to a patient's "quality of life." This is a term that has become prominent in recent years in health psychology and medicine. Just what does it mean? When we refer to **quality of life** in the context of serious and chronic illness, we are talking about the extent to which symptoms and treatment affect a person's physical, social, cognitive, and emotional functioning. Further, we are interested in how the person *prioritizes* and *values* these functions. In this way, we can develop a more complete understanding of the impact the condition and treatment are having on the person's life.

It may seem obvious that quality of life would be a primary concern in the treatment of people with serious and/or chronic illness. However, this has not always been the case. This is because some treatments that actually might alleviate some of the medical causes of the disease can have very negative effects on other aspects of a patient's life. If the treatment plan is focused solely on biological factors, such as tumour size, it is easy to lose sight of the price the patient is paying for that treatment in a more holistic sense. This is especially true for cancer patients, who can often be subjected to treatments producing side effects that are worse than the symptoms of the disease.

Two issues become important when quality of life is made a priority as a treatment outcome. First, those providing treatment must be sensitive to the *tradeoff* between duration of life and quality of life. Second, the patient must be an integral member of the decision-making team, because quality of life is primarily a *subjective* phenomenon (Osoba, 1990). Let's look more closely at each of these issues.

The Tradeoff between Duration and Quality of Life

Regarding serious illness, treatment efficacy is often defined by the extent to which the treatment prolongs the life of the patient. For example, a person with throat cancer may have surgery that will prolong his or her life by 5 years. Without the surgery, he or she will probably live 1 year. Thus, the treatment is deemed reasonably effective because it has the potential to prolong the person's life by 5 years. Of course, after the surgery, which will very possibly involve the removal of the person's larynx, he or she will have to use a pros-

FOCUS ON RESEARCH 11-1 Using the Time Tradeoff Technique to Calculate Treatment Utility

At Northwestern University in Chicago, Elizabeth Calhoun (Calhoun, 1998) uses something called the **time tradeoff technique**, or TTO, to assess patients' views of various treatment options. When using the TTO technique, patients are given two choices based on how long they can expect to live and what their lives will be like. Essentially, they must choose between a period of time with various side effects from a treatment, or a *shorter* period of time in their current state of health, often called "time without symptoms or toxicity" (Cole, 1998). For example, a patient might be told that she could live 12 months after treatment, but with side effects, or she could live 9 months without symptoms or toxicity. In subsequent steps, the choices are changed such that the number of months of life without treatment are reduced, let's say to 7 months, then 5 months, and so on. Presumably, at some point, the patient is going to say that she would rather have the 12 months of life with side effects than the short period of time in comfort. The **utility** of the treatment is calculated simply by creating a fraction, with the numerator being the symptom- and toxicity-free duration that caused the patient to choose treatment and the denominator being the duration with side effects.

For example, let's say a woman with ovarian cancer chooses 9 months of comfortable life with no treatment over 12 months of life with treatment side effects. She is then asked if she would choose 7 months of no-treatment comfortable life over the treatment option and its side effects. Let's assume she says she would. The researcher would keep reducing the no-treatment duration until the patient decided that the best option had become the treatment option. In other words, the tradeoff between 12 months of treatment-assisted life and a shorter period of toxicity-free life tips in favour of treatment. Let's say the woman said she would rather live 12 months with treatment side effects than 3 comfortable months foregoing treatment. The utility of this particular treatment would be 3/12 or 0.25, which is not very high. Of course, if the woman never chose the treatment option, stating in effect that she would rather die now than go through the treatment, the utility of that treatment would be zero for her.

In this example, we used 12 months as the time frame for the treatment option. This can be lengthened or shortened depending upon the patient's prognosis, but the process stays the same. When described in cold numerical terms as we have done here, it is easy to lose sight of the fact that the person is making very difficult life-and-death decisions. Still, with this in mind, the time tradeoff technique helps practitioners develop an understanding of what the patient considers to be the costs or value of a given treatment. In so doing, it involves the patient clearly in the decision-making process.

thetic device in order to talk. Their voice will not resemble his or her own and will sound almost robot like. Also, there will be high levels of postoperative pain. In this case, the tradeoff is clear—5 years with an artificial voice and pain versus 1 year with his or her own voice and much less pain. The fact that the two options are clear does not make the decision an easy one, however.

The point of the example, of course, is that this decision must be based primarily on quality of life. If the person is an opera singer who cannot stand the thought of having a mechanized voice, then his or her quality of life would be compromised so severely by the surgery that it ceases to be a viable option. On the other hand, if the patient has a granddaughter who is getting married in 18 months and the patient dearly wants to be at the wedding, surgery is a good option because his or her quality of life is defined in terms of the

FIGURE 11-1 Treatment and Quality of Life

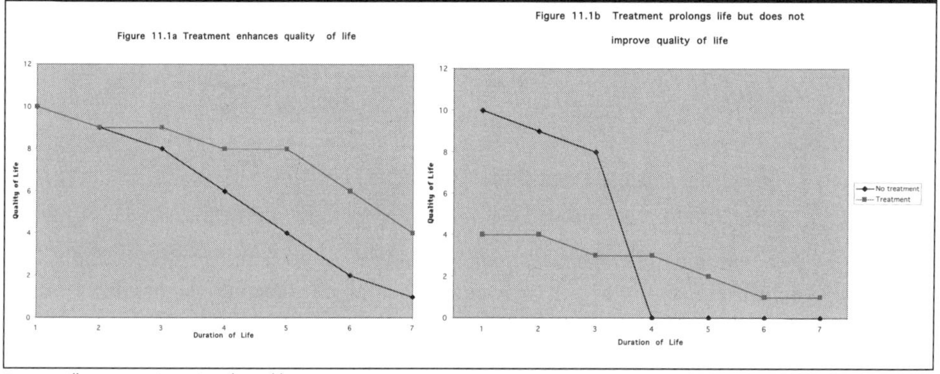

Source: Albertsen, P. (1998). Adapted by permission.

wedding rather than his or her voice. (Focus on Research 11.1 presents an arithmetic representation of the tradeoff decisions associated with treatment and quality of life.)

Figure 11.1 presents a graphic representation of what practitioners and patients must consider (Albertsen, 1998). In Figure 11.1a, the decision is quite straightforward. The therapeutic gain from the treatment is realized immediately from the time of treatment, as indicated by the distance between the treatment and no treatment lines at the start of the graph. Also, this gain is maintained for 7 years, and the duration of life is equivalent with or without treatment. This would be analogous to the types of treatment gains typically found in coronary bypass surgery or angioplasty for older patients. The decision based on Figure 11.1b is more difficult. Without treatment, the patient could live a high quality life for approximately 3 years. With treatment, she would live at least twice as long but at a much lower quality of life. It is not until those lines cross, at about 3.5 years, that any therapeutic gain is realized by the treatment. This graph would be indicative of the kinds of decisions some cancer patients must make.

Quality of Life as a Subjective Phenomenon

No one can decide what another person's quality of life is. It must be measured **phenomenologically**, that is, by asking the person directly to report on the phenomenon. In this respect, quality of life is like freedom. If someone says she is free, then she has freedom, regardless of whether she lives in an oppressive regime or on a deserted island. To illustrate this, consider the following conversation between a physician and her patient:

Patient: If I have this operation, will I be able to play competitive tennis again?

Physician: No. It will give you at least 5 more years of life, but your mobility will be restricted so that tennis would be very difficult.

Patient: Then I don't want the operation.

Physician: Because of tennis?

Patient: Yes.

Physician: But it's only a game!

For the physician, the notion that someone would rather not live than live without tennis is unthinkable, as it may be for you. However, what the physician thinks or what you and I think are irrelevant, because this is a quality of life decision, which is subjective.

Most of the quality of life questionnaires in use today acknowledge the subjectivity of the phenomenon when they ask respondents to indicate not only if they are able to perform a given function, but also how *important* the function is to the person. A good example is the Functional Assessment of Cancer Therapy (FACT) scales (Cella et al., 1993). After completing each subscale that assesses such things as emotional or physical well-being, the respondent is asked how important emotional well-being is to him or her.

There are others who have argued that the use of these scales, even when they do ask questions about importance, do not account for the subjectivity of quality of life (Clark, 1998). This is because the person designing the scale chose what functions should be tapped and also the language with which these functions would be described. This is like putting words in the patient's mouth. To remedy this, some researchers are conducing focus groups with cancer patients to learn how these patients talk about their disease (e.g., Clark, 1998). When this is done, patients bring up things that are not featured in most scales, which tend to be quite biomedical in their focus. For example, 30 to 40 percent of a group of prostate cancer patients said they regretted their treatment choice (Clark, 1998), which is something that isn't explored in quality-of-life questionnaires as a rule. Another consideration when measuring quality of life is whether the assessment is **multidimensional** or **global**. The scales we have been discussing have been multidimensional in that they assess different aspects of quality of life, such as physical, emotional, and social functioning. A global approach would require just one question, for example, "How would you rate your quality of life today?" (Gough, Furnval, Schilder, & Grove, 1983). Generally, multidimensional approaches are favoured because they allow for an assessment of how an illness is affecting specific areas of a person's life.

DEATH AND DYING

Obviously, one of the most traumatic aspects of serious illnesses is that they are life threatening. People die from them. For this reason, any attempt to help people cope with chronic and serious illnesses must address the prospect of premature death; in some cases, this prospect is very real.

Patients' Reactions to Death

Our thinking about death and the process of dying has been influenced greatly by the foundational work of psychiatrist Elizabeth Kübler-Ross (Kübler-Ross, 1969). Through her work, we moved from the belief that dying people did not want to know or talk about their death to the realization that they *did* know and *did* want to talk about important issues their impending death gave rise to. Another important contribution was her theory identifying a series of possible reactions a person might experience when facing his or her own death. When her theory was first published, it was presented as a stage theory, which is to say that the reactions were postulated to occur in a particular sequence (Kübler-Ross, 1969). Now, it is believed that the reactions she identified may be common to many patients but that not all patients experience all reactions, or even in a particular order.

The first reaction identified by Kübler-Ross is **denial**. As we have seen throughout this chapter, denial is a defence mechanism we call upon when we are confronted with novel and severe trauma. The news that one is about to die certainly fits in that category. When people receive this news, they may think the physician is not being serious, or that some mistake has been made. They may make long-range commitments, ignoring the fact that their prognosis indicates they will not be alive to keep them.

Anger is a reaction that often follows denial. The patient might get angry at the medical system for being "incompetent" and "for all its fancy equipment and pills" being unable to prevent the patient from dying. He or she might get mad at the unfairness of it all. The anger may diffuse to family and friends. The dying person may lose patience with them for not being helpful enough or trying to be too helpful, regardless of what they are actually doing. This can be difficult for family and friends to understand. A person may also respond by **bargaining**, trying to do things that will buy more time. Perhaps the person will volunteer for research or make strong commitments in terms of religiosity or spirituality.

We have discussed **depression** quite extensively in this chapter, so it will come as no surprise to learn that Kübler-Ross identifies it as a common reaction to dying. Depression is common and understandable, but it is still problematic because it often means the person gives up, thus unduly hastening death.

Finally, there is **acceptance**. If and when a person reaches this point, he or she is likely to be at peace. Perhaps death is viewed as a relief. In fact, the patient might be considerably more peaceful than family and friends who are preparing for bereavement. It is worth noting that acceptance is emotionally different from depression. Acceptance tends to come later than depression in the dying process and is not accompanied by a sense of despondency.

Group therapy for people with serious illnesses must confront participants' feelings regarding death. If not, it is very possible that some of the people will die without a very important sense of reassurance allowing them to die peacefully and, as people who work in palliative care might call it, successfully. When patients do talk about death, a number of issues emerge (Block & Billings, 1995). There are concerns about physical and psychological suffering and that they will lose their decision-making capacity at a time when they feel they must make important decisions. Seriously ill patients are also concerned about the possible suffering of their friends and family. These patients may also worry about the relationship they have with their primary-care physician and other medical staff. In addition, existential and spiritual issues can be very important.

Given these issues and concerns, what are the most important assurances therapists can give to seriously ill group members? Certainly, global assurances like, "Everything will be just fine" won't be very helpful. However, Molyn Leszcz and Pamela Goodwin, from the University of Toronto and Mount Sinai Hospital, respectively, have identified some key assurances that can be made (Leszcz & Goodwin, 1998). These include assurance that the person will not die lonely or alone, that the person's wishes will be respected, and that every effort will be made to minimize physical suffering. Of course, for wishes to be respected they must be clearly communicated, which can only be done if the group doesn't collude to avoid discussions about death, fearing that discussing death will somehow bring it on (Leszcz & Goodwin, 1998).

Bereavement and Grief

It is also important to consider the family, friends, and loved ones who are left to cope with the patient's death. They are coping with **bereavement**, which is the loss of someone close to them. **Grief** is a common psychological response to bereavement. The bereaved are clearly an at-risk population (Yalom & Vinogradov, 1988). They suffer higher death rates and suicide rates than the rest of the population. They have a higher incidence of depression and substance abuse, and they have more medical problems. For these reasons, many grieving people either seek grief counselling or are sent for it. If they seek it themselves, the success of the intervention is significantly greater (Allumbaugh & Hoyt, 1999).

There are a number of possible approaches that can be taken in grief therapy (Allumbaugh & Hoyt, 1999). The therapist may pick one or a combination of them, depending on the needs of the participants and the preferences of the therapist. For example, there is the **psychodynamic approach**, in which the therapist becomes a temporary substitute for the diseased as the bereaved person addresses unfinished issues related to mourning. There is the **client-centred approach**, in which the therapist offers nurturance and empathic understanding, paraphrasing the feelings of the person rather than prescribing solutions to him or her. With the **cognitive approach**, the therapist tries to expose dysfunctional or irrational beliefs. For example, the bereaved person might think that his life is effectively over now that his wife has died. By thinking this way, he is ignoring the support offered by his friends and family and is discounting all the things he can still do in his life. Another approach is **behavioural**, in which the therapist and bereaved person focus on problem solving, using goal setting and skill learning to help the person cope with his or her loss. Research indicates that grief counselling does help people cope with loss, although, as we mentioned, it is more effective when the clients choose to go rather than being sent.

KEY TERMS

chronic condition
acute illness
episodic illness
lifetime statistics
oncology
sites of cancer
metastasized
intrusive memories
emotion-focused coping
problem-focused coping
disfigurement
radical surgery
radiation therapy
chemotherapy
adjuvant therapy
anticipatory nausea
antiemetic medication
family-oriented care
social support
help-intended communication
monitors
blunters
social comparison
insulin-dependent diabetes (Type I)
non-insulin dependent diabetes (Type II)
hypoglycemia
mycardial infarction (MI)
coronary artery bypass graft (CABG)
angioplasty
myocardial ischemia
cardiac invalidism
cardiac arrest
angina
holistic rehabilitation programs
cognitive reappraisal and restructuring
human immunodeficiency virus (HIV)
acquired immune deficiency syndrome (AIDS)
serotonin reuptake inhibitors
antiretroviral medications
protease inhibitor
quality of life
time tradeoff technique
treatment utility
phenomenological
multidimensional measures of quality of life
global measures of quality of life
denial
anger
bargaining
depression and dying
acceptance
bereavement
grief
psychodynamic approach
client-centred approach
cognitive approach
behavioural approach

C h a p t e r 12

EXERCISE AND SPORT

Chapter Outline

Key Questions

1. How would you rate the balance in your own life with regard to the mental, physical, social, motivational, and spiritual well-being dimensions discussed in this chapter?
2. What are the five forms of exercise and which do you practise?
3. How might the model of self-efficacy be applied to explain the development of a skill in your own life in which you have achieved a high level of competency?
4. If you have ever had an injury in sport, exercise, or another activity how did it affect you psychologically?
5. Have you had one or more concussions in your life? If yes, how can they be categorized according to grade?
6. How would you describe your own behaviour with regard to adherence to health-enhancing activities? What factors affect people's adherence?

Donna had been a fitness instructor for 3 years. For the most part, she loved her work. She was an active person herself, and she couldn't imagine another job that would allow her to stay fit and active like this one did. She was also an upbeat person, and the people who attended her classes seemed to appreciate that about her.

There were times, however, when the job was quite frustrating. Some of Donna's clients were very dedicated. They never missed an aerobics class. Most, though, were very hit and miss. When she got frustrated, Donna would think about the dozens of people who would come to one or two of the first classes of a season and then never come back. They had invested money in the class (not to mention in their exercise clothes). They had seemed very committed at the beginning. But then they would disappear, never to be seen again.

Donna wondered if it was something about her. Could she be more enthusiastic? More outgoing? A better role model? Probably not. All of Donna's fitness instructor colleagues had the same problem. And whenever Donna went to a garage sale, there always seemed to be some fairly new piece of exercise equipment for sale—a stair-climber, a rowing machine. Donna simply couldn't figure out why so many people start exercise programs but can't stay with them.

It has been suggested that the most important issue in health care and well-being in the coming years will be the personal choices individuals make. This chapter is about choices and the decisions individuals make with regard to exercise and sport. Many of us will admit that the first commitment in our daily schedule that we won't follow through on when the demands for time begin to overwhelm us is exercise and sport. We make statements such as,

"I won't be able to go for a run today as I have too much work to do" or, "I will need to cancel my squash game this evening as I need to spend some time with my family." The implication is, of course, that we have no choice in the matter. In the examples given, it is the fault of our job and our family that we will not exercise today. Many of us are not even prepared to take responsibility for the decision. We need to blame it on someone else. It is a matter of priority and exercise and sport are often low on our priority list. Does it occupy a space in our day-timer? Or, is it more a vague sense of something I will do if time allows and, if it doesn't, I can always do it tomorrow?

EXERCISE AND QUALITY OF LIFE

In this chapter, we discuss issues relevant to both exercise and sport while recognizing that one can attach quite different meanings to these two terms. Hays (1999) points out that although exercise and sport may have different implications, the two fields are clearly related. The effect of exercise is usually considered a concern within the field of sport psychology. She suggests that **sport psychology** is focused on the influence of psychological factors on sport behaviour, whereas **exercise psychology** is concerned with the influence that sport and exercise have on psychological behaviour. Hayes states that, "Exercise psychology attends to the body-to-mind relationship, whereas sport psychology is directed toward the mind-to-body relationship" (Hays p. 240). Gauvin and Spence (1995) define exercise as "leisure activity (as opposed to occupational physical activity) undertaken with a specific external objective, such as the improvement of fitness, physical performance, or health, in which the participant is advised to conform to recommended mode, intensity, frequency, and duration of such activity" (p. 435). The purpose of the activity is important in this definition. If we go to the gym to ride a stationary bike or play basketball to improve our fitness, this is considered exercise; whereas, if walking is part of our work (e.g., a postal worker), this is not considered exercise as it is not being done to improve our fitness. Understanding the intention of the activity appears important in determining whether or not it is exercise. We can push a hand-mower, shovel snow, or chop wood to either get some exercise or to cut the grass, clear the driveway, or get some wood for the fire. The intention is different, but the outcome is the same. Conversely, **physical activity** can be a part of either leisure or work activities, as it is defined in terms of bodily movements produced by skeletal muscles (Casperson, Powell, & Christenson, 1985). Whether it is purposeful or without intention, it involves the expenditure of energy. **Physical fitness** refers to physiological functioning and has been described in relation to attributes we have that influence the ability to perform physical activity (Casperson et al.). Different forms of physical fitness have been identified (Kaplan, Sallis, & Patterson, 1993). These include cardiorespiratory endurance, muscular endurance, muscular strength, body composition, and flexibility.

It has been suggested (Eysenck, Nias, & Cox, 1982) that typical definitions for **sport** are too inclusive, and that it is difficult to make distinctions between activities such as games, recreation, play, leisure activity, and sport. LeUnes and Nation (1989) review different definitions of sport and conclude that specific properties emerge. They include the recognition that defining sport will involve some ambiguity, rules or limits, a sense of history, an aspect of winning and losing, and an emphasis on physical exertion in the context of competition (p. 11). These authors suggest that such definitions fall short in that they do not speak to the spirit of "sport for all", a broader-based concept that returns us to a more inclusive definition. It is our sense that such a definition, which includes the youngster playing recreational sport for the first time and the professional athlete who entertains others and makes his or her living in sport, is most appropriate.

We begin this chapter with a personal journey that involves the choices that one individual, Peter, made when confronted with ill health. His story is true and has been observed by one of the authors over a period of approximately 4 years. Initially, Peter was observed in the gym to be like so many others. He was somewhat overweight but not significantly so. He was heavily muscled and had an intensity that would make one think he was an ex-athlete of some significance, such as an NHL hockey player or a CFL football player. A friendship between Peter and the author developed over time and grew between sit-ups, curls, bench presses, and extended periods on the treadmill and exercise bike. As Peter states, "our contact is unique." Between huffs and puffs, discussion revealed that Peter was exercising for a reason. He had suffered a heart attack and had been presented with choices about the direction he wanted his life to take. His story, in a highly personalized, very courageous, and slightly edited version, is presented below.

CASE 12-1 Peter's Story

March 4, 1995 is a very memorable day in my life. It had been a busy Saturday for me. In the morning I exercised at a local gym and in the afternoon I did some yard work. In the evening I worked on some files in my home office. At approximately 9:30 p.m., I asked my wife Brenda if she would make me a cup of tea, as I was feeling the strain of the work and I wanted to take a break. Brenda called to let me know the tea was ready, and I went downstairs to get it. I was feeling tired and experiencing some pain in my back. I was also short of breath, which I attributed to my morning exercise and the stress of the evening's work. I decided to have a hot bath to see if that would ease the discomfort in my back. Brenda commented that I looked peaked and pale and that a bath would probably be beneficial. I began running the bath, although by this time I was feeling quite nauseous. I got into the bathtub and the pain, rather than dissipating, actually became more intense. I had also developed a severe headache to go along with the now excruciating pain in my back. I got out of the bath and spoke with my wife, who said I was a shade of gray-green. I remember feeling faint to the point that I thought I might lose consciousness.

At this point, Brenda suggested that she take me to the hospital, which we decided to do. We arrived there very quickly, although I do not remember much of the trip. The hospital admissions staff asked a few questions upon my arrival and seemed to know that I was experiencing a heart attack. The rest is history. At about midnight, the resident physician informed me that I had had a heart attack. The words "heart attack" scared the living hell out of me. I was moved up to the critical care unit early on Sunday morning. I was being given morphine intravenously and my blood pressure was constantly monitored. My wife had gone home to explain the events of the previous evening to our two children, and on Sunday morning my family arrived at the hospital. It must have been a shock for them to see me in this state. My 8-year-old son was very disturbed, and I could see the tears welling up in his eyes. A person beside me had passed away and was being removed from the ward. My son asked, "Does this mean you are going to die too?" The question hit me hard and I too began to cry. In fact, we all had a darn good cry together and finished up with a family hug. I told my son, "I will be here for a long time, so don't you worry."

I left the hospital on March 10, 1995. It was my daughter's tenth birthday and I wanted to be home for it. To do so, I had to prove to the hospital staff that I could walk up a flight of stairs and around the ward. This may seem a mundane physical task; however, I can assure you that it was very tiring for an individual in my condition. I was able to spend the evening with my daughter, although not as an active participant. It just felt great to be home.

The next year was an emotional roller coaster. I was not sure if I was going to live or die and it wore a hole through my soul. A full year passed and my emotions were so torn that I descended into a deep funk, known as "depression." Depression was an unfamiliar word for me and caused me great anguish. I was prescribed an antidepressant that took away my spark for life. I had discussions with my family physician, and he suggested I get physically fit again. I had always been a physical person; however, in the last year I had abandoned this for fear I would have another heart attack. After talking with my physician, I started going back to the gym. I thank him for helping me get back on track. I weighed 226 pounds at this time and was completely out of shape.

The exercise certainly helped. After about a year, my weight had dropped to 219 pounds; however, I was at the point where I could not see any significant differences in the way I felt. This continued over the next 2 years. My weight remained between 217 and 219 pounds. My diet included more of the good foods I was supposed to eat. I ate more vegetables and fruits and less meat. Despite these changes, my diet still consisted of many high fat and high calorie foods. In mid-1998, we bought a Sheltie pup. He provided me with the incentive to walk twice a day. He is also a great friend of mine. Funny how an animal can change your disposition. When I come home from work the first thing to greet me is my barking, spirited friend.

In late 1998, I saw an advertisement in the Vancouver Sun. St. Paul's Hospital was looking for volunteers to participate in an atherosclerosis-reversal program. I immediately replied to the advertisement and, when I did not hear back, called insistently. There was no way I was not going to be a participant in a program that could reduce my risk of atherosclerosis. I was accepted into the program and started in January 1999.

The first step was to be interviewed by the coordinator, who described the objectives of the program. Reversing my disease was right up my alley, so I became an active participant. I then met the nurse clinician. She further described the program and directed me to the first of my tests. These were concerned with stress and blood. The stress test measured my overall level of fitness and the blood tests measured cholesterol, triglycerides, and homocysteine. These initial tests served as a baseline for subsequent tests. By far the most important role of the nurse was that she provided inspiration to improve. Most patients like me need a positive light, a friendly face, and a person who can be trusted if we are to see improvements. She provides this inspiration on each and every visit.

I next met the dietician, who weighed me and measured the circumference of my hips and waist. I learned that these are very critical measurements. The waist-to-hip ratio should be less than 0.9 to 1.0. I weighed 217 pounds on my first visit and today am 198 pounds. My waist-to-hip ratio is between 0.85 and 1.0. These are solid improvements over a short period of time. I consume about 30 grams of fat per day, whereas before I entered the program I probably consumed approximately 100 grams of fat per day. Do I feel better? You bet! Did I learn anything? You bet! I learned that I could eat a low fat diet that was extremely tasty. It also included some of my favourite foods (e.g., sushi, salmon, chicken, certain cuts of pork, and any vegetable). The most difficult change was giving up the vast amounts of beef I used to consume. I now miss it only on occasion. The dietician wants to see me make improvements. Her suggestions and coaching have made me believe that one can be creative in creating healthy food choices.

My next contact was the exercise specialist, who developed a program to fit my needs. I typically do about 45 minutes of cardiovascular training and 45 minutes of weight training 5 days per week. I review the progress I am making on my monthly visits and she suggests alternatives or new exercises to help me achieve the results I want. She also uses calipers to measure my body fat. Each time I have improved. My goal is to achieve a body fat count of 15 per cent. I will attain this goal. I feel extremely fortunate to have been chosen to be a part of this program and to have the benefits of experts who advise me on lifestyle, diet, exercise, and mental well-being. I have also put together my own thoughts on how to win against a disease when the odds may not be in your favour.

Through trial and error, I have arrived at the following recommendations: (1) share your beliefs with the ones you love (e.g., your partner and your children); (2) choose positive friends and discard the negative ones; (3) change your lifestyle, be healthy, read and share information with those who need and want it; (4) take time for yourself; (5) relax, relax, relax; (6) thank those who make a difference in your life; and (7) make new friends. In summary, I believe changes can be made if we want them to. Sometimes we are forced, or perhaps blessed, through adverse health situations into changing our lifestyle.

Exercise and the Five Components of Health

Peter's story demonstrates in a rather compelling manner the reality, and in his case the necessity, of lifestyle change. For Peter, the alternative was unacceptable given the enthusiasm he displays for life and love of his family. The choices he faced and the decisions he made illustrate many issues of concern in the area of exercise and sport. Greenberg and Pargman (1989) describe a health-illness continuum that is anchored by four points: death, illness, health, and perfect health. It is remarkable to think that Peter has moved from the extremes of the continuum in so short a time. To have been faced with the very real possibility of death and to now be moving between health and perfect health demonstrates the power of personal change processes. It should be noted that, for Greenberg and Pargman, the extremes of the continuum, represented by death and perfect health, are connected by units, each of which is made up of five components of health: mental, physical, emotional, social, and spiritual. Regardless of the position an individual occupies on the continuum, wellness is a function of the balance experienced among the five components. The goal is to be well rounded in all areas.

Pargman (1998) suggests that those involved in sport and exercise need to appreciate how physical activity can contribute to wellness. It is important to invest not only in this or any other area disproportionately, but rather in a manner that enhances balance and therefore wellness. One assumes that each of these areas influences and is influenced by the others. This principle of reciprocity is clearly indicated in Peter's story, in which growth in all five areas is evident. Not only has he moved a significant distance on the continuum of health and illness, he has achieved a greater sense of balance in his life. Clearly, his physical health has improved dramatically. This is a matter of objective record, and improvements in this regard are evident whenever he visits the clinic for another round of tests.

Conversations with Peter reveal that in the other four areas he feels that his life has improved in very positive ways. Mentally, he is more focused and self-confident. This is most obvious in his work, where he has experienced an increase in commitment to and energy for his job. Emotionally, Peter describes himself as being more stable and less reactive. He exudes a sense of optimism that is infectious and wonderful to observe. Socially, he is active, involved, and fun to be around. He seeks out rather than avoids social experiences. Although he may not describe spiritual changes in his life, it is obvious that things have happened. By his own admission he has in some sense been "reborn." Although these four components of health (mental, social, emotional, and spiritual) are subjective and therefore more difficult to quantify, Peter would suggest that these are the most important elements of change for him as they reflect the quality of his life. They represent the aspects of change that he is aware of and directly affect his daily living. He has discovered the joy of what Csikszentmihalyi (1997) has described as **active** compared to **passive leisure**. The former is described as an extremely positive experience that is associated with activities such as hobbies, playing a musical instrument, and exercise. He states that when people engage in activities such as these, they "tend to be more happy, motivated, concentrated, and more often in flow than in any other part of the day. It is in these contexts that all the various dimensions of experience are most intensely focused and in harmony with one another" (p. 39). He suggests that improving one's quality of life is based upon organizing our life to provide those activities that provide the most rewards—the one's that make us the happiest. This is something Peter has discovered.

Rates of Exercise

It has been recommended that ideally we should have at least 30 minutes of moderate exercise every day (Pate, 1995). Although an appropriate program of exercise has long been recognized as part of a prescription for physical and psychological health, it is clear that many individuals do not get sufficient exercise and that for those who initiate a program of exercise the levels of continued adherence are low. A frequently cited statistic in this regard has been provided by Dishman (1988). His research indicates that 50 percent of those who begin a structured exercise program discontinued it within the first 6 months. Kirschenbaum (1997) reports that, depending on the definition one uses to define exercise, from 5 to 25 percent of American adults are involved in regular, vigorous exercise. We will return to the issue of adherence later; however, the incidence of exercise behaviour is something that should be examined now.

Based on data collected in 1996/97, Statistics Canada (1999) reports that 57 percent of Canadians over the age of 15 years exercise three or more times a week, with the highest percentage being for those in the 15 to 19 years of age group and the lowest in the 65 years of age and over group. Exercise in this instance includes activities that are considered to be vigorous (e.g., calisthenics, jogging, racquet sports, brisk walking, dance) and that continue for a period of at least 15 minutes. Some would suggest that this is a somewhat generous definition; however, it does allow us to examine exercise involvement according to age and gender in Canada. The percentage of Canadians who exercise three or more times per week is slightly higher for women, at 58 percent, compared to 56 percent for men. The highest percentage, at 73 percent, is seen in men 15 to 19 years old, whereas the lowest, at 47 percent, is for women over 65 years old. Twenty-two percent of the sample indicated that they exercised less than once a week or never. With regard to specific forms of exercise, data obtained by Statistics Canada in the National Population Health Survey in 1994/95 indicate that when Canadians are asked to list the physical activities they have engaged in during the past 3 months, walking (61.1%) is the most frequently chosen of the 19 activities listed. This is followed by home exercise (25.2%), bicycling (25.2%), swimming (23%), running or jogging (13.6%), weight training (11.2%), fishing (10.7%), and baseball or softball (10.1%).

The inclusion of fishing as a physical activity indicates how far the definition can extend. It is interesting to speculate as to whether some of the activities on the list are uniquely Canadian and as such are influenced by seasonal restrictions. Winter activities such as skating (8.5%), ice hockey (4.8%), downhill skiing (4.4%), and cross-country skiing (2.9%) obtained relatively low scores compared to some other activities. Obviously the point in the year at which Canadians are asked about their physical activity in the previous 3 months will greatly affect their responses. It is also possible that this same source of variation will influence regional variations in exercise activity. The 1994/95 data indicated that those living in British Columbia were more likely to engage in regular exercise at 30 percent compared to the rest of the Canadian provinces, for which the figure was 20 percent or lower. It is interesting to note that in 1997 Canadians indicted they watched television almost 23 hours per week (Statistics Canada, 1999).

A report by King, Boyce, and King (1999) summarizes information obtained on three occasions (1989/90, 1993/94, and 1997/98) comparing the health of Canadian adolescents to that of those in 10 European countries. Over this period, there was a decline in the percentage of Canadian adolescents who exercised two or more times outside of school hours. However, this was balanced by an increase in those who were involved in intensive exercise of more than 4 hours per week. It is suggested that this may be due to a movement toward more structured activities such as team or club activities which, although they may occur less frequently, involve more organization and participation time. Across all three data points, boys were more likely to exercise than girls. Of the 11 countries involved, Canadian youth were ranked at the mid-range with regard to their physical activity level. Again, it is interesting that 20 to 30 percent of the adolescents indicated that they watched television 4 or more hours per day. It was also noted that there were marked increases in playing computer games over this time period. This was particularly the case for boys. For example, 40 percent of grade 9 boys indicated they played computer games more than 4 hours per week, compared to 7 percent of girls in the same grade.

THE FIVE FORMS OF EXERCISE

It is obvious that exercise and physical activity can be expressed in many different forms; however, physiologically there are five forms of exercise. Three of them, **isometric**, **isotonic**, and **isokinetic**, are based on the principle of resistance, which involves placing demands on, or overloading, the muscles to affect both muscle strength and endurance. Isometric exercise involves contraction of a muscle group against an immovable object without movement in the body. This may seem counterintuitive, as there is no noticeable body movement; however, the contraction of the muscles improves muscle strength, although it does little for endurance. Isotonic exercise is the form of exercise most of us associate with weightlifting or "bodybuilding." This involves using weights or calisthenics to place tension on the muscle by shortening or lengthening the muscle group. Most of the exertion occurs in one direction. Over time it can be expected that such a program will improve both muscle strength and endurance. Isokinetic exercise is the most efficient method of developing muscle strength and endurance as it involves placing tension on a muscle group through a complete range of motion. The difficulty is that training in this area requires specialized, often expensive equipment designed to vary the load placed on the muscle group according to muscle strength and position.

The two other forms of exercise are **aerobic** and **anaerobic**. Given that the word *aerobic* means "with oxygen", these can be defined in terms of the relationship between exercise and oxygen use. In anaerobic exercise, intense effort is expended over a short period of time. The oxygen taken in is less than the oxygen required, so that a deficit needs to be made up. A sprint to first base in a softball game, an all-out effort to catch a thrown football, or even an attempt to demonstrate how fast we can still run the 100-yard dash on a track can leave us "gasping for air." Conversely, aerobic exercise involves an increased consumption of oxygen over an extended period of time. The oxygen being taken in is sufficient to replace that being used. Therefore, although the exercise may be strenuous it does not result in an oxygen deficit. It is the sustained nature of aerobic exercise that produces the health benefits associated with it, as the intensity and duration of the exercise stimulates the cardiovascular, pulmonary, and muscular systems, improving the efficiency with which the body uses oxygen. Common forms of aerobic exercise include jogging, swimming, cycling, cross-country skiing, paced walking, and activities done in a fitness facility— "aerobics" classes, working out on equipment like an exercise bike, a treadmill, a rowing machine, or a stairmaster. Sports associated with high levels of aerobic fitness include soccer, ice hockey, basketball, marathon running, and triathlons.

PSYCHOLOGICAL BENEFITS OF EXERCISE AND SPORT

The psychological and physical benefits of sport and exercise have been widely documented in both the empirical and lay literature. At this point in our examination of these phenomena, it seems appropriate that we examine some of the claims that have been made in support of involvement in these activities. Central to this discussion is the integration of mind and body. As Mahoney (1996) points out in the foreward to a recent text on exercise and sport psychology, "The body is back and so is the mind. They are not separate realms. They never were" (p. xv). He suggests that psychology is in the midst of a "phase transition", in which new paradigms are being established that recognize the complexity of the mind-body integration. He believes that, "One of the areas where such integrations and elaborations are particularly evident is that of exercise and sport psychology" (p. xv). Individuals who exercise frequently often make statements that indicate they believe their commitment to such activities has an impact on their psychological well-being. We hear positive comments such as, "I exercise because it helps me cope with the stress of my work"; or "When I run I leave the world behind and go into the zone"; "I love to see how far I can push myself in the gym" ; or, "Exercise makes me feel good about myself." On the downside, comments like, "If I don't get my workout in, I get depressed"; or, "I need to exercise every day" are not uncommon. Pargman (1998) suggests that, "People feel better about themselves when they believe they look better" (p. 116). The at times embarrassing presence of floor-to-ceiling mirrors in gyms and fitness centres supports this contention.

Although anecdotal enthusiasm for the psychological benefits of exercise exists, some concerns have been raised about methodological issues in the empirical evaluation of this relationship (Kircaldy & Shephard, 1990; Morgan, 1997; Pargman, 1989). One such concern has to do with the choice of experimental and control groups. The initial health status of the experimental group (i.e., whether they are depressed, anxious or recovering from a physical illness) will affect the impact of an exercise program and therefore the degree to which the results can be generalized. How an exercise program affects one mentally would be expected to be somewhat dependent on an individual's psychological starting point. A control group that is excluded from participation in an exercise program may not provide the appropriate comparison for a group that is assigned to an exercise condition and receives ongoing support to continue participation. Adherence to exercise programs has already been mentioned as a problem and may result in difficulties in evaluating those who remain in compared to those who drop out of an exercise program. To what extent are those who persist with an exercise program already committed to a personal change process that makes the particular physical activity they are involved in irrelevant? (Prokop et al., 1991.)

Evaluation of change may be difficult using standard clinical measures, particularly those originally designed to assess psychopathology rather than the more subtle changes one might expect through becoming involved in an exercise program. In this regard, the work of Ostrow (1996), who has provided us with an extensive directory of psychological tests appropriate to the sport and exercise field, is important.

Exercise and Sense of Self

Despite concerns such as these, there is an increasing body of evidence to support a correlation between involvement in physical activity and improvements in psychological health. For example, it has been postulated that participation in physical activity inproves one's *self-concept*. In 1981, Folkins and Syme reviewed the existing research regarding physical fitness training and improvements on psychological variables related to perceptions of the self. The conclusion was that only about 15 percent of the studies reviewed were of an acceptable standard; however, those that were indicated that physical fitness training results in improved mood, work behaviour, and self-concept. They concluded that the "personality research with the highest payoff has been that which focuses on self-concept" (p. 380). What may be most important is the perception of change, which may occur quite independently of changes in physical fitness. This position was also supported by the research of Jasnoski, Holmes, Soloman, and Aguiar (1981).

Reviewing the literature on self-esteem and exercise 6 years later, Sonstroem (1997) came to essentially the same conclusion about research on self-esteem. Although a positive relationship between exercise and self-esteem is indicated, methodological flaws somewhat limit the conclusion that can be drawn. However, as Brannon and Feist (2000) have summarized, "It may not be necessary to know the exact variables responsible for improved self-esteem as long as increased feelings of self-worth and self-confidence are associated with an exercise program" (p. 491). The implication is that exercise may indirectly influence one's self-esteem. Brannon and Feist conclude that, "Participation in an exercise program is strongly associated with feeling good about oneself" (p. 491). We're sure that Peter would agree with this position.

It is interesting to note that numerous tests have been constructed to measure concepts related to perceptions of the self. The development of these tests suggests that many of those who work in the exercise and sport field believe that not only does a relationship exist between involvement in these activities and the participant's psychological state, but that it can be objectively measured in a manner that demonstrates acceptable levels of validity and reliability. Some examples are provided here to give a sense of the different ways in which this relationship is viewed.

The Exercise Identity Scale (Anderson & Cychosz, 1994) was designed to "assess the extent to which exercise is descriptive of one's concept of self" (Ostrow, 1996, p. 245). *The Physical Self-Description Questionnaire* (Marsh et al., 1994) assesses an individual's sense of physical self-concept. *The Self-Acceptance Scale for Athletes* (Waite, Gansneder, & Rotella, 1990) is designed to be a sport-specific measure of individual differences in the perception of self-acceptance, defined as "the valuing and feeling good about oneself regardless of one's shortcomings or failures as an athlete" (p. 266). *The Physical Estimation and Attraction Scales* (Sonestroem, 1978) proposes to assess "(a) self-perception of physical fitness and athletic ability, hypothesized to be a component of global self-esteem (estimation) and (b) interest in vigorous physical activity (attraction)" (Ostrow, 1996, p. 255). Finally, the *Elite Athlete Self Description Questionnaire* (Marsh, Hey, Johnson & Perry, 1997) was constructed to assess components of self-concept in elite athletes. The authors developed the test based on an intuitive model that proposes that self-concept in an elite athlete is made up of six components: skill level, body suitability, aerobic competence, anaerobic competence, mental competence, and performance.

Exercise and Cognitive Functioning

Exercise has also been examined in regard to its impact on information processing and cognitive functioning (Etnier et al., 1997; Nideffer & Sharpe, 1978; Pargman, 1998; Tomporowski & Ellis, 1986). Does involvement in exercise have the facilitative effect on one's mental abilities that those who engage in exercise and sport frequently report? Does the ability to remember or discriminate improve? Based on their review of the existing literature, Tomporowski & Ellis (1986) concluded that the results to that point were inconsistent, which is attributed mainly to a lack of a coherent methodology for examining the issue. They acknowledge that there is research indicating a facilitation of cognitive functioning both during and after physical activity, while some research suggests either no effect or even an impairment of cognitive abilities due to exercise. They provide a possible explanation for this discrepancy that is quite appealing. The suggestion is that exercise, due to its affect on the central nervous system, will initially improve attentional processes. However, as the intensity or duration of the exercise increases, this will be negated by the effects of increasing muscular fatigue. The implications for the assessment process are obvious. Tomporowski and Ellis propose that, "The dominant state determines the ability of subjects to perform tests of cognition. Thus, it may be possible for exercise to either facilitate or impair performance on the same cognitive test depending on the level of physical fitness of the subject and the point at which the subject is tested" (p. 344).

The recent meta-analysis by Etnier and colleagues (1997) further explores this relationship. They reviewed 134 relevant studies and concluded that exercise and fitness have a small yet positive impact on cognitive functioning. However, they also suggest that this may not reflect a difference that appears to exist for the impact of chronic, as compared to acute, exercise. The indication is that exercise administered in an acute manner will have little impact on cognition, whereas chronic exercise that produces gains in fitness will improve cognition. This conclusion "would support the physiological mechanisms as explanations for the beneficial effects of exercise or fitness upon cognition" and "would suggest that the adoption of a chronic exercise program may be a useful intervention for enhancing cognitive functioning" (p. 267).

Exercise and Mood

An extensive body of literature has looked at the impact of exercise and physical activity on mood states, with the primary focus being on anxiety and depression. With regard to the anxiolytic (anxiety-reducing) and antidepressant effects of exercise, there are methodological issues such as the use of anecdotal versus empirical evidence, the assessment of mood state, the actual effect-size found, the representativeness of the data, and the mechanisms used to explain the findings. Despite these concerns, there is evidence that exercise is effective in reducing anxiety in some people (Hackfort & Spielberger, 1989; Landers & Petruzzello, 1994; McAuley, Mihalko, & Bane, 1996; Petruzzello et al., 1991; Raglin & Morgan, 1987). This effect applies in particular to state, as compared to trait, anxiety. The mechanism by which physical activity produces an anxiolytic effect is not clear. Morgan, who has been concerned with the effect of exercise on mood states for many years, has suggested that exercise provides a distraction or "time out" from the pressures and anxieties of daily living (Bahrke & Morgan, 1978). For many of us, this model will have considerable intuitive appeal. Our exercise time is a period of the day when we can leave the world behind. We are removed from our obligations or are at least less aware of them, are often inaccessible to others, are completely focused on the task before us, and are absorbed in the process.

To return to our friend Peter, he recently acknowledged with frustration that what bothers him most about his exercise sessions is when he is disturbed by club members who know he is in the exercise room and want to discuss issues related to his duties as chairman of a club committee. He makes statements such as, "This is *my* time, why don't they leave me alone?" or, "Don't they understand that I am occupied with my exercise program and do not want to be disturbed?" In this context, exercise serves as a distraction and can clearly be a very effective one; however, many activities can fulfill this function if this is all that is required. Is there a moderating effect that is unique to exercise? Tate and Petruzzello (1995) have demonstrated a differential pattern of anxiety responses for those engaged in exercise compared to those in a resting control condition. Research by McAuley, Mihalko, & Bane (1996) indicates that anxiety levels increase during exercise and then decrease significantly following exercise. There is a concern expressed by these authors that anxiety and arousal are confounded in the measurement of state anxiety. Research by Rejeski, Hardy, & Shaw (1991) indicates that anxiety decreases in a linear fashion during exercise, whereas arousal increases during exercise and decreases noticeably following exercise. This seems a reasonable position and helps explain what appears to be confusing results. It should be noted that in the directory of tests for exercise and sport there are 31 tests described to assess anxiety in a wide variety of exercise and sport situations.

The impact of exercise on depression has been the subject of research for a considerable length of time, with the implication being that those who exercise are less depressed than those who don't. As in research discussed previously, methodological problems limit the conclusions that can be drawn. However, there is evidence that physical activity can decrease *non-clinical* depression (e.g., Brown, Ramirez & Traub, 1978; Jasnowski, Holmes, & Banks, 1988; Stein & Motta, 1992). With regard to clinically depressed individuals, initial research by Griest and his colleagues examined the effect of running as a treatment and reported decreased levels of depression in those involved in a running program (1984). With regard to *clinical* depression, exercise is an effective treatment. Reviews by Martinson (1990, 1993, 1994), Martinson and Morgan (1997) and North, McCullagh, and Tran (1990) have indicated that exercise is effective in comparison to psychotherapeutic techniques; that both aerobic and anaerobic exercise are effective treatments for depression; that exercise has *not* been shown to be effective with severe depression; that fitness levels are lower for clinically depressed individuals; and that there is no evidence that exercise can prevent relapse.

There are other areas in which the psychological impact of exercise and sport has been evaluated. Perhaps the most obvious of these would be with regard to stress, where it has been indicated that physical activity may buffer the effects of stress (this topic was considered more specifically in Chapter 5 on stress and coping). Other areas are new and still developing. For example, a recent study by Lox, McAuley, and Tucker (1995) reported that individuals at various stages of HIV-1 infection benefited both psychologically and emotionally from involvement in an exercise program.

PHYSICAL BENEFITS OF EXERCISE AND SPORT

The physical benefits of exercise can be expressed in different ways. For some, this may be expressed as a high level of fitness and the physical appearance that goes with it. For others, it may mean the absence of disease and the promotion of health and longevity. For still others, it may simply be the expression of an optimistic, positive lifestyle that is highly desirable in comparison to the alternative. A study by Kavussanu and McAuley (1996) showed that highly active individuals are significantly more optimistic and less pessimistic than inactive individuals. Numerous studies have demonstrated the positive benefits of exercise, some of which have been enormous undertakings. For example, the longitudinal research of Blair and colleagues (1989) examined the role of physical fitness on mortality rates in over

10 000 men and 3 000 women over an average of 8 years. Exercise appeared to reduce the risk of mortality from all causes, particularly cardiovascular disease and cancer. Some of the benefits attributed to physical activity include improved cardiovascular functioning and a reduced risk of cardiovascular disease; improved muscle strength and endurance; increased cardiorespiratory fitness; improved flexibility; improved weight control and fat metabolism; improved sleep; prevention of bone density loss; a reduction in poor health habits such as cigarette smoking and alcohol consumption; reduced risk of injury; and increased energy. There are others; however, what is important to each one of us is that since higher levels of physical fitness translate into decreased mortality and increased longevity, any deterioration in health will take on tremendous significance in our life. The limitations and costs imposed by ill health may be devastating. If involvement in exercise and sport can decrease such events, they assume a most important status in our culture. The description Peter provided us of his experience underscores this position very powerfully. For the purposes of this discussion, we will focus our attention on the important benefits attached to exercise and sport in the prevention of cardiovascular disease.

Since the 1950s, considerable evidence has accumulated to demonstrate that those who are physically active are less likely to develop and die from coronary heart disease (CHD). Miller, Balady and Fletcher (1997) have stated recently that "a sedentary lifestyle carries approximately the same risk for the development of coronary artery disease as the more traditional risk factors of cigarette smoking, hypertension, and hypercholesterolemia" (p. 220). Early research examined the presence of CHD in individuals according to their occupation and the level of physical activity required in their work (Kahn, 1963). Individuals whose work involved a high level of physical activity appeared to be at a decreased risk for CHD (Brand, Paffenbarger, Scholtz, and Kampert (1979). The next level of evaluation involved the comparison of physically active and inactive individuals according to measures of energy expenditure. The most influential of these is the Harvard Alumni Study carried out by Paffenbarger and his colleagues. They assessed men who had graduated from Harvard University over a 50-year period according to their weekly expenditure of energy and divided them into two groups, high and low activity. They reported that men who were physically active had a 25 percent lower mortality rate from any cause and were 36 percent less likely to die from CHD (Paffenberger, Wing, & Hyde, 1978). The Framingham Heart Study evaluated CHD in both men and women and found that when the very active as compared to the very inactive groups were compared with regard to CHD, the risk for the latter group was approximately three times greater (Dawber, 1980). Also, exercise rehabilitation has been found to significantly decrease mortality in survivors of myocardial infarction (Haskell et al., 1994). Miller, Balady, and Fletcher (1997), after an extensive review of the literature, provide a series of summary statements that suggest a very positive role for exercise in the prevention and rehabilitation of cardiovascular disease.

It should be noted that the possible protective role played by physical activity with regard to stroke and cancer is still emerging. With stroke, there is evidence that physical activity provides protection, particularly for those who are middle-aged and beyond (Abbot, Rodriguez, Burchfiel, & Curb, 1994). The impact of physical activity in protecting against cancer appears positive, particularly for men. For example, Lee, Paffenberger, and Hsieh (1992) reported that participants in the Harvard Alumni Study who were physically active were much less likely to develop prostate cancer than those who were inactive. Support for this position is found in research by Wannamethee, Sharpe, and Macfarlane (1993), who report that physically active men are less likely to die of cancer.

STAYING WITH AN EXERCISE PROGRAM

Despite the many psychological and physical benefits attached to exercise, a disturbingly small percent of individuals exercise on a regular basis, as we have seen. For those who do exercise, a significant issue is **non-adherence**, an inability to stay with an exercise program. The most frequently cited statistic in this regard is based on the work of Dishman (1988) who reports that approximately 50 percent of those involved in a physical activity program drop out within the first 6 months. This seems a paradox, as we think of ourselves as being in the midst of an exercise and sports boom. Fitness centres are everywhere, fitness equipment is easily available and we frequently dress in casual exercise clothes. Sports participation seems to be increasing, particularly through the recreational and master's sports movements. One need only think back to what the situation was like 20 years ago to appreciate how far we have come.

Taylor (1994) believes that the avoidance of exercise and sport is not difficult to understand, pointing out that exercise is initially somewhat aversive and offers few immediate rewards. The environment can be unappealing, the activities monotonous, progress often slow, a lack of expertise may be obvious, and social comparison with experienced exercisers can be unpleasant. The first experience in an aerobics course or an exercise room can be most threatening. The obvious comparison to those with expertise may be quite aversive. With regard to sports involvement, a lack of skills development and knowledge of rules combined with an often highly competitive environment can be a threat to self-esteem.

To a large extent, the positive benefits of exercise and sport emerge with time and will ultimately outweigh the initial impediments. It seems simplistic to suggest that the dilemma is that to become involved in exercise and sport for the longterm, an individual needs to persist for a long time. Zifferblatt (1975) suggested some time ago that the likelihood of compliance is directly related to the visibility of the cues or reasons as to why the individual should comply. When the reasons are vague or ambiguous the likelihood of compliance is low, whereas if they are specific, relevant, or salient the likelihood of compliance is high. The implication of this is that initial experiences in exercise and sport often do not provide enough reasons as to why one should continue. They may become obvious in time, but it will take time. Most of us can relate to self-doubts such as, "Am I really making any progress?", "Is this enjoyable?", "How do you work this machine?", or "I look ridiculous compared to that person."

To better understand the factors affecting adherence to physical activity, numerous theoretical models have been used to help better understand the issues involved. Many of these were introduced in Chapter 1 and include include the health belief model (Becker & Maiman, 1975); the theory of reasoned action (Ajzen & Fishbein, 1980); the theory of planned behaviour (Ajzen, 1985); self-efficacy theory (Bandura (1977); the transtheoretical model (Prochaska and DiClemente, 1983); and the relapse prevention model (Marlatt and Gordon, 1980). It is important to note that these models were developed in the context of other behaviours and that it is still not clear how relevant they are to physical activity. Important predictors of adherence include physical proximity to the exercise area, availability of time, spousal support, group size and constitution, socioeconomic status, choice of exercise, and injury (LeUnes and Nation, 1989). It seems that the issue of salience is most important here. Why should I do this? What are the reinforcements I receive and what rewards await me as a consequence of my sustained commitment to physical activity?

Kirschenbaum (1998) has proposed, in a rather innovative manner, that involvement in sport and the models that sport psychology have developed provide a strategy for increasing adherence to physical activity. Given the indications provided above that health psychologists have achieved only modest success in this regard (Dishman and Buckworth, 1997), it seems reasonable to consider Kirschenbaum's proposal. In a recent book, Kirschenbaum (1998) used a self-regulatory model to identify seven steps designed to improve athletic performance. He believes that this model is similar to that used by health psychologists to increase adherence and that sport can be used as a target for exercise adherence. By focusing on the commitment many individuals have to sport, psychologists can design strategies to increase adherence to exercise. The energy expended in sport can be considerable, and the modification of existing patterns could result in even greater expenditures. For example, individuals could be encouraged to run to and from the gym to play basketball rather than drive their car.

It is interesting to note that professional athletes often ride an exercise bike for an extended period of time after a competition, as it simulates the fitness demands of an overtime period and leads to improved levels of anaerobic fitness. Kirschenbaum suggests that, "Not only could we target extant interest in sport as a goal in health psychology, but we could use sport psychology interventions to maximize involvement in such sports. These interventions could help participants enjoy their sports more fully, thereby sustaining their involvement in them" (p. 17). The extraordinary commitment that many individuals display for their sport can be used to indirectly increase their levels of physical activity and produce physical and psychological health benefits.

PSYCHOLOGICAL FACTORS AFFECTING PERFORMANCE IN EXERCISE AND SPORT

One of the most widely cited psychological variables thought to affect performance in the sport and exercise realm is **self-efficacy**, a construct that has been clearly articulated in the work of Bandura (1977, 1986, 1990). He defines perceived self-efficacy as "people's judgement of their capabilities to organize and execute courses of action required to attain designated types of performances. It is concerned not with the skills one has but with judgements of what one can do with whatever skills one possesses" (Bandura, 1986, p. 391). It is important to distinguish self-efficacy, a situation-specific belief that reflects an individual's perception of his or her ability to succeed at a particular task at a specific time, from self-confidence, which reflects a global trait associated with overall performance expectations. As Bandura (1990) points out, "confidence" as a colloquial term is an idea that permeates sport; however, it does not indicate direction. An individual can be quite confident that they will be unsuccessful, whereas self-efficacy involves the affirmation of performance capabilities. The implication of the theory is that, given that an individual has the required skills and appropriate incentives are in place, it will predict actual performance. Performers in all fields are frequently told that all they need is a "little more confidence" in their ability and they will realize their goals. So persuasive is this fascination with the confidence that one has in their skills that it is often held out as the deciding factor in determining the outcome of one's actions. Individuals who have highly developed technical and physical skills often fall short of their goals simply because they are unable to use these skills in the relevant context, whereas those with limited technical and physical abilities often achieve well beyond their, and others', expectations because they believe in themselves.

Every one of us can relate to those times when we thought we were well prepared for an event only to find our performance deteriorating due to what we often describe as a "loss of confidence." As Jackson and Csikszentmihalyi (1999) have observed in discussing the challenge-skills (CS) balance, "It is not the objective skills that become critical in the CS balance, but rather how one perceives one's skills in relation to the relevant challenges. It is important to realize that what you *believe* you can do will determine your actual experience more than your actual abilities" (p. 17).

How far will this belief system take us? For many there is almost a mystical quality to experiencing the upper reaches of performance achievements, or what Bandura (1989) has described as "transcendent accomplishments." Bruce Jenner, the decathlon champion at the 1976 Olympic games held in Montreal, described the transformation he underwent during the competition: "A strange feeling began to come over me...I started to feel that there was nothing I couldn't do if I had to. It was a feeling of awesome power, except that I was in awe of myself, knocking off these p.r.'s (personal records) just like that. I was rising above myself, doing things I had no right to be doing" (Jenner, 1976, p. 77).

This sense of transcendence is often expressed in terms of physical barriers that are seen as unattainable. The most famous of these would be the 4-minute mile. Considered a physical impossibility and even life-threatening , it became commonplace following the remarkable performances by Roger Bannister and John Landy at the Commonwealth Games in Vancouver in 1954 when they became the first individuals to run the mile in under 4 minutes in competition. Prior to 1954, it is reported that over 50 medical journals contained articles indicating that it would not be possible for a human run a mile in under 4 minutes. Within the next year, four more runners broke the 4-minute barrier. Obviously, the athletes who followed so quickly in breaking the same barrier did not change physically or technically in this short timeframe. What was now different was their belief that it could be done. What had been overcome was a mental limitation, not a physical one. Bannister in describing the experience of breaking the 4-minute mile states, "The moment of a lifetime had come. There was no pain, only a great unity of movement and aim. The world seemed to stand still, or did not exist. The only reality was the next two hundred yards of track under my feet. The tape meant finality–perhaps extinction" (Bannister, 1955, p. 213–14). Bannister has predicted that humans will run the mile in 3.5 minutes.

Of course, what is being described here is not self-confidence in the true sense, as this is a global trait that reflects on expectations of overall performance. Rather, what is being described is the situation-specific set of beliefs reflected in Bandura's theory of self-efficacy. Successful performers are well aware of this difference. They honestly acknowledge that the specific skills they have developed in a particular activity do not generalize to other activities in any significant way. They have situation-specific, state skills. Despite this recognition of the specificity of their skills, they still identify their belief in themselves as being "confidence" rather than "self-efficacy" , because this is the language they know. To say that a great athlete "oozed self-confidence" is clearly more understandable than saying he "oozed self-efficacy." For our part, we impose trait qualities on performers and often demand, and are often disappointed when we don't receive, excellence in areas outside of their skill domain. We should not be surprised when the sports icon we have come to admire so much on the basketball floor, skating rink, or baseball diamond turns out to be a disappointment as a public speaker. Self-efficacy theory would say to us, "What did you expect, she is a tennis player not a figure skater", or in an even less domain-specific manner, "He is a basketball player not a public speaker."

Researchers in the area (e.g., Bandura, 1989; Feltz, 1988; Hardy, Jones, & Gould, 1996) have indicated that the exercise and sport field is an excellent arena in which to study self-efficacy. It provides a microcosm of relevance and immediacy in which to examine the phenomena. Bandura (1990) speaks specifically to the role of self-efficacy in the context of athletic performance. He points out that athletes develop their skills to a high level of expertise and are often asked to execute these skills under situations of extreme stress against individuals who are also highly skilled. Skills performed with remarkable ease in practice often become fragile or break under the pressure of competition, often due to self-doubt. Minimal differences in skill execution will be reflected in significant differences in outcome. Successful athletes believe in their ability to focus on the task, ignore distractions, deal with mistakes and failures, cope with fatigue and pain, and ultimately in their ability to perform to the best of their ability in the particular circumstances in which they find themselves. They display what Bandura (1990) has termed the "development of resilient self-efficacy."

Bandura (1986) has identified four sources of efficacy expectations: **performance accomplishments**, **vicarious experience**, **verbal persuasion**, and **emotional arousal**. Performance accomplishments or enactive attainments are considered to be the most influential source of self-efficacy, as they are based on actual experiences of mastery. Success experiences raise self-efficacy and failure decreases it, although factors such as the perceived difficulty of the task, the effort expended, adverse external circumstances, and the temporal sequencing of events will affect the strength of the relationship. For example, early failure experiences may decrease self-efficacy, although initial setbacks, if eventually mastered as the result of commitment and effort, can strengthen one's belief that even the most difficult of obstacles can be mastered. Improved self-efficacy will incorporate occasional failures with ease and will generalize to other situations, although the degree of similarity to the original task will determine the extent of the generalization process.

Vicarious experience, which is gained through observing or visualizing others perform a skill, can alert one to one's own capabilities and raise the observer's sense of self-efficacy. How many times have we said to ourselves, "If they can do it, so can I", or to someone else, "Watch me first? If I can do it, so can you." We follow the ski instructor down the hill, observing their every move, or we watch the tennis instructor's serve and then try to duplicate it. We rely on these models to increase our sense of our own capabilities and teach us better ways to do things. Of course, if we observe failure at a task in an individual whom we feel similar to in terms of competency this may serve to decrease our own sense of capability. Although important in determining self-efficacy expectations, vicarious experiences are seen to be weaker than actual performance experiences. They may, however, confirm a sense of inability or, perhaps more important, cause one to persist despite performance failures, to ultimately achieve success. We can all identify those moments when we persisted at a task despite repeated failure simply because we observed success in someone else and believed that eventually we would be able to do it. Our sense of determination is derived from our belief that, like the model, we will ultimately be successful.

Verbal persuasion refers to the commonly used strategy of attempting to persuade others or ourselves that the capability exists to achieve a desired outcome. Although considered a weaker strategy than performance accomplishments and vicarious experience, verbal persuasion can result in sustained and increased effort. However, the utility of this strategy is predicated on a sense of realism. To promote an unrealistic sense of competence in an individual who does not possess the necessary skills will likely result in a performance failure that serves to decrease one's sense of self-efficacy and trust in future attempts at verbal persuasion. This might express itself in statements such as, "You told me the last time it would be okay and that I wouldn't fall and look what happened, disaster. Not only did I hurt myself, I embarrassed myself in front of my friends. I'm never going to believe you again." Those involved in teaching others clearly have to be cautious as to how they use persuasion to improve performance. If it serves to remove self-doubts and allows existing skills to emerge, then it has served its purpose. However, if the results of an individual's actions serve to disconfirm your persuasive abilities, your credibility will be undermined.

The final, and least powerful, source of efficacy expectations is emotional arousal or physiological state. This implies that individuals evaluate their capabilities according to their assessment of their physiological state. For example, high levels of arousal may be perceived as debilitating and predictive of failure and result in a spiralling decrease in self-efficacy. The optimal level of arousal to perform a particular task will depend not only on the nature of the task but on the causal inferences made about the arousal itself. Arousal may be interpreted positively or negatively according to the attributions one makes about their physiological state. Strategies for modifying arousal levels, such as relaxation techniques or mental rehearsal routines, will allow an individual to modify his or her arousal levels in the desired direction. It seems that the high level of arousal we experience prior to engaging in a particular task might be interpreted either with anxiety and foreboding or with excitement and anticipation, depending on the attributions we make about our physiological state.

There is a substantive research literature supporting the framework provided by self-efficacy theory in relation to performance in both exercise and sport. Research that demonstrates improved self-efficacy as a function of participation in exercise includes that of Bozoian, Rejeski, & McAuley, 1994; Michalko, McAuley, & Bane, 1996; McAuley, 1991; McAuley & Corneya, 1992; McAuley, Schaffer, & Rudolph, 1995; Rudolph & Butki, 1998. In the sport domain, self-efficacy has been demonstrated to be an important discriminating factor in research such as that of Doyle, Landers, & Feltz, 1980; Feltz, Bandura, & Lirgg, 1989; George, 1994; Gould, Weiss, & Weinberg, 1981; Mahoney & Avener, 1977; Mahoney, Gabriel, & Perkins, 1987; Weiss, Wiese, & Klint, 1989.

In the directory of tests, there are 12 tests that are specifically related to the measurement of self-efficacy. For example, the *Exercise-Specific Self-Efficacy Scale* (McAuley, 1991) is designed to "examine individuals' perceived capabilities to exercise in the face of barriers to participation" (Ostrow, 1996, p. 246). The *Physical Fitness Self-Efficacy Scale* (Bezjak & Lee, 1990) assesses "participants' perceived competence and confidence in performing tasks involving components of health-related physical fitness" (p. 501). Other tests relate to specific activities such as running, diving, basketball free throws, gymnastics, swimming, tennis, coaching, and a team's collective capabilities.

We will now examine in more detail some of the developments in the sport psychology field that have implications for health psychology and reflect on our overall concern in this chapter for the choices individuals make regarding their health behaviour. There are two principle areas of concern in sport psychology. One is performance enhancement as it relates to the development of psychological skills that can be used to optimize athletic performance. The second has to do with the clinical realm and issues of a clinical nature, such as depression or an eating disorder that may compromise an athlete's performance. An area of concern in this regard is injury, which will be discussed shortly.

We will focus initially on psychological skills as they can be applied to sport and life. This is important, for it recognizes that sport skills are utilized in a context that allows for their extension to life outside of sport. They are not only sport skills, they are life skills, and their utility extends beyond the domain of sport. This position is often recognized anecdotally by coaches who are aware of their impact on others, particularly young athletes, and view themselves as teachers of life skills. They frequently attach more importance to this component of their work than they do to the development of sports skills. Danish, Pettipas, and Hale (1993) have developed a psychoeducational model for sport psychology that focuses specifically on the teaching of life skills, which they describe as "life development intervention." They suggest that sport is an effective and accessible analogy for the teaching of life skills.

It is obvious that most young athletes will not go on to a career in sports; for these people, "growing up means further defining their identity, discovering other skills and interests, and, it is hoped, applying some of the valuable principles learned during sport participation to their adult pursuits. These transferable behaviors and attitudes are called *life skills*" (Danish, Nellen, and Owens, 1996). An area of specific concern in this program is helping young people make appropriate decisions with regard to health-enhancing, as opposed to health-compromising, behaviours. Smith (1999) has addressed the assumption that sports skills will generalize beyond the athletic environment. He examines factors that improve the generalization of coping skills into two situations outside of sport, academic exams and physical or sexual assault. He indicates that the generalizability of sports skills should not be assumed and should be an issue of focal concern.

In describing psychological skills training in sport, a distinction is sometimes made between **psychological skills** and **psychological methods** (Vealey, 1988). This assumes that concerns such as arousal or attentional control relate to psychological skills and that issues such as relaxation, goal-setting, or imagery are psychological methods; the latter serve to develop the former. Others have suggested that the distinction should be made between "basic psychological skills", which can be used on their own, and "advanced psychological skills" , which the former can be a component of (Hardy, Jones, & Gould, 1997). In this discussion, we will focus on the basic skills, with the assumption that they can be used as the components of a psychological skills training program that can be applied both within and outside the sport and exercise domain. It should also be recognized that these skills have application within models of stress management that have been adapted for sport. Examples of these would be Kirschenbaum's (1997) self-regulatory model, Meichenbaum's (1975) stress-inoculation training, Smith's (1980) cognitive-affective stress management training, and Suinn's (1972) visuomotor behavior-rehearsal program. However, it has been shown that rather than using specific programs such as these, the component skills of a psychological training program should be taught and used according to individual needs (Hardy, Jones, and Gould, 1997).

Relaxation

The ability to relax is an essential skill in coping with the pressure of athletic performance. Most individuals will acknowledge some degree of performance anxiety in anticipation of the demands of a task. **Relaxation skills** inprove one's ability to reduce anxiety to manageable levels, such that energy can be used to positively influence performance. Many of us experience "butterflies" prior to a performance, which is not a problem if we can teach them to "fly in formation." Relaxation skills assist in this process. It is also recognized that effective performance is effortless and automatic, which is more likely to occur in a relaxed state (Taylor, 1996; Kirschenbaum, 1997). Many successful athletes have developed relaxation skills on their own. Through a process of trial and error, they have arrived at a set of strategies that work for them. However, there may be limitations to their ability to relax under pressure. In this regard, relaxation is viewed as a learned skill that needs to be applicable to the performance circumstances. For example, we might acknowledge that watching television or reading a book is relaxing; however, these activities, which are external to the individual, are not applicable to a performance situation. In this context we are describing an internal response usually described in either physical or mental terms.

The most widely practised form of relaxation in sport would be variations on the technique of progressive muscular relaxation (PMR) pioneered by Jacobson (1938). It involves focusing attention on different muscle groups within the body (e.g., the biceps, shoulders, or stomach) and progressing systematically through the entire body. Initially in the training of PMR, the individual is encouraged to tense the muscle briefly before relaxing it on command. Jacobson felt that this was necessary to allow one to learn the distinction between tension and relaxation. With training, the tensing is eliminated and muscle groups are combined such that what previously took 30 minutes to accomplish can be achieved in a period as short as 30 seconds. The individual has learned what Benson (1976) has termed the "relaxation response." It is important that as familiarity with the technique increases, the ability to relax is generalized to the relevant performance domain. It seems that PMR is most effective in coping with the somatic or physiological components of anxiety, whereas strategies such mental rehearsal and the management of self-talk may be more appropriate to coping with cognitive anxiety. Within sports it is also recognized that proper breathing is an effective strategy for increasing levels of relaxation and successfully coping with anxiety. The deep, rhythmical breathing associated with relaxation can quickly be replaced by the shallow, staccato breathing associated with tension and anxiety. Training in breath control can be most helpful in inducing and maintaining states of relaxation (Nideffer, 1985).

Self-Talk

Self-talk is a term used in sport psychology to examine the ways that people think. What do athletes say to themselves either internally or externally? It is frequently the observation that athletes talk to themselves a great deal, sometimes constantly and very negatively. Monitoring an athlete's self-talk gives us an opportunity to evaluate their perceptions and beliefs. We can identify cognitive distortions and irrational ways of thinking that might disrupt performance. It has been reported that patterns of self-talk can distinguish successful from unsuccessful performers (e.g., Mahoney and Avener, 1977; Orlick and Partington, 1988).

Positive self-talk is associated with successful performances and negative self-talk with poor performances. Williams and Leffingwell (1996) have identified different functions that self-talk can serve in sport, including correcting bad habits, focusing attention, modifying activation, increasing self-confidence, increasing efficacy, and maintaining exercise behaviour. With regard to correcting bad habits, self-talk could be used to correct faulty technique. A tennis player could be encouraged to consciously say, "Follow through" each time they hit the ball, in an attempt to correct their tendency to cut the stroke short. The emphasis is on "to do" rather than "not to do." To focus attention, an athlete might say, "Watch the ball" or "execute." In modifying activation, the athlete might want to increase or decrease their arousal levels. Their self-talk might take the form of "relax" or "let go", as opposed to "push" or "work". Self-confidence may involve changing the tendency to call oneself a "loser" to saying "yes" to oneself.

With regard to exercise behaviour it has been suggested by Gauvin (1990) that those who continue have positive and motivating self-talk in comparison to the negative self-talk of non-exercisers. Once inappropriate patterns of self-talk have been identified, the concern is to modify this behaviour in the appropriate direction. This involves a restructuring process that replaces maladaptive cognitions with those that are more adaptive.

In this context, the work of Ellis (1975) is most relevant. His work on rational emotive behavior therapy (REBT) involves the modification of irrational thoughts. Ellis attributes this view to Epictetus, a Greek philosopher who 2 000 years ago commented that, "Humans are not affected by events but by the view they take of them." Ellis identifies patterns of faulty reasoning, including absolute thinking in which events are viewed in all-or-none terms such as "I must always do well." Overgeneralization involves drawing global conclusions on the basis of single events, for example, "I am never going to win a match." Catastrophization involves viewing minor concerns as disasters, for example, "Losing that match is the end of my career." In REBT, irrational beliefs are actively disputed and individuals learn to substitute more rational ways of thinking. It is interesting that Ellis (1994) provided an invited address to Division 47, Exercise and Sport Psychology, at the 1993 American Psychological Association convention. His presentation was concerned with "The Sport of Avoiding Sports and Exercise." He believes that those who avoid exercise and sport have a low frustration tolerance that may be combined with a fear of failing. He states that, "REBT helps them to discover and dispute their grandiose demands and absolutist musts" (p. 258). Ellis describes an intensive REBT program designed to help avoiders transform their inhibitions into healthy choices. In sport psychology, athletes are encouraged to restructure their self-talk and focus their attention on the task or process in a positive manner (e.g., Kirschenbaum, 1997; Rushall, 1984). It has been stated simply as "focus on the process and let the outcome take care of itself."

Imagery

Ninety-nine percent of Canadian athletes who participated in the 1984 Olympic Games indicated that they used imagery techniques to improve their performance (Orlick and Partington, 1988). Some of these athletes indicated that they used imagery techniques for up to 3 hours in preparation for competition. There is a difference between *imagery* and *mental rehearsal* (Jones, Hardy, & Gould, 1997). The latter is a sensory experience that is performed in the absence of external stimuli, whereas mental rehearsal is a technique that involves the use of imagery to mentally practise a skill.

A distinction is made between **internal** and **external imagery** (Mahoney and Avener, 1977). In external imagery, the individual is a third-person, passive, external observer of their actions. Internal imagery is a much more active experience, in which the individual imagines being inside their body experiencing a situation as close to reality as possible. Several explanations have been given for the mechanisms underlying the relationship between imagery and performance (Gould and Damarjian, 1996). The psychoneuromuscular theory suggests that imagery causes the actual motor pattern to be rehearsed and therefore practised. Symbolic learning believes that imagery provides the opportunity to symbolically practise an event. As one athlete said, "It felt like *déjà vu*, like I had done it before."

With regard to an imagery training program, Gould and Damarjian (1996) make several recommendations, which include the following: "Practise imagery on a regular basis, use all senses to enhance image vividness, use both internal and external perspectives, facilitate imagery through relaxation, use videotapes or audiotapes to enhance imagery skills, develop coping strategies through imagery, emphasize dynamic kinesthetic imagery, imagine in real time, use imagery in practise and competition" (p. 48). Reviews of the literature such as that of Feltz and Landers (1983) indicate that mental rehearsal is better than no practice, that the combination of mental rehearsal and physical practise is most effective, and that the effects are greater for cognitive as compared to motor tasks.

More recently, Driskell, Copper, and Moran (1994) carried out a meta-analysis of the literature and concluded that mental practice has a "positive and significant effect on performance" (p. 481). They acknowledge, however, that given that it is an effective strategy for improving performance, it is less effective than physical practice. They suggest that this makes it most appropriate for difficult or dangerous training situations, for situations in which opportunities for physical practise are minimized, and simply as a strategy for supplementing normal training routines.

Goal-Setting

The final psychological skill we will discuss in this section is goal-setting, a motivational strategy for improving performance. It also represents one of the most widely researched areas in the field, as considerable research in goal-setting in industrial and organizational fields has been applied to sports. The history of research on goal-setting provided by Locke and his colleagues, beginning with his important paper in 1968, has been influential. Several important consistencies emerged from this. These indicate that higher levels of performance are achieved through difficult compared to easy goals, specific goals compared to general goals or no goals, and a combination of both short-term and longterm goals (Locke, 1968; Locke and Latham, 1985; Locke and Latham, 1990).

Two different goal perspectives have been identified (Duda, 1992), **ego orientation** and **task orientation**. The former is focused on success and failure, with success often coming at the expense of others. Those people subscribing to the former like to win. The latter describes individuals who derive their satisfaction from the sense of competence they experience as they improve. Their focus is on effort and their *own* performance rather than that of others. These are not independent positions, and successful performers often make use of both of them (White & Duda, 1991).

Three different types of goals have been described in the literature (Hardy, Jones, & Gould, 1996). **Outcome goals** are concerned with the results or outcomes of events and usually involve comparisons to others. These goals might be expressed as a need to finish first in a race, with even second being equated to losing. **Performance goals** describe an outcome that can be achieved independently of others' performance; a novice marathoner may describe a desire to run his next race in under 4 hours. **Process goals** focus on specific processes that a performer will be concerned with during a performance. A tennis player may indicate that during a match he intends to run down every ball, get to the net whenever he can, and use a script to help manage his self-talk.

Weinberg (1996) provides a set of goal-setting principles based on his review of the relevant literature. They are, "Set specific goals, set realistic but challenging goals, set both long- and short-term goals, set goals for practise and competition, 'ink it, don't think it', develop goal-achievement strategies, set performance goals, set individual and team goals, provide support for goals, provide for goal evaluation" (p. 11).

This review of psychological skills training has focused on four of the basic skills that are fundamental to understanding the more complex issues involved in concerns such as attentional control, emotional control, confidence and self-efficacy, motivation, and coping with stress. For any one of us, a particular skill may have more relevance at a particular time than at another. What works for one individual may not work as well for another. As we discussed earlier, these are not skills unique to exercise and sport but rather extend into other domains; however, in the sport and exercise context, they can be useful in helping us to improve our performance and, most important, enjoy ourselves. All indications are that we are more likely to continue to engage in exercise and sport if we enjoy ourselves. When asked for the ten reasons why they play sports, children always indicate that their number one reason is to have "fun" , with winning usually occupying the number ten position.

ATHLETIC INJURY

The final issue we will consider in this chapter is of a more clinical nature and relates to the psychological consequences of injury in sport and exercise. Clearly, athletic injury is an event that occurs with an extremely high frequency. Most of us will remember an injury we experienced in the context of sport or exercise and could identify some of the psychological consequences of this event. We are also made very aware through the media of the injuries that regularly sideline our sports heroes. Sometimes these are acute and sometimes they are chronic. The physical and psychological impact of these injuries is usually minimal; however, at times they can be very serious, extremely costly, and even career threatening.

Ultimately, a particular individual's reaction to a sports injury is a complex issue and will depend on numerous factors. These include the nature and severity of the injury, the role and importance of sport in the individual's life, and the response of the individual's support network. For example, with regard to the latter issue athletes often state that the attention they receive from coaches and other support staff decreases dramatically when they are injured. Attention is given to those who can compete rather than those who can not. It is also the case that an injured individual can be a vicarious reminder of what can happen and that the uninjured do not want them around, as they find their presence disturbing. Those who are injured are also made painfully aware of what they are missing. One injury that has received considerable attention over the past few years is concussion. In some ways, it is as if we have suddenly realized how much a concussion can affect an individual's life. We will provide a

BOX 12-1 Concussion

Athletes often describe it as "having your bell rung", while to the health professional it is known as a **closed head injury** or **concussion.** With disturbing frequency we read in our newspapers of the athlete whose career has been threatened by a blow to the head. One of the authors noted that within a 1 week period, he read accounts in the sport pages of concussion affecting the performance, and even careers, of two NHL hockey players, an NFL quarterback, a major league baseball player, a world cup rugby player, and an NBA basketball player. The latter, after suffering a concussion during an NBA basketball game, stated, "The last thing I remember is checking into the game, then the next thing I remember is lying on the table and them asking me if I remember things. A long time elapsed between them. That's the scary part about it...that your mind can be altered like that" (Kingston, 1999).

Concussion is a bruising of the brain that represents a most serious sports injury. It can result in severe neurocognitive deficits, permanent disability, and even death. There is evidence that even mild concussion can result in neuropsychological impairments (Macciocchi et al., 1996). Concussions are commonly described according to two types. An **acceleration-deceleration injury** occurs when an immobile head is hit by a moving object or a moving head hits an immobile object. A **rotational injury** usually results from a blow to the side of the head. Another concern in concussion is **second-impact syndrome.** This results when an athlete who has suffered a concussion returns to activity too soon and receives another blow to the head, which can result in much greater trauma to the brain than that initially experienced. **Post-concussion syndrome** is a term frequently seen in the press today. This describes a set of symptoms such as memory problems, difficulties in concentration, and complaints such as headaches, dizziness, and irritability.

It is important to remember that concussions can be experienced without losing consciousness, and that there is no visible physical evidence of concussion. The usual signs and symptoms of concussion include: any period of loss of consciousness; confusion and inability to focus attention; disorientation; slurred or incoherent speech; delayed verbal and motor responses; inappropriate emotional behaviour; memory deficits; and lack of coordination. Other signs include complaints such as headaches, dizziness, ringing in the ears, nausea/vomiting, impaired vision, seeing stars, and sensitivity to light.

Three grades of concussion have been identified. A **Grade One** concussion does not involve a loss of consciousness, although the athlete may display transient confusion. The athlete should be taken out of the activity and examined for post-concussive symptoms. They can return to the activity if any abnormalities or symptoms have cleared within 15 minutes. A **Grade Two** concussion also does not involve a loss of consciousness; however, the concussion symptoms persist beyond the 15-minute period. The athlete should be taken out of the activity and not allowed to return. They should be seen the same day by a medical professional and should only return to their sport after 1 asymptomatic week and neurologic clearance by a physician. A **Grade Three** concussion involves any loss of consciousness, brief or prolonged. The athlete may need to be taken to hospital by ambulance if still unconscious or if there are other concerns such as neck pain. A neurologic evaluation is required initially and further assessment will be necessary to determine when the athlete can return to their sport. Multiple concussions of any grade will further complicate the recovery process. The decision to return to activity should always be based on a physician's evaluation.

Concussion represents a serious problem in the sport and exercise field. It is estimated that 24 000 individuals will experience a closed head injury within the next year in British Columbia and that 20 percent of these will be sports related (Iverson, 1998). With increasing public awareness of this problem, we have become more concerned to better understand the nature of concussion and, most importantly, to focus on the prevention of brain injury.

closer look at this potentially devastating injury to help us better understand the phenomenon and become more aware of issues related to treatment and prevention.

When individuals experience a sports injury, a wide range of emotions may be experienced, such as anger, disbelief, frustration, fear, anxiety, guilt, panic, loneliness, and depression. A number of models have been proposed to help us better understand the psychological processes associated with an athletic injury. They can be divided into essentially two different approaches, those that focus on stages of reaction and those that take a cognitive appraisal position. The former assumes that individuals will pass through a series of stages in the same order. They derive initially from the model developed by Kübler-Ross (1969) to explain the experience of death and dying. She described five stages an individual who is dying goes through: denial and isolation, anger, bargaining, depression, and acceptance. In this context, the injury is considered to be similar to death and, indeed, many who suffer a debilitating injury view it this way. This model has been adapted to sport by Astle (1986) and Lynch (1988), who provide strategies for assisting those who will be involved in the psychological rehabilitation of the injured person. The cognitive appraisal approach views an injury in the context of a stress and coping model (Brewer, 1994). An individual's emotional and behavioural responses to an injury will be determined by their personal appraisal of the event and their choice of coping strategies.

Brewer, Raalte, and Linder (1991) describe what they consider to be the primary responsibilities of a psychologist working with an injured athlete within a sports medicine context. The first involves an initial assessment of the individual's psychological status. The second is to facilitate, where necessary, communication between the physician and the athlete. The third is to provide the athlete with psychological skills to assist in the coping and rehabilitation process. These skills might include several we have discussed previously, such as relaxation training, goal-setting, imagery and mental rehearsal, and cognitive restructuring. The fourth responsibility of the psychologist is to facilitate and provide social support for the injured athlete. The psychologist may be involved in actively seeking the assistance of others to develop a support network. The role of the psychologist is being increasingly recognized as a crucial component in the intervention of injuries that occur in the context of sport and exercise.

We have come a long way in our discussion of sport and exercise and, as we bring this chapter to a close, it seems appropriate to return to our friend Peter. Time has passed for him as well—it has been 1 year since he began his rehabilitation program. He was asked to provide an update and the following is what he had to say.

CASE 12-2 Peter's Story: An Update

The main purpose of the atherosclerosis-reversal program is to show that over a 2-year period, artherosclerosis can be reversed. Changes must come from within. There must be a personal motivating factor that drives us to achieve some predetermined desired result. One of my personal challenges is to maintain a high level of fitness. This is easier said than done. I document my fitness routine daily. I identify what I do and for what duration. To help me stay motivated from an exercise point of view, I envision that my heart is a muscle like any other muscle, and that it can benefit from exercise. I see my heart getting stronger ever day. I have a picture in my mind of the heart—blood gushing through unrestricted. As mentioned, I measure my results daily. I compare to make sure I am progressing and I push a little harder if I feel I am slipping. My current body fat is now at 16 percent. The goal for someone my age is between 17 and 23 percent. My personal goal is 15 percent. I recently completed a stress test as a comparison to the test I had a year ago. The results have been very positive. The stress test involves walking on a treadmill in 3-minute intervals. At each interval, the speed is increased, as is the elevation. I have increased my time by close to 2 minutes. This is a significant improvement. My other objective results are excellent. For example, my blood pressure is 117 over 71 as compared to 140 over 90 a year ago. My resting heart rate is 68 beats per minute. My hip-to-waist ratio is 0.9. My weight has decreased by 30 pounds. I have been told that I now have the physical fitness level associated with someone in their thirties. This means more to me than anything else and proves that hard work pays off. I progress by continually measuring against my initial goals. I can then alter the course by stretching the objectives. I push myself as hard as I do because I believe there is a cure for my disease.

Most important, though, my mental outlook has improved. I keep abreast of new techniques and routines and challenge myself to experiment. A routine that never changes allows the muscles and mind to stagnate and stop growing. I continuously read, and discuss materials with friends at the gym. They provide me with the positive comments that encourage me to keep going. Make sure you keep feeding your good friendships. As with exercise, make sure the diet is also new and changing. It is too easy to slip back into old habits. I try to create a new menu every week that consists of low fat, low sugar items. I invite input from my family, as without their continuous support the program would not work. The goal of the program is to maintain a consumption of 2 000 calories each day, with a limit of 30 grams of fat per day. I have met this objective easily. The motivator here is purely ego. I get compliments as I have lost 30 pounds. When I receive compliments, I get even more motivated. I still experience some disappointments. This is a big challenge for me. When a goal is not met I review my progress to date, see where I fell short of the program, and take corrective actions. I will get there some day. There are times when I become so engrossed in the program that I lose focus on my family and friends. Every now and then I need a reality check. This comes primarily from my kids. They are my barometers. Remember that it is family first, health second, and that everything else is somewhere down the list. My wife has provided support that has allowed me to continue to improve. I thank her dearly for this. I will close by saying that the friendships I have developed, the support I have received from these people, has contributed more to my success than any one thing. I thank you all.

KEY TERMS

sport psychology
exercise psychology
physical activity
physical fitness
sport
active leisure
passive leisure
isometric exercise
isotonic exercise
isokinetic exercise
aerobic exercise
anaerobic exercise
self-efficacy
performance accomplishments
vicarious experience
verbal persuasion
emotional arousal
non-adherence
psychological skills
psychological methods
relaxation skills
self-talk
internal imagery
external imagery
ego orientation
task orientation
outcome goals
performance goals
process goals
closed head injury
concussion
acceleration-deceleration injury
rotational injury
second-impact syndrome
post-concussion syndrome
grade-one concussion
grade-two concussion
grade-three concussion

Chapter 13

HEALTH VIEWED FROM BROADER PERSPECTIVES

Chapter Outline

What is Medical Geography?

A Brief History of Medical Geography

Medical Geography Today

Methods in Medical Geography

Understanding Malaria from the Standpoint of Medical Geography

Key Questions

1. Generally, what are some of the other ways social scientists study health and health care?
2. What is epidemiology and how many different ways can we interpret epidemiological data?
3. What are some of the concepts central to the way sociologists view health and health care?
4. How do medical anthropologists collect data and what are their areas of study?
5. How can we best determine the relationship between health and the geographic location of the people we are studying?
6. What are some examples of Canadian university programs at which broader perspectives on health are studied?

When Rose Wong's father was diagnosed with prostate cancer, she decided to make a study of the disease. She learned that the incidence of prostate cancer has risen rather dramatically in the last 10 years, and she wanted to know why that was. Concerning her father's treatment, she was pleasantly surprised to find that the health care system in their province was well-coordinated. At each step of his treatment, the health care professionals seemed well aware of what Rose's father had been through and was about to go through. She came to believe that this level of organization and understanding actually saved lives.

From the time of his diagnosis, it became clear that there were many other things to consider besides Mr. Wong's prostate gland. There was a local support group, providing advice, information, and an opportunity to meet with others who were dealing with the disease. And there were language and cultural issues to consider. Rose's father was much more comfortable speaking Cantonese than English. Also, there were important family rules to take into account. As busy as Rose was with her own life, she had a clear obligation to help her father with transportation and translation, since her mother didn't drive and didn't speak English very well.

There were difficult times during treatment, when Mr. Wong felt weak and confused regarding what was being done and why. There was also the worry that the cancer would spread. However, the Wong family coped quite well, drawing strength from their family and a health care system that is well structured and available to all.

In Chapter 1, we introduced the biopsychosocial approach to the understanding of health. Everything we have introduced subsequently reflects that approach. Health must be understood from microscopic and macroscopic perspectives. Back in Chapter 1, we introduced Alan, who had suffered a heart attack. When we asked questions regarding the cause of his heart attack, the answers came from a variety of levels. There was his blocked artery, his personality, his lifestyle, his culture, and even the economic ideology that supports high-fat food. In the current chapter, we are going to focus our lens at the macroscopic level, looking at culture, environment, and society. To do this, we will introduce medical anthropology, medical geography, and medical sociology.

These are the broadest versions of the social component of the biopsychosocial approach. They are vital because health psychologists must develop a facility for multidisciplinary analysis. When one of the authors of this text started doing research in a large suburban hospital in the Greater Vancouver area, he discovered that one-third of the patients were Indo-Canadians and that most of these were traditional Sikhs. Did this matter? Of course it did. At the time, the author was doing research on the effects of hospital visits and was working in the maternity department (Poole & Ting, 1995). Indo-Canadian patients were getting more than twice as many visitors as other patients were getting. Having a baby is very much a cultural experience. Very quickly, the people conducting the study realized that they were doing work that was as much anthropological as it was psychological.

This brings us to our opening example, Rose Wong and her father. Take a moment to think about all the different levels of analysis featured in that example. There is the family, which is, in many ways, a culturally defined institution. There is the health care system, which is defined by a country's political ideology, which, in this case, favours socialized medicine. There are economic issues, since this system is expensive. There are organizational aspects, which means the system must have a hierarchy and a good means of communication. And, of course, there is the geographic environment. As Rose investigates possible causes of prostate cancer, she may well find that many researchers believe the rising incidence of all cancers is linked to environmental toxins.

It is because of all these factors that anyone studying health psychology must also know something about bigger pictures — geography, sociology, and anthropology. Indeed, the list does not stop there. Economics, history, and many other disciplines in the social sciences and humanities provide valuable insights into people's health and the health care system. We begin our exploration by introducing **epidemiology**, which literally means the study of epidemics. Today, it refers to many health-related statistics that chart rates and locations of occurrence, from accidents to diseases.

EPIDEMIOLOGY

We have said that epidemiology is the study of incidence rates and locations of health-related phenomena. Epidemiologists chart *patterns* of health and disease (primarily disease) across populations and geographic areas, studying the origin and distribution of health problems (Cockerham, 1998). It is truly biopsychosocial in nature. People working in the field include everything from sociologists to physicians to meteorologists (for such things as air pollution data). Psychologists also work with epidemiological data.

The Language of Epidemiology

To do their work, epidemiologists often start with a single case then trace back to its starting point. From there, they determine how widespread the problem has become. They then try to identify factors shared by all people with the problem. The goal is to identify causes so the problem can be either eliminated or at least controlled. In doing this work, epidemiologists use terminology that health psychologists should get to know.

For example, a **case** is one instance of the problem. The **incidence** is the number of new cases of the problem in a set period of time. For example, if an epidemiologist says that there were 30 cases of X reported in the past 2 weeks, that would be called an incidence rate. Epidemiologists use incidence rates to determine whether a problem is on the rise or if it is waning. The word "outbreak", as in an "outbreak of influenza", often refers to incidence rates. On the other hand, **prevalence** refers to the total number of cases that exist at any given time, including existing and new cases. **Point prevalence** refers to prevalence at a given point in time. **Lifetime prevalence** refers to the total number of people who have ever had the problem, even if the problem went away or if they died from it. Cancer rates are often reported in terms of lifetime prevalence, which presents the proportion of people who have ever had the disease. Cancer rates are often reported as proportions of the population, for example, the number of cases found per 100 000 people.

The Statistics of Epidemiology

Epidemiologists rely heavily on ratios and proportions to report their findings. The most basic ratio is as follows:

$$\frac{\text{Cases}}{\text{Population}}$$

In other words, epidemiologists try to ascertain the total number of cases of a given problem in an entire population. They then convert this into a *proportion* by multiplying that ratio times 100 000, if that is the proportion they are using.

Epidemiologists call this a **crude rate** because it is population wide. However, it is more common to report **age-specific rates**, which, as the term implies, present the prevalence of a certain problem for a particular age range. One of the most common age-specific rates is **infant mortality rate**, which is the number of deaths of all infants under 1 year of age. Infant mortality rate is calculated as follows:

$$\text{Infant mortality rate} = \frac{\text{Total number of infant deaths in 1 year}}{\text{Number of live births}} \times 100\,000$$

The Steps Involved in Epidemiological Research

The first step in epidemiological research is to establish a pattern of the problem and identify **agents** (Cockerham, 1998). These are the means by which a problem spreads. There are five types of agent: biological, nutritional, chemical, physical, and social/behavioural. Table 13.1 presents these agents along with the academic discipline most often associated with each.

TABLE 13-1 Agents of Disease and Related Disciplines

Agent	Example	Discipline
Biological	Bacteria	Medicine
Nutritional	Saturated fats	Medical anthropology Health psychology Nutritional sciences
Chemical	Air/water pollutants	Medical geography
Physical	Climate and geography	Medical geography
Social/behavioural	Socioeconomic status and lifestyle	Medical sociology Medical anthropology Health psychology

After an agent has been identified, epidemiologists look for **hosts**. These are the carriers of the agents. In human disease, human hosts are those people who are must susceptible to a given agent. Epidemiologists can determine if a given agent is travelling through a certain age group, or perhaps through people who have been in a certain area, or who have possibly consumed contaminated water (see Box 13.1).

BOX 13-1 John Snow: The First Epidemiologist

In 1854, John Snow traced the spread of a deadly and prevalent disease in London known as *cholera*. He discovered that cholera was transmitted through the water supply. From this discovery, he traced much of the contaminated water back to a source called the Broad Street pump. The pump was closed down, and that brought an end to one of London's worst health epidemics.

The story of John Snow illustrates the three main steps in epidemiology. First, he identified the *agent*, which was bacterial. Second, he found the *vehicle*, which was the water supply and then those who consumed that water passing the bacteria to one another. These were the people who were the *hosts*. Finally, he proposed a control measure, the closing of the Broad Street pump, which stopped the problem by affecting the vehicle and hosts, thus containing the agent.

There are other ways that agents are transmitted in addition to using hosts. For example, there are **vectors**. These are living organisms that can transfer an agent from one host to another (Prescott, Harley, and Klein, 1999). A good example of a vector is the *Anopheles* mosquito, which carries malaria. Also, there are **vehicles**. These are non-living media involved in the transmission of an agent (Prescott, Harley, and Klein, 1999) (see the example in Box 13.1 of London's water supply, which was the vehicle for transmission of a disease known as cholera). Biologists and epidemiologists describe transmission by way of vehicles as being water-borne, food-borne, or air-borne, depending upon the vehicle. For example, tuberculosis adheres to dust and then becomes air-borne (Prescott, Harley, and Klein, 1999).

The third and final step epidemiologists employ is to propose strategies for control of the agent. Then, the steps start again to see if there are other agents and hosts or if the control measures have worked. Of course, proposed control measures don't always get implemented. If the agent is an effluent being dumped into a river and there are no legislative measures to stop this from happening, the profit motive of the company doing the dumping will prevail over the will of the epidemiological recommendation.

The Four Eras of Epidemiology

In Box 13.1, we describe the early epidemiological work of John Snow, who worked in London in 1854. From that date to the present, epidemiology has gone through four distinct eras, as defined by the types of agents and hosts that have become prevalent (Susser & Susser, 1996, cited in Cockerham, 1998). As we describe these eras, think about how health promotion programs would change in each.

The first era was called the **sanitation era**, which spanned the early part of the nineteenth century. This was the era of John Snow. One way to confirm that bacteria were the cause of the world's plagues was to trace the spread of those plagues. It was the poor who were most likely to be hosts, due in large part to their unsanitary living conditions. Epidemiologists were able to contradict the notion that the upper class were somehow less susceptible by virtue of their superiority. The truth was that they did not have to live near open sewers and drainage systems.

The second era was the **infectious disease era**, which spanned the late nineteenth and early twentieth centuries. You may remember our discussion of changing patterns of illness in Chapter 1. We pointed out that the leading causes of death in 1900 were respiratory diseases (influenza and pneumonia) (Sexton, 1979). The hosts in this era were people who were susceptible to bacteria and viruses that were spread by human contact.

The era of the latter part of the twentieth century has been called the **chronic disease era**. As we have pointed out on a number of occasions throughout this book, it is lifestyle that increases people's susceptibility to these diseases. The era we are moving into in the twenty-first century is called the **ecoepidemiological era**. As the name implies, the primary agents in this era are chemical in nature. Now and in the future, epidemiologists will be tracking the toxins in our environment as sources of health problems.

Tracing the Spread of AIDS: An Example of Epidemiology in Action

Now that you have been introduced to the methods of epidemiology, we'll turn to an application of those methods in the study of one of the most serious health problems of our century — acquired immune deficiency syndrome (AIDS). The first known cases of AIDS began emerging in New York, San Francisco, and Los Angeles in 1979 (Cockerham, 1998). These cases attracted attention, in part, because they were defined by rare forms of cancer, such as Kaposi's sarcoma, and a particular type of pneumonia called *Pneumocystis carinii*. By 1981, physicians' reports were coming into the Centers for Disease Control in Atlanta, Georgia, and epidemiologists went to work identifying hosts and agents (Cockerham, 1998). At this time, the *prevalence* was about 50 cases. However, through the early 1980s, the *incidence* rate began to skyrocket. Within 3 years, the number of cases went from 50 to over 4 900 in the United States. By 1995, the number had risen to over 500 000 (Cockerham, 1998).

At first, it was thought that the *agent* was a drug used by some gay men to enhance sexual experience, but interview data ruled this out when it revealed that men who used the drug were not infected with AIDS (Cockerham, 1998). Then, when a number of intravenous drug users and one transfusion patient (a baby in San Francisco) contracted AIDS, the search for an agent became biological; namely epidemiologists started suspecting a virus. The tracing of sexual partners as *hosts* supported this hypothesis.

This tracing of sexual partners of those first showing symptoms of AIDS in North America led, eventually, to one person. This was the so-called "patient zero", a flight attendant from Canada named Gaetan Dugas (Taylor, 1999). After being located, Dugas estimated that he had had 2 500 sexual partners in the 10 years prior to being identified (Taylor, 1999).

An analysis of the AIDS epidemic in central Africa, where five to twenty percent of adults in cities are infected (Cockerham, 1998), illustrates how sociological and anthropological factors explain epidemiological data. In Africa, unlike North America, AIDS is spread primarily through sexual intercourse among heterosexuals. The economy of central Africa is such that there are many male migrant workers (Cockerham, 1998). Their movement from place to place facilitates the spread of the virus. In general, women in central Africa do not have the power to demand condom use or abstinence. From this analysis, we can see that economic, geographic, social, and cultural factors explain the proliferation of AIDS in central Africa (Cockerham, 1998).

In Canada, the total number of confirmed AIDS cases from the onset of the epidemic to December 31, 1998 was 16 236. During that time, there were a total of 43 347 positive HIV tests. These cases were reported to the Laboratory Centre for Disease Control (LCDC) at Health Canada from all provinces and territories. The good news is that since 1993, the number of AIDS cases reported to the LCDC has steadily declined. In 1998, the annual number of reported AIDS cases was 279, compared to 1 751 in 1993 (Laboratory Centre for Disease Control, Health Canada web site, 1999, www.hc-sc.gc.ca).

The epidemiological picture is quite different, however, among Canada's aboriginal population. When delay of reporting is taken into account, epidemiological data show a sharp increase in AIDS cases among Canada's aboriginal persons, according to the LCDC (1998). The LCDC also reports the proportion of AIDS cases in Canada attributed to aboriginal persons has risen from 2 percent in 1989 to 10 percent in 1996/97. You may remember that in Chapter 11 we reported that aboriginal persons with AIDS also tend to be younger than their non-aboriginal counterparts, with 30 percent of aboriginal people with AIDS being under the age of 30 years, compared to 19 percent of non-aboriginals with AIDS being under the age of 30 years (Health Canada web site). In addition, the proportion of women with AIDS is greater in our aboriginal population (16% versus 7%).

What conclusions can we draw from these statistics? Certainly, we know that it is premature to relax our attempts at health promotion regarding AIDS and, in particular, with Canada's aboriginal population.

Other Uses of Epidemiological Statistics

Epidemiological data can also uncover positive outcomes. Take, for example, the story of Roseto, Pennsylvania. In the 1970s, heart attack mortality rates for men in the United States were 3.5 per 1 000 people (Plotnik, 1989). However, in Roseto, only one man in 1 000 died of a heart of attack. This could not be attributed to diet, smoking, or exercise, none of which was particularly impressive for Rosetan males. The difference was in the closeness of the community and the cohesiveness of the families (Greenberg, 1978). In fact, when men moved away from Roseto, their incidence of heart attack mortality rose (Plotnik, 1989). Thirty years worth of prospective research has documented the gradual breakdown of Roseto's cohesion and the concomitant rise in heart attack mortality (Wolf, 1997). This epidemiological work underscores the importance of *social support* in health.

How can we best interpret epidemiological data? Are the trends identified by such studies attributable to biological agents? Peculiarities of the geography? Cultural practices? Differences in socioeconomic status? Geopolitical events? Behavioural or social factors? The answer is often "Yes" to all of these possibilities. As such, epidemiology serves as a perfect introduction to health-related substrates in the other social sciences. Let's look at some of those now.

MEDICAL SOCIOLOGY

Sociology is "the study of social causes and consequences of behaviour" (Cockerham, 1998, p. 1). Sociologists study groups, institutions, and society. According to Clarke (1996), **medical sociology** is "the study of the ways the institutionalized medical system constructs what it deems to be illness out of what is recognized as signs and symptoms, and constitutes its response to such 'illness' through the treatments it prescribes" (p. 16). The term "medical sociology" was used as early as 1894 by Charles McIntire (Cockerham, 1998).

An interesting distinction has been made between sociology *in* medicine and sociology *of* medicine (Strauss, 1957). The term **sociology in medicine** refers to sociological research that has been motivated by a particular medical problem. In this context, sociologists work *within* the health care setting, conducting research in areas such as epidemiology and health promotion, trying to explain epidemiological data and affect changes to those trends. The **sociology of medicine** refers to a sociological critique of a health care system, perhaps as it acts as an agent of social control or as a propagator of an ideology such as capitalism.

While this is an interesting distinction that helps people outside the field of sociology understand some of the different work medical sociologists do, it is also problematic. This is because, in modern medical sociology, the "of/in" distinction has become necessarily blurred

(Cockerham, 1998). This blurring is in response to the argument that, to work effectively *in* a health care system, one must also *analyze* it in terms of its effectiveness, strengths, and weaknesses. Whether the same sociologists who work within the health care system can be expected to objectively critique it is an open question.

Health psychologists, who tend to study health-related phenomena on a more individual level, can work well with medical sociologists. For example, in Chapter 3 we explored psychoneuroimmunology (PNI), which is the study of the ways in which our psychological states might affect our health. Research in PNI reveals physiological reasons why stress can be unhealthy. It focuses on the cellular level; specifically, the workings of the immune system. But what about some of the causes of that stress? Knowing what you know about PNI, would it surprise you to learn that illness tends to follow unemployment trends? Probably not. However, as soon as we introduce trends of this type into the analysis, we are no longer working at a microscopic level. Now we are working at the level of medical sociology.

Why is there a moratorium on silicone breast implants? Is it because of a biomedical discovery or because of mass social action? Medical sociologists would say that this development is due more to the latter than the former (Clarke, 1996). In her book, *Health, Illness, and Medicine in Canada*, Juanne Clarke (1996) applies prominent sociological theories to health and health care. A close look at some of those applications will provide us with a good overview of what medical sociology is all about.

Talcott Parsons' Notion of the Sick Role

Sociologists who study social structures and institutions tend to adopt a theoretical perspective called **structural functionalism**. According to this perspective, society is best understood by analyzing its systems and the way they interrelate. Sociologists adopting this perspective would call something like unemployment rates **social facts**. They would argue that most of these social facts stem from social structure. For example, employment may be related to economic structures like capitalism or a government's legislation.

One offshoot of this analysis that is quite relevant to health is the study of *roles*. Roles are sets of behaviours, attributes, and expectations that are institutionally defined. For example, the institution of *family* yields roles of *father, mother, daughter, son,* and so on. According to well-known sociologist Talcott Parsons (1951), the medical institution has created something called the **sick role**. People who legitimately adopt the sick role are temporarily exempt from their other roles. This is because they could not perform those roles adequately if forced to do so, and so the sick role was created to prevent social breakdown. We say that people adopting the sick role are *temporarily* exempt because the role is defined in such a way that people can't opt out of their other roles indefinitely and keep the social organization functioning. Therefore, one defining characteristic of the sick role is that it can't be assumed indefinitely. Anyone who tries to do so will be given a different label, like malingerer, for example.

Roles carry with them certain rights and duties. People adopting the sick role have two duties. First, they must be trying to get well. Second, they should seek technically competent help and cooperate with the prescribed regimen. If someone were to shirk one of these duties, he or she would lose the rights of the sick role. There are two of these. First, as we have said, a person adopting the sick role is temporarily exempt from other responsibilities. Second, the person is not responsible for his or her condition, and so can't be blamed for his or her incapacitation.

Parsons' notion of the sick role has come under some criticism. For example, the reality is that the extent to which a person is held responsible for his or her condition varies by condition. Also, with today's emphasis on health promotion and healthy lifestyles, people are being held more personally responsible for their health. This should mean that fewer people can legitimately adopt the sick role. Also, some people associate certain diseases with a person's moral worth. Perhaps the best example of this is HIV/AIDS (Altman, 1986). This would mean that people with such diseases would have a more difficult time adopting the sick role. Indeed, it is generally the case that people with socially stigmatized diseases (such as sexually transmitted diseases) are not afforded sick-role status (Clarke, 1996).

You will remember that one "duty" is that people must be trying to get well to be given sick-role status. But what about those people who may want to get well but cannot? These people must make longterm adaptations and in so doing fit into another role, such as "disabled", or "impaired", or "chronically ill."

Sociologists refer to a person's **master status**. This is the status that reflects the person's most prominent position in society. This may stem from such things as his or her occupation, family role, or position in the community. A person's disease status should not become his or her master status, because the sick-role status normally intervenes. However, because AIDS is stigmatizing and chronic, people with this disease often find that their disease status does become their master status. Disease status overwhelms other aspects of their identity, and this can make coping with the disease all the more difficult.

Criticism of the sick role construct has also been levelled at the duty concerning cooperation with technically competent help. This could mean that to be granted sick-role status, a person must accept the biomedical model. Sociologists call this model **allopathic medicine**, which is a form of medicine that attempts to cure sickness by creating conditions in the body that oppose the disease (Clarke, 1996). According to this duty, people seeking what are currently called complementary or alternative treatment would not be afforded the sick role. If allopathic medicine becomes the gatekeeper of sick-role status, then the already powerful medical establishment becomes even more powerful.

Indeed, from the perspective of structural functionalism, the medical establishment is seen as an agent of social control. There are at least two forms that this control takes. First, allopathic medicine dictates the conferring of sick-role status. Second, from this perspective, sickness is viewed as a form of deviation from the norm, and sick people need to be brought back to that norm. In what often is called Western society, the medical establishment holds the responsibility for doing this. As an indication of this, think of conditions that are viewed today as illnesses that were once considered to be religious or legal transgressions (hint: some of the best examples come from psychiatry).

Conflict Theory and the Righting of Injustices

Another school of thought in sociology argues that structures do not simply exist; rather, they exist in *conflict*. This is an important assumption of **conflict theory**. This theory has a long history in medical sociology. As early as 1845, Fredrich Engels, a collaborator with Karl Marx, made the point that inequality in living conditions and the emergence of capitalism in England had negative effects on people's health. To maximize profits, companies paid their workers poorly, forcing them to live in slums. These living conditions became breeding grounds for infectious diseases such as typhoid. Conflict theory, then, would be very useful when trying to understand socioeconomic differences in health status.

Modern multinational corporations have been accused of exploitation in a manner that is not dissimilar. Clarke (1996) points out that the largest-ever cluster of anencephalic babies (babies born without a brain) has been found recently just across the border in Mexico along the Rio Grande. Clarke also points out that toxic waste dumps by multinational corporations in that area exceed United States standards by up to 53 000 times. Other companies may take advantage of less stringent regulations regarding the use of pesticides, thus affecting the food supply for all of North America.

Proponents of conflict theory might also argue that the state tends to deflect responsibility for ill health away from political ideology or governmental responsibility and focus it on the individual. Health then becomes a "commodity with a certain value in the marketplace" (Clarke, 1996, p. 28). These theorists would argue that research conducted by and funded by institutions within that marketplace, like pharmaceutical companies, cannot be expected to produce findings that are self-critical, hence the need for health-related research from the social sciences and humanities. Later in this chapter, we will describe some university-based programs doing this type of research in Canada.

Symbolic Interactionism: Uncovering Subjective Meaning in Health and Health Care

Sociologists also take a more microscopic look at social factors by analyzing the interactions between people and by interviewing people to determine the meaning they attach to events. When these researchers adopt the perspective of **symbolic interactionism**, they are assuming that people's interpretations of their interactions and the events of their lives go well beyond the actual words used or, in the case of health-related events, the diagnosis they are given. As is the case with much of sociology, another assumption here is that reality is **socially constructed** rather than objective. In other words, we piece together our version of the world by interacting with others and construing our own interpretation of that world.

Medical sociologists using symbolic interactionism often use **transcript analysis** in their research. As the term implies, they record interactions then transcribe them to paper. They are also interested in the pauses between turns, which can be very meaningful in an interaction between a physician and a patient. Another research method is the in-depth interview. For example, a person with arthritis may be interviewed at length to determine the meaning the person attaches to having that illness. It may be associated with aging, frustration, loss of control, or being pitied by others. The possibilities are numerous. The point is that it is the *person with the illness* who determines the meaning.

Researchers adopting this approach make a distinction between disease and illness. **Disease** refers to the physical pathology. **Illness** refers to the subjective experience of having that pathology. From this perspective, it is possible for two people to have the same disease but different illnesses. This distinction is rarely made in medical settings. It is the *illness* that sociologists try to understand. For example, two people with very similar tissue damage from a heart attack may have very different subjective experiences as a result. One may be motivated to re-prioritize his life and make the most of each day; another might live each successive day in fear and become an invalid unnecessarily.

Psychologists who use the theory of reasoned action, introduced in Chapter 1, may do well to consider the tenets of symbolic interaction. You may remember that one important component of the theory of reasoned action is social norms — that collection of beliefs regarding what other people would do and would want us to do. Sociologists would remind us that, by interacting with others to establish these social norms, we are also constructing a social reality. The person then decides on a course of action based on this constructed meaning of the problem.

Feminist Theory as Applied to Health and Health Care

In Chapter 8, we discussed gender issues related to health care, specifically from the perspective of the practitioner. We could have adopted a more sociological perspective on those issues by applying **feminist theory**. In terms of health care, feminist theory focuses on at least three important topics. First, it makes salient the fact that women's health concerns are both biologically and socially different from men's. For example, stress-related medical conditions are different for women because the causes of their stress can be different. Women's stress is more likely to stem from **role strain**, in which a woman is expected to perform two or more roles that compete for her time and, in addition, may be in conflict with one another. This is compounded by the social fact that women still find themselves in subdominant positions, with little control compared to men.

A second topic concerns the fact that socially constructed meanings of health experiences have historically been male dominated. For example, one measure of the seriousness of an illness is the number of days a person misses from work. This is fairly easy to assess if that work takes place outside the home and is salaried. On the other hand, "days missed" are harder to quantify when the work is being done in the home. Traditionally, this situation has applied to women more than to men. More to the point, women may well argue that, when it comes to tasks like child-rearing, there is no such thing as a "day missed", regardless of one's health.

Third, we know that the health care system has been male dominated. This can make it more difficult for women to find practitioners who can empathize with and legitimize their health concerns. Feminists have been vocal in their attempts to raise awareness regarding these three issues and to change the health care system accordingly. As a result, feminist theory has had a tangible impact on health care and, indeed, on health psychology.

As we mentioned in Chapter 8, there has been a "feminization" of the medical profession brought about, in part, by growing numbers of female practitioners. This trend has engendered a greater emphasis on prevention than cure. In addition, more attention is being paid to the feelings of the patient. Symbolic interactionists with a feminist background might say that by allowing patients to express their feelings, practitioners are learning more about the subjective *meaning* patients ascribe to their conditions. At this point, it appears that female practitioners are more inclined to explore emotion-related aspects of health with their patients than male practitioners (Roter & Hall, 1998). The difference between males and females in terms of the exploration of emotions related to health is not attributed to assumptions that females are "more emotional." Rather, it a result of females being better at talking about emotions than men are. Sociologists would say that this difference is the product of institutional expectations regarding roles.

While feminist theory is relatively new compared to other theoretical perspectives in sociology, women's contributions to our understanding of the sociology of medicine are not. In fact, the first woman to graduate from an American medical school, Elizabeth Blackwell, wrote on medicine and society in 1902 (Cockerham, 1998).

Summary

Now that you have been introduced to medical sociology, think of the ways in which health psychologists and medical sociologists can collaborate. In what ways are the two similar? In what ways are they different? Clearly, they share a mutual concern for the improvement of health, as the World Health Organization defines health — not just the absence of disease, but the ability to live a life of reasonable quality. We hope that you can appreciate how sociologists and psychologists differ in their **unit of analysis**. For psychologists, it is the individual, for sociologists, it is people in groups, organizations, and societies. This isn't to say, of course, that psychologists aren't interested in social phenomena. However, the "bottom line" for psychologists tends to be how these phenomena affect the individual.

Medical sociologists and health psychologists can collaborate very effectively in the area of health promotion. While psychologists know things about attitude formation and persuasion, sociologists know things about demographic trends. Both are needed to fashion an effective program in health promotion. We move now to another potential partner for the health psychologist, the medical anthropologist.

MEDICAL ANTHROPOLOGY

It is a penetrating glimpse into the obvious to state that health beliefs and health behaviours are influenced by culture. In fact, we could go so far as to say that health beliefs are cultural beliefs. Activity levels, diet, and medical practice are dictated by cultural norms. The question isn't whether there is a connection between culture and health, the questions are much more complex. How do different cultures approach health issues? What can we learn from other cultures in this regard? How can we fashion a health care system in Canada that takes cultural differences into account? These are the questions of **medical anthropology**, which is the study of culture and health.

In the example that opened this chapter, we met Mr. Wong, who had recently been diagnosed with prostate cancer. We learned that Mr. Wong's family was very important in this story, and that the members of that family had strong and clear obligations regarding Mr. Wong's experience with the disease and all it entailed. The role that a family plays in cases such as these is very much dictated by cultural norms. While sociologists might be interested in the subjective meaning a person places on a disease experience, anthropologists are interested in how that meaning is defined by one's cultural affiliation.

Of course, anthropologists do not just study the cultural experiences of people who come to their countries. They also have a long history of travelling around the world to study different cultures. From these studies, anthropologists have learned about a wide variety of health practices and beliefs (Pelto & Pelto, 1997). By studying the health and health habits of different cultures, anthropologists have learned that certain diseases common to North America, such as heart disease and certain cancers, are virtually unheard of in other parts of the world. With this knowledge, we can learn about the causes of disease and ways to prevent them.

In the mid-twentieth century, medical anthropologists were documenting medical practices in other cultures, but they did not attempt to use that knowledge to solve health problems across cultures (Hill, 1991). The emphasis at that time was on the extent to which Western medicine was encroaching on non-Western cultures and how, in spite of this, some non-Western cultures persisted in what was then called non-scientific beliefs. Research at this time was descriptive in nature, and researchers stayed away from making applications of their findings. Then, after World War II, applied anthropology came into prominence as a way of solving problems in areas such as nutrition and international aid (Hill, 1991). In these contexts, researchers were looking at ways in which indigenous peoples consumed Western medical services. The goal here wasn't to learn from other cultures so much as it was to help people from non-Western cultures reduce the incidence of disease.

In this way, medical anthropologists were helping medical practitioners spread knowledge around the non-Western world. More recently, medical anthropologists have been studying medical institutions as cultures in and of themselves. A good example of this was discussed in Chapter 8 when we introduced Sinclair's account of medical school (Sinclair, 1997).

Ethnography: The Principle Research Tool of Medical Anthropology

One of the best ways to develop an appreciation for medical anthropology is to look at the ways in which anthropologists gather their data. The primary method is called **ethnography**. It is a research method intended to provide considerable detail. The objective of ethnography is to create portraits that are as complete and accurate as possible. Of course, these portraits are usually of cultures. As such, ethnography requires immersion within a culture and exhaustive data collection. Ethnographic data may be quantitative, but are more likely to be qualitative in nature.

Ethnography takes on three main forms (Trotter, 1991). These are direct observation, participation in life experience, and in-depth interviewing. The first two forms are often combined to become **participant observation**. This is a technique that is used in a number of social science disciplines. As the term implies, it involves *becoming a member* of the group being observed. The advantages are twofold. First, a skilled participant observer will earn the trust of the people being observed. As we will see later in this section, trust is an essential component of ethnographic research. Second, by participating, the researcher can gain first-hand experience. To illustrate these advantages, imagine being in another country and being invited to an important dinner. Could you learn about that dinner without eating any of the food? Perhaps, but not nearly as much as if you actually *ate* it. Also, what would your hosts think of you if you declined to eat what they had prepared? Would they trust you and let you into their confidence? Not likely.

In medical anthropology, however, it can be difficult to participate, especially if you are studying a hospital culture. You may remember from our discussion of the psychology of hospital stays in Chapter 6, we actually adopted an anthropological approach when we introduced the hospital as a distinct culture. From this perspective, one good way to learn about that culture is through ethnography — observation and interview. This can't be done in a day. To fully understand a culture (and a hospital is no exception) anthropologists recommend spending at least 1 year in that setting (Hill, 1991).

Perhaps one of the most fascinating things about anthropology, and that is particularly relevant to medical anthropology, is that it is the study of cultures both very distant from the anthropologist's own experience *and* those close to home. Because of this, anthropologists attempt to get to know distant cultures as though they were their own, and they also study their own cultures as if they were new to them. This is what anthropologists mean when they say they must make the *strange familiar* and the *familiar strange*. Medical anthropologists who study hospitals must start by making the familiar strange.

There are a number of approaches anthropologists can take when they observe and interview (Trotter, 1991). They can be **passive** and remain completely "arm's length"; they can be **adaptive** and try to fit in without drawing attention to themselves; they can be **interactive** by trying to become a communicating member of the group they are studying; or they can be **intrusive** and have an effect on the group they are studying. All four of these approaches apply to the work of medical anthropologists, whether they are studying hospitals, medical schools, or health practices of other cultures.

Let's look at some examples of how these approaches may manifest themselves in actual research. In the mid-1970s, Michael Agar published what was called a street ethnography of drug use. In this work, urban street life was the culture under study. To do this, Agar had to live on the street, become adaptive for his own well-being, interact with street drug users, and probably collect data at times that changed some aspects of street life for a while. Agar (1976) pointed out that dyadic relationships (i.e., between two people) are either symmetrical or asymmetrical. Asymmetrical relationships are what he calls one-up/one-down. Most street drug users are in the one-down position in relation to dealers and others in society. When Agar entered the street drug culture, he entered one-down, as a learner among the users. Gradually, he became even-up in his relationships with them as he learned the ways of the street culture.

Contrast this with a psychologist's approach to this work. This might involve surveys or individual interviews that might or might not be conducted on the street. Medical anthropologists would argue that the only way to truly learn about street drug use is to get close to that experience. Clearly, this isn't easy work. In fact, handbooks for anthropologists (medical or otherwise) often begin with advice regarding personal comfort and safety (e.g., Hill, 1991).

Important Steps in Ethnographic Research

Obviously, the first steps in conducting ethnographic research are to define the problem or objectives and make plans regarding basic necessities (Trotter, 1991). For example, an ethnographer must secure permission to enter another culture. This applies to hospital-based research as well as to the study of other cultures. There is some challenging political work to be done to secure permission to intrude on a hospital unit for an extended period of time, especially if the staff feel they are being judged. The medical anthropologist can assure them that, though they are being studied, they are not being judged. However, this isn't always as reassuring as it might be, considering the person who sanctioned the study (probably a hospital administrator) may be very interested in the results of the study. In this regard, the challenges faced by medical anthropologists are not unlike those of health psychologists doing hospital-based research. You may remember that we discussed these in Chapter 2, when we introduced research methodology.

Once permission has been secured and other details have been ironed out, the next step is what anthropologists call **field entry** (Trotter, 1991). This is when the medical anthropologist actually shows up and starts collecting data. Field entry can be difficult because anthropologists are deviants in their own research milieu. They must begin very carefully and "gently", beginning with what anthropologists call **social mapping** (Trotter, 1991). Social mapping involves "charting the waters" before full-scaled intrusion takes place. Social mapping usually takes two forms, observation and homework. The former is straightforward enough. It implies that the researcher must be passive before intrusive, and try to learn about relationships and rules by watching. Homework refers to early interviews and reading that give the medical anthropologist a sense of such things as the chain of command, the unwritten rules, and the types of questions that can and can't be asked.

As an example of social mapping, imagine doing research in a maternity department of a large urban hospital. Among the nursing staff, there is a head nurse and another nurse who is second in command. The head nurse takes great pride in the professionalism of her staff and isn't afraid to use her authority to maintain high standards. In fact, no significant decision is made in the department without her approval. As a medical anthropologist studying the birth experiences of patients from various cultures, would you have to put in valuable time establishing a rapport with this head nurse? Of course.

And then there is the second-in-command. It turns out that this nurse has a marvelous manner with patients, such that, if she suggests to a patient that she take part in your study, the chances are very good the patient will. Another ally? Again, of course. We could complicate this hypothetical scenario by saying that the head nurse and second-in-command battle for power in the department, but since this is your first ethnography we won't. The point here is that the process of getting to know all of these social facts is what social mapping in hospital-based medical anthropology is all about.

Once the medical anthropologist has done adequate social mapping, he or she must then decide whom to interview to find out what the culture is like. Anthropologists call these people **informants**. The term may conjure up underground police work, but that is not a particularly apt comparison. This is because the anthropologist does not make value judgments about the behaviour being observed or the information being gleaned.

Informant selection, as it is called, can be difficult. This is because the medical anthropologist is trying to find someone who is typical, articulate, and informed (Trotter, 1991). If the informant isn't typical and informed, the information is not representative of the culture. Also, the informant must be articulate enough to communicate this information. This usually isn't a problem when working with medical practitioners, but it can be with patients. In fact, it is often the case that a patient who is actually comfortable and articulate in an interview is a different kind of health care consumer from one who is not. The problem with practitioners is that they must be willing and able to express things in non-medical language, unless the medical anthropologist is well versed in medical terminology. People with that willingness and ability might not be typical either.

Random selection of informants is possible for something like hospital research. How, though, can this be done when studying something like the health concerns of prostitutes? What is more likely in an important study of this nature is that the medical anthropologist will get those who are willing and able to cooperate, then perhaps they will get others to participate in a kind of chain approach.

Once it has been established just where the information will be coming from, the medical anthropologist then must sustain the project in the field. This requires that a high level of trust be established, and the researchers may be tested early in this regard by the group being studied (Trotter, 1991). Medical anthropologists can establish trust by creating **dyadic relationships**. In other words, they form one-on-one working relationships with group members. They can also adopt a sustainable role. They become "the person doing that study." An important example of this is the wearing of hospital photo identification. We have found that this increases the degree to which hospital staff sees a researcher as belonging. We have also found that when research assistants were required to don operating room scrubs as part of their work, their adoption of a sustainable role was made easier.

Finally, the researchers must **exit the field** (Trotter, 1991). In so doing, they must think carefully about what they are leaving behind and what debriefing should be done with the people who participated in the study. One study of a hospital's maternity department resulted in the modification of visiting rules for that department (Poole & Ting, 1995). Other follow-up activities included meetings with nurses in the department to get their interpretation of the study's findings and research presentations to nursing staff in the entire hospital.

Data Collection Techniques in Ethnographic Research

Medical anthropologists will use techniques that are not common in psychology but that are very useful all the same. One example is **free listing** (Trotter, 1991). Researchers using this technique will ask a participant to list all the example of a phenomenon they can think of. For example, a nurse may be asked to list all the ways he or she knows that a patient is in pain. This could yield some interesting answers that might not be immediately obvious to psychologists, such as "gripping the bed sheets." Researchers can then compare these lists between participants and roles. From the above example, it would be interesting to learn if nurses or physicians gave you the longest lists, and just what each list contained.

Scaling can also be used. In this case, concepts are placed along a continuum. For example, some cultures conceptualize illnesses as being either "hot" or "cold" (see, for example, Weller, 1983). People from rural Guatemala might call measles a cold disease and rheumatism or a stomach ache hot (Weller, 1983). These conceptualizations have important implications for the way people interpret the cause of a disease and the cures they believe will work. Other helpful scales may measure such things as perceived severity and contagion (Trotter, 1991).

Another technique used by medical anthropologists is **decision modelling** (see for example, Garro, 1998). As the term implies, this technique involves the charting of decision-making processes, both for individuals and groups. Anthropologists could use decision modelling to determine how people from various cultures interpret and act upon symptoms. They could also use this technique to determine the extent to which something like the health belief model is culturally universal (Garro, 1998). In other words, do considerations of perceived threat enter into the decision-making process for all cultures? Anthropologists might also look at something like the theory of reasoned action and remind us that "reason" varies from culture to culture; what is rational in one is not necessarily so in another.

Other techniques include **focus groups**, in which groups of people are asked to discuss specific questions. This technique is appropriate for the assessment of a health promotion program. The advantages are that a great deal of data are generated, and the data are in the participants' own words. Anthropologists will also use **surveys** and **network analysis** (Trotter, 1991). Network analysis borrows from sociology in that it is a study of the interrelationships among the people being studied.

Pluralistic Health Care Practices

Now that you have an understanding of the methods medical anthropologists use in their research, let's look at some of the phenomena they study and the analysis they provide. In so doing, you will see that they explain differences in health by citing cultural differences. These cultures can be in more remote parts of the world, or can be created within Western society — the best example being the culture of medicine.

Knowledge and Belief

In Western medicine, a distinction is often drawn between *knowledge* and *belief*. Knowledge refers to an awareness of what we hold to be scientific fact; it is our understanding of "the truth." For example, a person might have the knowledge that certain mosquito bites can cause malaria (Pelto & Pelto, 1997). Belief, on the other hand, refers to what are sometimes called "traditional ideas." The implication here is that these beliefs are wrong, perhaps born out of superstition or folklore. An example would be that certain diseases are caused by spirit possession (Pelto & Pelto, 1997). Pelto and Pelto also make the point that beliefs can be considered beneficial by Western medicine, but this is mostly due to coincidence. In other words, the behaviour that is engendered by the belief just happens to be healthy.

Further, we often think of medical knowledge as being rational and cultural beliefs as being irrational. However, this delineation may be quite arbitrary. For example, high-tech procedures that are hallmarks of medical knowledge, such as kidney dialysis or organ transplant, carry with them a less rational, somewhat arbitrary set of eligibility criteria (Hunt & Mattingly, 1998).

Anthropologists do not accept this distinction. Instead, they tend to view medical "knowledge" as another set of beliefs. All cultures, including Western medicine, have explanatory models (Kleinman, 1980). These models usually share similar components. Some components are associated with causal attributions, for example, etiology, time and mode of onset of symptoms, and pathophysiology. Others deal with the predicted course of the sickness and still others with treatment. According to Kleinman (1980), all cultures address these components, though some focus more on one component than another. Anthropologists, then, view Western medicine as one explanatory model.

A culture, medical or otherwise, is a *system* of beliefs. In other words, beliefs are linked to one another. For example, health beliefs may be linked to religious beliefs, moral beliefs, and beliefs about social structure. For example, in some cultures, when people get sick the illness is considered to be isolated in one person. That is generally the Western view. In other cultures, however, if one family member has symptoms, the whole family is considered ill.

This means that new or foreign beliefs must be incorporated into the entire system rather than simply supplanting the old beliefs if they are to be adopted at all (Pelto & Pelto, 1997). This is very important to keep in mind when people with Western medical training enter other cultures to provide medical assistance. It also applies to situations in which members of Canada's diverse cultures consume medical services. When new health beliefs are incorporated into a cultural system, the result is what are called **pluralistic health care practices** (Pelto & Pelto, 1997, p. 151). This means that a person uses a combination of health practices from his or her own culture and from other cultures, when deemed appropriate. Pelto & Pelto (1997) call this a combination of "indigenous and cosmopolitan health care resources" (p. 151).

Anthropologists argue that this pluralistic approach is much more common than an all-or-nothing adoption of Western medical practices. Acknowledgment of this eliminates the need for competition between Western and non-Western medicine. Medical anthropologists become the bridge builders between these cultural belief systems. From this perspective, there is no such thing as "alternative" medicine. The term, anthropologists may argue, implies that there is the "truth", in the form of medical *knowledge*, and there are alternatives to that truth, in the form of belief-driven practices. The term *alternative* medicine, therefore, assumes a false distinction between knowledge and belief.

This argument does not assume that Western medicine is ineffective but rather that the legitimacy of people's beliefs regarding other health practices, and the possible efficacy of those practices, must be acknowledged if we are to provide health care in a pluralistic society.

So, how do people make health-related decisions and choices in this pluralistic system? When do they use "cosmopolitan" practices and when do they opt for "traditional" ones? When Pelto and Pelto (1997) came up with their decision model, they identified four factors affecting these decisions: cultural, geographic, psychological, and sociological. This means that health-related decisions in a pluralistic context depend upon the strength of the cultural beliefs in the various systems, geographic realities that may affect opportunities to seek different types of health care (think of Canada's indigenous peoples living in the north, hundreds of kilometers from the nearest "cosmopolitan" practitioner), and factors that might be best understood by biopsychosocial models such as the health belief model. Indeed, this form of decision modelling yields what we might call a multidisciplinary health belief model composed of all these components rather than just the psychological ones.

James Young (1981) has created just such a model by identifying the following factors that predict which health belief system will be followed in a given situation. First, the system chosen must match the seriousness of the health condition. This does not necessarily mean that Western medicine will always be chosen for more serious conditions, although it might more commonly be the case. Second, there is the *knowledge* of either traditional or Western remedies. Closely related to this, and very reminiscent of the health belief model, is the perceived efficacy of the various choices. Finally, there is the availability of the choices and resources that allow for choice, such as money and transportation.

We can see from Young's model that the decision to pursue a particular treatment type involves more than just cultural beliefs. This is why health decisions of people in a rural Mexican community had little to do with their beliefs about the "hot" or "cold" nature of their illness (Young, 1981). When we apply Young's model, we don't view people as passive manifestations of cultural beliefs. Instead, they are active decision-makers choosing from a wide array of options for their health, or at least as wide an array as their circumstances will allow. It is important to note that people from Western cultures fit this description as well. A good example is the rapid growth in popularity of a remedy such as ginseng.

Also, by adopting a decision-making model such as Young's, medical anthropologists move from a study of global cultural beliefs to applied research focused on specific health conditions, because a person's behaviour will differ from condition to condition. This form of applied research is called **focused ethnographic study** (Pelto & Pelto, 1997, p. 155). This form of research looks at specific conditions and the beliefs and behaviours associated with it within a given culture. The World Health Organization has developed an entire research protocol using focused ethnographic study to learn how various cultures deal with acute respiratory infection.

An example of this research is the work of Gittelsohn, Silla, and Sanneh, (1991, cited in Pelto & Pelto, 1997). These researchers interviewed mothers in The Gambia before the mothers took their children in to see a health care worker. The children were suffering from respiratory ailments that concerned the mothers enough to seek treatment. To get a sense of the mothers' beliefs, they were asked if they could recognize rapid breathing in their children. The vast majority of mothers could. The researchers then took note of the number of times the mothers, without being prompted, mentioned rapid breathing as a worrisome symptom. It turned out that mothers mentioned rapid breathing between 20 and 50 percent of the time, but that it was rarely a motivation to seek treatment.

These were important questions, because rapid breathing in children is a symptom of pneumonia, which, if not treated, could be fatal. Subsequently, mothers were trained to recognize this type of breathing and, presumably, they came to accept the importance of doing so. Thus, beliefs regarding the importance of recognizing and reporting fast breathing were incorporated with existing beliefs about respiratory infection. For example, the mothers generally thought that a persistent cough was a clear reason for a clinic visit and the majority of mothers thought it was the most serious of symptoms (Gittelsohn, Silla, & Sanneh, 1991).

Other anthropologists have argued that serious illness is an important manifestation of culture because it demands action (Hunt & Mattingly, 1998). In particular, serious illness demands the application of what anthropologists and members of the culture might call "practical wisdom" (Hunt & Mattingly, 1998, p. 268). These authors stress the need to find the best combination of different types of reasoning to maximize treatment effectiveness. Arguably, this need could be applied to any patient-practitioner interaction. A practitioner's recommendations must "make sense" to a patient to be adopted. This means that the recommendations must fit with the patient's belief system. A good example would be visiting rules in a hospital's maternity department. Many maternity departments place restrictions on the number of visitors and the hours of those visits. This is done to facilitate the running of the department and allow mothers to get rest and learn to care for their newborns. However, for many cultures, the birth of a child is an occasion that must be marked by visits from many family members and friends. The result is a clash between hospital personnel and visitors where no one is satisfied. And the new mother usually doesn't get rest anyway!

Amniocentesis

In the prenatal diagnostic process called amniocentesis, fluids are analyzed to identify potential genetic abnormalities in the developing fetus. Anthropologist Rayna Rapp (Rapp, 1993) studied the processes involved in this identification and, more important, the way abnormalities were communicated to pregnant women. Perhaps the most interesting, though difficult, cases are those in which uncertainty exists regarding prognosis. Rapp documents one case in which the abnormality in question was an unusual one, for which there was no clear findings in the literature. The mother-to-be was informed of this abnormality and given the medical opinion that her baby would not be normal. After being told this, she chose to continue the pregnancy and have the baby. When the baby was born, she agreed to let the physicians follow the course of his development, since so little was known about the genetic abnormality he possessed.

According to Rapp's account, the decision to continue the pregnancy upset the genetic counsellor because of the likelihood of abnormality. However, the decision needed to be understood in terms of the woman's life circumstances, cultural beliefs, and psychology. The woman was opposed to abortion on religious grounds and was supported in her decision by her mother-in-law. It was her husband's second marriage and, at age 37, the woman wanted a child.

The point of this example isn't to judge whether the woman's decision was right or wrong. Rather, it is to provide an understanding of the ways medical, psychological, and anthropological factors combine to shape such decisions.

Medicine as Business

Medical anthropologists and economists would agree that any analysis of health and health care must acknowledge that many health-related decisions have monetary implications. These might not be so evident to the average Canadian patient, who rarely makes direct payment for medical services, but that does not negate the fact that medicine is big business, in this country and elsewhere. With this in mind, how would you answer the following question: why did the number of prostatectomies (removal of the prostate gland) for benign prostatic hyperplasia (enlarged prostate gland) in the United States increase from 191 000 in 1965 to 410 000 in 1987? As we stated earlier in this chapter, there are many possible explanations for this epidemiological fact. The anthropologist might forward an answer that emphasizes economics, if economic concerns were central to the culture in question. This happens to be the case in the United States (McDade, 1996).

First, we should consider the biomedical nature of benign prostatic hyperplasia (BPH). The prostate gland, a walnut-sized gland surrounding the urethra, tends to enlarge as men age. According to Begun (1993), this enlargement is not linked to prostate cancer. There are, however, possible problematic symptoms associated with enlargement of the prostate. These include waking in the night to go to the bathroom and discomfort when urinating. The mortality rate for BPH is 3 deaths per 100 000 men. The most common physical test for BPH is the digital exam, in which the physician uses touch to estimate the size of the gland (a common but less-than-popular component of most general physical examinations for men). Any change in the incidence of BPH or improvement in diagnosis would help explain the marked increase in the related surgery.

There might be psychological reasons for this increase as well. As prostate cancer becomes more widely publicized, men become more aware of the need for early detection and therefore may pay more attention to their urinary symptoms and get tested more often.

The anthropological economic explanation would cite the fact that, in the United States, approximately 38 percent of all operations performed by urologists are prostatectomies

FOCUS ON RESEARCH 13-1 Taking Medicine because There is No Time to be Sick

A mother takes 2 days off work to look after family members who have the flu. Then, to no one's surprise, she comes down with the flu. However, rather than taking more time off work, she takes antidiarrheal medication and goes to work. She needs the medicine because she can't afford to take any more time off work. There is no time for her to be sick.

Cold symptoms? No time to let them run their course. Decongestants and analgesics keep us going because we don't have time to be sick.

If this sounds familiar, then you have experienced what Nancy Vuckovic (1999) discovered in her ethnographic study of women's use of over-the-counter (OTC) medicine. According to Vuckovic, most people live in a state of "time famine" (p. 51). There is always more to do than there is time to do it in. This time famine is built on the Western notion that time is "unidirectional and unrecoverable" (p. 52). It keeps marching on and once gone, you can't get it back. Not all cultures view time this way, although it is true that it makes time a very valuable commodity. This is especially true for cultures that also value productivity, which tends to be the case in most Western societies. People living in these societies may take medications, not because they need them to recover from illness, but because they need to recover *quickly*. Medications, then, become a time saving strategy that increases our capacity to produce.

To investigate this, Nancy Vuckovic conducted interviews over an 18-month period with women in 40 American households. With work schedules in and out of the home, daycare arrangements, dance classes, soccer practices, mealtimes, bedtimes, and a host of other responsibilities, these women confirmed that a time famine definitely existed for them. Vuckovic learned further that this hectic pace increased the women's susceptibility to acute and chronic illness, thus increasing the need for so-called time-saving medication.

In their interviews, the women told Vuckovic they took medication, not just because of a "reluctance to feel uncomfortable" (p. 55), but because of their "impatience with illness" (p. 55). One participant said that she took Tylenol for a headache so that she could keep going. Another reported that she took OTC medication to mask symptoms rather than take the time to see her physician.

In many cases, children don't have time to be sick either. Vuckovic found that children are more likely to be given medication to reduce a fever if they get that fever in mid-week rather than on the weekend. As one mother put it, she gives her children medicine, sends them to school, goes to work, and hopes she doesn't get a call from the school. So much for the sick role! Of course, it is doubtful that these mothers would send their children to school if they thought the medicine would not make their children feel better. Nor would they deny their children medicine on the weekend if the symptoms were creating undue discomfort for the children. Nevertheless, the consumption of OTC medication is affected significantly by the time pressures of the circumstance.

Many OTC medications are formulated to acknowledge the time famine that has made them so necessary. Remedies are "fast acting" or perhaps feature a "non-drowsy" formula that allows the person to take the medicine and keep producing in a society that demands productivity. Vuckovic concludes by calling these OTC medications "commodities of efficiency" (p. 62), like microwave ovens and drive-through fast-food outlets.

(Holtgrewe, 1990; cited in McDade, 1996). Also, there has been an 88 percent increase in the number of urologists in the United States between 1965 and 1990 (McDade, 1996). In other words, if we view urology as a business, it is in that business' best interest to diagnosis BPH and remove prostate glands. Consistent with this explanation, McDade (1996) points out that diagnosis of BPH in the United States is two to three times that of Scotland or Japan, even though enlargement of the prostate is not believed to differ across cultures.

It is not our intention here to assess the validity of McDade's analysis. We introduce it, rather, to provide an example of one of the ways in which anthropologists might explain epidemiological data.

MEDICAL GEOGRAPHY

We have said that epidemiological statistics can sometimes be explained by looking at geography. In other words, health trends are influenced by the place in which we find those trends. Are there environmental toxins? Is there overcrowding? Questions like these provide the rationale for journals like *Health and Place* and for symposia like the *International Symposium in Medical Geography*, which is held every 2 years and alternates between European and North American locations.

What is Medical Geography?

In an editorial written on the occasion of the first anniversary of *Health and Place*, North American Associate Editor Michael Hayes provided some useful general definitions of the field of medical geography (Hayes, 1996a). Hayes, from Simon Fraser University, stated that medical geographers study "differences in health and health care in specific places" (p. iii). He also made another important point: "All conceptions of human health involve some notion of a dynamic interplay between people and their environments" (p. iii). In other words, we cannot study health or improve it without acknowledging that everyone's health is *situated* in some environmental context. It isn't enough for health psychologists to identify ways to persuade Canada's population to have regular physical examinations and cancer screening procedures without also exploring the possibility that the nearest medical facility might be 250 kilometers away.

Medical geography is linked to health promotion and to what is generically known as "population health" (Evans, Barer, & Marmot, 1994). This later term has become a kind of catch-all phrase to describe health-related research conducted in the social sciences and humanities. Another related term that has come into the discourse is "social determinants of health." Both terms refer to a level of analysis that goes beyond individualism. When health psychologists focus on cognitive, affective, and behavioural issues relevant to health, they rarely need to draw maps to conduct their analysis. The "map" is the person — what he or she does, thinks and feels. In **population health**, as the term implies, the unit of analysis is a segment of the population, or possibly the entire population. The maps are more literal, showing parts of a geographic area. We will look at these maps more closely in a moment.

A Brief History of Medical Geography

To chart the development of medical geography as a discipline, we must go back to the year 1850. At that time, some people thought that a geographical approach to medicine would yield insights into the *causes* of disease. However, germ theory was dominant, and so there was less emphasis placed on macroscopic, distal causes. Also, it appears that the link between microbiology and geography had not yet been explored. For these reasons, medical geography took a back seat to microbiological investigation.

One of the first publications to start changing this dominance was published in 1850 by physician Daniel Drake (Barrett, 1996; Drake, 1850–1854). Drake's book documented his own research, which featured considerably more detail and rigour than any previous attempts to chart disease over geographic areas. The geographic areas included much of the interior of North America, though Drake started his analysis in the city of Cincinnati. His own words demonstrated his tie with medical geography when he called his work "an attempt to present an account, etiological, symptomatical, and therapeutic, of the most important diseases of a particular portion of the earth; not of a state or political division, for it is indirectly, and to a very limited extent only, that civil divisions can originate varieties in the character of disease" (Drake, 1850–1854, Vol. 1, p. 2, cited in Barrett, 1996, p. 796).

Historically, a distinction has been made between *medical geography* and *geographical medicine* (Barrett, 1996). **Medical geography** is a subdiscipline of geography. The main focus is place, and the health of those in it. For example, medical geographers might study the health of people living in urban ghettos. The emphasis of **geographical medicine**, which is a subdiscipline of medicine, is somewhat different. In this case, the main focus is a disease, with secondary interest in geography. For example, students of geographical medicine might investigate which areas of the world are prone to a disease like malaria. This distinction reminds us that people enter this area with primary training in either geography or medicine. The emergence of interdisciplinary teams, however, should make the distinction unnecessary.

Medical Geography Today

It has been argued that medical geography is going through an "identity crisis" (Hayes, 1996b, p. 787) and that the term no longer adequately captures the breadth of activity in the field. Also, the term "medical geography" implies a focus on biomedical outcomes that a more general term like "health geography" does not. The latter term apples a definition of health that goes beyond absence of illness to acknowledge the ability to perform daily functions and enjoy a reasonable quality of life. Indeed, people working in the field may be more likely to refer to it as "the geography of health and health care."

That debate aside, the *Sixth Annual Symposium in Medical Geography*, held in 1994 in Vancouver, addressed a range of topics that help define the field as it is seen today. Some of these topics included environment and health, housing and health, access to health care, and physician practice patterns. The Canadian government publication *Health Reports* features epidemiological data relevant to all of these topics. Examples include such papers as "Mortality in Metropolitan Areas" (Gilmour and Gentleman, 1999) and "Use of Postal Codes and Addresses in the Analysis of Health Data" (Wilkins, 1993).

Another topic of interest is the extent to which people **age in place**. In other words, when people retire, do they stay where they are or do they move? Is the Saskatchewan bumper sticker that reads, "There's more of us in B.C." really true? You may wonder what this has to do with health. The medical geographer would have a quick answer. Have you ever been to Vancouver Island? If so, you will know that there are communities in that part of the country made up predominantly of retirees. For the most part, the health care facilities closest to these facilities were not designed in anticipation of this influx. As a result, people living in mid-island communities like Parksville and Qualicum Beach must often make the trip to Nanaimo or further still to Victoria for vital medical care. Of course, this also has the potential to create longer waiting times for appointments and treatments.

Medical geographers are also interested in health-related differences between urban and rural dwellers. We typically think of "the country", with its lower population density, cleaner air, and slower pace of life, as being healthier than the city. However, this isn't entirely the case. As we saw with the Vancouver Island retirees, access to health care is usually much better in urban areas. Also, remote rural areas might not feature the levels of social support that are available to urban dwellers.

All of these topics challenge the widely held view that disease is located solely within the body. However, epidemiologists talk about "human hosts" of disease. This implies that there are non-human hosts, which of course there are (animals carrying rabies are one example). Remember also that there are inanimate vehicles of disease. Diseases *travel* in numerous ways. Taking all this into account, it may be helpful to think about diseased *places* as well. While they might not use the exact term, medical geographers help us think in these ways.

Indeed, medical geographers may tell us that we need to expand our conceptualization of *place*. It is more than a physical locale or geographic site. It is also more than a set of coordinates on a map. The boundaries of place can be physical, as in mountain ranges, coastlines and climates, political, as in national borders, anthropological, as in distinct cultural enclaves, and economic, as in neighbourhoods in urban and suburban areas. Medical geography invites us to consider all of these conceptions of place and more.

Methods in Medical Geography

One of the main concerns of medical geography is the quantitative study of disease distributions and patterns of health care provision over geographically defined areas. This quantitative study is called **spatial analysis** (Gatrell & Bailey, 1996). When medical geographers use spatial analysis, they may present their data in the form of maps. A more specialized version of this is called **spatial data analysis** (Gatrell & Bailey, 1996). Researchers using this technique look at the outcome of some process working in a defined space. Spatial data analysis is more than a straightforward description of patterns. It attempts to chart the effect of some factor or factors affecting health patterns.

Maps presenting spatial data analysis might present more complex information than disease patterns. They might also chart the presence of toxin-producing industries, climatic characteristics, and so on. That way, people reading the map can assess relationships between factors and disease patterns.

There are a number of different methods involved in spatial data analysis. For example, there are **visualization methods**. The most common type is maps, which have been called "atlases of disease" (Gatrell & Bailey, 1996, p. 844). One type of map presents what is called a **point pattern**, where points on the map indicate disease prevalence, either in absolute terms or as a ratio of the population (such as rate per 1 000 people). More complex maps may use shading, in which one type of shading indicates *morbidity* rates and another indicates *mortality*.

Exploratory methods provide interpretations of the maps by describing relationships and illustrative patterns. Exploratory methods might identify *clusters* of disease and link them to possible geographic markers (Gatrell & Bailey, 1996). Earlier in the chapter, we discussed research showing a cluster of anencephalic babies along the Rio Grande river in Mexico. That pattern could be identified by mapping and exploratory methods, showing points clustered along the river.

Another method, called **quantitative modelling**, allows medical geographers to *predict* patterns. This method would use maps that chart predictor and outcome variables, such as asthma prevalence and some measure of air quality, such as ozone levels. If the researchers could track the patterns of poor air quality, say in a valley near an urban area such as the Fraser Valley in Greater Vancouver, they could then predict asthma incidence rates as the patterns of air quality improved, worsened, or moved because of changes in climate or industry.

Understanding Malaria from the Standpoint of Medical Geography

Malaria is a disease that is a serious problem in over 90 countries, encompassing 40 percent of the world's population (WHO, 1998). As we discuss this problem, try to develop an appreciation for the contribution that medical geography can make to our understanding and control of malaria. Also, think about the staggering scope of this disease. In Chapter 11, we talked about chronic and serious illnesses that are common in the Western world — cancer, heart disease, and AIDS, for example. None of these health problems comes close to the morbidity and mortality rates of malaria. Finally, as you read this section, think about the ways researchers from a variety of disciplines can work together to solve the problems brought on by malaria. The statistics and analysis we provide here were derived primarily from a World Health Organization Fact Sheet on malaria (WHO, 1998).

The Scope of Malaria

Malaria is responsible for over 1 000 000 deaths per year. Every 30 seconds, a child dies of malaria, with 3 000 children under the age of 5 years dying every day from the disease. When a child is fatally inflicted with malaria, they often die within 72 hours of infliction.

The Geography of Malaria

Over the past 50 years, the geographic area covered by malaria has decreased. However, recent developments are causing it to begin spreading again. Ninety percent of all cases of malaria are found in the sub-Saharan region of Africa. The disease hits the poor more than any other disease.

As we mentioned earlier in the chapter, the vector for malaria is the *Anopheles* mosquito. Remember that a vector is a word epidemiologists use to describe living organisms that can transfer an agent from one host to another. This means that patterns of malaria spread are linked to factors that affect the breeding of the mosquito. These include such obvious things as climate changes. Global warming and El Niño have increased the number of *vector breeding* sites for the agent carrying mosquito.

Geography is also linked to economics, and so economic development affects malaria's spread. A current example is the Amazon, which is experiencing changes in land use with road building and logging. Agricultural and irrigation projects are also associated with the spread of the disease. Armed conflicts affect spread as well, primarily by creating mass movements of refugees from more to less affected areas. Also, there is something called **airport malaria**, which refers to the growing number of cases of malaria brought home by international travellers. In any one of these areas, the problem is made worse if there is a decline in health services.

Medical geographers can map all these patterns along with the factors associated with them, like economic development, weather patterns, international travel rates, and quality of health services. They can also map areas in which attempts have been made to control the disease and chart changes over time as a result of these attempts.

There are at least three effective strategies for controlling malaria. There are behavioural strategies, like sleeping under bednets treated with a naturally occurring insecticide such as *pyrethrum*. This is important because the mosquitoes transmitting the disease tend to come out after dark. Second, there are educational strategies. One survey found that half of the people surveyed in Ghana did not know malaria was transmitted by mosquitoes. Third, there are biomedical disease management strategies. Medicines such as chloroquine do an effective job of preventing the disease and curbing its symptoms if contracted. A review of these three strategies indicates ways in which people from a variety of disciplines can come together to help control malaria. Such a collective effort represents health promotion on a global scale.

BOX 13-2 Health Studies Centres and Institutes at Canadian Universities

We have made the point repeatedly in this chapter that health psychologists must develop an awareness of the ways other disciplines study health-related issues. This implies that health psychologists should work *together* with people from other disciplines. In this section, we provide some examples of research and teaching centres in Canada that feature the interdisciplinary study of health; this will help you develop an appreciation for the sorts of initiatives undertaken. Also, we include them to provide you with some ideas regarding the types of further education and training you may want to pursue in health-related areas. This is not an exhaustive list; rather, it is a sampling.

The York University Centre for Health Studies

The York University Centre for Health Studies (YCHS) is an interdisciplinary research unit that also conducts seminars and supports a variety of health-related programs. Examples include the National Network on Environments and Women's Health, the Hanna Institute for the History of Medicine, and the National Institute on Aging Project. The Centre has been in existence since 1990, bringing together researchers from law and the social, health, and environmental sciences.

Centre for Applied Health Research (University of Waterloo)

Housed within Waterloo's Faculty of Applied Health Sciences, the Centre for Applied Health Research supports research in disease and injury prevention and health promotion. Research areas include such topics as smoking prevention, cancer prevention, social networks and quality of life, health care services, environmental health, and social determinants of health.

Department of Community Health Sciences (University of Manitoba)

The Department of Community Health Sciences is housed within the Faculty of Medicine at the University of Manitoba. The department's mission statement is to "... contribute to the physical, psychological, cultural, social and economic well-being of the people of Manitoba, Canada, and the world" (departmental web site). To achieve this objective, the department works to ensure that teaching in the Faculty of Medicine has a "population health and critical appraisal perspective and preventive focus where appropriate" (departmental web site). Specific units include the Alcohol and Tobacco Research Unit, the Manitoba Centre for Health Policy and Evaluation, and the Occupational and Environmental Medicine Unit, to name a few.

Department of Social Studies of Medicine (McGill University)

The Department of Social Studies of Medicine, which is an academic unit within McGill's Faculty of Medicine, brings together three disciplines — anthropology, history, and sociology. The department is described as a bridge between the Faculty of Medicine and the Faculty of Arts. The department offers undergraduate courses in the history of medicine, the anthropology of medicine and the medical humanities and social sciences. Degrees are offered at the undergraduate and master's levels.

University of British Columbia Health Care and Epidemiology: Health Economics and Policy Program

This program is part of the Department of Health Care and Epidemiology, housed in the Faculty of Medicine. The program is multidisciplinary, with five areas of health research: Health Technology Assessment, Human Health Resources, Health Information, Health Policy Research, and the Program in Population Health. The latter two areas have the closest links to social science research. The groups working in these areas consist of economists, epidemiologists, and representatives from other disciplines. Recent research from the Health Policy Research Group has investigated hospital waiting lists, child health issues, pricing of and access to physician services, community income levels and access to health care, health care and the elderly. The Program in Population Health integrates work from genetics, medicine, epidemiology, sociology, political science, economics and policy analysis.

McMaster University: Centre for Health Economics and Policy Analysis (CHEPA)

The Centre for Health Economics and Policy Analysis (CHEPA) is part of the Faculty of Health Sciences at McMaster University. This program is interdisciplinary with its major focus on health economics and policy. Its objective is to develop and apply methods to evaluate costs, risks, and benefits of health, health services, and population health. Its mandate is research, training, and education.

The Health Psychology Research Group at Simon Fraser University

The Health Psychology Research Group conducts research in the areas of social determinants of health, psychological impact of medical procedures, and communication in medical settings. The group engages in a wide variety of projects. Some current examples include a study of social support among prostate cancer patients, an assessment of the psychological consequences of various anesthetic induction techniques for children in day surgery, an investigation of the needs of brain tumour patients' caregivers, and a comprehensive descriptive study of concussion among adult rugby players.

KEY TERMS

epidemiology
case
incidence
prevalence
point prevalence
lifetime prevalence
crude rate
age-specific rates
infant mortality rate
agents
hosts
vectors
vehicles
sanitation era
infectious disease era
chronic disease era
ecoepidemiological era
sociology
medical sociology
sociology in medicine
sociology of medicine
structural functionalism
social facts
sick role
master status
allopathic medicine
conflict theory
symbolic interactionism
socially constructed reality
transcript analysis
disease
illness
feminist theory
role strain
unit of analysis
medical anthropology
ethnography
participant observation
passive observation
adaptive observation
intrusive observation
field entry
social mapping
informants
dyadic relationships
exiting the field
free listing
scaling
decision modelling
focus groups
surveys
network analysis
pluralistic health care practices
focused ethnographic study
population health
medical geography
geographical medicine
aging in place
spatial analysis
spatial data analysis
visualization methods
point pattern
exploratory methods
quantitative modelling
airport malaria

Chapter 14

THE FUTURE OF HEALTH PSYCHOLOGY

Chapter Outline

Key Questions

1. What are the main challenges that health psychology will face in the future?
2. What is complementary and alternative medicine?
3. What are the attitudes toward complementary and alternative medicine?
4. Why do people use complementary and alternative medicine
5. What are some examples of current health psychology research programs at Canadian universities?
6. How is health psychology research funded, how is this changing, and why are these changes important?

Everything seemed quite new for Suzanne—new office, new position as Director of a new Health Studies program at her university. It promised to be an interesting job. While her background in health psychology would certainly be an asset, in some ways, it was just a beginning. The Health Studies program was designed to bring together medical scientists and social scientists to study health. As Director, Suzanne would need to develop an understanding of the contributions the other disciplines would make to the program. Further, she would have to ensure that her own discipline, psychology, continued to make significant contributions. For Suzanne, this meant doing good research that provided convincing evidence of the link between psychology and health.

On her desk, Suzanne had spread out a collection of newspaper articles documenting the case of Tyrell Dueck, a boy from Saskatchewan who had died of cancer when he was 13 years old. In addition to being a tragic story, Suzanne was struck by the many elements of her Health Studies program that the story illustrated. There was, of course, the medical perspective. A young boy is diagnosed with cancer and modern medicine prescribes a treatment. But there is much more than medicine in Tyrell's story. There is religious belief, alternative medicine, ethics, and a host of other perspectives.

For reasons of religion, Tyrell's parents refused the treatment prescribed by oncologists, which would have involved chemotherapy and possible leg amputation. A

Saskatchewan court ordered them to follow the oncologist's treatment but they refused. Instead, they took Tyrell to a clinic in Tijuana, Mexico, where he received treatments using laetrile and shark cartilage. Unfortunately, the treatments were unsuccessful and Tyrell returned home, where he died in a Saskatchewan hospital.

As Suzanne worked her way through the collection of articles on this story, she contemplated the ways in which her Health Studies program could provide analysis. There is the relationship between treatment and belief. There is the power of medical science and the controversies surrounding unproven treatment options. And there is the large issue of ethics. Suzanne concluded that people in her program would have no trouble finding important things to study, now and in the future.

In this chapter, we gaze into our crystal ball to predict future directions for health psychology. These predictions are based on extrapolations of trends in health and health care, and on the research that is being actively pursued in Canada and elsewhere.

THE ONGOING CHALLENGE OF PROVIDING PROOF

Some of the findings in health psychology and psychology in general could be called common sense. Stress is bad for your health. Exercise is generally good. People who believe that they are in control of their lives enjoy better health and recovery rates than people who do not share this belief. Some may feel that it is unnecessary to prove common sense empirically. However, psychologists would disagree for a number of reasons.

First, even if a phenomenon does seem straightforward, we need to know the extent of this phenomenon. *How* toxic is stress? *What kinds* of stress are particularly bad? Why do some people cope with ostensibly stressful situations better than others? How do people establish a sense of control in medical situations where most of their control is taken away from them? Why do people differ in their control beliefs? These are just a few of the questions that need to be answered for seemingly "common sense" findings. Second, not all common sense findings are as simple as they look. Stress isn't always unhealthy, especially if the person involved approaches life with a sense of *hardiness*. This is an approach to life's events that is characterized by a sense of commitment, challenge, and control. Providing patients with information about their condition and the procedures they are about to go through usually helps them cope, but not always. Sometimes the provision of information contradicts the patient's coping strategy, which in the case of *blunters* is to avoid information about their condition.

Third, some things that we think are common sense are wrong. For example, we might think that the more serious a person's condition, the more likely the person is to follow a prescribed regimen. But this isn't always the case. People with high blood pressure, which could be life threatening, might be less likely to follow advice to change their lifestyles than are people with ear infections who are told to take an antibiotic.

For these reasons, we must continue to find proof that relationships exist between psychological state and health, and that psychology can help improve health care. Whether the phenomenon appeals to common sense or is counterintuitive, health psychology as a discipline will grow only as its credibility grows, and that will come from theories supported by strong evidence. This evidence must take a number of forms.

For one, it must appeal to people who understand health from a biomedical perspective. Health psychologists must continue to do research using health indicators as outcome variables. Morbidity and mortality rates, recovery rates, and other measures of health status need to be included if our work is going to attract the attention and support of physicians and others trained in biomedical analysis.

Much of the research in health psychology has looked at patients' self-reports of coping and quality of life. These are important measures, but from a biomedical perspective they are often viewed as indirect biproducts of "real" health measures. Health psychologists must continue to make the case that these self-report measures are as important to well-being as cell counts. Indeed, many physicians are considering quality of life to be an important, if not *the most* important treatment outcome. The question then becomes how quality of life is defined. In the search for answers to this question, health psychologists have much to contribute.

It is vital, then, that health psychologists provide empirical findings that are either biomedical in nature or are linked in convincing ways to well-being. However, it would be a mistake to stop here. Though the biomedical perspective is an important and powerful one in health, it is not the only perspective. As we saw in Chapter 13, there are broader perspectives that health psychologists need to understand and contribute to. It is one thing to demonstrate that psychological principles can be applied to improve health *one person at a time*. It is something else again to say that such principles can be used to improve the health of *populations*.

How can health psychologists do this? One way is through the application of social psychological theories in persuasion to health promotion. This requires an interdisciplinary approach, in which psychologists work with sociologists and anthropologists (among others) to produce programs that target the right groups, appeal across cultures, and feature strategies that are likely to affect attitudes and behaviours. To prove the effectiveness of these kinds of interventions requires different kinds of data. We must look to epidemiological data and other broad survey techniques for our proof.

Regardless of the nature of our data, health psychologists, like all scientists, must use sound methodology. Psychological research in applied settings will never be as controlled as biomedical "bench work" with *in vitro* cultures. Still, psychologists make important strides forward with every prospective design that replaces a retrospective one, and every study that features random assignment compared to participant self-selection. There are many times when these are unattainable ideals, but we must strive for them nonetheless.

COMPLEMENTARY AND ALTERNATIVE MEDICINE: A CALL FOR PROOF

The story of Tyrell Dueck reminds us that not everyone embraces the Western medical establishment. The use of medical treatments that are not the product of what has been called conventional medical science continues to grow in popularity. As we look to the future of health psychology, we must consider the role that psychologists can play in understanding people's decisions to use these treatments. In addition, we can help explain some of the potential effects of these treatments. The first step is to understand the issues that surround complementary and alternative medicine and to become intelligent consumers of research in the field.

Treatments Not Commonly Found in Western Medicine: Terminology

A number of different terms have been used to identify treatments that fall outside normative Western medical practice. Each carries its own set of connotations and implied set of values. As such, the terminology of the area makes for a good starting point.

We have used the terms "complementary and alternative medicine" in the heading to this section. They are a pair of terms that are commonly used to describe the area; the acronym is CAM. Although the terms are used together, they do not mean the same thing. *Complementary treatment* is used in conjunction with allopathic treatment. You may remember from Chapter 13 that allopathic treatment attempts to cure sickness by creating conditions in the body that oppose the disease (Clarke, 1996). It is decidedly biomedical in nature. This definition of complementary treatment implies that patients must be aware of potential interactions between the allopathic treatment and the complementary one, since they are being used simultaneously.

Alternative treatment is the term given to treatments that are not allopathic. This would indicate that the patient has either rejected allopathic treatment, given up on it, or perhaps is ignorant of it. Some may infer that the term "alternative" carries a certain attractive value, as in "viable alternative", or even "better alternative." In keeping with this, it has been suggested that proponents of such treatments were the ones to coin the term (Beyerstein, 1997). In contrast, others may consider the term to be pejorative, implying that such treatments are not mainstream and, as such, are marginalized. In other words, the implication is that they are not your best choice, but are an "alternative."

Others make the distinction between "traditional" and "non-traditional" treatments. However, this distinction is usually rejected by anthropologists because it implies that there is a single tradition, that being allopathic medicine, and that nothing else has a tradition. This contradicts the fact that some remedies called "alternative" have been around for centuries. Still others delineate between "conventional" and "unconventional therapy" (UT). Some authors have argued that unconventional is the least pejorative of all the terms used to describe these treatments (Fitch et al., 1999). Not everyone interprets the word "unconventional" in neutral terms, however.

Finally, it has been suggested that the most useful dichotomy is between treatments that work and those that don't. From this point of view, other terms such as alternative, unconventional, traditional, or the less-often used term "frontier" , are unnecessary.

The conclusion that we can draw from this dilemma is that there is probably no single term that everyone is going to be comfortable with regarding such therapies. We have chosen the CAM approach because, at the very least, those terms draw a useful distinction between treatment followed in conjunction with or instead of allopathic regimens. It turns out that the names people choose represent only one of the controversial aspects of CAM. Before we explore the main debates in detail, though, we should get some idea of how commonly CAM is used.

How Prevalent is the Use of Complementary and Alternative Medicine?

If complementary and alternative therapies were rarely used, they would not be such an important topic of discussion. However, there is growing evidence that these treatments are quite widely used. For example, 37 percent of Canadian women reported using what the authors called unconventional therapies for breast cancer (Campion, 1993). Another study found that 39 percent of head and neck cancer patients used complementary therapy and that 23 percent of them had used it specifically for their cancer (Warrick et al., 1999).

A study of brain tumour patients in southern Alberta found that 24 percent of them were using complementary therapy (Verhoef et al., 1999). Interestingly, these researchers became interested in CAM when they discovered that some of their patients had a distinctive orange colour on their hands. It turned out that these patients were using beta carotene as a complementary treatment. A study of 366 pediatric cancer patients in British Columbia between 1989 and 1995 revealed that 42 percent of the children had received alternative therapy (Fernandez et al., 1998). International research comparing CAM usage among people with inflammatory bowel disease showed that 68 percent of the patients in Los Angeles used CAM. This compared to 57 percent of the patients in Winnipeg, 32 percent in Stockholm, Sweden, and 31 percent in Cork, Ireland.

From all these studies, we can conclude that CAM is anything but rare. Indeed, it is likely that these figures represent an under-reporting of CAM use. A study in the United States estimated that just under 39 percent of alternative therapy use was being disclosed by patients to their physicians (Eisenberg et al., 1998, cited in Wong, 1999). In the southern Alberta study, 45 percent of the patients said their doctors were aware of the patients' alternative therapy use. This means that practitioners and health psychologists need to know more about CAM in terms of its perceived effectiveness and the reasons why patients pursue it. Perhaps this is one reason why a survey of all sixteen Canadian medical schools found that nine had alternative medicine education as part of a required course, six had it as an elective course, and seven explored alternative medicine through student-developed presentations (Ruedy, Kaufman, & MacLeod, 1999).

Some Examples of Complementary and Alternative Medicine

It is important to realize that CAM covers a very wide and diverse collection of treatments. These range from the conservative, such as certain lifestyle changes (exercise and relaxation training), to what Beyerstein (1997) has called the "patently absurd" (p. 149), such as crystal healing. Of the many substances that may be prescribed as part of CAM regimens, some are herbal (such as echinacea), some animal or vegetable derivative (such as shark cartilage or mushrooms), some macrobiotic, and others vitamin (as in the beta carotene used by brain tumour patients). Some other CAM procedures do not require the ingestion of substances. These include such treatments as acupuncture and various forms of homeopathy (Verhoef et al., 1999).

Currently, research assessing the effectiveness of these treatments is either scant or poor (or both). In 1998, Elizabeth Kaegi published a series of papers in the *Canadian Medical Association Journal* reviewing the research on six alternative treatments used by breast cancer patients. These papers were written in conjunction with the Task Force on Alternative

Therapies of the Canadian Breast Cancer Research Initiative (e.g., Kaegi, 1998a; 1998b; 1998c; 1998d). The work was given a mixed, if not entirely polarized, reception by the *CMAJ* readership. We'll say more about that later. For now, let's look at two of the papers to become a bit more familiar with two alternative treatments and the research done on them.

One of the treatments reviewed by Kaegi is called "714-X" (Kaegi, 1998d). It was developed in Canada by Gaston Naessens, following his theories of cancer development. The name for the treatment is derived from Naessens' name and birth date. The seven is for the seventh letter of the alphabet (G) and the fourteen for the fourteenth (N), thus representing Naessens' initials. The "X" represents the twenty-fourth letter in the alphabet, representing the year of Naessens' birth (1924). The 714-X treatment is not available in Canada for general therapeutic use but is allowed in some cases on compassionate grounds. It is used most by breast and prostate cancer patients (Kaegi, 1998d). Research assessing the effectiveness of 714-X does not yield strong scientific data proving its effectiveness. Rather, most support comes in the form of individual patient testimonials (Kaegi, 1998d).

In contrast to the rather small amount of research conducted on the effectiveness of 714-X, there has been a great deal of research on the vitamins A, C, and E and their potential role in the prevention and treatment of cancer (though considerably more on prevention than treatment) (Kaegi, 1998c). Since it is widely accepted that a diet rich in fresh fruits and vegetables reduces the risk of some cancers and that these foods contain vitamins A, C, and E, it seems reasonable to investigate the potential of supplements of these vitamins as cancer treatments. Also, high dosages of these vitamins rarely have serious toxic effects (Kaegi, 1998c). Further indirect support for their use in cancer treatment comes from studies that have reported an enhancement in immune functioning associated with them. These effects are more common for vitamins A and C than for E. It also must be noted, however, that the dosages required to bring about real therapeutic effects, as opposed to measurable immune system enhancement, might be too high to be practical. It appears that more research is required in this area.

Related to her series of research reviews, Kaegi also wrote a paper for the *CMAJ* entitled, "A Patient's Guide to Choosing Unconventional Therapies" (Kaegi, 1998e). Again, this paper generated debate among its readers. In it, Kaegi provided detailed advice for the potential consumer of what she called "unconventional therapies." For example, she cautioned people to do the research before choosing, to ask practitioners for their credentials, check for possible interactions with conventional therapy before committing to unconventional therapy, and to know one's comfort level regarding such therapy. This all seems like sound advice except that, for patients, doing the research isn't as easy as it sounds. Kaegi herself generally concluded that the research on the treatments she reviewed was still inconclusive. Others have argued that patients usually aren't assertive enough to ask for a practitioner's credentials or, if shown them, don't have the expertise to evaluate them (Tannock & Warr, 1998).

Who Uses Complementary and Alternative Medicine and Why

You may draw the conclusion that, given the paucity of current research proving the effectiveness of CAM, the only people who would use it would be those who aren't in a position to make educated choices. If you drew this general conclusion, however, you would be wrong. Warrick and colleagues' (1999) analysis of head and neck cancer patients found more use in patients who were younger, had postsecondary education, and were in upper income brackets. These findings are consistent with other similar analyses. In their study of brain tumour patients in southern Alberta, Verhoef and colleagues (1999) found that alternative therapy was more commonly used among younger patients.

Why do patients pursue alternative therapies? The reasons for using alternative therapies will, of course, vary considerably from person to person and from condition to condition. The Alberta brain tumour patients tended to talk about needing to take charge of their treatment, and pursuing alternative therapies provided them with the feeling they were doing that (Verhoef et al., 1999). Other studies have also found that increasing one's sense of personal control is a motivating factor in alternative treatment choice (e.g., Seidl & Stewart, 1998). Menopausal patients have said that some alternative therapies are more natural and holistic. On a related theme, these same patients expressed concerns with possible side effects and risks of allopathic methods. Still others reported that they have found CAM to be a more user-friendly environment (Seidl & Stewart, 1998).

Other research (Nam et al., 1999) indicates that people who attend support groups may be more likely to use complementary or alternative therapy. The study looked at men who either had prostate cancer or were considered at high risk for the disease, as defined by family history and abnormal prostate specific-antigen (PSA) scores. Among the high-risk men, 80 percent of those attending support groups were using complementary therapies, compared to 26 percent who were interviewed in a clinic. Of all the patients using CAM, 24 percent did not tell their urologist they were doing so.

One explanation for the effect of support group attendance on CAM usage might be that information on CAM is more available to support group attenders. Consistent with this possibility, another study of prostate cancer patients discovered that attenders of support groups were significantly more likely to cite fellow patients as their main source of informational support; whereas, non-attenders cited medical staff in this category (Poole et al., submitted for publication). A study of women with breast cancer reported that only 54 percent of the participants were satisfied with the available information on what the authors called unconventional therapies (Campion, 1993). It would be worthwhile to discover how this satisfaction differed for support group attenders and non-attenders. At present, there has been little research linking CAM usage and support group attendance. To complicate matters somewhat, there may be those who consider support group attendance to itself be a form of CAM.

Contentious Questions Related to Complementary and Alternative Medicine

We need look no further than to the reactions to Elizabeth Kaegi's *CMAJ* papers on alternative treatments for breast cancer to get a clear sense of the range of opinions in the medical community regarding complementary and alternative medicine. There is little doubt that Fernandez and colleagues (1998) were correct when they called discussions of CAM "highly polarized" (p. 1279). In fact, the worlds of Western medicine and CAM have been called "two solitudes" (Best & Herbert, 1998, p. 953). There are many questions concerning CAM that yield polarized answers. For example, should physicians be educated regarding the forms of CAM and the efficacy research that has been conducted? Should funding be provided for research into the effectiveness of CAM? Should patients pursue CAM? Should research be conducted to discover *why* patients use therapies for which evidence is scant or non-existent regarding their effectiveness?

To develop an appreciation of the divergence in practitioners' answers to these questions, consider the following positions. Tannock and Warr (1998) have stated that "...the decision to set aside funds to study 'complementary' cancer therapies...is in our opinion a big mistake" (p. 802). In response to the Tannock and Warr position, John Hoey, (1998) editor-in-chief of the *Canadian Medical Association Journal* wrote, "We need to construct bridges, not moats, between thoughtful and careful science and unconventional therapy" (p. 803). Let's look at the key questions associated with CAM and try to assess current opinions for each.

Should physicians be educated regarding the forms of CAM and the efficacy research that has been conducted? It is probably safe to say that the majority of physicians believe that they need to be reasonably well informed regarding the types of CAM and the nature of the research testing their effectiveness. This is because, as we have already seen in this section, a significant number of patients either use these treatments or are interested in them. Paradoxically, physicians may feel that their credibility is threatened if a patient asks a question regarding a therapy about which the physician knows little or nothing (Kent, 1997). It is also possible, though, that physicians may resent having to learn about alternative therapies, not because they are viable but because they feel their patients are unreasonably drawn to them.

Should funding be provided for research into the effectiveness of CAM? This is one of the most contentious issues associated with CAM, as indicated by the opinions expressed in the Tannock and Warr (1998) paper and the Hoey (1998) reply. Those who believe this research must be done fall into one of two camps. There are those who believe that virtually all unconventional treatments are ineffective and that this needs to be proven, and there are those who believe that some of these treatments may prove effective, and so we can leave no stone unturned in our search. Those in favour of this research accuse those opposed to it of pomposity and being fearful of change or of loss of "turf." On the other hand, those opposed to CAM efficacy research believe that we already have enough negative results from these therapies to know that they don't work. Thus, further research to confirm what we already know, just because there is a growing interest in the area among the lay population, represents a waste of precious research funds.

Where would health psychologists stand on this question? The answer depends on how complementary and alternative treatments are defined. If we are talking about such things as relaxation training and cognitive therapy to treat something like chronic pain, most if not all health psychologists would be strongly in favour of research testing these methods. On the other hand, if the treatment was shark's cartilage or healing crystals, we speculate that opinions would be less positive.

Should patients pursue CAM? In terms of ethics, this question takes us into murkier waters unless, of course, the treatment in question has been shown clearly to do more harm than good. However, to make this determination, we must conduct the very research that some physicians oppose. Typically, however, this question becomes difficult to answer because patients may be using treatments with little or no good evidence that they work or are harmful. Venturing into these unproven treatments may be a recipe for false hope, resulting in disappointment and/or depression, not to mention considerable expense. On the other hand, the reasons why patients show an interest in CAM are not entirely illogical. They can gain a feeling of control, especially when conventional treatments have proven ineffective. Health psychologists might say that these control-related cognitions that motivate an exploration of CAM are the very thoughts that are associated with better quality of life for those with a serious illness, regardless of the efficacy of the treatment (Helgeson, 1992). As such, patients should not be discouraged from this exploration.

Should research be conducted to discover why patients use therapies for which evidence is scant or non-existent regarding their effectiveness? For health psychologists, this is a much easier question to answer, and the response would be "yes." This is because the reasons why patients pursue CAM are primarily psychological in nature. In fact, health psychologists have theories that will provide comprehensive explanations for patients' interest in CAM. For this reason, health psychologists would say that research in this area should definitely be conducted. Later in this section, we will apply the theory of reasoned action to the seeking of complementary and alternative therapies. The products of this research will help health practitioners better understand beliefs and behaviours related to complementary and alternative medicine.

Given this rather complex set of questions and the diversity of opinions associated with them, it is not surprising to find the *Canadian Medical Association Journal* publishing, with the logo of the Canadian Cancer Society, Elizabeth Kaegi's (1998) article, "A Patient's Guide to Choosing Unconventional Therapies," as well as Tannock and Warr's (1998) comment that the article represents "a low point for both *CMAJ* and the Canadian Cancer Society" (p. 802). This mixed reaction is apparent among nurses as well. When Fitch and colleagues (1999) interviewed 20 nurses regarding their attitudes toward unconventional therapies, the prevailing opinions expressed were not negative. Rather, it was thought that more information on these therapies needs to be made available for patients and health care professionals. Also, the nurses were not generally critical of patients who sought such therapy. In contrast, 92 nurses in Finland expressed negative attitudes toward CAM, considering most of these methods to be unsafe and indicative of quackery rather than beneficial medicine (Salmenperae, Suominen, & Lauri, 1998). It must be noted that Fitch interviewed Canadian nurses, whereas Salmenperae, Suominen, and Lauri interviewed nurses in Finland. Also, Fitch distributed a guide to unconventional therapy to her participants before interviewing them.

Assessing Research in Complementary and Alternative Medicine

If we adopt the position that research into the effectiveness of complementary and alternative therapies should be conducted, then we must impose upon it the same standards of scientific rigour we would on any other research. It is unfortunate, indeed, that a considerable amount of research conducted to date in this area does not meet these standards. For example, a study may assess the effects of aromatherapy as a complementary therapy to conventional cancer treatment. In this study, the authors may report that the patients who used various aromatherapies experienced reductions in tension and other unpleasant effects of cancer treatment. However, such studies typically have no control group. Nor is there a group that is given aromas that were not expected to have any effects. Also, the sample size is usually small. This is not to say that aromatherapy cannot be helpful, but a study with these major flaws cannot assess this.

What questions should you ask to evaluate research in CAM? In a recent presentation at Simon Fraser University, Wallace Sampson, Stanford professor of medicine and editor-in-chief of *The Scientific Journal of Alternative Medicine*, provided some suggestions (Sampson, 1999). First, look for **evidential flaws**. As the term implies, these refer to the nature of the evidence provided. Be wary of subjective outcomes in the form of personal testimonials. There are many reasons why one person would report that an alternative treatment worked when it would not work for someone else. Also, pay attention to the size of the differences reported. If there is a control group, how much better did the treatment group fare? Are the differences clinically significant? If there isn't a control group, at least there should be pre- and post-test comparisons. How much improvement did these comparisons demonstrate? Remember that even pre- and post-test designs should have a control group. Finally, has the evidence been replicated? If so, how many times?

The issue of control groups needs further elaboration. Some studies do have control groups, but they do not match the treatment group very well. For example, they may be self-selected because they refused alternative treatment. Indeed, to be convincing, treatment studies must feature randomized assignment to treatment and control groups. They should also be conducted by researchers and practitioners who are blind as to which group a patient may be in. If the study features a pre-test baseline measure, check the duration of this measurement period. This is called a **run-in period**. In most well-conducted medical studies, this period is about 2 weeks. In poorly run studies, baseline measures may be taken only once, making them susceptible to reliability problems. In other words, the patient might have been doing very badly on that particular day, increasing the likelihood that an improvement would be found, even if it was only the result of the normal ups and downs of the illness.

At the other end of the timeline, be critical of studies that stop their analysis prematurely. Investigators may say that they ran a treatment over a 6-month period, but the best results occurred at the 2-month period, and these are the ones that get reported. By the end of the 6-month treatment period, the treatment group's advantage has disappeared.

Sampson also talks about **theoretical flaws**. These refer more to the underlying logic of the design and the research process than the nature of the evidence. For example, does the design produce evidence that is direct or indirect? If the intervention cannot be operationally defined, as in something like "healing energy", then we cannot assess its direct effect on a medical or psychological condition. Similarly, some research is guilty of errors of causality. Watch for a third factor that might explain the effect.

As we have stated, all research with biomedical outcomes, whether testing "conventional" or "unconventional" treatments, must be subjected to this analysis. This does not mean, however, that research on CAM should be rejected out of hand because it isn't easily explained by existing biomedical paradigms. Medical anthropologists would say that it is illogical to claim, in effect, that, "If our science can't explain it, it must be bad science."

Reported Benefits of Complementary and Alternative Medicine

When the standards of scientific rigour outlined in the previous section are applied, few complementary or alternative therapies have shown a proven benefit. Still, this does not mean that people don't feel that they have benefitted from some of these therapies. One of the reasons for this is the **placebo effect**. These are effects that are based on patients' beliefs rather than on the direct medicinal properties of the treatment. All treatments, regardless of how conventional, are affected by the extent to which the patient thinks they will work. For this reason, simply paying attention to a patient tends to be at least somewhat therapeutic. This is why research into CAM needs control conditions in which patients receive similar attention, even believing they are getting the alternative therapy in question when they are getting a placebo instead. This way, we can tease out the placebo effect from the reported benefit. This is not to say that the placebo effect isn't real. If a patient reports benefit then at some level there *is* benefit.

Patients using alternative therapies that have been proven generally ineffective may also be susceptible to something called **illusory correlation**. This means that, when two events seem to vary coincidentally, we think they are related causally. Patients with serious or chronic illness will often experience improvements and setbacks in their condition in the natural course of the disease. If an improvement coincides with a treatment, the patient will causally associate the two (Beyerstein, 1997).

Both placebo effects and illusory correlation are more likely if the patient believes that the treatment will work. But then, conventional treatments are also more likely to be effective if the patient believes they will work. This makes this a difficult area to assess, especially when one considers the growing body of evidence cited in Chapter 3 on psychoneuroimmunology, indicating relationships between psychological state and physical functioning. Remember also that health psychologists cannot and do not claim that the beneficial effects of all complementary and alternative therapies are attributable solely to psychological or coincidental factors. Rather, we are referring here to therapies that have been proven ineffective by research that controls for things like placebo and common fluctuations of conditions.

Decision Models and Theories Applied to the Decision to Use Complementary and Alternative Medicine

Here's a good essay question for an exam: How can the health belief model be used to explain why some people use complementary and alternative therapies and others do not? Interestingly, there is very little literature that applies the theory in this way. To answer the question, let's look at Table 14.1 to remind ourselves of the components of the theory.

TABLE 14-1 The Health Belief Model

General Belief	A Health Threat Exists		A Behaviour Will Affect the Threat	
Related Beliefs	Beliefs regarding personal vulnerability to the threat	Beliefs about the severity of the consequences	The belief that a course of action will actually work or not	The assessment of the costs and benefits associated with this action

On the left side of the model, we have general beliefs about the health threat. Specifically, the person has beliefs about vulnerability and severity. In the case of seriously ill patients, this side of the model is quite clear. These patients know they are vulnerable because of their diagnosis and the treatment they have gone through. This means that, unless the person is working very hard at denial, the vulnerability is quite salient. So too would beliefs about severity be quite clear. For cancer patients who have not had success with conventional therapy, the severity of their situation increases. For people who are dealing with conditions that are not life threatening, the severity beliefs obviously would not be as strong.

This means that, for cancer patients whose disease is progressing, at least half of the health belief model would predict that they would pursue alternative therapies. Let's look at the other side of the model. On the right side, we have beliefs about the behaviour, which in this case, involves using the treatment. Here is the most interesting side of the model in relation to CAM. First, there are the beliefs about the efficacy of the treatment. Will it work? In light of the information we have presented thus far in this section on CAM, this may well be a difficult question to answer definitively. It is this very uncertainty that makes this decision such an interesting one psychologically. We know that if the person does not think the treatment will work, then he or she is unlikely to try it. However, if the person believes there is a chance it will work, we then move to the last consideration—the assessment of costs and gains.

Here again, people may well be in a quandary. With little research to guide them, they cannot confidently assess the costs or gains. Is the treatment potentially toxic? Will it interact poorly with current conventional treatment if used in a complementary way? It may be difficult to know. In some cases, the patient believes the costs of the therapy are small compared to the potential gains. You may hear people say, "What have I got to lose? It can't hurt me and it might help." This is classic cost/gain thinking. Of course, this doesn't take monetary costs into account. One concern that physicians have is that their patients will waste large sums of money on untested therapies. From the patient's perspective, however, if they believe that the severity of their current condition is grave, then the cost/gain decision becomes an easier one. If they feel their prognosis is hopeless with conventional medicine, then even potentially toxic alternatives may look attractive from a cost/gain perspective.

Still, the patient is left with considerable uncertainty. At times like this, we often look to the opinions of others to help reduce the uncertainty (Festinger, 1954). To analyze this step, we need to expand our model to include an important element from the theory of reasoned action—subjective norms. Table 14.2 reminds us of the two components that are relevant here. First, there are the beliefs about what other people would do and what they would want us to do. Second, there is the motivation (or lack thereof) to do what others would want us to do. For a decision that features this much potential uncertainty, these can become very important considerations. This explains why prostate patients (either cancer or high-risk) are much more likely to use CAM if they attend a support group (Nam et al., 1999). The support group increases the chances that the person will be exposed to subjective norms favouring CAM use. Presumably, the more supportive the person perceives the group to be, the more motivated he or she will be to follow the norm.

TABLE 14-2 Subjective Norms as Defined in the Theory of Reasoned Action

Subjective Norms	
Beliefs regarding what other people think regarding the behaviour	Motivation to do what other people think should be done

The value of the health belief model is that it helps answer a question often asked by physicians: Why do patients pursue a particular alternative therapy when there is no evidence that it will work or even if there is evidence that it doesn't work? The answer is that beliefs about the efficacy of the treatment are only part of the decision equation. Admittedly, even the model does not shed a great deal of light on situations in which people whose prognosis is not bleak still pursue treatments that are proven to be expensive, ineffective, and toxic. However, the model would also predict that such people are quite rare compared to those who pursue CAM because their beliefs about its efficacy are just positive enough to move them to a cost/gain analysis.

FOCUS ON RESEARCH 14-1 Deciding to Use Alternative Therapies

Women in Toronto who were coping with the symptoms of menopause were interviewed regarding their use of alternative therapies (Seidl & Stewart, 1998). The study included 13 women whose average age was 52.6 years. Reasons for using alternative therapy were consistent with the health belief model. In terms of their cost/gain analysis, the women using alternative therapy stated the belief that the treatment was safe and somewhat helpful. In terms of subjective norms, those using the therapy reported confidence in the advice they received from non-physicians but were not motivated to follow their physician's advice because some of the participants perceived their physicians to be disinterested or negative regarding alternative therapy.

In another study, (Boon et al., 1999) breast cancer patients ranging in age from 41 to 73 years met in focus groups to discuss why they did or did not use alternative therapy. The researchers confirmed that these decisions were made without the benefit of much research evidence supporting or discrediting alternative therapies. The women's reasons for using or not using these therapies fit well within the cost/gain component of the health belief model. Women who used an alternative therapy believed that it could do little harm, and so any gain at all would tip the balance in favour of the therapy. In contrast, women who did not use alternative therapy did not believe that it would work and believed that it could be harmful.

When we compare the reasons provided by the women in these two studies, we find some similarities and some differences. Those pursuing alternative therapy, whether they were dealing with menopause or breast cancer, did so because they felt the potential gains would outweigh the costs. However, the menopausal women were more likely to cite a disenchantment with the conventional medical system than were the breast cancer patients. The sample sizes do not allow us to conclude that this is a trend among menopausal women. Rather, the two studies point out some of the different reasons why people may choose CAM.

SOME CANADIAN RESEARCH PROGRAMS: THE SEARCH FOR PROOF

When we started writing this book, we asked various health psychologists working in Canadian universities to send us some of their research papers. Our hope was that this would give us a "snapshot" of the types of work being done across the country. This did turn out to be the case. In this section, we want to show you this snapshot so that you will get an idea of several research programs that are either quite new or are well established in Canadian health psychology. The key word here is "program." We are not describing isolated studies in this section. Instead, we are looking at research representing a number of years of investigation into some aspect of health psychology. As you read through the descriptions, try to get a sense of the programmatic nature of the work. It is possible that some of these programs are where the future lies in terms of Canadian research in the discipline and, perhaps, for yourself if you are interested in being a part of that future. The list is not intended to be exhaustive. It is, rather, a sampling.

Studying the Relationship between Psychological State and the Cardiovascular System

A considerable amount of research has been conducted investigating possible relationships between psychological states and cardiovascular health. Wolfgang Linden and his colleagues at UBC have conducted a significant portion of this research, focusing much of their attention on what is called **cardiovascular reactivity**. This refers to acute cardiovascular changes in response to some stimulus, often a stressor of some kind. This acute reactivity is believed to be related to chronic hypertension (high blood pressure) and, therefore, risk for coronary heart disease (CHD). In other words, one explanation for the relationship between stress and CHD is that some people have cardiovascular systems that react much more dramatically than others in the face of stressors. Also, this reactivity may be predicted by psychological factors. If these factors can be identified, then interventions can be implemented to affect them and thus further reduce risk of CHD. This is just the sort of work Wolfgang Linden and his colleagues have been doing for much of the 1990s.

In the early 1990s, Linden and others (Linden, Chambers, Maurice, & Lenz, 1993) had students wear monitors to measure their blood pressure at various points in their day. These readings were then correlated with psychosocial variables such as hostility and social support. They found that women's systolic blood pressure was significantly correlated with their social support (systolic blood pressure is the larger of the two numbers, usually reported before diastolic pressure. For example, in a reading of 120/70, the 120 would be systolic and the 70 diastolic). For men in this study, their levels of hostility were significantly related to their heart rates and overall blood pressure. These findings are independent of other physical predictors of blood pressures such as age, alcohol consumption, and body fat.

Given this finding, the next step should be to assess the effects of interventions designed to moderate psychosocial factors and thus improve cardiovascular health. This is just what Linden and Chambers did in 1994 when they published a meta-analysis of 166 studies on the topic. The purpose of their meta-analysis was to compare non-drug treatments of hypertension to drug treatments. Non-drug treatments included such things as weight reduction, exercise, and cognitive-behavioural therapy. They discovered that these non-drug treatments were generally as good as drug treatments in reducing systolic blood pressure. It is important to note that drug therapies are typically introduced when blood pressure is quite high; indeed, higher than for non-drug treatments, which are usually introduced before drug therapy. Linden and Chambers controlled for these initial blood pressure levels when they did their analysis.

Several years later, Linden, Stossel, and Maurice (1996) conducted another meta-analysis, this time comparing different treatments for patients with coronary artery disease. The two treatment types were: (1) a standard treatment, consisting of medication, exercise, and diet regulation; and, (2) this standard treatment plus psychosocial interventions, including such things as relaxation training and group counselling. Again, it was found that the addition of psychosocial treatment improved outcomes in terms of reduced psychological distress, systolic blood pressure, heart rate, and cholesterol levels. Further, groups receiving the standard treatment only had higher recurrence of cardiac problems and mortality rates.

Still another meta-analysis showed that autogenic training also helped reduce angina pectoris (chest pain) and hypertension (Linden, 1994). **Autogenic training** is a form of cognitive-behavioural intervention in which the person learns a set of six formulas intended to enhance relaxation and vascular dilation. These include repeating to oneself such phrases as, "My arm is very heavy" to improve relaxation and, "My arm is very warm" to improve vascular dilation.

At about this same time, Linda Turner, Wolfgang Linden, and others (Turner et al., 1995) pilot-tested a program of their own that featured stress management and exercise. They compared a group involved in this program to a group that did exercise only, measuring blood pressure reactivity in patients who had heart disease, as indicated by myocardial infarction (MI) or coronary artery bypass graft (CABG). Though the study had a small sample size due in part to a fairly high dropout rate, the exercise plus stress management program was found to be superior to exercise alone in reducing blood pressure reactivity.

The next logical step was to control the nature of the stressor and manipulate some psychosocial factor. Two studies did this. In one, researchers from universities in California, New York, and British Columbia collaborated to measure the effect of different forms of social support on cardiovascular reactivity (Christenfeld et al., 1997). In this study, people gave a speech in one of three conditions. In one, they talked to a neutral stranger. In another, they talked to a supportive stranger. In a third, they talked to a friend. It was found that systolic blood pressure reactivity was lower when the speech was given in front of a supportive stranger or a friend than in front of a neutral stranger. The next study looked at the other side of the coin, creating conditions in which people were non-supportive rather than supportive (Earle, Linden, & Weinberg, in press). This time, one group of participants was verbally harassed as they did mental arithmetic tasks. The harassed women showed higher heart rates. The harassed men showed the greatest increase in diastolic blood pressure. All harassed participants, regardless of sex, showed greater general stress reactivity in the form of an elevated cortisol response. Cortisol is a product of autonomic reactivity; specifically, the link between the hypothalamus, the pituitary gland, and the adrenal gland.

Linden's more recent work, in conjunction with colleagues including Thomas Rutledge at Toronto Hospital and Andrea Con at St. Paul's hospital in Vancouver, focuses on psychological aspects of treatment for and recovery from heart disease. One study (Rutledge & Linden, forthcoming) features an investigation of psychological factors that might inhibit standard drug treatment regimens for ischemic heart disease. This is heart disease that involves a blockage of blood flow. Patients received common anti-ischemic drugs or a placebo condition. These conditions were compared to a baseline condition without drugs for number of ischemic episodes, treadmill performance, blood pressure, and post-treatment angina. It was found that daily baseline stress levels impaired drug treatment effects for number of ischemic episodes, treadmill time, and post-treatment angina. Also higher scores on a measure of hostility were related to smaller improvements in blood pressure during drug therapy. It is interesting to note that, despite the fact that psychological factors can interfere with drug treatment for these patients, less than 50 percent of treatment programs include psychosocial interventions, though that number appears to be increasing (Rutledge & Linden, in press).

Finally, Con, Linden, Thompson, and Ignaszewski (in press) compared psychological responses of men and women recovering from coronary artery bypass graft (CABG). While previous studies had looked at the psychological aspects of men's recovery from CABG, comparisons between men and women had not been made. It was discovered that women were more likely to experience greater depressive symptoms and that these symptoms were positively correlated with their reports of pain. For men, pain and functional impairment were negatively correlated with social support.

Studying the Working Lives of Health Care Practitioners

In Chapter 8, we cited the work of Astrid Richardsen and Ron Burke at York University, who conducted an extensive survey of Canadian physicians to investigate their stress levels and the factors that predicted their stress. As you may remember, the researchers discovered that 38 percent of those responding described their practice as being very or extremely stressful (Burke & Richardsen, 1990). Also, physicians cited time pressure as a significant contributor to this stress (Richardsen & Burke, 1991). Ron Burke has also worked with Ester Greenglass at York to learn about the ways nurses cope with changes to their work.

In two papers (Greenglass & Burke, 1997; 1999), these researchers explored the nature of nurses' psychological responses to hospital restructuring in Ontario. In that province, as has been the case in most of Canada, "restructuring" has meant "downsizing." While some of this downsizing is the result of improvements in medical technology and pharmaceutical science, much is the result of governmental decisions to decrease spending. Greenglass and Burke wanted to know if these cutbacks and related changes were affecting nurses' anxiety levels or their job-related anger and hostility.

Greenglass and Burke (1997) have described the extent of hospital restructuring in Ontario in the 1990s. There were 10 hospitals targeted to be closed in the Toronto area and it was estimated that 10 000 health care workers would lose their jobs in the province. These workers feel the stressful impact on two simultaneous fronts—their workload goes up as does the threat that they will lose their jobs. Such changes are hard enough for any job sector to deal with, but it is especially hard for those in health care, where caring for others is the main objective and the workers know that cutbacks could severely compromise their ability to provide that care. Greenglass and Burke cite a nursing survey indicating that 81 percent of 20 000 nurses in Ontario believe that downsizing and budget cuts have yielded unsafe conditions for patients (Dialogue on Health Reform, 1996, cited in Greenglass and Burke, 1997).

In their research, Greenglass and Burke surveyed over 1 300 nurses. They asked them to document such things as their current workload, the upkeep of their hospital, the extent of restructuring they had encountered and the impact this had on health care and staff moral, and their understanding of the hospital's future plan. This last variable also included an assessment of the nurses' involvement in that planning. Psychological variables studied included measures of state and trait anger, hostility, anxiety, depression, and self-efficacy as well as other variables.

They discovered that evidence of cutbacks, in the form of budget cuts and layoffs, was prevalent at almost all the hospitals in which respondents worked. These cuts and layoffs were significantly correlated with anxiety and depression. Interestingly, anxiety was negatively correlated with the amount of involvement the nurses said they had in the hospital restructuring process. Anger was positively correlated with their reports of job deterioration ($r = .29$), perceived impact of restructuring ($r = .33$), and workload ($r = .35$). Anger was negatively correlated with the amount of information that the hospital disseminated to the nurses ($r = -.12$).

In that same sample, Greenglass and Burke (1999) looked at the impact of these variables on role conflict. In Chapter 13, we introduced this as role strain, referring to a situation in which someone is expected to perform two or more roles that compete for the person's time and, in addition, may be in conflict with one another. Greenglass and Burke discuss two types of role conflict for nurses, the majority of whom are female. They called one **work-family conflict** and the other **family-work conflict**. The former refers to the extent to which work obligations interfere with family obligations; the latter refers to the reverse. Greenglass and Burke were able to construct a model using multiple regression that accounted for 20 percent of the variance in work-family conflict. The elements of the model included demographic variables, job-related variables (such as whether the nurses worked full- or part-time), perceived stressors, and individual resources (such as self-efficacy). Of these variables, stressors accounted for the most variance in work-family conflict (13 percent). These stressors were measured in terms of the amount of hospital restructuring. What this all means is that hospital restructuring brought on by budget cuts increased the likelihood that nurses would have work-related obligations interfere with family life. This suggests that such restructuring will have effects that reach beyond the hospital workplace.

Studying the Social Psychology of Sexual and Reproductive Health

Given that sexual behaviour is usually social in nature, it makes sense that there are social psychological factors affecting things like safer sex practices and general sexual and reproductive health. William Fisher and his colleagues at the University of Western Ontario and elsewhere have looked at some of these factors. For example, they have reviewed literature that has assessed the ways different types of dyadic relationships are related to AIDS risk behaviour (Misovich, Fisher, & Fisher, 1997).

You might assume that people in longterm, stable relationships are less likely to engage in sexual behaviour that puts them at risk for AIDS. However, Misovich, Fisher, and Fisher (1997) argue that this is not necessarily the case. Being in a trusting, longterm relationship may be psychologically rewarding, but it is not a guarantee against AIDS. The only way such a relationship is safe is if both partners are "tested and true" — tested in that they are sure they are HIV negative, and true in that they will definitely remain monogamous.

These authors suggest that this monogamy is not common enough in modern relationships to allow us to generalize regarding the safety of longterm relationships when it comes to sexual health.

Misovich and colleagues (1997) state that there are at least two kinds of monogamy that are common today. One is **serial monogamy**. This means that a person stays exclusively with one partner for a time, and then may move on to another partner. At no time are there two simultaneous relationships; over the course of time, however, there are multiple partners. The other kind is what the authors call **realistic monogamy**. This is defined as serial monogamy plus occasional transgressions. The important point is that sexual activity is often unprotected in each scenario and, because there are steady partners involved, sex is more frequent. In fact, the only way that these longer-term relationships can be low risk in terms of AIDS is if partners honestly admit to any violations of monogamy and then are both re-tested for HIV. The investigators' conclusion is that people in longterm relationships may actually be at greater risk for HIV infection.

Misovich and colleagues (1997) provide evidence, albeit indirect, in support of this conclusion. For example, in the mid-1990s the Centers for Disease Control in Atlanta reported that the incidence of HIV related illness increased rapidly among persons infected heterosexually. It has also been shown that single men having more than one recent sexual partner were twice as likely as men in monogamous relationships to use condoms (Tanfer et al., 1993, cited in Misovich, 1997). Another study found that heterosexual men and women in their late twenties tended to say that they always used a condom with casual partners and never with their relationship partners (McKusick, Hoff, Stall, & Coates, 1991, cited in Misovich et al., 1997).

Fisher and colleagues have also explored other aspects of reproductive and sexual health (Fisher et al., submitted for publication). In one study, they surveyed over 400 women attending an obstetrics and gynecology outpatient clinic to determine sexual and reproductive health as well as incidence of sexual coercion and partner abuse. These patients were also asked whether they had discussed these problems with their physicians. In this way, the researchers got a measure of problem prevalence and the patient-physician dialogue (or lack thereof) regarding these problems.

Fisher and colleagues discovered that 25 to 30 percent of single women had multiple sex partners during the preceding year, yet fewer than 25 percent of these women said a condom was always used. In fact, less that 20 percent of single, non-pregnant women with more than one sexual partner said they always used condoms. Seventy-one percent of single, non-pregnant women said they had discussed condom use with their physicians.

In terms of sexual coercion and partner abuse, 22 percent of all women said they had had sexual contact with someone against their will due to verbal threats. Ten percent of these women said this occurred before the age of twelve years. Twenty-three percent said they had been forced to have sexual contact against their will due to physical force. Seven percent of these were before the age of twelve years. Unlike condom use, which the majority of women discussed with their physicians, sexual coercion is discussed much less frequently. Only 33 percent of women said they had discussed incidents involving verbal threats with their physician, and 37 percent said they had discussed physical force. One conclusion from this research could be that physicians would underestimate the incidence of coercion and abuse in their patients' lives due to patients' decisions not to discuss these things with them.

CASE 14-1 Pains of the Mind Felt in the Gut

Sue-Ann first started experiencing symptoms while she was driving her car. The portion of her seat belt that went across her lap seemed to be pushing into her right side as though caused by something in her coat pocket. But there wasn't anything in her coat pocket. Sometimes the sensation was faint; other times it was as though there was some internal inflammation and swelling. Sue-Ann thought little of this until things started to get worse. She would feel bloated at times, and other times she would feel cramps in her lower abdomen.

Then one day she was talking on the phone at work. The conversation was with a colleague who seemed to be good at coming up with problem after problem but never with any solutions. As the conversation went on, Sue-Ann's cramping in her intestinal tract got worse and worse until finally she found herself doubled over trying to cope with it. When this happened, she decided enough was enough and she called her GP for an appointment.

Sue-Ann's GP ordered a series of tests to rule out anything serious like cancer. The tests showed that she did not have cancer, but the symptoms persisted, especially when things were particularly demanding at work. Her doctor told her that she had functional dyspepsia, which was caused by a narrowing of the intestine where the large and small intestine meet. Sue-Ann's physician said that she could prescribe medicine but that the best treatment would be the adoption of an exercise plan that featured continuous exercise, like jogging. Also, she should find ways to relax more.

Studying Affective Distress and Physical Health

We talk of having "butterflies" in our stomach when we are tense. If you have ever had this sensation and thought that stressors and anxiety in your life were having an adverse effect on your gastrointestinal system, you may well have been right. Ron Norton and colleagues at the University of Winnipeg and the Regina Health District (Norton et al., forthcoming) have studied the relationship between affective distress and what are called functional gastrointestinal (FGI) disorders. They have found a relationship between certain kinds of affective distress and specific gastrointestinal functions. In other words, the functional dyspepsia experienced by Sue-Ann in Case Study 14.1 could very well be brought on by stress and anxiety.

This is an important area of research, because it has been shown that FGI symptoms, from esophageal to anorectal, are quite common. One study of over 5 000 people in the United States found that 69 percent of them had experienced symptoms of at least one FGI disorder (Drossman et al., 1993, cited in Norton et al., in press). Other research in Switzerland has shown that stomach complaints are significantly related to depression and intestinal complaints to anxiety (Hochstrasser and Angst, 1996, cited in Norton et al., forthcoming).

With this in mind, Norton and colleagues surveyed 127 university students with a mean age of 20 years regarding their FGI symptoms and affective distress. They discovered that, independent of any experiences with anxiety or depression, 51 percent of the students reported

FGI disorders. This means that they reported symptoms that met diagnostic criteria and lasted for at least 3 months. In addition to measuring incidence of anxiety and depression, the researchers also assessed **anxiety sensitivity**. This refers to the extend to which people fear anxiety-related symptoms because they believe these symptoms will have serious social, physical, or psychological consequences. Anxiety sensitivity can be called a "fear of fear." In addition to discovering that FGI disorders were quite prevalent among this sample of young adults, Norton's team found that anxiety sensitivity was significantly related to an FGI disorder known as *functional dyspepsia*, which is experienced as an uncomfortable disruption of functioning of the intestinal tract.

The FGI study assumed that psychological states would have an impact on physical functioning. Asmundson and colleagues (1998) looked at the reverse—the possibility that work-related injury could result in post-traumatic stress disorder (PTSD). Of course, the process doesn't stop there, because PTSD can then affect pain experience and recovery. In a study that included 121 injured workers who had been referred for rehabilitation, Asmundson and colleagues identified prevalence of PTSD and other psychological factors that were predictors of PTSD. Most of the participants (81 percent) reported current and chronic pain. The investigators found that 35 percent of their sample displayed current symptoms of PTSD. Also, PTSD frequency was correlated with scores on the Beck Depression Inventory ($r = .57$) and the Anxiety Sensitivity Index ($r = .49$). Research linking PTSD and chronic pain is necessarily correlational, and so we cannot draw firm conclusions regarding causal links. However, a number of studies of accident victims have shown that chronic pain and PTSD commonly coexist. For example, Chibnall and Duckro (1993, cited in Asmundson et al.) found that 29 percent of motor vehicle accident sufferers referred to a pain clinic for headaches met PTSD criteria. Taken collectively, this research indicates that PTSD, which is related to psychological states such as depression and anxiety sensitivity, can be a problem for people recovering from injury.

Graduate Research in Community Health at the University of Northern British Columbia

The University of Northern British Columbia offers graduate degrees in psychology and in community health. Through the community health program, students (some of whom are health care practitioners returning for continuing education) can work in interdisciplinary settings to study pressing health issues. Two such issues are First Nations health and cancer screening behaviour.

The Health Belief Model and First Nations Health Care

We have seen elsewhere in this book (Chapter 11 on serious illness and Chapter 13 on medical anthropology) that the health concerns of First Nations peoples are unique compared to those of the rest of the population. The prevalence of some medical conditions is greater and, it has been argued, sociological and anthropological reasons can be cited to explain why the need for aboriginal health care is greater than it is for some of the other segments of the population (Verde, 1999). For these reasons, much research is needed on First Nations health status and behaviours.

There is evidence that First Nations people underuse health care for prevention or early care, which results in more prolonged treatment that might have been avoidable (Verdes, 1999). The health belief model might be useful in trying to understand First Nations patterns of health care usage (see Table 14.1 for a brief summary of the model). Specifically, First Nations males and females may differ from non-natives (and from each other) in their beliefs about vulnerability and severity. Also, it is very possible that the costs or barriers associated with using the health care system are different for native and non-native Canadians. It is precisely these possibilities that Domingos Verdes investigated in his graduate work (Verdes, 1999).

What barriers may exist for First Nations people when it comes to using the health care system? Verdes points out that there are quite a few. One is trust. Given that First Nations people have experienced a history in which they suffered exploitation and abuse, it wouldn't be surprising to find that they don't have a great deal of trust in yet another non-native institution—the health care system. Also, there are cultural barriers made more significant by a health care system that isn't always culturally sensitive. For example, First Nations people may have different interactional styles, such as engaging in less eye contact, that might be misinterpreted by non-native practitioners. Also, there may be differences in cultural values, as one culture values competitiveness and individualism while the other values codependence and collectivism. Related to this is a possible language barrier. Finally, there may be perceptions of racism, with First Nations people believing that practitioners have negative opinions of them.

It is also possible that these barriers affect males and females differently. For example, income and transportation difficulties might be more prevalent for females than males. Males, on the other hand, might believe they are not susceptible to disease in order to preserve an image of strength.

Verde tested these possibilities by administering a questionnaire to 100 members of the Nisga'a First Nation, along the Northwest coast of British Columbia. He found that elements of the health belief model did predict frequency of health care usage at a clinic serving the area. For females, frequency of usage was related to having a family physician, age, financial barriers, and perceived susceptibility. Interestingly, frequency of usage was not related to child care, cultural differences, trust in modern medicine, transportation or perceived racism. For males, usage was related to the amount of health knowledge the men had, as well as perceived cultural differences. Verdes concluded that for this community at least, the health belief model can be used to understand First Nations health care usage.

Social and Cultural Factors Influencing Women's Participation in Cancer Screening Services. Research has been conducted to measure participation rates of First Nations women in cervical cancer screening programs. It has been discovered that these participation rates are low, in spite of the fact that mortality rates due to cervical cancer are high among First Nations women (Deschamps et al., 1992, cited in Bryant, 1999). There are a number of reasons for this lack of participation, some of which might be encompassed by the health belief model as applied by Verdes (1999). Other social and cultural reasons have been cited as well. For example, Deschamps and colleagues discovered that there was a lack of knowledge among First Nations women about the Pap test and its importance. Related to this are reports by First Nations women that they feel embarrassed about the procedure. Also, there can be a lack of continuity of care due to a high turnover rate among physicians in aboriginal communities. Finally, Clarke and colleagues (1998, cited in Bryant, 1999) have pointed out that the clinics can be culturally insensitive.

For her graduate research, Bryant used data from the 1994 National Population Health Survey to analyze the use of cancer screening among 416 women in the Prince George area. She found that participation rates were generally high, as they have been across the province of British Columbia. However, the lowest participation was among immigrant women, single women, and women with less education. Also, older women were less likely than younger women to have mammograms and Pap tests. Bryant concluded that health promotion campaigns must be aware of these groups in which underuse is more common and try to target information to them.

FUNDING HEALTH PSYCHOLOGY RESEARCH

In this section, we will describe major changes to the ways health psychology research is being funded in Canada. In fact, these changes apply to all health-related research. We know that you might not be at a stage in your academic career when you will be applying for research funding. Nevertheless, you are currently reading a very important section of this book. The reasons for this are numerous.

First, the nature of funding that a country provides for health research says a great deal about the extent to which government values the health of its citizens, and you need to have an understanding of the Canadian situation. Second, the types of health research that are funded indicate the way determinants of health are construed; if all the research money went to biomedical researchers, this would be a clear statement that psychosocial factors are not considered important. Fortunately, this is not the case in Canada. Instead, the program that we are going to describe stems from the acknowledgment that there are numerous determinants of health and that we need to do research that investigates all of these in a coordinated way.

This leads to another reason for this section. As a student of health psychology, you not only need to know something about the *methods* that psychologists have used to generate the knowledge documented in a text of this kind, you also need to know something about the *means*. There will be very few findings reported in this book (or any other like it) that were not generated by funded research. Knowledge of this nature doesn't just happen. It results from time-consuming research that is paid for by someone who thinks it is valuable. The fact that new programs are emerging in this country to fund multidisciplinary research in health says something very important about the country. Finally, as a taxpayer, you are the "someone" who is providing the funding. It is important, therefore, to know how that funding is being managed and allocated.

Rationale for a New Funding Structure for Health-Related Research in Canada

Canada has experienced a "brain drain" in recent years—an alarming number of our highly trained researchers are leaving the country. For the most part, they are going to the United States, lured by higher salaries and better research opportunities. Nowhere is this more true than in health research. In a presentation to the Standing Committee on Finance Roundtable on Research, the president of the Coalition for Biomedical and Health Research, Dr. Barry

McLennan, pointed out that for every seven investigators that leave Canada, only one returns (McLennan & Gauthier, 1998). McLennan cited a C.D. Howe Institute study estimating the costs of this brain drain to the Canadian economy to be approximately $1.68 billion per year. If about one-third of this is health-related, this means a loss of $560 million per year. Stopping the brain drain would pay for a significant increase in health-related funding—one of the main reasons for the problem in the first place!

Canada's health care system is touted as one of the best in the world. Its maintenance requires more than just money. It needs well-coordinated research that can be translated into better health care practices and improved quality of life for Canadians. As we have seen throughout this book, this research is challenging because we must acknowledge the multiple determinants of health. We must explore everything from molecules to communities. In fact, those extremes are mentioned in the description of Canada's new health research funding structure, the Canadian Institutes for Health Research (CIHR).

In its attempt to improve the coordination of health-related research and encourage multidisciplinary approaches to that research, the CIHR offers new opportunities to health psychologists. To quote the CIHR web site, "CIHR is committed to bringing health researchers from the social sciences and humanities into a strong, national network to collaborate with scientists from other health research disciplines" (www.mrc.gc.ca/cihr-icrs). In other words, the CIHR has the potential to do the kinds of things we were talking about at the beginning of this section—to improve health research and send clear messages regarding the value of this research and the importance of investigating multiple determinants of health. Let's take a closer look at the CIHR to get an idea of what it proposes to do.

The Canadian Institutes for Health Research

In 1998, a task force was struck to investigate ways in which health research funding could be improved in Canada. At that time, the majority of government funding was supplied by the Medical Research Council (MRC) and the National Health Research and Development Program (NHRDP). Other councils supplying health research funding included the Social Sciences and Humanities Research Council (SSHRC) and the Natural Sciences and Engineering Research Council (NSERC). These agencies worked well for some time. However, it was difficult to coordinate multidisciplinary research because biomedical researchers were typically applying to one agency and social science and humanities researchers to another. The task force, therefore, proposed the CIHR. This bit of history is important, because it shows that the CIHR was proposed by researchers and practitioners, not politicians. In October of 1999, Health Minister Allan Rock announced the creation of specific CIHR programs, with application deadlines of January and February 2000.

To be perfectly practical, the excitement over these developments was not based entirely on the announcement of a new structure. It was probably generated primarily by the promise of significant increases in funding. The recommendation was that health research should be funded to the tune of $750 million annually. The current budget for the Medical Research Council is $267 million. The federal government allocated an additional $65 million for health research in 2000/01, and another $175 million for the following fiscal year. These are the kinds of numbers that attract the attention of researchers.

The Four Theme Areas of the Canadian Institutes for Health Research

In an attempt to focus and coordinate health research, the CIHR has identified four theme areas. One is basic biomedical research. Examples would be genetic research and microbiological research. A second theme is applied clinical research. Examples include searches for cures for specific diseases, as well as research that applies the findings from basic research. A third theme is research on health care systems and services. Research on this theme may test a rehabilitation program or investigate ways of delivering health care in ways that are more cost effective. The final theme is society, culture, and health of populations. In this area, research would look at social and behavioural determinants of health as well as community programs and cultural factors affecting the use of the health care system.

The creation of the CIHR represents a transition from a group of separate funding agencies to one unified program. As we pointed out earlier, before the CIHR, health-related research was funded by a number of different agencies, including the MRC, SSHRC, and NSERC. In addition to being less coordinated, it was very possible for health related research to "fall between the cracks" in this divided system. For example, a psychologist might submit a grant proposal to MRC for a study looking at communication between physicians and patients. That council might think that it wasn't "really medical" and so send it to SSHRC. By this time, granting decisions would have already been made for that year's SSHRC competitions, and the project wouldn't get funded.

The Nature of the Canadian Institutes for Health Research

At the heart of the CIHR concept is a series of institutes based on health-related topics. The plan is to have 10 to 15 of these across the country. They will be "virtual" in nature, so that funding will not be spent on buildings to house them. In the language of funding, CIHR states that the funding is not for "bricks and mortar." When the CIHR is fully operational, researchers will apply directly to the relevant institute for funding. In so doing, they become affiliated with the institute. This provides the added advantage of expanding networks of communication between researchers working in similar fields. To further increase the likelihood of this, institutes will be encouraged to organize conferences on their designated topic. It is also hoped that the institutes will be able to more efficiently prioritize research needs and help researchers develop joint projects with colleagues across the country. For example, a researcher looking at social support among prostate cancer patients in Nova Scotia could be linked to others doing work with support groups and other prostate patients across the country. This would greatly increase the sample size of the study and the possibility that important findings would be translated into helpful interventions on a national scale.

With these examples in mind, the goals of the institutes become readily apparent. They will be designed to integrate health research into Canada's health care system on a national level where appropriate, coordinate research on a national level, and help Canadians get the best benefits of the research (both human and economic). Some possible examples include an Institute of Aging, of Immunology and Infectious Diseases, and of Public and Population Health.

The First Programs from the Canadian Institutes for Health Research

To make the transition from the old to the new system of funding, the established agencies have put together what is called a "suite of new transitional programs." The nature of these programs provides evidence of new thinking regarding the way health research can be conducted, which is very relevant to health psychologists. When we look at each program, try to imagine ways in which the work of psychologists could be supported.

One of the new transition programs is called the Community Alliance for Health Research (CAHR). The hallmark of this program is the formation of partnerships between community groups and university-based researchers. Such partnerships are not new. However, the difference in this case is that the community groups will be expected to be fully involved in the formulation of research plans, disseminating findings, and applying the outcomes of the research. One goal is to "enhance mutual learning among community groups and researchers" (CIHR web site). Another goal is to enhance the relevance of the research.

Consider the implications of this program for our prostate cancer researchers. Now, instead of measuring social support by asking permission to go into support groups and clinics, the researchers would enlist the involvement of the support group executive in *designing* the study in the first place. Other teams could be formed to investigate ways to improve health care delivery to remote communities. The possibilities are numerous. This program came into operation in April 2000.

Another program is called the Interdisciplinary Health Research Teams (IHRT). This program provides funding for groups of five or more researchers forming an interdisciplinary team that addresses a single health issue. In addition to being interdisciplinary, the team must have members from at least two institutions. You can see from these rules that CIHR wants to encourage collaboration more than competition between institutions. Also, the multidisciplinary stipulation of the program opens the door for research that adopts the biopsychosocial model, which has been so prominent in this book.

The CIHR, then, invites Canadian health researchers to acknowledge the many factors affecting health and to work together across institutions and disciplines to study these factors, improve the health of Canadians, and keep our health care system highly regarded. It is hoped that this new funding structure will bring health psychologists into the picture even more prominently when it comes to health-related research in the years to come.

BOX 14-1 Canadian Health Data on the Internet

As a nation, Canada does a very good job of collecting health-related data. We took advantage of these resources in the course of writing this book, often accessing them on the Internet as we wrote. Because of this comprehensiveness and convenience, we thought you might also want to be privy to a number of the sources we found so helpful.

Statistics Canada: The People

Perhaps the most comprehensive source of health-related statistics can be found on the Statistics Canada web site (www.statcan.ca). When you visit the site, you will discover that statistics are divided into four large sections: "The People", "The Land", "The Economy", and "The State." It is "The People" that you should explore for health statistics. You will learn that only select data are available free on the site. There is much more that can be ordered. Still, even within the free material there is a wealth of information on the status of Canadians' health and their patterns of usage of the health care system. If you are referencing this material, make a note of the catalogue number that usually appears at the bottom of each chart.

Health Canada

Closely related to Statistics Canada is Health Canada (www.hc-sc.gc.ca). Here again, there is a wealth of information on the health of Canadians. It is not all statistical. Some of it takes the form of articles and other documents. They are organized alphabetically from "Aboriginal Health" all the way to "Youth."

Canadian Institute for Health Information

The Canadian Institute for Health Information has offices in Ottawa, Toronto, Edmonton, and Vancouver. Its main function is to bring together health-related information from Statistics Canada, Health Canada, The Hospital Medical Records Institute, and other organizations. As such, it is a convenient web site to use as a starting point for a general search for information (www.cihi.ca).

The Canadian Institutes for Health Research

We have already discussed the CIHR in this chapter. This is the web site where we found much of our information (www.mrc.gc.ca/cihr-icrs).

KEY TERMS

evidential flaws
run-in period
theoretical flaws
placebo effect
illusory correlation
cardiovascular reactivity
autogenic training
work-family conflict
family-work conflict
serial monogamy
realistic monogamy
anxiety sensitivity

Glossary

A-Delta Fibres The afferent peripheral fibres that are associated with transmitting sharp, distinct pain.

Acceleration-Deceleration Injury A type of concussion that occurs when an immobile head is hit by a moving object or a moving head hits an immobile object.

Acceptance The final stage of Kübler-Ross' theory of death and dying in which the person achieves a peaceful acceptance of his or her own death.

Accounting for Variance Using correlations and other statistics to identify predictor variables that account for differences in some outcome variable.

Acquired Immune Deficiency Syndrome (AIDS) A disease that develops as a result of the human immunodeficiency virus (HIV). The body's compromised immune system makes it susceptible to a host of other infections.

Acquired Immunity Protection against an antigen as a result of prior exposure to the antigen, either by having contracted the disease or by receiving an inoculation that presents the body with a non-toxic dose of the antigen.

Active Leisure A positive experience that is associated with activities such as hobbies, playing a musical instrument, and exercise.

Active-Passive Model A patient is unable to participate in his care or to make decisions for his own welfare because of his medical condition.

Acupuncture An ancient Chinese pain control technique that involves the insertion of fine needles to create stimulation to the peripheral nerves.

Acute Illness An illness with a defined beginning and end.

Acute Pain Pain that lasts less than 6 months and serves to warn of impending tissue damage or the need for convalescent rest.

Acute Stressor A stressor that is immediate in its duration and proximity.

Adaptive Observation An approach used by anthropologists when gathering data in which they try to fit to the observational setting without drawing attention to themselves.

Addiction The state of being physically or psychologically dependent on a substance.

Addictive Smokers Smokers who develop a psychological dependence on smoking and are keenly aware when they are not smoking.

Adherence The degree to which patients carry out the behaviours and treatments that physicians and other health professionals recommend.

Adjunctive Methods Treatments that complement biomedical regiments, such as behaviour therapies.

Adjuvant Therapy Therapy used in conjunction with other therapy.

Adrenal Cortex The outer portion of the adrenal gland that provides hormones to the body at times of stress. These hormones assist with the provision of energy and increase blood pressure, but they can adversely affect the body's ability to resist disease and recover.

Adrenal Medulla The central portion of the adrenal gland that secretes catecholamines (containing both adrenaline and noradrenaline) when the hypothalamus initiates the stress response.

Advanced Illness A stage of illness at which death is imminent.

Advanced Practice Nursing Nursing that includes teaching, consultation, and research within a specialty area where superior clinical skills and judgment are acquired through a combination of experience and education.

Aerobic Exercise Exercise that involves the increased consumption of oxygen over an extended period of time, such as jogging.

Affect A psychological term for emotion.

Affective Disorder One of a number of psychological disorders involving emotion, including depression, mania, and bipolar disorder.

Afferent (sensory) Neurons Nerve cells that conduct impulses from a sense organ to the central nervous system, or from lower to higher levels in the spinal cord and brain.

Age-Specific Rates The prevalence of a certain problem for a particular age group. An example would be infant mortality rates.

Agency-Provided Support Social support that is provided by agencies and organizations that have been formed to fill the void when naturally occurring support is either lacking or unavailable.

Agents The means by which a problem spreads or the factors that must be present for a disease to occur.

Aging in Place A topic of interest to medical geographers that focuses on whether people stay where they are or move when they retire.

Airport Malaria Malaria brought home by international travellers.

Alarm The initial phase of Selye's General Adaptation Syndrome in which the body mobilizes its defences against a stressor.

Alcohol Dependency Syndrome Model A theory that suggests that at certain times and for a variety of reasons people do not exercise control over their drinking and this leads to problem drinking.

Alcohol Myopia A drinker's decreased ability to engage in insightful cognitive processing.

Alexithymia A tendency to interpret arousal in purely physical terms without feeling the emotion that others would associate with that arousal.

Allopathic Medicine A form of medicine that attempts to cure sickness by creating conditions in the body that oppose the disease.

Alternative Treatment A treatment that is used instead of allopathic treatment.

Anaerobic Exercise Exercise such as sprinting in which intense effort is expended over a short period of time, developing an oxygen debt.

Analysis of Variance (ANOVA) A method used to compare differences in groups' means when there are more than two groups in a study.

Anger A reaction that often follows denial when we are confronted with novel and severe trauma as identified by Kübler-Ross.

Angina Chest pain.

Angioplasty A procedure in which a bubble-like device is inserted into the artery at the point of the blockage, thus expanding the artery and allowing for better blood flow.

Anorexia Nervosa An eating disorder that is characterized by a dramatic reduction in food intake and extreme weight loss due to an extreme fear of gaining weight.

Anticipatory Nausea Nausea that is felt before a chemotherapy treatment begins, explained in terms of classical conditioning.

Antiemetic Medication Medication intended to reduce nausea and vomiting.

Antigens Microorganisms that are foreign to our physiology.

Antimicrobial Substances Chemicals created by the immune system that kill antigens.

Antiretroviral Medications (e.g., AZT) Medication that is significantly prolonging the lives of people living with AIDS.

Anxiety Sensitivity The extent to which people fear anxiety-related symptoms because they believe these symptoms will have serious social, physical, or psychological consequences.

Applied Discipline A science that attempts to solve real-life problems.

Applied Research An area of research designed to solve real-world problems.

Appraisal Delay The time it takes a person to decide that a symptom is a sign of illness.

Asymptomatic Conditions that are not accompanied by palpable symptoms or sensations.

Attitude A cognition in which a person evaluates some object or idea.

Attributions The explanations people give for events such as their successes and failures.

Autogenic Training A form of cognitive behavioural intervention in which the person learns a set of six formulas intended to enhance relaxation and vascular dilation.

Aversion Therapy Therapy that includes the pairing of a behaviour that one is attempting to eliminate with some unpleasant stimulus so that the undesired behaviour will elicit negative sensations.

B Lymphocyte Cells Cells that, when re-encountering a specific pathogen, produce an antibody designed to eliminate the pathogen.

Baby Talk Simplistic explanations or the use of descriptive words that would usually be used with small children.

Bargaining A response, identified by Kübler-Ross, that may occur when a person is confronted with novel and severe trauma, includes trying to do things that will buy more time.

Basic Research In psychology, an area of research where the primary goal is to learn about psychological processes like memory or sleep patterns.

Behavioral Health An interdisciplinary subspecialty within the framework of behavioural medicine that is concerned with the maintenance of health and the prevention of illness and dysfunction in currently healthy individuals.

Behavioral Medicine A branch of medicine concerned with the relationship between health and behaviour. The focus is usually on remediation.

Behavioural Approach An approach used in grief therapy in which the therapist and bereaved person focus on problem solving, using goal-setting and skill-learning to help the person cope with loss.

Behavioural Delay The time that elapsed between the decision to seek medical care and the person acting on this decision by making an appointment.

Behaviourist One who believes that most behaviour is learned as opposed to innate.

Beliefs as Person Variables Pre-existing notions, both personal and cultural, that influence appraisal, and thus stress, by determining the meaning given to the environment.

Benign Appraisal A cognitive process by which an event is appraised to involve outcomes that are positive and may enhance well-being.

Bereavement Emotions attendant upon the loss of a close friend or loved one.

Biobehavioural Model A theory that maintains that people use and come to depend on the effects of nicotine to regulate cognitive performance and emotional affect.

Biofeedback The use of techniques designed to provide individuals with visual or auditory feedback on particular physiological responses that they want to modify.

Biofeedback The recording of physiological measures through electronic instruments and providing the individual with immediate feedback concerning their physiological state in an attempt to modify physiological processes.

Biomedical Model An approach suggesting that health is best understood in terms of biology.

Biopsychosocial Approach A model that suggests that biological, psychological and social factors are all involved in any given state of health or illness.

Biopsychosocial Communication Pattern Communication patterns between a physician and patient that include a balance of psychosocial and biomedical topics.

Blind Procedure To avoid experimenter bias, people who collect data are unaware of the hypothesis or at least unaware of the group into which a participant has been placed.

Blunters A term used to describe people who avoid information in their attempt to cope with illness and its accompanying challenges.

Blunters A term used by some to describe people who avoid information in their attempt to cope with illness and its accompanying challenges.

Box Scale A scale on which people rate and report their pain by choosing the number that best indicates the degree of pain that they are experiencing from a series of numbers in boxes ranging from "no pain" on the left to "worst pain imaginable" on the right.

Bulimia Nervosa An eating disorder that involves recurrent episodes of binge eating followed by purging.

Burnout A condition that is similar to compassion fatigue and includes symptoms of physical exhaustion, depersonalization of patients, and feelings of discouragement and low accomplishment.

C-Fibres The afferent peripheral fibres that are associated with transmitting diffuse, dull, or aching pain.

Cadavers Corpses, bodies that have been donated to a medical school for first-year medical students to dissect.

Carcinogenic Cancer-causing.

Cardiac Arrest The cessation of the heart.

Cardiac Invalidism The curtailing of activity levels far more than required by disease status because of anxiety related to a possible subsequent heart attack.

Cardiovascular Reactivity Acute cardiovascular changes in response to some stimulus, often a stressor of some kind.

Caring The role that most lay people think is the primary task of nurses.

Case One instance of a medical problem.

Case Studies In-depth narratives that usually focus on one person (or in some cases, compare two or more individuals). Individual histories, symptoms, specific reactions or treatment outcomes might be included.

Cell-Mediated Immunity The use of cells that directly attack infected cells and antigens.

Central Control Trigger In the gate control theory of pain, a specialized system of large-diameter, rapidly conducting fibres that activate selective cognitive processes that then influence, by way of descending fibres, the opening and closing of the gate.

Central Nervous System The division of the nervous system that is composed of the brain and the spinal cord.

Central Route to Persuasion The use of logic, facts, and reason to affect someone's attitude.

Centrally Acting Analgesics Pain-killing medications that operate on the central nervous system by imitating the effects of the body's endogenous pain relief system.

Challenge A type of appraisal in which, though an event is perceived to be stressful, the focus is one of positive excitement and the potential for growth.

Chemotherapy Treatment used in addition to surgery and/or radiation therapy when it is suspected that cancer has metastasized, or to help prevent it from doing so.

Chronic Condition A condition that doesn't go away or get better.

Chronic Disease Era The era of the latter part of the twentieth century in which lifestyle increased people's susceptibility to chronic diseases.

Chronic Intractable Benign Pain Continuous pain that varies in intensity.

Chronic Pain Pain lasting for longer than 6 months.

Chronic Progressive Pain Continuous pain that gradually intensifies as a person's condition worsens.

Chronic Recurrent Pain Intermittent intense episodes of acute pain followed by relief.

Chronic Stressor A stressor that is longterm.

Client-Centred Approach An approach in grief therapy in which the therapist offers nurturance and empathic understanding, paraphrasing the feelings of the person rather than prescribing solutions.

Clinical Nurse Specialist A nurse with a master's or doctoral degree in nursing and extensive experience in a given clinical specialty.

Closed Head Injury (concussion) A bruising of the brain that can result in severe neurocognitive deficits, permanent disability, and even death.

Coercive Power The mediation of punishment by the physician in the form of withholding praise or services to promote patient adherence to medical recommendations.

Cognitive Appraisals People's determinations as to whether or not an event is stressful.

Cognitive Approach An approach used in grief therapy in which the therapist tries to expose dysfunctional or irrational beliefs so that they may be changed.

Cognitive Reappraisal and Restructuring Therapy, sometimes used with cardiac patients, in which they learn to think differently about the things that tend to make them angry and they also learn some behavioural changes such as learning to control their voice tone and breathing.

Cognitive Restructuring A therapeutic intervention aimed at changing people's stress-prone interpretations of events.

Cognitive Restructuring A technique whereby maladaptive, stress-producing cognitions are identified and replaced with ones that are more appropriate.

Cognitive Transactional Models Models that emphasize the relationship that exists between a person and his or her environment and the appraisal that the individual makes of the situation.

Cohort The group that is followed over time in longitudinal research.

Collectivist One who considers himself as part of a greater whole and who considers his individualism as less important than his allegiance to the group.

Compassion Fatigue A lack of energy among health care professionals, particularly nurses, who are constantly working in an environment in which suffering is common.

Complementary Treatment Treatment that is used in conjunction with allopathic treatment.

Compliance The degree to which patients carry out the behaviours and treatments that physicians and other health professionals recommend.

Concussion (a closed head injury) A bruising of the brain that can result in severe neurocognitive deficits, permanent disability, and even death.

Conflict Theory A theory that suggests social structures do not simply exist; rather, they exist in conflict.

Confounding Variables Uncontrolled variables that can affect the dependent variable or outcome of a study.

Consumerist Communication Pattern The use of the physician as a consultant who answers questions rather than being the one who asks them.

Continuing Medical Education (CME) Ongoing education for practitioners.

Continuity of Care A designated staff person, usually a nurse, takes primary responsibility for a patient during his or her hospital stay.

Control Group Participants in a study who don't receive the manipulation (the dependent variable).

Coping Strategies that an individual employs to deal with stresses caused by ever-changing demands of the environment.

Coping Goal The objective of a coping response (which is usually to reduce the impact of stress).

Coping Outcomes The specific outcomes of a coping response.

Coping Response An intentional physical or mental act that is initiated in response to a stressor.

Coping Styles Patterns in the way people deal with difficult situations.

Coronary Artery Bypass Graft (CABG, commonly called bypass surgery) A procedure in which healthy arteries from other parts of the body, often the legs, are grafted into the coronary artery system to bypass blocked arteries.

Correlation Matrix A table that presents all possible correlations among a group of variables.

Correlational Research The use of statistical analyses to determine if variables covary.

Cost-Gain Belief The assessment of the costs (such as effort, discomfort, embarrassment, or inconvenience) associated with an action compared to the benefit of the behaviour to your health.

Counter-Balancing The changing of the order of the administration of questionnaires when more than one survey is completed so that researchers can assess possible order effects.

Covary Changing together. If two phenomena covary, then they go up and down together, or as one increases, the other decreases correspondingly.

Creative Non-Adherence The intentional modification or supplementing of a recommended treatment regimen by the patient.

Credible Knowledgeable and believable.

Critical Period (of fetal development) The period when the fetus is developing most rapidly and is at greatest vulnerability.

Cross-Sectional Research Comparing two or more groups that differ according to stage of life.

Crude Rate A ratio used by epidemiologists to denote the proportion of cases in an entire population.

CTD "Circling the Drain" A term used among some physicians to describe a patient who is about to die.

Curing The role that most lay people think is the primary task of physicians.

Curvilinear Relationship A relationship between two phenomena that, when graphed, produces a U shape or inverted U shape.

Cytotoxic T Cells Cells that directly attack infected cells and antigens.

Danger Control Constructive behavioural changes focused on problem solving, which can proceed without fear when the danger is health-related.

Day Care Patient A person who goes to the hospital for a procedure or test that is more involved than, for example, routine radiography, but does not stay overnight.

Day Care Surgery A person has surgery in the hospital but does not remain overnight.

Decision Modelling A data collection technique used by medical anthropologists that involves the charting of decision-making processes, both for individuals and groups.

Dehumanization/Depersonalization The taking away of one's sense of individuality.

Dehumanize The tendency to see people as objects or body parts rather than human beings.

Delayed Gratification The term used by behaviourists to describe a situation in which there is a time lag between a behaviour and its reinforcement.

Demand Characteristics Beliefs held by people when they know that they are in a psychology study as to what is expected of them or how they are "supposed" to respond.

Dementia A term that refers to a group of diseases that are characterized by a progressive and usually irreversible decline of cognitive abilities.

Demographic Related to personal variables such as age, culture, socioeconomic status, employment status, marital status and gender.

Denial A coping strategy in which people deny that distressing events exist or that negative emotions are being felt.

Dependent Variable In an experiment, the variable that is hypothesized to be measurably affected by the manipulation of the independent variable.

Descriptive Research Research that is conducted primarily to measure the extent to which certain phenomena exist.

Descriptive Statistics The data from descriptive studies that tend to be in the form of frequency distribution, group means, correlations and qualitative anecdotal summaries.

Diathesis-Stress Model A model that suggests that illness results from an interaction between certain personality characteristics and environmental stressors.

Discharge Planning A process in which post-hospital care is organized and risks, such as social problems and lack of support, are assessed.

Discriminant Function Analysis A method that can be used to determine how well a combination of variables predicts that someone belongs to a certain category, such as those with a particular illness.

Disease Physical pathology.

Disease Model (of problem drinking) A theory that suggests that alcoholism is a disease resulting from the physical properties of alcohol.

Diseases of Adaptation Health problems that are the result of the impact of longterm neurological and hormonal changes present because of ongoing stress.

Distraction A pain management technique in which the person focuses attention on something other than the sensation of pain.

Do Not Resuscitate Order An order, which is the responsibility of the physician, indicating that CPR and other interventions are not to be used if the patient stops breathing.

Doctor-Centred Consultations Consultations in which physicians tend to ask questions that require only very brief answers.

Double-Barrelled Item When one survey item actually makes two statements or asks two questions.

Drive Reduction Theory A theory that suggests we are driven to reduce the tension brought about by deprivation or other aversive states.

Dyadic Relationships One-on-one working relationships between group members.

Eco-Epidemiological Era The era of the twenty-first century in which the primary epidemiological agents are chemical and/or environmental in nature.

Ego Orientation A goal perspective that focuses on success and failure with success often coming at other people's expense.

Electroencephalograph An instrument that assesses pain by measuring electrical activity in the brain.

Electromyograph An instrument that assesses pain by measuring electrical activity in muscles.

Electromyographic (EMG) Biofeedback Biofeedback that measures muscle tension.

Embryonic Stage The period from approximately 2 to 8 weeks after conception during which the developing organism is most vulnerable to teratogens.

Emotion-Focused Coping Coping by focusing on ways to reduce the emotional impact of the disease; reducing the discomfort of a problem without trying to solve the problem; a strategy used to cope by controlling the emotional response to an event.

Emotional Arousal A source of efficacy expectation by which individuals assess their emotional level and evaluate their capabilities accordingly; for example, high levels of emotion may be thought to be debilitating and predictive of failure.

Emotional Support Support provided by people who take the time to understand our fears and frustrations, who help calm us during anxious times, who help bring our moods up, or distract us from our worries.

Endocrine System A system of the body that controls glandular responses to stress, albeit more slowly than the nervous system but whose effects associated with it can persist for weeks.

Endogenous Opioids Opiate-like substances produced within the body that regulate pain.

Enumerative Assay A lab test done to count cells (typically white blood cells) as they exist in the bloodstream.

Environmental Tobacco Smoke (secondhand smoke) Smoke that is in the air we breathe because of others smoking.

Epidemiologists Those who study patterns of illness across populations and geographic areas, focusing on the interrelationship of the status of health and demographic factors.

Episodic Illness An illness with a defined beginning and end.

Ethanol (ethyl alcohol) The alcohol used in beverages.

Ethnography A research method that is intended to provide considerable detail or to create portraits, usually of cultures, that are as complete and accurate as possible.

Eustress A positive, yet stressful experience.

Euthanasia The deliberate ending of a patient's life to relieve suffering.

Event Uncertainty The inability to predict the probability of an event which, as a result, increases the stress response.

Evidential Flaws In research, flaws in the nature of the evidence provided.

Evoked Potentials Electrical responses produced by stimuli.

Exercise Psychology The study of the influence that sport and exercise have on one's psychology and behaviour.

Exhaustion An end point identified by Selye in his General Adaptation Syndrome in which the body experiences fatigue and immunocompromise because of the severity or duration of a stressor.

Exiting the Field The final activities as anthropologists leave the location of study involving such activities as debriefing of the people who participated in the study.

Expanded Biomedical Communication Patterns Communication patterns that include numerous closed-ended medical questions and moderate levels of biomedical and psychosocial exchange between the physician and patient.

Experimental Group Participants in a study who receive the manipulation (the independent variable).

Experimenter Bias When a person who knows the hypothesis interacts with participants or interprets qualitative data and this knowledge affects participant's responses or qualitative data interpretation.

Expert Power The increased likelihood that a patient will adhere to medical recommendations.

Explanatory Research A form of research that is designed to discover relationships between phenomena, often in the form of cause and effect.

Exploratory Methods A method used by medical geographers in spatial data analysis to provide interpretations of the maps by describing relationships and illustrative patterns of disease.

Extended Parallel Process Model A model that suggests that low fear messages stimulate neither fear nor danger control; whereas, high fear messages stimulate fear control and danger control if the message is accompanied by an effective behavioural recommendation.

External Imagery A technique in which an individual is a third-person, passive, external observer of their actions.

External Reinforcement The encouragement and praise needed by rehabilitation patients from physiotherapist, friends, family, and other practitioners for their successes.

External Validity The extent to which study results can be generalized to real-life settings.

Face Validity The extent to which an item on a questionnaire appears to be directly measuring what it intends to measure.

Factor In factor analysis, the result of grouping together variables that correlate with one another.

Factor Analysis A statistical process in which variables that are correlated with one another are combined to form a larger category such as "health beliefs" or "social support."

False Positive Results that indicate abnormality when none exists.

Family Orientation In comprehensive cancer care, the family becomes the patient because for virtually every cancer patient there is a family and a collection of close friends who are also affected by the disease.

Family-Work Conflict The extent to which family obligations interfere with work obligations.

Fear Appeals The attempt to change people's behaviour by presenting frightening accounts of what could happen to them if they continue a given behaviour or if they don't adopt a behaviour.

Fear Control Reducing the discomfort of a situation without addressing the source of danger.

Fear of Death among Physicians The extent to which a patient's life threatening condition is a source of stress for physicians.

Fear of Restriction Anxiety experienced due to the inability to move because of being in a small enclosed space.

Fear of Suffocation Anxiety experienced due to the belief that one might die from the inability to breathe.

Feminist Theory of Health Theory that focuses on the fact that women's health concerns are both biologically and socially different from men's.

Feminization of Medicine The trend toward increased proportions of female physicians in the profession.

Fetal Alcohol Effects (FAE) The term used to describe children who have some of the characteristics of fetal alcohol syndrome.

Fetal Alcohol Syndrome (FAS) A set of symptoms including low birth weight and retarded subsequent growth, subnormal intelligence, and certain facial characteristics that has been linked to excessive prenatal alcohol consumption.

Fetal Stage The stage of prenatal development from approximately 8 weeks until birth.

Field Entry When a medical anthropologist first starts collecting data, after permission has been secured and other details have been ironed out.

Field Experiments Experiments that take place in the actual setting in which the application is to be made.

Fight or Flight Response The body's complex autonomic reaction when faced with a perceived threat.

First-Order Partial Correlation Correlations between two variables that take into account the possibility that both variables may be correlated with a third variable they share in common.

Focal Infection An infection that remains in one area of the body but sends toxins to other parts of the body.

Focus Group A data collection technique in which groups of people are asked to discuss specific questions.

Focused Ethnographic Study A study that looks at specific conditions and the beliefs and behaviors associated with them within a given culture.

Free Listing A data collection technique frequently used by medical anthropologists that asks participants to list all the examples of a phenomenon that they can think of.

Frustrated Battleaxe A common stereotype in nursing based on erroneous generalizations that are exploited in some get-well cards.

Functional Tests of Immunity Tests done to assess the immune system "at work."

Gate Control Theory A theory that suggests that a neural mechanism in the dorsal horns of the spinal cord acts like a gate that can increase or decrease the flow of nerve impulses from peripheral fibres to the central nervous system thereby influencing the sensation of pain.

General Adaptation Syndrome The three-stage response of the body to stressors as identified by Selye, which include alarm, resistance, and exhaustion.

Geographical Medicine A subdiscipline of medicine in which the main focus is a disease, with secondary interest in geographical patterns of the disease.

Germ Theory An approach that suggests that many illnesses are caused by the activity of microorganisms such as bacteria.

Germinal Stage The earliest stage of prenatal development, lasting from conception to about two weeks.

Gestational Diabetes A temporary condition affecting 2 to 4 percent of all pregnant women.

Global Assessment of Quality of Life A general or overall assessment of quality of life without focusing on specific aspects.

Glucocorticoids Substances released by the adrenal glands upon stimulation from the sympathetic division when one is under stress.

Goal-Setting A motivational strategy for enhancing performance.

GOK ("god only knows") A term used among some physicians to describe a condition that cannot be definitively diagnosed.

Grade One Concussion A concussion that does not involve a loss of consciousness, although the athlete may display transient confusion.

Grade Two Concussion A concussion in which the symptoms persist beyond the 15-minute period but does not involve a loss of consciousness.

Grade Three Concussion Any concussion that involves a loss of consciousness whether it is extremely brief or prolonged.

Gradient of Reinforcement The greater the lag time between a behaviour and a reinforcer, the weaker the behaviour.

Grief Deep sorrow, usually in response to bereavement.

Grounded Theory A research method in which the theory is developed as data are collected.

Guidance-Cooperation Model The patient seeks advice from the physician and answers the questions that are asked but the physician is responsible for determining the diagnosis and treatment.

Guided Imagery A form of relaxation that relies on distraction in which the participant is told to imagine a calm, peaceful, and pleasant image.

Habit In terms of health behaviour, any behaviour that becomes part of a person's routine and, therefore, is likely to persist.

Habitual Smokers Smokers who smoke without the awareness that they are doing so.

Hallucinogens Drugs that dramatically affect perception, emotions, and mental processes and can result in hallucinations.

Handwarming A strategy related to thermal biofeedback in which migraine headache sufferers can learn to bring blood to their hands, which reduces the pain caused by dilated cranial blood vessels.

Hardiness An approach to life's events that is characterized by a sense of commitment, challenge, and control.

Harm/Loss A type of stressful appraisal at the time of the initial evaluation of a situation (primary appraisal) which involves significant physical or psychological loss.

Health Belief Model A model that analyzes health behaviour in terms of the belief that a health threat exists and the belief that a given course of action will affect the threat.

Health Promotion Strategies intended to maintain or improve the health of large populations.

Health Promotion Mechanisms Encouragement to look after one's self and each other and make the environment healthier by reducing pollution, improving safety, and so on.

Health Psychology The compilation of all that psychology has to offer to the diagnosis and treatment of illness as well as people's attempts to maintain health and well-being.

Help-Intended Communication Communication that includes support, especially emotional support.

Helper T Cells (T lymphocytes) Cells that produce substances called interleukins that speed the division of B lymphocyte cells.

Holistic Rehabilitation Programs A program in which all aspects of the participant's life are addressed, from diet to exercise to psychological well-being.

Homeostasis The dynamic physiological response on the part of the body to maintain a stable internal state in spite of the demands of the environment

Hospital Separation A measure of hospital usage calculated as an overnight hospital stay for one person.

Hosts In the language of epidemiology, carriers of agents.

Human Immunodeficiency Virus (HIV) A virus that gradually breaks down the body's immune system, making it susceptible to a host of other infections and eventually resulting in AIDS.

Humoral Immunity The process by which cells called B lymphocytes produce specific antibodies that attack specific antigens.

Hypnosis An altered state of consciousness.

Hypoglycemia Low blood sugar.

Hypometabolic State A state of the body in which the heart slows, blood pressure drops, breathing is slow and easy, muscle tension decreases, and blood flow shifts.

Hypothalamus A portion of the brain that initiates the stress response in both the nervous system and the endocrine system.

Idiographic Approach Method in which individual cases are looked at on an in-depth basis.

Illness The subjective experience of having a disease.

Illness Delay The time taken between recognizing that one is ill and deciding to seek medical care.

Illusory Correlation When two events appear to vary coincidentally, we mistakenly think that they are related causally.

Imagery A sensory experience that is performed in the absence of external stimuli.

Immune System Memory The ability of certain immune system cells to adapt to an antigen, to remember the antigen when it encounters it again and to work to eliminate it.

Immunocompetence The extent to which our immune system is functioning properly to ward off microorganisms.

In Vitro Outside the body.

In Vivo Inside the body.

Incidence The number of new cases of a problem in a set period of time.

Inclusion Criteria Those characteristics that make a person eligible for a study.

Incommunication Stage A period in ICU during which a patient is either unconscious or barely conscious.

Independence The ability to perform one's activities of daily living without help.

Independent Variable In an experiment, the variable that the researcher manipulates to determine its effect on the dependent variable.

Individualist One who focuses on independence and self-reliance rather than placing group needs above his or her own.

Infant Mortality Rate The number of deaths of all infants under one year of age, typically presented as a rate per 100 000 births.

Infectious Disease Era An era that spanned the late nineteenth and early twentieth centuries during which time the leading causes of death were respiratory diseases.

Inferential Statistics Statistics that allow inferences to be drawn regarding real differences between groups in the population and about cause-effect relationships. Explanatory studies provide this kind of statistic.

Informants Those interviewed by medical anthropologists conducting ethnographic research.

Information–Motivation–Behavioural Skills Model A theory that maintains that there are a number of steps that one must go through to successfully achieve safe sex practices.

Informational Power The presentation of information or knowledge by a physician to promote patient adherence to medical recommendations.

Informational Support The provision of information that might include such things as treatment options or typical recovery times from a treatment or injury.

Informed Consent A consent that enables a person to know enough about a research project to make a reasonable decision regarding participation.

Innocent Angel A common stereotype in nursing based on erroneous generalizations which are exploited in some get-well cards.

Instrumental Treatment Treatment for which there is little interaction between practitioner and patient (e.g., surgery, anesthesiology).

Insulin-Dependent Diabetes (Type I) A condition in which a person produces very little or no insulin and as a result is required to take insulin on a daily basis, usually by way of self-administered injection.

Interaction When variables combine to produce an effect that is different from the effect of either variable alone.

Interactional Model Any scientific explanation that assumes an outcome is the result of two or more variables interacting to affect that outcome.

Interactive Observation An approach used by anthropologists when gathering data, in which they try to become a communicating member of the group that they are studying.

Interleukins Substances produced by T lymphocytes that speed the division of B lymphocyte cells.

Internal Imagery An individual imagines being inside his or her body experiencing a situation as close to reality as possible.

Internalization The changing of one's pattern of beliefs to accommodate the beliefs advocated by the health care practitioner.

Internship A labour-intensive training period the first year after a person graduates from medical school.

Interpersonal Small Talk Talk engaged in by a technologist during a procedure that has nothing to do with the procedure but passes the time and establishes rapport.

Intrusive Memories Unwanted thoughts, often visual in nature, that are related to memories that the patient has about cancer and death.

Intrusive Observation An approach used by anthropologists when gathering data in which they have an effect on the group that they are studying.

Invasiveness A measure of the extent to which hospital procedures, in a physical sense, involve piercing the skin or entering the body with instruments or, in a psychological sense, have the potential to cause embarrassment.

Irrelevant Appraisal A cognitive process by which an event is appraised to have no implications for the individual's well-being.

Isokinetic Exercise Exercise that involves placing tension on a muscle group through a complete range of motion.

Isometric Exercise Exercise that involves the contraction of a muscle group against an immovable object without movement in the body.

Isotonic Exercise Exercise that involves using weights or calisthenics to place tension on the muscle through the shortening or lengthening of the muscle group.

Job Strain Model A model that suggests a job with high strain is one that includes high demands and low control.

Lay Referral System An informal network of non-practitioners who offer their interpretation of symptoms well before any medical treatment is sought.

Learned Helplessness A state in which a person, because of experience with previously uncontrollable stressful situations, learns to do nothing about a new stressor, rather than trying to cope constructively with it.

Legitimate Power Power derived by virtue of the appointed position a person holds in a system.

Lifetime Prevalence The total number of people who have ever had a particular medical problem.

Lifetime Statistics A person's chance of getting a particular disease at any time during his or her life span.

Limbic System A system of the brain that is responsible, in part, for emotion in the stress response.

Line of Best Fit The line drawn through a scatterplot that comes closest to as many data points as possible.

Linear Relationships Statistical relationships between two variables that, when graphed, are best described by a straight line.

Local Anesthetics Pain-relieving chemicals that can be applied topically but are much more effective when injected at the site where the pain originates.

Localized Infection An infection that is confined to a defined site.

Lock-Out Interval The time period between allowable dosages, when patient controlled analgesia is used. A device is set by a practitioner to control this period.

Locus of Control The extent to which one believes that the events of his life are controlled internally, by himself, or externally by outside forces.

Longitudinal Research Following one group over time to chart their changes.

Lyse Destroy.

Main Effects Model Any scientific explanation that assumes an outcome is the result of the effects of one variable only.

Malignant Neoplasms Cancerous growths that may be treated by radiation and chemical therapy.

Master Status A sociological term referring to the status that reflects the person's most prominent position in society.

Matching Groups When it is not possible to assign people randomly to groups, researchers must find control group subjects that match the experimental group subjects as closely as possible to reduce confounding variables.

Medical Anthropologists Those who study the interrelationship of the status of health and cultural factors.

Medical Delay The time between the person making an appointment and first receiving medical care.

Medical Geography The study of the health-related impact of differences in environments.

Medical Geography A subdiscipline of geography in which the main focus is place and the health of those in it.

Medical Jargon Technical language used by a physician that is sometimes unintelligible to the patient.

Medical Level (of health promotion) Promotion in which the orientation is disease based and the goal is disease treatment.

Medical Sociologists Those who study the interrelationship of the status of health and demographic factors as well as the relationship between social systems and health.

Meditation A technique of stress reduction that includes attention to the process of thought rather than the outcome.

Meditation A form of relaxation in which the patient attempts to focus attention fully on a single thought or image.

Memory B Cells A particular kind of B lymphocyte cell that develops a "memory" for a specific antigen after being exposed to it and acts only on that antigen by producing antibodies and immunoglobulins.

Mental Rehearsal A technique that involves the use of imagery to mentally practise a skill.

Metastasized Spread (frequently used to denote the spread of cancer).

Microorganisms In terms of the immune system, the relevant forms include bacteria, viruses, parasites, and fungi.

Mind-Body Dualism The belief that the mind and body are separate entities working independently of one another.

Mitogen A relatively harmless substance that stimulates immune cell activity as though the immune cell were acting against an invading cell or antigen.

Mixed Management Model of Care The preparation of a patient for eventual death while at the same time providing life-sustaining treatments.

Modelling A technique used to reduce stress associated with fear-provoking situations, in which observing a model coping well with a situation facilitates a similar response by the observer in a similar situation.

Monitors A term used to describe people who seek information in their attempt to cope with illness and its accompanying challenges.

Mood State A transient or short-term experience of emotion.

Motion Artifacts Distortions to an MRI image caused by a patient's movement.

Multilevel Explanations Explanations that use medical jargon followed by further explanation of the medical jargon using everyday language.

Multidimensional Assessment of Quality of Life An assessment that includes specific aspects of quality of life, such as physical, emotional, and social functioning.

Multidimensional Health Locus of Control Scale (MHLC) A scale that measures health-specific control beliefs.

Multidisciplinary Pain Management Program A program to manage pain that involves an interdisciplinary team often including physicians, psychologists or psychiatrists, physical therapists, and occupational therapists.

Multiple Correlation The correlation between the value a combination of variables would predict for the outcome variable and the actual value of that outcome variable.

Multiple Regression A statistical method in which a group of variables is combined to predict, as best as possible, some outcome.

Multiple Regulation Model A theory that maintains that the physiological effects of nicotine interact with the psychological functions of smoking to produce addiction.

Multiple-Infarct Dementia A dementia that is the result of a series of small strokes.

Mutual Aid A responsibility to family, friends, loved ones, and even society as a whole when it comes to health and safety.

Mutual Participation Model The physician and patient make joint decisions about every aspect of care.

Myocardial Infarction (MI) Heart attack caused by lack of blood flow to the heart.

Myocardial Ischemia A lack of blood flow to the heart muscle.

Narrowly Biomedical Communication Pattern Communication pattern characterized mainly by biomedical talk, closed-ended medical questions, and very little discussion of psychosocial issues.

Natural-Killer (NK) Cells Cells that have the specific job of "seeking and destroying" cells that are infected, cancerous, or altered in some other way.

Natural Observation Method used in observational research that is global in nature. It attempts to determine generally what is going on in a given situation or context.

Naturally Occurring Support The support we find from friends, relatives, coworkers, and others in our own social networks.

Negative-Affect Smoker A smoker who smokes to reduce negative affect such as anxiety, distress, fear, or guilt.

Negative Correlation As one variable increases, the other variable decreases.

Neoplasms New growths.

Network Analysis A study of the interrelationships among a group or groups of people.

Neuromatrix Theory An extension to the gate control theory, with greater emphasis placed on the brain's role in pain perception.

Nicotine Fixed Effect Model A theory that maintains that nicotine produces addiction because of its paradoxical capacity to simultaneously produce feelings of mental alertness and relaxation.

Nicotine Gum Gum used by some people when they are attempting to stop smoking that provides small amounts of nicotine when it is chewed.

Nicotine Patch A bandage-like patch that releases a small continuous dose of nicotine into the body's system. It is used by some people when they are attempting to stop smoking.

Nicotine-Regulation Model A theory that proposes that smokers develop an optimal level of nicotine in their bodies and then smoke to maintain this level and avoid withdrawal symptoms.

Nicotine-Replacement Therapy A technique to help one stop smoking that provides some form of nicotine to replace that previously obtained through smoking.

NK-Cell Cytotoxic Activity Assay A test in which the proliferation and effectiveness of NK cells is measured after they have been exposed to diseased cells.

NK-Cell Lysis The destroying of tumour cells by exposing them to NK cells.

Nociceptors The afferent nerve endings that respond to pain stimuli.

Nomothetic Approach Method in which large groups are analyzed through statistics such as averages or correlations.

Non-Discrepant Responses Responses by the physician to the patient using the same sophistication of vocabulary that the patient used when asking his or her question.

Non-Insulin-Dependent Diabetes (Type II) A condition in which a person does not produce enough insulin or is not able to use the insulin effectively. Although the person does not have to take insulin, he or she is still required to regulate diet, and some are required to use oral medication.

Non-Invasive A term to describe any procedure that does not include piercing the skin or entering the body with an instrument.

Non-Specific Immunity General protection against antigens, rather than against one specific antigen.

Non-Adherence (related to exercise) The inability to stay with an exercise program.

Non-Adherent Does not follow the advice of the health professional.

Norm Expectations regarding behaviour and beliefs, usually communicated by way of consensus.

Novelty The extent to which an individual's previous experience with a situation influences the appraisal process.

Nurse Practitioner A nurse who often works in rural, remote settings frequently performing functions that would be performed by a physician if available.

Observational Research Method in research by which data about phenomena are collected by observing those phenomena without trying to manipulate them. It is usually descriptive in its purpose.

Occupational Rituals Behaviours that indicate one has been socialized into a profession. For nurses, these are communicated through interaction with other nurses.

Oncology The study and treatment of cancer.

Onset Control The belief that the onset of an illness can be controlled or avoided. The greater this belief, the greater the depression when an illness reoccurs.

Operant Pain Pain that is reinforced by a person's environment.

Operational Definition A statement that explains how an abstract concept or phenomenon is going to be measured concretely in a given study.

Outpatient A person who goes to the hospital for a procedure or test but does not stay overnight.

Outcome Goals Goals that are concerned with the results or outcomes of events and usually involve comparisons to others.

Outcome Studies Studies designed to measure the effect of an intervention or program.

Outcome Variable In correlational research, the measure of the phenomenon the researcher is trying to understand or predict.

Pain Behaviours Alterations in behaviour by a person experiencing pain to either reduce the pain or to prevent it from getting worse.

Pain Threshold The point at which the intensity of a stimulus is perceived as painful.

Pain Tolerance The duration of time or intensity at which a person is willing to endure a stimulus beyond the point where it began to hurt.

Palliative Care Care intended to maintain quality of life as best as possible for a patient who is in the advanced stage of an illness. The focus is the control of pain and other symptoms as opposed to the cure of the illness.

Palliative Treatment Treatment designed to relieve suffering but that is not expected to lead to a cure or remission.

Pancreas A gland that secretes insulin and glucagon as a function of blood sugar levels. The latter stimulates increases in blood sugar, which is an energy source during stress.

Panels The name that The National Population Health Survey uses for the groups that they follow longitudinally.

Pap Test or Pap Smear A test done to screen for cervical cancer.

Parallel-Response Model A model that suggests that recipients of fear-arousing messages focus on either fear control or danger control or some combination of the two.

Parasympathetic The component of the autonomic system that reestablishes homeostasis in the system and promotes the reconstructive process following a stressful experience.

Partial Correlation A correlation between two variables that takes into account possible correlations that they might have with a third variable.

Partialling Out A statistical process by which a correlation between two variables takes into account correlations those variables may have with a common third variable.

Participant Modelling A technique used to reduce stress in which, subsequent to an individual observing a model coping with an anxiety evoking situation, the person is encouraged to engage in the behaviour while receiving reassurance from the model.

Participant Observation Becoming a member of the group one is observing.

Passive An approach used by an anthropologist when gathering data where they stay completely at "arm's length."

Passive Leisure A positive experience that is associated with lack of activity (e.g., listening to music, daydreaming).

Passive Smoking The breathing of environmental tobacco smoke.

Pathogens Antigens that have the potential to create disease.

Patient-Controlled Analgesia (PCA) The patient controls analgesic administration independently.

Patient Delay The period between an individual's first awareness of a symptom and treatment for that symptom.

Patient-Centred Consultations Consultations with physicians that tend to include more open-ended questions by the physician.

Pattern Theory A theory that suggests that there is no separate system for perceiving pain and that the receptors for pain are shared with other senses such as the sense of touch.

Perceived Behavioural Control The belief that a specific behaviour is within one's control.

Performance Accomplishments (enactive attainments) Actual experiences of mastery, considered to be the most influential source of self-efficacy.

Performance Goals Goals that describe an outcome that can be achieved independently of others' performances.

Periaqueductal Gray Area An area of the midbrain which, when electrically stimulated, resulted in rats being pain free.

Peripheral Nervous System The division of the nervous system that is made up of the somatic nervous system and the autonomic nervous system (which is further divided into the sympathetic and the parasympathetic nervous systems).

Peripheral Route to Persuasion Attempts to affect attitude by way of an appeal to emotion and general impression.

Peripherally Acting Analgesics Non-narcotic medications that decrease pain by reducing inflammation at the site of tissue damage. They also inhibit the synthesis of neurochemicals in the peripheral nervous system that facilitate the transmission of pain impulses.

Person Variables Variables, most importantly commitments and belief, that interact with situation variables to affect the appraisal of a situation in terms of its stressfulness.

Personal Efficacy The belief that we are able to succeed at a given task.

Personal Factors in Stress People with high self-esteem, a clear sense of control, and who try to find ways to make their job more manageable are better able to cope with the stressors of their job.

Personal Resources Resources that are available to people in their own lives that help them reduce the potential for stressful events and help them to cope with stressful situations as they occur.

Personality A person's collection of attributes and behavioural tendencies that are consistent over time and across a variety of situations.

Persuasion The attempt to change people's attitudes and beliefs.

Phagocytes White blood cells that consume antigens.

Phagocytosis The process by which white blood cells attach themselves to antigens, ingest them, kill them, and then digest them.

Phenomenologically According to a person's own report on the phenomenon.

Physical Activity The expenditure of energy, either purposely or without intention, as a result of bodily movements produced by skeletal muscles as part of leisure or work activities.

Physical Therapy Therapy involved in the rehabilitation of muscle, bone, joint, or nerve disease.

Physician Impairment A state in which stress-related symptoms interfere with the physician's ability to perform his or her job.

Pituitary Gland A gland located in the brain that is described as the master gland because of its controlling effect on other glands by way of the hormones it secretes. Most of these hormones have an indirect impact on stress.

Placebo Condition Participants of an experimental group are given general attention but not the specific intervention that constitutes the independent variable.

Placebo Effect When participants of an experimental group improve because of attention and not because of anything inherent in the nature of the intervention; the effects that are based on patients' beliefs rather than the direct medicinal properties of the treatment.

Pluralistic Health Care Practices The use of a combination of health practices from one's own culture and some from other cultures when deemed appropriate.

Point Pattern Points on one type of map used in spatial data analysis in medical geography to indicate disease prevalence either in absolute terms or as a ratio of the population.

Point Prevalence Prevalence of a health problem at a given point in time.

Population Health Health concerns in which the unit of analysis is a segment of the population or possibly the entire population.

Positive-Affect Smoker A smoker who smokes because of the positive affect (e.g., to increase stimulation, to relax, or to gratify sensorimotor needs).

Positive Correlation As one variable increases or decreases so does another.

Post-Concussion Syndrome Symptoms experienced subsequent to a concussion, such as memory problems, difficulties in concentration, headaches, dizziness, and irritability.

Practical Support (tangible support) Help with the demands of daily living, such as getting meals and rides to the doctor.

Predictability A characteristic of the environment that allows an individual to prepare for an event and therefore reduce the stress involved.

Predictor Variables In correlational research, the variables that are used to predict or explain variance in some outcome.

Presbyopia A defective condition of accommodation of one's eyesight in which near objects are indistinct.

Prevalence In epidemiology, the total number of cases that exist at any given time.

Primary Appraisal The initial evaluation of a situation.

Primary Care The same nurse cares for a patient throughout his or her stay in the hospital.

Primary Care Physicians Those physicians in general and family practice.

Primary Prevention The establishing and maintaining of appropriate health behaviors to decrease susceptibility to disease.

Problem-Focused Coping Coping by actively addressing the stressors associated with a disease such as cancer and its treatment.

Problem-Based Learning (PBL) Learning in which students work in groups to solve the problems posed by actual cases.

Problem-Focused Coping The altering of a situation or the creating of conditions in which stress and danger are reduced; a rational approach that involves changing the situation by defining the problem, looking at alternative solutions, evaluating the implications of the alternatives, and choosing the best one to act on.

Procedure-Based Information Information give by a technologist at the time of a procedure that addresses what will be done and why it will be done.

Process Goals Goals that focus on specific processes that a performer will be concerned with during a performance.

Prognosis A prediction of how a medical condition will change in the future.

Progressive Illness A condition that will continue to worsen in spite of treatment.

Progressive Muscular Relaxation (PMR) A technique in which a person achieves relaxation by flexing and gradually relaxing muscle groups.

Proliferate To reproduce one's self.

Prospective Research Participants are disease free or newly diagnosed with an illness at the outset of the research. Predictor variables are measured and the participants are monitored to see how their health progresses and how this progression is related to predictor variables.

Protease Inhibitors Medication that is significantly prolonging the lives of people living with AIDS.

Psychodynamic Approach An approach used by a therapist in grief therapy in which he or she may become a temporary substitute for the deceased as the bereaved person addresses unfinished issues related to mourning.

Psychoeducational Care When applied to the postoperative period, the provision of information regarding self-care practices, further procedures, and typical patterns of recovery.

Psychological Methods (in sport) Issues such as relaxation, goal-setting, or imagery. These are used to develop psychological skills.

Psychological Skills (in sport) Arousal or attentional control implemented to enhance performance.

Psychoneuroimmunology (PNI) The study of the relationship between psychological states and the functioning of the immune system.

Psychosocial Communication Pattern A communication pattern that includes a substantial amount of psychosocial exchange between the physician and patient.

Public Health Level (of health promotion) Promotion in which the orientation is behavior based and the goal is disease prevention.

Qualitative Methods Techniques in research that rely on verbal description.

Quality of Life The extent to which symptoms and treatment affect a person's physical, social, cognitive, and emotional functioning.

Quantitative Methods Techniques in research that attempt to express phenomena numerically.

Quantitative Modelling A method that uses maps that chart predictor and outcome variables, thus allowing medical geographers to predict patterns.

Quasiexperimental Designs Studies that are conducted in real-life settings but where there is control over the variables.

Radiation Therapy A form of cancer treatment in which radiation is used to shrink or destroy tumours.

Radical Surgery Cancer surgery that requires the removal of a considerable amount of normal tissue.

Random Assignment An experimental procedure in which participants are placed randomly in either the control or experimental group.

Random Clinical Trial Studies Participants are randomly assigned to treatment conditions in a study measuring a health-related intervention.

Reactance Behaving counter to recommendations in response to a feeling that one has lost personal control over their own health behaviors; the non-compliant behaviors and attitudes of patients who perceive hospital rules and regiments to be unacceptable challenges to their freedom.

Reactivity Hypothesis An hypothesis that states that people whose sympathetic divisions are more reactive would be more likely to experience immunosuppression when under stress.

Readaptation Stage A period in ICU when a patient can sense a struggle to recover and recognizes his or her dependence on machines.

Realistic Monogamy Serial monogamy plus occasional transgressions.

Reality Shock The reaction to the discrepancy between a training environment and an actual work environment.

Reappraisal A continuous experience in which existing appraisals of situations are changed or modified on the basis of new information.

Referent Power Power as a result of referring to a particular person or group with whom the patient desires to identify.

Reflexion Stage A period during which a patient who was in ICU tries to piece together his recent experience.

Relaxation Skills One's ability to reduce anxiety to manageable levels so that the energy can be used to positively influence performance.

Relaxation Techniques Strategies based on the principle that we cannot be relaxed and tense at the same time.

Reliability The extent to which a measurement device can be expected to obtain repeatable and thus trustworthy readings over a series of identical trials.

Repression A coping strategy in which people ignore distressing events or push them to the unconscious.

Residency A period of further training after internship, in which physicians encounter a rather sudden increase in accountability.

Resistance A set of physiological responses that allow a person to deal with a stressor.

Resistance The second phase of Selye's General Adaptation Syndrome in which the body mobilizes its resources over an extended period of time if the source of stress moves from acute to chronic.

Respondent Pain Pain that occurs in response to noxious stimulation or tissue damage.

Response Efficacy The perception that a threat-reducing strategy will work.

Retrospective Research Participants' histories are traced back to find variables that would possibly explain how they came to have a given condition.

Reward Power The mediation of rewards, either tangible or intangible, by a physician to promote patient adherence to medical recommendations.

Role Strain Stress as a result of the demands of multiple social roles, such as health care practitioner and family member.

Roles Sets of behaviours, attributes and expectations that are institutionally defined.

Rotational Injury A type of concussion resulting from a blow to the side of the head.

Run-In Period The duration of the pre-test baseline measurement period in treatment studies.

Salivary or Secretory Immunoglobulin A (sIgA) An antibody that exists in saliva and mucous and represents one of the body's first lines of defence against antigens.

Sampling Bias Some variable or factor is shared by the people who take part in a study that makes them different somehow from the population that the researchers are studying.

Sanitation Era An era that spanned the early part of the nineteenth century, during which time disease spread, most likely with the poor as the hosts, due in large part to unsanitary living conditions.

Scaling A data collection technique in which participants are asked to place concepts along a continuum.

Scatterplot A figure used in correlational research that shows the plotting of the pairs of values for two variables.

Second Impact Syndrome The result when an athlete who has suffered a concussion returns to activity too soon and receives another blow to the head that can result in much greater trauma to the brain than that initially experienced.

Secondary Appraisal A person's evaluation of his or her ability to cope with a situation subsequent to the initial evaluation of the nature of the event.

Sedatives Medications, such as barbiturates, that affect pain indirectly by reducing patient anxiety and helping the patient to sleep.

Sedentary Behaviour Never exercising or exercising less than once per week.

Self-Efficacy An individual's perception of his or her ability to succeed at a particular task at a specific time.

Self-Awareness Model A theory that suggests that drinking inhibits the use of normal, complex information-processing strategies, such as memory and information acquisition, making people less self-aware.

Self-Blame A person's perception that he or she is responsible for a given problem.

Self-Care Behaviours such as exercise, diet, voluntary screening, and regular medical check-ups that one does to promote one's health.

Self-Management Strategies Strategies used to help people overcome the environmental conditions that perpetuate smoking.

Self-Reinforcement Praising oneself or rewarding oneself for accomplishments.

Senile Dementia Dementia that is officially referred to as "diseases of the Alzheimer's type."

Sensation-Based Information Information given by a technologist at the time of a procedure that includes what a procedure will feel like or sound like and how long it will last.

Sensitivity (of medical tests) The ability of a test to identify correctly those who have the disease.

Sensorineural Hearing Loss Hearing loss that is a result of disturbances of the nervous system of the inner ear.

Serial Monogamy A person stays exclusively with one partner for a time and then moves on to another partner.

Serial-Position Effect The likelihood that when a person is presented with a series or list, the items at the beginning and end are more apt to be remembered.

Seroconversion The production of antibodies by memory B cells when exposed to a specific previously encountered and remembered antigen.

Serotonin Reuptake Inhibitors (SSRIs) Psychotropic medication such as Prozac.

Sex Symbol A common stereotype in nursing based on erroneous generalizations that are exploited in some get-well cards.

Shape Modify or adjust a rehabilitation program for a particular person and goal.

Shiatsu Massage A deep massage conducted with movements such as friction, percussion, and pettrisage to release the flow of energy blockages according to the underlying belief of this treatment.

Sick Role A status when temporarily, legitimately adopted exempts people from their other roles because they could not perform those roles adequately if forced to do so.

Sites of Cancer Types of cancer as defined by the location of the tumour.

Situation Variables Variables that interact with person variables to influence the appraisal of a situation.

Social Comparison People look to the opinions and experiences of others to determine what is right and wrong, normal and abnormal, and then use this information to help with decision making.

Social Fact A term used by sociologists to denote a factor that is the result of social structure, for example, unemployment.

Social Factors in Stress The elements of a person's social network, such as family, friends and coworkers, that affect one's ability to cope with job stressors.

Social-Learning Model This theory, when applied to drinking behaviour, proposes that people drink because they experience positive reinforcement for doing so or because they observe others drinking and model the behaviour.

Social Mapping The careful field entry preparation conducted by anthropologists that includes both observation and homework regarding the culture to be studied.

Social Support A collection of interpersonal resources that we have at our disposal to help us avoid or cope with difficult times in our lives.

Socially Constructed Reality The assumption that we piece together our version of the world by interacting with others and construing our own interpretation of that world.

Socioemotional Care Interactions that help patients maintain a sense of optimism and psychological well-being.

Socioenvironmental Level (of health promotion) Promotion for which the orientation is toward social change and health public policy.

Sociology The study of social causes and consequences of behaviour.

Sociology in Medicine Sociological research that has been motivated by a particular medical problem.

Sociology of Medicine The sociological critique of a health care system.

Spatial Analysis The quantitative study of disease distributions and patterns of health care provision over geographically defined areas.

Spatial Data Analysis A technique in which researchers look at the outcome of some process working in a defined space with an attempt to chart the effect of some factor or factors affecting health patterns.

Specific Immunity Protection against a particular antigen.

Specificity The ability of a test to identify correctly those who do not have the disease.

Specificity (of immune system cells) Certain immune system cells will remember an antigen and respond only to the remembered antigen.

Specificity Theory of Pain A theory that suggests that pain is an independent sensation and that there are specific pain receptors, pain fibres, routes of transmission, and centres in the brain that register and interpret only one kind of stimulus.

Sport An activity that involves rules or limits, a sense of history, an aspect of winning and losing, and an emphasis on physical exertion in the context of competition.

Sport Psychology The study of the influence of psychological factors on sport behaviour.

Statistical Significance A measure of the likelihood that a given research result was caused by chance.

Stimulant A drug that increases alertness, decreases appetite and the need for sleep, and may produce intense feelings of euphoria and a strong sense of well-being.

Stimulation-Produced Analgesia (SPA) Freedom from pain as a result of electrical stimulation.

Stress The non-specific mental or somatic result of any demand upon the body.

Stress-Buffering Hypothesis A theory that posits that social support has an indirect effect and acts as a buffer to protect individuals from the negative effects of stress.

Stress-Inoculation Training A technique designed to help people cope effectively with stressful events. It includes reconceptualizing events in less stressful ways, improving coping strategies, and applying the reconceptualized cognitive and behavioural approach to relevant stressors.

Stress Intrusion Scores A measure of the impact a stressful event has on a person's life.

Stress-Management Techniques Techniques that have been developed specifically to help people cope with stress either directly or indirectly.

Stress Response A response that reflects a spontaneous emotional or behavioral reaction to stress, rather than a deliberate attempt to cope.

Stressful Appraisal A cognitive process by which an event is appraised to involve harm/loss, threat, or challenge at the time of the primary appraisal.

Structural Functionalism In sociology, a theoretical perspective that suggests society is best understood by analyzing its systems and the way that they interrelate.

Subjective Norms Beliefs regarding what others think we should do and the extent to which we are motivated to go along with these people.

Suppressor T Cells (CD8) Cells that stop the production of antibodies after the antigen has been destroyed.

Surveys A data collection technique that involves the use of open- or closed-ended questions or a rating scale.

Swedish Massage Slow, gentle stroking movements to warm and relax tissue and stimulate blood circulation.

Symbolic Interactionism In sociology, an assumption that people's interpretations of their interactions and the events of their lives go well beyond the actual words used or, in the case of health-related events, the diagnosis that they are given.

Sympathetic (nervous system) The system responsible for the "fight or flight" changes when triggered by the hypothalamus (e.g., faster heart beat, increased blood pressure).

Systematic Desensitization A technique developed to help people cope with fear and anxiety that combines relaxation plus gradual exposure to the fear-inducing stimulus.

Systematic Observation Method used in observational research that focuses on targeted behaviours. It is intended to discover the frequency or specific forms of a phenomenon.

Systemic Infection An infection that spreads to affect a number of areas of the body at once.

T Lymphocytes (helper T cells) Cells that produce substances called interleukins that speed the division of B lymphocyte cells.

T-Test A statistic used that compares two means to determine if the difference between them is due to the independent variable or due to chance.

Task Orientation A goal perspective in which individuals derive their satisfaction from the sense of competence that they experience as they improve. Their focus is on effort and their own performance rather that that of others.

Team Narcotics Pain-killing medications that operate on the central nervous system (the brain and the spinal cord) blocking the transmission of pain signals.

Technical Care Activities involving prescribed medical procedures, independent of the psychological needs of the patient.

Temporal Uncertainty Lack of knowledge as to when an event will occur, which could result in stress.

Tension-Reduction Hypothesis An hypothesis that maintains that people drink alcohol because of its tension-reducing properties.

Teratogen An agent that causes a birth defect (e.g., viruses or medications).

Theoretical Basis Research in which the hypotheses and methods are justified by referring to established theory. This is frequently the case in explanatory research.

Theoretical Flaws Flaws related to the underlying logic of the design and the research process of a study.

Theory of Planned Behaviour A theory that posits that behaviour is preceded by intention and that our intention is influenced, not only by subjective norms and beliefs about the efficacy of the behaviour, but also by the belief that one is actually capable of performing the behaviour.

Theory of Reasoned Action A theory that posits that behaviour is preceded by intention and that our intention is influenced by beliefs about the behaviour and subjective norms.

Therapeutic Rituals In nursing practice, primarily activities that deal with patient-nurse interactions, for example, the administration of medication and bathing of patients.

Thermal Biofeedback Biofeedback that measures temperature and blood flow.

Thermography The measuring of skin temperature to estimate autonomic nervous system functioning and pain, particularly the emotional components of pain.

Third Variable A variable that correlates with two other variables and, because of this, creates an artificial correlation between those two variables.

Threat A type of stressful appraisal at the time of the initial evaluation of a situation (primary appraisal) that involves the anticipation of situations of harm or loss.

Thyroid Gland A gland that is important in the stress response because of its production of thyroxine, which increases blood pressure and respiration rate and affects mental processes.

Time Tradeoff Technique (TTO) A technique used to assess patients' views of various treatment options, in which they choose among those options based on length and quality of life associated with each.

Timing of Events Events that occur other than at the appropriate or "usual" time in the life cycle may be appraised as more stressful.

Tolerance (of immune system cells) Although immune system cells remember and respond to a remembered antigen, they do not react to the body's own cells.

Total Institution Any institution, such as a hospital, that takes control of virtually every aspect of a person's day-to-day life.

Tranquillizers Medications such as diazepam (Valium) that affect pain indirectly by reducing patient anxiety.

Transcendental Meditation (TM) A technique of meditation to reduce stress introduced by Maharishi Mahesh Yogi in the late 1950s.

Transcript Analysis The recording of interactions followed by their transcription on paper. This is often used by medical sociologists adopting a symbolic interactionism perspective.

Transcutaneous Electrical Nerve Stimulation (TENS) A pain control technique that involves placing an electrode on the surface of the skin and applying electrical stimulation.

Treatment Utility Calculated by creating a fraction with the numerator being the symptom and toxicity-free life expectancy at which the patient chooses treatment and the denominator being life expectancy with treatment-related side effects.

Type A Behaviour Pattern Behaviours include impatience, time urgency, aggressiveness, hostility, and competitiveness, originally believed to be predictive of coronary heart disease.

Type C Personality A cancer-prone personality typified by passivity.

Uncertainty A significant source of stress for physicians because medicine is not a precise science and the consequences of medical decisions are uncertain.

Unit of Analysis A term used to describe the nature of a discipline's ultimate focus, ranging from the individual to society.

Unobtrusive A form of observation such that the dynamics or the nature of the interaction the investigator is hoping to observe is not changed by that observation.

Upper Respiratory Infection (URI) One of a collection of illnesses such as colds, coughs, and bronchitis.

Validity The extent to which a test measures what it claims to measure.

Vectors In epidemiology, living organisms that can transfer an agent from one host to another.

Vehicles In epidemiology, non-living media involved in the transmission of an agent.

Verbal Persuasion A commonly used strategy of attempting to persuade others or ourselves through the use of words that the capability exists to achieve a desired outcome.

Verbal Rating Scale (VRS) A rating scale in which people are asked to describe their pain by choosing the phrase that most closely resembles the pain that they are experiencing.

Vicarious Experience Experience that is gained through observing or visualizing others perform a skill, which can alert one to one's own capabilities and raise one's sense of self-efficacy.

Viral Challenge Studies Studies in which volunteer subjects are intentionally exposed to controlled dosages of viruses related to upper respiratory infection and to environmental stressors to measure the clinical progression of the virus and the response of the immune system.

Visual Analog Scale (VAS) A scale on which people rate and report their pain by marking a point on a line anchored on the left by the phrase "no pain" and on the right by a phrase like "worst pain imaginable."

Visualization Methods One of the methods used by researchers in spatial data analysis to portray their data (e.g., maps.)

Vulnerability Physically, the adequacy of an individual's resources; psychologically, when that which is valued by the individual is threatened.

Withdrawal The unpleasant symptoms people experience when they stop using a substance on which they have become dependent.

Work-Family Conflict The extent to which work obligations interfere with family obligations.

References

Abbott, B., Ippoliti, C., Bruton, J., Neumann, J., et al. (1999). Antiemetic efficacy of granisetron plus dexamethasone in bone marrow transplant patients receiving chemotherapy and total body irradiation. *Bone Marrow Transplant, 23(3)*, 265–269.

Abbott, R.D., Rodriguez, B.L., Burfiel, C.M., & Curb, J.D. (1994). Physical activity in older middle-aged man and reduced risk of stroke: The Honolulu Heart Program. *American Journal of Epidemiology, 139*, 881–893.

Abramson, L., Garber, J., & Seligman, M.E.P. (1980). Learned helplessness in humans: An attributional analysis. In J. Garber & M.E.P. Seligman (Eds.), *Human helplessness: Theory and applications* (pp. 3–34). New York: Academic Press.

Achterberg, J., Kenner, C., & Lawlis, G.F. (1988). Severe burn injuries: A comparison of relaxation imagery and biofeedback for pain management. *Journal of Mental Imagery, 1*, 71–87.

Ader, R. (Ed.) (1981). *Psychoneuroimmunology*. New York: Academic Press.

Agar, M. (1976). One-up, one-down, even-up. Some features of an ethnographic approach. *Addictive Diseases: An International Journal, 2*, 619–626.

Agras, W.S., Schneider, J.A., Arnow, B., Raeburn, S.D., & Telch, C.F. (1989). Cognitive-behavioral and response-prevention treatments for bulimia nervosa. *Journal of Consulting and Clinical Psychology, 57*, 215–221.

Ajzen, I. (1985). From intentions to actions: A theory of planned behaviour. In J. Kuhland & J. Beckman (Eds.), *Action-control: From cognitions to behavior* (pp. 11–39). Heidelberg, Germany: Springer.

Ajzen, I. (1991). The theory of planned behavior. *Organizational Behavior and Human Decision Processes, 50*, 179–211.

Ajzen, I., & Fishbein, M. (1980). *Understanding attitudes and predicting social behaviour*. Englewood Cliffs, NJ: Prentice-Hall.

Akil, H., Watson, S.J., Young, E., Lewis, M.E., et al. (1984). Endogenous opioids: Biology and function. *Annual Review of Neuroscience, 7*, 223–255.

Alaranta, H., Rytökoski, U., Rissanen, A., Talo, S., et al. (1994). Intensive physical and psychosocial training program for patients with chronic low back pain: A controlled clinical trial. *Spine, 19*, 1339–1349.

Alberta Alcohol and Drug Abuse Commission (1999, December 31). Beyond the ABCs: Information for professionals. Http://www.gov.ab.ca/aadac/addictions/beyond/beyond

Albertsen, P. (1998, November). A competing risk analysis of outcomes associated with men treated conservatively for clinically localized prostate cancer. Paper presented at the Cancer Care: Quality of Life and Outcomes Symposium, Chicago, Illinois.

Aldwin, C.M. (1994). *Stress, coping and development: An integrative perspective*. New York: Guilford Press.

Alexander, C.N., Robinson, P., Orme-Johnson, D.W., Schneider, R.H., & Walton, K.G. (1994). The effects of transcendental meditation compared to other methods of relaxation and meditation in reducing risk factors, morbidity, & mortality. *Homeostasis, 35*, 243–263.

Allumbaugh, D.L., & Hoyt, W.T. (1999). Effectiveness of grief therapy: A meta-analysis. Journal of Counseling *Psychology, 46*, 370–380.

Aloise-Young, P.A., Hennigan, K.M., & Graham, J.W. (1996). Role of the self-image and smoker stereotype in smoking onset during early adolescence: A longitudinal study. *Health Psychology, 15*, 494–497.

Alonso, J., Black, C., Norregaard, J.C., Dunn, E., et al. (1998). *Medical Care, 36*, 868–878.

Alter, C.L. (1996). Palliative and suportive care of patients with pancreatic cancer. *Seminars in Oncology, 23*, 229–240.

Altman, D. (1986). *AIDS in the mind of America*. New York: Anchor Press/Doubleday.

Amelang, M. (1997). Using personality variables to predict cancer and heart disease. *European Journal of Personality, 11*, 319–342.

American Pain Society (1999).

Http://www.ampainsoc.org/

Anand, B.K., & Chhina, G.S. (1961). Investigations on yogis claiming to stop their heart beats. *Indian Journal of Medical Research, 49*, 90–94.

Anand, B.K., Chhina, G.S., & Singh, B. (1961a). Studies on Shri Ramand Yogi during his stay in an air-tight box. Indian *Journal of Medical Research, 49*, 82–89.

Anand, B.K., Chhina, G.S., & Singh, B. (1961b). Some aspects of electroencephalographic studies in yogis. *EEG and Clinical Neurophysiology, 13*, 452–456.

Anda, R., Williamson, D., Jones, D., Macera, C., Eaker, E., Glassman, A., & Marks, J. (1993). Depressed affect, hopelessness, and the risk of ischemic heart disease in a cohort of U.S. adults. *Epidemiology, 4*, 285–294.

Andersen, B.L., Cacioppo, J.T., & Roberts, D.C. (1995). Delay in seeking a cancer diagnosis: Delay stages and psychophysiological comparison processes. British Journal of Social Psychology, 34, 33–52.

Andersen, M.R., & Urban, N. (1997). Physician gender and screening: Do patient differences account for differences in mamography use? *Women and Health, 26(1)*, 29–39.

Anderson, D.F., & Cychosz, C.M. (1994). Development of an Exercise Identity Scale. *Perceptual and Motor Skills, 78*, 747–751.

Anderson, E.A. (1987). Preoperative preparation for cardiac surgery facilitates recovery, reduces psychological distress, and reduces the incidence of acute postoperative hypertension. *Journal of Consulting and Clinical Psychology, 55*, 513–520.

Anderson, K.O., Bradley, L.A., Young, L.D., McDaniel, L.K., & Wise, C.M. (1985). Rheumatoid arthritis: Review of psycholgical factors related to etiology, effects, and treatment. *Psychological Bulletin, 98*, 358–387.

Andersson, A., & Holmgren, E. (1975). On acupuncture analgesia and the mechanism of pain. *American Journal of Chinese Medicine, 3,* 311–334.

Andrasik, F., Blanchard, E.B., Arena, J.G., Saunders, N.L., & Barron, K.D. (1982). Psychophysiology of recurrent headaches: Methodological issues and new empirical findings. *Behavior Therapy, 13,* 407–429.

Antepohl, W., & Herzig, S. (1999). Problem-based learning versus lecture-based learning in a course of basic pharmacology: A controlled randomized study. *Medical Education, 33*, 106–113.

Antoni, M.H., August, S. LaPerriere, A., Baggett, H.L., Klimas, N., et al., (1990). Psychological and neuroendocrine measures related to functional immune changes in anticipation of HIV-1 serostatus notification. *Psychosomatic Medicine, 52*, 496–510.

Arborelius, E., & Bremberg, S. (1992). What can doctors do to achieve a successful consultation? Videotaped interviews analyzed by the 'consultation map' method. *Family Practice, 9*, 61–66.

Arborelius, E., & Thakker, K.D. (1995). Why is it so difficult for general practitioners to discuss alcohol with patients? Family *Practice, 4*, 199–422.

Aronoff, G.M., Wagner, J.M., & Spangler, A.S. (1986). Chemical interventions for pain. *Journal of Consulting and Clinical Psychology, 54*, 769–775.

Ary, D.V., & Biglan, A. (1988). Longitudinal changes in adolescent cigarette smoking behavior: Onset and cessation. *Journal of Behavioral Medicine, 11*, 361–382.

Asmundson, G.J.G., Norton, G.R., Allerdings, M.D., Norton, P.J., & Larsen, D.K. (1998). Posttraumatic stress disorder and work-related injury. *Journal of Anxiety Disorders, 12*, 57–69.

Astle, S.J. (1996). The experience of loss in athletes. *Journal of Sports Medicine and Physical Fitness, 26*, 279–284.

Atkinson, J.M. (1993). The patient as sufferer. *British Journal of Medical Psychology, 66(2)*, 113–120.

Auerbach, S.M., Martelli, M.F., & Mercuri, L.G. (1983). Anxiety, information, interpersonal impacts, and adjustment to a stressful health care situation. *Journal of Personality and Social Psychology, 44*, 1284–1296.

Azar, B. (1999, February). Sex differences in pain reports may be smaller than previously thought. *APA Monitor*, p. 7.

Badgley, R.F. (1994). Health promotion and social change in the health of Canadians. In Pederson, A., O'Neill, M., & Rootman, I. (Eds.), *Health promotion in Canada: Provincial, national and international perspectives* (pp. 200–239). Toronto, ON: Saunders.

Bahrke, M.S., & Morgan, W.P. (1978). Anxiety reduction following exercise and meditation. *Cognitive Therapy and Research, 2,* 323–334.

Baider, L., Cooper, C.L., & Kaplan De Nour, A. (Eds.), (1996). *Cancer and the family.* Chichester, England: Wiley.

Bain, D.J.G. (1979). The relationship between time and clinical management in family practice. *Journal of Family Practice, 8,*

551–559.

Baker, C., & Melby, V. (1996). An investigation into the attitudes and practices of intensive care nurses toward verbal communication with unconscious patients. *Journal of Clinical Nursing, 5*, 185–192.

Baker, L.H., Cooney, N.L., & Pomerleau, O.F. (1987). Craving for alcohol: *Theoretical processes and treatment procedures. In Treatment and prevention of alcohol problems: A resource manual* (pp. 183–202).

Baker, S.A., Morrison, D.M., Carter, W.B., & Verdon, Michael, S. (1996). Using the theory of reasoned action (TRA) to understand the decision to use condoms in an STD clinic population. *Health Education Quarterly, 23*, 528–542.

Bakker, A.B., Buunk, B.P., Siero, F.W., van Den Eijnden, R.J.J.M. (1997). Applications of a modified health belief model to HIV preventive behavioral intentions among gay and bisexual men. *Psychology and Health, 12*, 481–492.

Balla, J.I. (1982). The late whiplash syndrome: A study of an illness in Australia and Singapore. *Culture, Medicine and Psychiatry, 6*, 191–210.

Bandura, A. (1977). Self-efficacy: Toward a unifying theory of behavior change. *Psychological Review, 84*, 191–215.

Bandura, A. (1989). Human agency in social cognitive theory. *American Psychologist, 44*, 1175–1184.

Bandura, A. (1990). Perceived self-efficacy in the exercise of personal agency. Journal of *Applied Sport Psychology, 2*, 128–163.

Bandura, A. (1991). Self-efficacy mechanism in physiological activation and health-promotion behavior. In J. Madden IV (Ed.), *Neurobiology of learning, emotion, and affect* (pp. 229–269). New York: Raven Press.

Bandura, A. (l986). *Social foundations of thought and action: A social cognitive theory*. Inglewood Cliffs, New Jersey: Prentice-Hall.

Bannister, R (l955) *The four-minute mile*. New York: Dodd, Mead.

Barber, J. (1986). Hypnotic analgesia. In A.D. Holzman & D.C. Turk (Eds.), *Pain management: A handbook of psychological treatment approaches*. New York: Pergamon Press.

Barbounis, V., Koumakis, G., Hatzichristou, H., Vassilomanolakis, M., Tsoussis, S., & Efremidis, A. (1999). The anti-emietic efficacy of tropisotron plus dexamethasone in patients treated with high-dose chemotherapy and stem cell transplantation. *Support Care Cancer, 7(2)*, 79–83.

Barling, N.R., & Moore, S.M. (1996). Prediction of cervical cancer screening using the theory of reasoned action. *Psychological Reports, 79*, 77–78.

Baron, R.S., Cutrona, C.E., Hicklin, D., Russell, D.W., & Lubaroff, D.M. (1990). Social support and immune function among spouses of cancer patients. *Journal of Personality and Social Psychology, 59*, 344–352.

Barraclough, J., Pinder, P., Cruddas, M., Osmond, C., Taylor, I., & Perry, M. (1992). Life events and breast cancer prognosis. *British Medical Journal, 304*, 1078–1081.

Barrett, F.A. (1996). Daniel Drake's medical geography. *Social Science and Medicine, 42*, 791–800.

Barron, C., Houfek, J.F., & Foxall, M.J. (1997). Coping style, health beliefs and breast self-examination. *Issues in Mental Health Nursing, 18*, 331–350.

Barton, J., Chassin, L., Presson, C.C., & Sherman, S.J. (1982). Social image factors as motivators of smoking initiation in early and middle adolescence. *Child Development, 53*, 1499–1511.

Battle, E.K., & Brownell, K.D. (1996). Confronting a rising tide of eating disorders and obesity: Treatment vs. prevention and policy. *Addictive Behaviors, 21*, 755–765.

Bauchner, H., Vinci, R., Bak, S., Pearson, C., & Corwin, M.J. (1996). Parents and procedures: A randomized controlled trial. *Pediatrics, 98*, 861–867.

Baum, A., & Posluszny, D.M. (1999). Health psychology: Mapping biobehavioral contributions to health and illness. Annual *Review of Psychology, 50*, 137–163.

Baxter, N., Cohen, R., & McLeod, R. (1996). The impact of gender on the choice of surgery as a career. *American Journal of Surgery, 172*, 373–376.

Bearison,D.J., Sadow, A.J., Granowetter, L., & Winkel, G. (1993). Patients' and parents' causal attributions for childhood cancer. *Journal of Psychosocial Oncology, 11*, 47–61.

Beck, A. (1963). Thinking and depression: 1. Idiosyncratic content and cognitive distortions. Archives of General Psychiatry, 9, 324–333.

Beck, A. (1976). *Cognitive therapy and the emotional disorders*. New York: International Universities Press.

Beck, K.H., & Frankel, A. (1981). A conceptualization of threat communication and protective health behavior. Social *Psychology Quarterly, 44*, 204–217.

Becker, M.H. (1974). The health belief model and sick role behavior. Health Education *Monographs, 2*, 409–419.

Becker, M.H. (1979). Understanding patient compliance: The contributions of attitudes and other psychosocial factors. In S.J. Cohen (Ed.), *New directs in patient compliance*. Lexington, MA: Heath.

Becker, M.H., & Janz, N.K. (1987). On the effectiveness and utility of health hazard/health risk appraisal in clinical and nonclinical settings. *Health Services Research, 22*, 537–551.

Becker, M.H., & Maiman, L.A. (1975). Sociobehavioral determinants of compliance with health care and medical care recommendations. *Medical Care, 13*, 10–24.

Beckman, H.B., & Frankel, R.M. (1984). The effect of physician behavior on the collection of data. *Annals of Internal Medicine, 101*, 692–696.

Beecher, H.K. (1959). *Measurement of subjective responses*. New York: Oxford University Press.

Begun, F.P. (1993). Epidemiology and natural history of prostate cancer. In Lepor, H, & Lawson, R.K. (Eds.), *Prostate disease* (pp. 257–268). Philadelphia: W.B. Saunders.

Beisecker, A. & Beisecker, T. (1990). Patient information-seeking behaviors when communicating with doctors. *Medical Care, 28*, 19–28.

Belar, C.D. (1997). Clinical health psychology: A specialty for the 21st century. *Health Psychology, 16*, 411–416.

Bem, S.L. (1974). The measurement of psychological androgyny. *Journal of Consulting and Clinical Psychology, 42*, 155–162.

Ben-Sira, Z. (1976). The function of the professional's affective behavior in client satisfaction: A revised approach to social interaction theory. *Journal of Health and Social Behavior, 17*, 3–11.

Ben-Sira, Z. (1980). Affective and instrumental components in the physician-patient relationship: An additional dimension of interaction theory. *Journal of Health and Social Behavior, 21*, 180–180.

Benson, H. (1975). *The Relaxation Response*. New York: William Morrow.

Benson, H., Beary, J.F., & Carol, M.P. (1974). The relaxation response. *Psychiatry, 37*, 37–46.

Bergh, K.D. (1998). The patient's differential diagnosis. Unpredictable concerns in visits for acute cough. *Journal of Family Practice, 46*, 153–158.

Berkley, K.J. (1997). Sex differences in pain. *Behavioral and Brain Sciences, 20*, 371–380.

Berkman, L.F., & Syme, S.L. (1979). Social networks, host resistance, and mortality: A nine-year follow-up study of Alameda County residents. *American Journal of Epidemiology, 109*, 186–204.

Berkman, L.F., Breslow, L., & Wingard, D. (1983). Health practices and mortality risk. In L.F. Berkman & L. Breslow (Eds.), *Health and ways of living: The Alameda county study*. New York: Oxford University Press.

Bernstein, D.A., & Borkovec, T.D. (1978) *Progressive relaxation training: A manual for the helping professions*. Champaign, Illinois: Research Press.

Bernstein, D.A., & Given, B.A. (1984). Progressive relaxation: Abbreviated methods. In R. Woolfolk and P. Lehrer (Eds.), *Principles and practice of stress management*. New York: Guilford Press.

Best, A., & Herbert, C. (1998). Two solitudes of complementary and conventional medicine. Where are we going? *Canadian Family Physician, 44*, 935–955, 960–962.

Beyer, J.E., & Wells, N. (1989). The assessment of pain in children. Pediatric *Clinics of North America, 36*, 837–855.

Beyerstein, B. (1997). Alternative medicine: Where's the evidence? *Canadian Journal of Public Health, 88*, 149–152.

Bezak, J.E., & Lee, J.W. (1990). Relationship of self-efficacy and locus of control constructs in predicting college students' physical fitness behaviors. *Perceptual and Motor Skills, 71*, 499–508.

Biegel, D.E., Sales, E., & Schulz, R. (1991). *Family caregiving in chronic illness*. Newbury Park, CA: Sage.

Biglan, A., Duncan, T.E., Ary, D.V., & Smolkowski, K. (1995). Peer and parental influences on adolescent tobacco use. *Journal of Behavioral Medicine, 18*, 315–330.

Biglan, A., McConnell, S., Severson, H.H., Bavry, J., & Ary, D. (1984). A situational analysis of adolescent smoking. *Journal of Behavioral Medicine, 7*, 109–114.

Birk, L. (Ed.) (1973). *Biofeedback: Behavioral medicine*. New York: Grune and Stratton.

Birmingham, C.L., Muller, J.L., Palepu, A., Spinella, J.J., & Anis, A.H. (1999). The cost of obesity in Canada. *Canadian Medical Association Journal, 160*, 483–488.

Birnbaum, M.H., Wong, R., & Wong, L.K. (1976). Combining information from sources that vary in credibility. *Memory and Cognition, 4*, 330–336.

Blackwell, B. (1972). The drug defaulter. *Clinical Pharmacology Therapy, 13*, 841.

Blackwell, B. (1997). From compliance to alliance: A quarter century of research. In B. Blackwell (Ed.), *Treatment compliance and the therapeutic alliance* (pp. 1–15). Amsterdam: Harwood Academic Publishers.

Blair, S.N., Kohl, H.W., Paffenberger, R.S., Clark, D.G., Cooper, K.H., & Gibbons, L.W. (1989). Physical fitness and all-cause mortality: A prospective study of healthy men and women. *Journal of the American Medical Association, 262*, 2395–2401.

Blanchard, C.G., Albrecht, T.L., Ruckdceschel, J.C., Grant, C.H., Hemmick, R.M. (1995). The role of social support in adaptation to cancer and to survival. *Journal of Psychosocial Oncology, 13*, 75–95.

Blanchard, E.B. (1977). Behavioral medicine: A perspective. In R.B. Williams and W.D. Gentry (Eds.), *Behavioral approaches to medical treatment*. Cambridge, Massachusetts: Ballinger.

Blanchard, E.B. (1987). Long-term effects of behavioral treatment of chronic headache. *Behavior Therapy, 18*, 375–385.

Blanchard, E.B., & Andrasik, F. (1985). *Management of chronic headaches: A psychological approach*. New York: Pergamon Press.

Blanchard, E.B., & Haynes, M.R. (1975). Biofeedback treatment of a case of Raynaud's disease. *Journal of Behavior Therapy and Experimental Psychiatry, 6*, 230–234.

Blanchard, E.B., & Young, L.B. (1973). Self-control of cardiac functioning: A promise as yet unfulfilled. *Psychological Bulletin, 79*, 145–163.

Blanchard, E.B., Andrasik, F., Guarnieri, P., Neff, D.F., & Rodichok, L.D. (1987). Two-, three-, and four-year follow-up on the self-regulatory treatment of chronic headache. *Journal of Consulting and Clinical Psychology, 55*, 257–259.

Blanchard, E.B., Appelbaum, K.A., Guarnieri, P., Morrill, B., & Dentinger, M.P. (1987). Five year prospective follow-up on the treatment of chronic headache with biofeedback and/or relaxation. *Headache, 27*, 580–583.

Blendon, R.J., Aiken, L.H., Freeman, H.E., & Corey, C.R. (1989). Access to medical care for black and white Americans: A matter of continuing concern. *Journal of the American Medical Association, 261*, 278.

Block, A. (1997). Controlling the costs of pain-related disability. *Journal of Pain and Symptom Management, 13*, 1–3.

Block, S.D., & Billings, J.A. (1995). Patient requests for euthanasia and assisted suicide in terminal illness: The role of the psychiatrist. *Psychosomatics, 36*, 445–457.

Bloom, F.E., Lazerson, A., & Hofstadter, L. (1985). *Brain, mind, and behavior*. New York: Freeman.

Bloom, J.R., & Kessler, L. (1994). Emotional support following cancer: A test of the stigma and social activity hypothesis. *Journal of Health and Social Behavior, 35*, 118–133.

Boey, K.W. (1999). Distressed and stress resistant nurses. *Issues in Mental Health Nursing, 20*, 33–54.

Boldt, J., Thaler, E., Lehmann, A., Papsdorf, M., & Isgro, F. (1998). Pain management in cardiac surgery patients: Comparison between standard therapy and patient-controlled analgesia regimen. *Journal of Cardiothoracic and Vascular Anesthiology, 12*, 654–658.

Booth, M.J. (1998). Nurse anesthetist reaction to the unexpected or untimely death of patients in the operating room. *Holistic Nursing Practice, 13*, 51–58.

Boroditsky, R., Fisher, W., & Sand, M. (1996). The 1995 Canadian contraception study. *Journal SOGC, 18 Supplement*, 1–31.

Boscarino, J.A. (1997). Diseases among men 20 years after exposure to severe stress: Implications for clinical research and medical care. *Psychosomatic Medicine, 59*, 605–614.

Bottomley, A., Hunton, S., Roberts, G., Jones, et al., (1996). A pilot study of cognitive behavioral therapy and social support group interventions with newly diagnosed cancer patients. *Journal of Psychosocial Oncology, 14*, 65–83.

Botvin, G.J., & Willis, T.A. (1985). Personal and social skills training: cognitive-behavioral approaches to substance abuse prevention. In C.S. Bell & R. Batties (eds.), *Prevention research: Deterring drug abuse among children and adolescents (NIDA Research Monograph 63)*. Washington, DC: U.S. Government Printing Office.

Botvin, G.J., Baker, E., Dusenbury, L., Tortu, S., & Botvin, E.M. (1990). Preventing adolescent drug abuse through a multimodal cognitive-behavioral approach: Results of a 3-year study. *Journal of Consulting and Clinical Psychology, 58*, 437–446.

Bouchard, L., & Renaud, M. (1997). Female and male physicians' attitudes toward prenatal diagnosis: A Pan-Canadian survey. *Social Science and Medicine, 44*, 381–392.

Bozoin, S., Rejeski, W.J., & McAuley, E. (1994). Self-efficacy influences feeling states associated with acute exercise. *Journal of Sport and Exercise Psychology, 16*, 326–333.

Bracegirdle, H. (1995). Children's stereotypes of visibly physically impaired targets: An empirical study. *British Journal of Occupational Therapy, 58*, 25–27.

Bradbury, K., Janicke, D.M., Riley, A.W., & Finney, J.W. (1999). Predictors of unintentional injuries to school-age children seen in pediatric primary care. *Journal of Pediatric Psychology, 24*, 423–433.

Bradford, R. (1997). *Children, families, and chronic disease: Psychological models and methods of care*. New York: Routledge.

Bradley, L.A. (1983). Coping with chronic pain. In T.G. Burish & L.A. Bradley (Eds.), *Coping with chronic disease: Research and applications*. New York: Academic Press.

Bradley, L.A., Young, L.D., Anderson, K.O., Turner, R.A., Agudelo, C.A., et al. (1987). Effects of psychological therapy on pain behavior of rheumatoid arthritis patients: treatment outcome and six-month followup. *Arthritis and Rheumatism 30*, 1105–1114.

Brady, J.V., Porter, R.W., Conrad, D.G., & Mason, J.W. (1958). Avoidance behavior and the development of duodenal ulcers. *Journal of the Experimental Analysis of Behavior, 1*, 69–72.

Brand, R.J., Paffenberger, R.S., Scholtz, R.I., & Kampert, J.B. (1979). Work activity and fatal heart attack studied by multiple logistic risk analysis. *American Journal of Epidemiology, 110*, 52–56.

Brandsma, J.M., Maultsby, M.C., & Welsh, R.J. (1980). *The outpatient treatment of alcoholism: A review and comparative study*. Baltimore: University Park Press.

Brannon, L., & Feist, J. (2000) *Health psychology: An introduction to behavior and health*. Belmount, California: Wadsworth/Thompson Learning.

Braun, B.L., Murray, D., & Sidney, S. (1997). Lifetime cocaine use and cardiovascular characteristics among young adults: the CARDIA study. *American Journal of Public Health, 87*, 629–634.

Brehm, J.W. (1966). *A theory of psychological reactance*. New York: Academic Press.

Brennan, A.F., Barrett, C.L., & Garretson, H.D. (1987). The utility of McGill Pain Questionnaire subscales for discriminating psychological disorder in chronic pain patients. *Psychology and Health, 1*, 257–272.

Brewer, B.W., Van Raalte, J.L., & Linder, D.E. (1991). Peak performance and the perils of retrospective introspection. *Journal of Sport and Exercise Psychology, 10*, 45–61.

Brewin, C.R., Watson, M., McCarthy, S., Hyman, P., & Dayson, D. (1998). Intrusive memories and depression in cancer patients. *Behaviour Research and Therapy, 36*, 1131–1142.

Brewster, A.B. (1982). Chronically ill hospitalized children's concepts of their illness. *Pediatrics, 69*, 355–362.

British Columbia Eating Disorder Association (1998). *School outreach program training manual*. Victoria, BC.

Britten,N., & Shaw, A. (1994). Patients' experiences of emergency admission: How relevant is the British government's Patients Charter? *Journal of Advances in Nursing, 19*, 1212–1220.

Brody, D.S., Miller, S.M., Leman, C.E., Smith, D.G., & Caputo, G.C. (1989). Patient perception on involvement in medical care: Relationship to illness attitudes and outcomes. *Journal of General Internal Medicine, 4*, 506–511.

Brousse, T. (1946). A psycho-physiological study. *Main Currents in Modern Thought, 4*, 77–84.

Brown, D.L. (1988). No pretending not to know. *Journal of the American Medical Association, 260*, 2720.

Brown, M.A., & Stetz, K. (1999). The labor of caregiving: A theoretical model of caregiving during potentially fatal illness. *Qualitative Health Research, 9*, 182–197.

Brown, R.S., Ramirez, D.E., & Taub, J.M. (1978). The prescription of exercise for depression. *Physician and Sportsmedicine, 6*, 35–45.

Brownell, K.D., & Cohen, L.R. (1995). Adherence to dietary regimens: 2. Components of effective interventions. *Behavioral Medicine, 20*, 155–164.

Bruch, H. (1973). Eating disorders. *Obesity, anorexia nervosa and the person within.*

New York: Basic Books.

Bruch, H. (1978). *The golden cage: The enigma of anorexia nervosa*. Cambridge. MA: Harvard University Press.

Bruch, H. (1982). Anorexia nervosa: Therapy and theory. *American Journal of Psychiatry, 139*, 1531–1538.

Brunton, P. (1972). *A search in secret India*. New York: Samuel Weiser.

Bryant, J. (1999). Social determinants of participation in preventive screening services in Prince George, British Columbia. Unpublished Master's Thesis, The University of Northern British Columbia.

Buckalew, L.W. (1991). Patients' compliance: The problem and directions for psychological research. *Psychological Reports, 68*, 348–350.

Buller, M.K., & Buller, D.B. (1987). Physicians' communication style and patient satisfaction. *Journal of Health and Social Behavior, 28*, 375–388.

Burack, J.H., Young, L.D., Anderson, K.O., Turner, R.A., Agudelo, C.A., et al. (1993). Depressive symptoms and CD4 lymphocyte decline among HIV-infected men. *Journal of the American Medical Association, 270*, 2568–2573.

Burack, R.C., & Carpenter, R.R. (1983). The predictive value of the presenting complaint. *Journal of Family Practice, 16*, 749–754.

Burgess, E.S., & Haaga, D.A.F. (1998). Appraisals, coping responses, and attributions as predictors of individual differences in negative emotions among pediatric cancer patients. *Cognitive Therapy and Research, 22*, 457–473.

Burke, R.J., & Richardsen, A.M. (1990). Sources of satisfaction and stress among Canadian physicians. *Psychological Reports, 67*, 1335–1344.

Burns, J.W., Johnson, B.J., Mahoney, N., Derleth, M., & Pawl, R. (1996). Sex differences in predictors of response to multidisciplinary treatment of chronic pain. *Pain Research and Management, 1(3)*, 149–154.

Burns, J.W., Sherman, M.L., Devine, J., Mahoney, N., & Pawl, R. (1995). Association between workers' compensation and outcome following multidisciplinary treatment of chronic pain: Roles of mediators and moderators. *Clinical Journal of Pain, 11*, 94–102.

Burnum, M.A., Timbers, D.M., & Hough, R.L. (1984). *Journal of Health and Social Behavior, 25*, 24–33.

Byrne, D. (1977). Social psychology and the study of sexual behavior. *Personality and Social Psychology Bulletin, 3*, 3–30.

Calderone, K. (1990). The influence of gender on the frequency of pain and sedative medication administered to post-operative patients. *Sex Roles, 23*, 713–725.

Calhoun, E. (1998, November). Reimbursement dilemmas for patients with refractory ovarian cancer. Paper presented at the Cancer Care: Quality of Life and Outcomes Symposium, Chicago, Illinois.

Calvillo, E.R. & Flaskerud, J.H. (1991). Review of literature on culture and pain of adults with focus on Mexican-Americans.J. *Transcult Nurs, 2(2)*, 16–23.

Calzavara, L.M., Bullock, S.L., Myers, T. Marshall, V.W., Cockerill, R. (1999). Sexual partnering and risk of HIV/STD among Aboriginals. *Canadian Journal of Public Health, 90*, 186–191.

Cameron, L., Leventhal, E.A., & Leventhal, H. (1995). Seeking medical care in response to symptoms and life stress. *Psychosomatic Medicine, 57*, 1–11.

Campion, E.W. (1993). Why unconventional therapies? *New England Journal of Medicine, 328*, 282–285.

Canadian Centre on Substance Abuse. (1999). Http://www.ccsa.ca/

Canadian Institute for Health Information. (1998). *National health expenditure trends, 1975–1998*. Ottawa.

Canadian Nurses Association. (1997a). Out in front—advanced nursing practice. *Nursing Now: Issues and Trends in Canadian Nursing, January, 1997*.

Canadian Nurses Association. (1997b) The future supply of registered nurses: A discussion paper, Ottawa, October, 1997.

Cannon, W.B. (1939). *The Wisdom of the Body*. New York: Norton.

Carlat, D.J., Camargo, C.A., Herzog, D.D. (1997). Eating disorders in males: A report on 135 patients. *American Journal of Psychiatry, 154*, 1127–1132.

Carlson, C.R., & Hoyle, R.H. (1993). Efficacy of abbreviated progressive muscle relaxation training: A quantitative review of behavioral medicine research. *Journal of Consulting and Clinical Psychology, 61*, 1059–1067.

Carlsson, C.P.O., & S j:olund, B.H. (1994). Acupuncture and subtypes of chronic pain: Assessment of long-term results. *Clinical Journal of Pain, 10*, 290–295.

Carney, R.M., Freedland, K.E., Veith, R.C., Cryer, P.E., Skala, J.A., Lynch, T., & Jaffe, A.S. (1999). Major depression, heart rate, and plasma norepinephrine in patients with coronary heart disease. *Biological Psychiatry, 45*, 458–463.

Carpenter, D.J., Gatchel, R.J., & Hasegawa, T. (1994). Effectiveness of a video-taped behavioral intervention for dental anxiety: The role of gender and need for information. *Behavioral Medicine, 20*, 123–132.

Carron, H., DeGood, D.E., & Tait, R.A. (1985). A comparison of low back pain patients in the United States and New Zealand: Psychosocial and economic factors affecting severity of disability. *Pain, 21*, 77–89.

Carson, B.S. (1987). Neurologic and neurosurgical approaches to cancer pain. In D.B. McGuire & C.H. Yarbro (Eds.), *Cancer pain management* (pp. 223–243). Philadelphia: Saunders.

Casperson, C.J. Powell, K.E., & Christenson, G.M. (1985). Physical activity, exercise, and physical fitness: Definitions and distinctions for health-related research. *Public Health Reports, 100*, 126–131.

Catania, J.A., Kegeles, S.M., & Coates, T.J. (1990). Towards an understanding of risk behavior: An AIDS risk reduction model (ARRM). *Health Education Quarterly, 17*, 53–72.

Catchlove, R. & Cohen, K. (1982). Effects of a directive return to work approach in the treatment of workman's compensation patients with chronic pain. *Pain, 14*, 181–191.

Cella, D. F., Tulsky, D. S., Gray, G., Saraflan, B., Linn, E., Bonomi, A., Silberman, M., Yellen, et al. (1993). The Functional Assessment of Cancer Therapy Scale: Development and validation of the general measure. *Journal of Clinical Oncology, 11*, 570–579.

Centers for Disease Control and Prevention (CDC). (1993). Cigarette smoking—attributable mortality and years of potential life lost—United States, 1990. *Morbidity and Mortality Weekly Report, 42*, 645–649.

Centers for Disease Control and Prevention (CDC). (1998). Deaths resulting from residential fires and the prevalence of smoke alarms—United States, 1991–1995. *Morbidity and Mortality Weekly Report, 47*, 803–906.

Chamberlain, J., Clifford, R.E., Nathan, B.E., Price, J.L., & Burn, I. Repeated screening for breast cancer. *Journal of Epidemiology and Community Health, 38*, 54–57.

Champion, V.L. (1990). Breast, self-examination in women 35 and older: A prospective study. *Journal of Behavioral Medicine, 13*, 523–538.

Champion, V.L. (1993). Instrument refinement for breast cancer screening behaviors. *Nursing Research, 42*, 139–143.

Chapman, C.R. (1984). New directions in the understanding and management of pain. *Social Science and Medicine, 19*, 1261–1277.

Chapman, C.R., & Syrjala, K.L. (1990). Measurement of pain. In J.J. Bonica (Ed.), *The management of pain* (2nd ed., pp. 580–594). Malvern, PA: Lea & Febiger.

Chapman, C.R., Casey, K.L., Dubner, R., Foley, K.M., et al. (1985). Pain measurement: An overview. *Pain, 22*, 1–31.

Chapman, S.L. (1991). Chronic pain: Psychological assessment and treatment. In J.J. Sweet, R.H. Rozensky, & S.M. Tovian (Eds.), *Handbook of clinical psychology in medical settings*. New York: Plenum.

Chapman, W.P. (1944). Measurements of pain sensitivity in normal control subjects and in psychoneurotic patients. *Psychosomatic Medicine, 6*, 252–257.

Charles, S.C., & Wilbert, J.R. (1985). Sued and nonsued physicians' self-reported reactions to malpractice litigation. *American Journal of Psychiatry, 142*, 437–440.

Charlton, A., Minagawa, K.E., & While, D. (1999). Saying "no" to cigarettes: A reappraisal of adolescent refusal skills. *Journal of Adolescents, 22*, 695–707.

Charnley, F. (1999). Occupational stress in the newly qualified staff nurse. *Nursing Standard, 13(29)*, 33–36.

Chasnoff, I.J., Landress, H.J., Barrett, M.J.E. (1990). The prevalence of illicit-drug or alcohol use during pregnancy and discrepancies in mandatory reporting in Pinellas County, Florida. *New England Journal of Medicine, 322*, 1202–1206.

Chaves, I.F., & Barber, T.X. (1976). Hypnotism and surgical pain. In D. Mostofsky (Ed.), *Behavioral control and modification of physiological activity*. Englewood Cliffs, NJ: Prentice-Hall.

Chen, J., & Millar, W.J. (1998). Age of smoking initation: Implications for quitting. *Health Reports, 9(4)*, 39–46.

Chen, J., & Wilkins, R. (1998). Seniors' needs for health-related personal assistance. *Health Reports, 10(1)*, 39–50.

Chen, J., Fair, M, Wilkins, R., Cyr, M. (1998). Maternal education and fetal and infant mortality in Quebec. *Health Reports, 10(2)*, 53–64.

Chen, J., Ng, E., & Wilkins, R. (1996). The health of Canada's immigrants in 1994–1995. *Health Reports, 7*, 42.

Cherny, N.I. (1996). The problem of inadequately relieved suffering. *Journal of Social Issues, 52*, 13–30.

Chilcoat, H.D., Dishion, T.J., & Anthony, J.C. (1995). Parent monitoring and the incidence of drug sampling in urban elementary school children. *American Journal of Epidemiology, 141*, 25–31.

Christenfeld, N., Gerin, W., Linden, W., Sanders, M., Mathur, J., Deich, J.D., & Pickering, T.G. (1997). Social support effects on cardiovascular reactivity: Is a stranger as effective as a friend? *Psychosomatic Medicine, 59*, 388–398.

Christianson, S. (1992). Emotional stress and eyewitness memory: A critical review. *Psychological Bulletin, 112*, 284–309.

Cinciripini, P.M., & Floreen, A. (1982). An evaluation of a behavioral program for chronic pain. *Journal of Behavioral Medicine, 5*, 375–389.

Cinciripini, P.M., Cinciripini, L.G., Wallfisch, A., Haque, W., & Van Vunakis, H. (1996). Behavior therapy and the transdermal nicotine patch: Effects on cessation outcome, affect, and coping. *Journal of Consulting and Clinical Psychology, 64*, 314–323.

Clack, G.B., & Head, J.O. (1999). Gender differences in medical graduates' assessment of their personal attributes. *Medical Education, 33*, 101–105.

Clark, J. (1998, November). Prostate cancer quality of life: Patient centered measures of health outcomes. Paper presented at the Cancer Care: Quality of Life and Outcomes Symposium, Chicago, Illinois.

Clark, J.H., MacPherson, B.V., & Holmes, D.R. (1982). Cigarette smoking and the external locus of control among young adolescents. *Journal of Health and Social Behavior, 23*, 253–259.

Clark, N.M., Gong, M., Schork, M.A., Evans, D., et al. (1998). Impact of education for physicians on patient outcomes. *Pediatrics, 101*, 831.

Clarke, H.F., Joseph, R., Dechamps, M., Hislop, T.G., Band, P.R., & Atleo, R. (1998). Reducting cervical cancer among First Nations women. *The Canadian Nurse, 94(3)*, 36–41.

Clarke, J.N. (1996). *Health, illness, and medicine in Canada, 2nd ed.* Toronto: Oxford University Press.

Coambs, R.B., Jensen, P., Her, M.H., Ferguson, B.S., et al. (1995). *Review of the scientific literature on the prevalence, consequences, and health costs of noncompliance and inappropriate use of prescription medication in Canada*. Ottawa, ON: Pharmaceutical Manufacturers Association of Canada (University of Toronto Press).

Coambs, R.B., Li, S., & Kozlowski, L.T. (1992). Age interacts with heaviness of smoking in predicting success in cessation of smoking. *American Journal of Epidemiology, 135*, 240–246.

Coates, R.J., Bransfield, D.D., Wesley, M., Hankey, B., et al. (1992). Differences between black and white women with breast cancer in time from symptom recognition to medical consultation. Black/White Cancer Survival Study Group, *Journal of the National Cancer Institute, 84*, 938–950.

Cockerham, W.M. (1998). *Medical sociology, 7th ed.* Upper Saddle River, NJ: Prentice Hall.

Cohen, G., & Eisdorfer, C. (1986). *The loss of self: A family resource for the care of Alzheimer's disease and related disorders.* New York: Norton.

Cohen, S. Tyrrell, D.A.J., & Smith, A.P. (1993). Negative life events, perceived stress, negative affect, and susceptibility to the common cold. *Journal of Personality and Social Psychology, 64*, 131–140.

Cohen, S., & Herbert, T.B. (1996). Health psychology: Psychological factors and physical disease from the perspective of human psychoneuroimmunology. *Annual Review of Psychology, 47*, 113–142.

Cohen, S., & McKay, G. (1984). Social support, stress, and the buffering hypothesis: A theoretical analysis. In Baum, A., Taylor, S.E., & Singer, J., (Eds.), *Handbook of psychology and health,* (Vol. 4, pp. 253–268). Hillsdale, NJ: Erlbaum.

Cohen, S., & Wills, T.A. (1985). Stress, social support, and the buffering hypothesis. *Psychological Bulletin, 98*, 310–357.

Cohen, S., Doyle, W.J., Skoner, D.P., Fireman, P., Gwaltner, J.M. Jr., & Newsom, J.T. (1995). State and trait negative affect as predictors of objective and subjective symptoms of respiratory viral infections. *Journal of Personality and Social Psychology, 68*, 139–169.

Cohen, S., Lichtenstein, E., Prochaska, J.O., Rossi, J.S., et al. (1989). Debunking myths about self-quitting. Evidence from 10 prospective studies of persons who attempt to quit smoking by themselves. *American*

Psychologist, 44, 1355–1365.

Colditz, G.A., Bonita, R., Stampfer, M.J., Willett, W.C., et al. (1988). Cigarette smoking and risk of stroke in middle-aged women. *New England Journal of Medicine, 318*, 937–941.

Cole, B. (1998, November). An overview of the Q-Twist method for evaluating trade-offs in clinical trials. Paper presented at the Cancer Care: Quality of Life and Outcomes Symposium, Chicago, Illinois.

College of Physicians and Surgeons of Ontario. (1996, January). Annual report of the complaints committee. *Members Dialogue.*

College of Physicians and Surgeons of Ontario. (1997 January/February). Annual report of the complaints committee. *Members Dialogue.*

COMMIT Research Group. (1995a). Community intervention trial for smoking cessation (COMMIT): I. Cohort results from a four-year community intervention. *American Journal of Public Health, 1995, 85*, 183–192.

COMMIT Research Group. (1995b). Community intervention trial for smoking cessation (COMMIT): II. Changes in adult cigarette smoking prevalence. *American Journal of Public Health, 1995, 85*, 193–200.

Compas, B.E., Haaga, D.A., Keefe, F.J., Leitenberg, H., & Williams, D.A. (1998). Sampling of empirically supported psychological treatments from health psychology: Smoking, chronic pain, cancer, and bulimia nervosa. *Journal of Consulting and Clinical Psychology, 66*, 89–112.

Con, A.H., Linden, W., Thompson, J., & Ignaszewski, A. (in press). The psychology of men and women recovering from coronary artery bypass surgery. *Journal of Cardiopulmonary Rehabilitation.*

Conger, J. (1956). Reinforcement theory and the dynamics of alcoholism. *Quarterly Journal of Studies on Alcohol, 17*, 296–305.

Conrad, K.M., Flay, B.R., & Hill, D. (1992). Why children start smoking cigarettes: Predictors of onset. *British Journal of Addiction, 87*, 1711–1724.

Coombs, R.H. (1998). Surviving medical school. Thousand Oaks, CA: Sage.

Coombs, R.H., & Fawzy, F.I. (1993). Surgeons' personalities: The influence of medical school. *Medical Education, 27*, 337–343.

Cooper, C.L., & Baglioni, A.J. (1988). A structural model approach toward the development of a theory of the link between stress and mental health. *British Journal of Medical Psychology, 61*, 87–102.

Cooper, Z. (1995). The development and maintenance of eating disorders. In K. Brownell & C. Fairburn (Eds.), *Eating disorders and obesity: A comprehensive handbook* (pp. 3199–206). New York: The Guilford Press.

Cooper-Patrick, L., Gallo, J.J., Gonzales, J.J., et al. (1999). Race, gender, and partnership in the patient-physician relationship. *Journal of the American Medical Association, 282*, 583–589.

Coser, R. (1962). *Life on the ward. East Lansing*, MI: Michigan State University Press.

Coser, R.L. (1962). *Life in the ward. East Lansing*: Michigan State University Press.

Cousins, N. (1979). *Anatomy of an illness.* New York: Norton.

Cousins, N. (1988). Intangibles in medicine: An attempt at a balancing perspective. *Journal of the American Medical Association, 260*, 1610–1612.

Cox, H. (1973). *The Seduction of the Spirit.* New York: Simon and Schuster.

Coyne, J. Aldwin, C., & Lazarus, R.S. (1981). Depression and coping in stressful episodes. *Journal of Abnormal Psychology, 90*, 439–447.

Cozby, P.C. (1993). *Methods in behavioral research, 5th ed.* Mountain View CA: Mayfield.

Craig, K.D. (1996). The back pain controversy—Reply. *Pain Research Management, 1*, 183.

Cramer, J.A., Mattson, R.H., Prevey, M.L., Scheyer, R.D., & Ouellette, V.L. (1989). How often is medication taken as prescribed? *Journal of the American Medical Association, 261*, 3273–3277.

Crook, J. (1982). Women and chronic pain. In R. Roy & E. Tunks (Eds.), *Chronic pain: Psychosocial factors in rehabilitation* (pp. 68–78). Baltimore: Williams and Williams.

Crook, J. (1993). Comparative experiences of men and women who have sustained a work related musculoskeletal injury. (Abstracts) 7th World Congress on Pain. Seattle: IASP Press.

Croyle, R.T., & Ditto, P.H. (1990). Illness cognition and behavior: An experimental approach. *Journal of Behavioral Medicine, 13*, 31–52.

Croyle, R.T., & Hunt, J.R. (1991). Coping with health threat: Social influence processes in reactions to medical test results. *Journal of Personality and Social Psychology, 60*, 382–389.

Croyle, R.T., & Uretsky, M.B. (1987). Effects of mood on self-appraisal of health status. *Health Psychology, 6*, 239–253.

Csikzentmihalyi, M. (1997). *Finding flow*. New York: Basic Books.

Cull, A. (1990). Invited review: Psychological aspects of cancer and chemotherapy. *Journal of Psychosomatic Research, 34*, 129–140.

Cullen, K.J., Knuimon, M.W., & Ward, N.J. (1993). Alcohol and mortality in Busselton, Western Austrralia. *American Journal of Epidemiology, 137*, 242–248.

Cunningham, J.A. (1999). Resolving alcohol-related problems with and without treatment: The effects of different problem criteria. *Journal of Studies on Alcohol*.

Cutler, R.B., Fishbain, D.A., Rosomoff, H.L., Abdel-Moty, E., et al. (1994). Does nonsurgical pain center treatment of chronic pain return patients to work? A review and meta-analysis of the literature. *Spine, 19*, 643–652.

Dahl, M. (1992). Nurses: An image change still needed. *Nursing Outlook, 33(2)*, 74–77.

Dalal, S. & Melzack, R. (1998). Potentiation of opioid analgesia by psychostimulant drugs: A review. *Journal of Pain and Symptom Management*.

Danish, S.J., Nellon, V.C., & Owens, S.S. (1996). Teaching life skills through sport: Community-based programs for adolescents. In J.L. Van Raalte and B. Brewer (Eds.), *Exploring sport and exercise psychology* (pp.205–225). New York: American Psychological Association.

Danish, S.J., Pettipas, A.J., & Hale, B.D. (1993). Life development intervention for athletes: Life skills through sports. *The Counseling Psychologist, 21*, 352–385.

Dantendorfer, K., Amering, M., Bankier, A., Helbich, T., Prayer, D., Youssefzadeh, S., Alexandrowicz, R., Imhof, H., & Katschnig, H. (1997). A study of the effects of patient anxiety, perceptions and equipment on motion artifacts in magnetic resonance imaging. *Magnetic Resonance Imaging, 15*, 301–306.

Dare, C. & Eisner, I. (1995). Family therapy and eating disorders. In K. Brownell & C. Fairburn (Eds.), *Eating disorders and obesity: A comprehensive handbook* (pp. 318–323). New York: The Guilford Press.

De Koninck, M., Bergeron, P., & Bourbonnais, R. (1997). Women physicians in Québec. *Social Science and Medicine, 44*, 1825–1832.

Deinzer, R., & Schüller, N. (1998). Dynamics of stress-related decrease of salivary immunoglobulin A (sIgA): Relationship to symptoms of the common cold and studying behavior. *Behavioral Medicine, 23*, 161–169.

Dembroski, T.M., & Costa, P.T. (1988). Assessment of coronary-prone behavior: A current overview. *Annals of Behavioral Medicine, 10*, 60–63.

Denissenko, M.F., Pao, A., Tang, M.-S., & Pfeifer G.P. (1996). Preferential formation of benzo[a]pyrene adducts at lung cancer mutational hotspots in P53. *Science, 274*, 430–432.

Dennis, C.R., Gardner, B., & Lim, B. (1975). Analysis of survival and recurrence vs. patient and doctor delay in treatment of breast cancer. *Cancer, 35*, 714.

Desbiens, N.A., Mueller-Rizner, N., Haniel, M.B., & Connors, A.F., Jr. (1998). Preference for comfort care does not affect the pain experience of seriously ill patients. The SUPPORT Investigators. Study to Understand Prognoses and Preferences for Outcomes and Risks of Treatment. *Journal of Pain and Symptom Management, 16*, 281–289.

Deschamps, M., Band, P.R., Hislop, T.G., Clarke, H.F., Smith, J.M., Ng, V., & Math, M. (1992). Barriers to cervical cytology screening in native women in British Columbia. *Cancer Detection and Prevention, 16*, 337–339.

Devine, E.C. (1992). Effects of psychoeducational care for adult surgical patients. A meta-analysis of 191 studies. *Patient Education and Counseling, 19*, 129–142.

Dialogue on Health Reform. (1996). Ontario Nurses Association.

Dickey, W.C., Dew, M.A., Becker, J.T., & Kingsley, L. (1999). Combined effects of HIV-infection status and psychosocial vulnerability on mental health in homosexual men. *Social Psychiatry and Psychiatric Epidemiology, 34*, 4–11.

DiFranceisco, W., Kelly, J.A., Sikkema, K.J., Somlai, A.M., Murphy, D.A., & Stevenson, L.Y. (1998). Differences between completers and early dropouts from 2 HIV intervention trials: A health belief approach to understanding prevention program attrition. *American Journal of Public Health,*

88, 1068–1073.

Dillbeck, M.C., & Orme-Johnson, D.W. (1987). Physiological differences between transcendental meditation and rest. *American Psychologist, 42*, 879–880.

Diltmar, S.S., Haughey, B., O'Shea, R.M., & Brasure, J. (1989). Health practices of nursing students: A survey. *Health Values, 13(2)*, 24–31.

DiMatteo, M.R. (1979). A social-psychological analysis of physician-patient rapport: Toward a science of the art of medicine. *Journal of Social Issues, 35*, 12–33.

DiMatteo, M.R. (1991). *The psychology of health illness, and medical care: An individual perspective*. Pacific Grove, CA: Brooks/Cole.

DiMatteo, M.R. (1994). Enhancing patient adherence to medical recommendations. *Journal of the American Medical Association, 271*, 79–83.

DiMatteo, M.R. (1995). Health psychology research: The interpersonal challenges. In Brannigan, G.G. & Merrens, M.R. (Eds.) *The social psychologists: Research adventures*. New York: McGraw-Hill, pp. 207–221.

DiMatteo, M.R., & DiNicola, D.D. (1982). *Achieving patient compliance: The psychology of the medical practitioner's role*. New York: Pergamon.

DiMatteo, M.R., Hays, R.D., & Prince, L.M. (1986). Relationship of physicians' nonverbal communication skill to patient satisfaction, appointment noncompliance and physician workload. *Health Psychology, 5*, 581–594.

DiMatteo, M.R., Linn, L.S., Chang, B.L., & Cope, D.W. (1985). Affect and neutrality in physician behavior: A study of patients' values and satisfaction. *Journal of Behavioral Medicine, 8*, 397–409.

Dimeo, F.C., Stieglitz, R.D., Novelli-Fischer, U., Fetscher, S., & Keul, J. (1999). Effects of physical activity on the fatigue and psychologic status of cancer patients during chemotherapy. *Cancer, 85*, 2273–2277.

Dinh, K.T., Sarason, I.G., Peterson, A.V., & Onstad, L.E. (1995). Children's perception of smokers and nonsmokers: A longitudinal study. *Health Psychology, 14*, 32–40.

DiNicola, D.D., & DiMatteo, M.R. (1984). Practitioners, patients, and compliance with medical regimens: A social psychological perspective. In A. Baum, S.E. Taylor, & J.E. Singer (Eds.), *Handbook of psychology and health: Vol. 4. Social psychological aspects of health* (pp. 55–84). Hillsdale, NJ: Erlbaum.

Dishman, R. K. (Ed.). (1988). *Exercise adherence: Its impact on public health*. Champaign, Illinois: Human Kinetics.

Dishman, R.K., & Buckworth, J. (1997). Adherence to physical activity. In W.P. Morgan (Ed.), *Physical activity and mental health* (pp. 63–80). Washington, DC: Taylor and Francis.

DiTomasso, R.A., & Kovnat, K.D. (1994). Medical patients. In F.D. Dattilio and A. Freeman. (Eds.), *Cognitive-behavioral strategies in crisis intervention* (pp.325–344). New York: Guilford Press.

Diverty, B. & Pérez, C. (1998). *The health of Northern residents. Health Reports, 9 (4)*, 49–58.

Dlin, B.M. (1980). The experience of surviving almost certain death. *Advances in Psychosomatic medicine, 10*, 111–118.

Donaldson, S.I., Graham, j.W., Piccinin, A.M. & Hansen, W.B. (1995). Resistance-skills training and onset of alcohol use: Evidence for beneficial and potentially harmful effects in public schools and in private Catholic schools. *Health Psychology, 14*, 291–300.

Doucet, M.D., Purdy, R.A., Kaufman, D.M., & Langille, D.B. (1998). Comparison of problem-based learning and lecture format in continuing medical education on headache diagnosis and management. *Medical Education, 32*, 590–596.

Doyle, L.A., Landers, D.M., & Feltz, D.L. (1980). Psychological skills in elite and subelite shooters. Paper presented at the North American Society for the Psychology of Sport and Physical Exercise, Boulder, Colorado.

Drake, D. (1850–1854). *A systematic treatise historical, etiological, and practical on the principal diseases of the interior valley of North America as they appear in the Caucasian, African, Indian, and Exquimaux varieties of its population, 2 volumes*. New York: Burt Franklin.

Drisckell, J.E., Copper, C., Moran, A. (1994). Does mental practice enhance performance? *Journal of Applied Psychology, 79*, 481–492.

Drossman, DA., Li, Z., Andruzzi, E., Temple, R.D., Talley, N.J., Thompson, W.G., Whitehead, W.E., Janssens, J., Funch-Jensen, P., Corazziari, E., Richter, J.E., & Koch, G.G. (1993). US householder survey of functional gastrointestinal disorders: Prevalence, sociodemography and health impact. *Digestive Diseases and Sciences, 38,*

1569–1580.

Drozda, D.J., Allen, S.R., Standiford, D.A., Turner, A.M., & McCain, G.C. (1997). Personal illness models of diabetes: Parents of preadolescents and adolescents. *Diabetes Education, 23*, 550–557.

Drummond, P.D., & Hewson-Bower, B. (1997). Increased psychosocial stress and decreased mucosal immunity in children with recurrent upper respiratory tract infections. *Journal of Psychosomatic Research, 43*, 271–278.

Duda, J.L. (1992). Motivation in sport settings: A goal perspective approach. In G. Roberts (Ed.), *Motivation in Sport and Exercise* (pp. 57–91). Champaign, Illinois: Human Kinetics.

Dudgeon, D., Raubertas, R.F., & Rosenthal, S.M. (1993). The Short-Form McGill Pain Questionnaire in chronic cancer pain. *Journal of Pain and Symptom Management, 8*, 191–195.

Dugan, J., Lauer, E., Bouquot, Z., Dutro, B.K., Smith, M., & Widmeyer, G. (1996). Stressful nurses: The effect on patient outcomes. *Journal of Nursing Care Quality, 10(3)*, 46–58.

Dumont, C., St. Onge, M., Fougeyrollas, P., & Renaud, L.A. (1998). Perceived burden in family caregivers with physical disabilities. *Canadian Journal of Occupational Therapy, 65*, 258–270.

Dunkel-Schetter, C. (1984). Social support and cancer: Findings based on patient interviews and their implications. *Journal of Social Issues, 40(4)*, 77–98.

Dunn, J., Steginga, S.K. Occhipinti, S., & Wilson, K. (1999). Evaluation of a peer support program for women with breast cancer—lessons for practitioners. *Journal of Community and Applied Social Psychology, 9*, 13–22.

Eagly, A.H., & Chaiken, S. (1993). *The psychology of attitudes*. New York: Harcourt Brace Jovanovich.

Earle, T.L., Linden, W., & Weinberg, J. (in press). Differential effects of harassment on cardiovascular and salivary cortisol stress reactivity and recovery in women and men. *Journal of Psychosomatic Research.*

Edwards, G., & Gross, M.M. (1976). Alcohol dependence: Provisional description of a clinical syndrome. *British Medical Journal*, 1058–1061.

Egbert, L.D., Battit, C.E., Weleb, C.E., Bartlett, M.K. (1964). Reduction of postoperative pain by encouragement and instruction of patients. A study of doctor-patient rapport. *New England Journal of Medicine, 270*, 825–827.

Eifert, G.H., Hodson, S.E., Tracey, D.R., Seville, J.L., & Gunawardane, K. (1996). Heart-focused anxiety, illness beliefs, and behavioral impairment: Comparing healthy heart-anxious patients with cardiac and surgical inpatients. *Journal of Behavioral Medicine, 19*, 385–400.

Eisenberg, D.M., Davis, R.B., Eltner, S.L., Appel, S., Wilkey, S., Van Rompay, M., et al. (1998). Trends in alternative medicine use in the United States 1990–1997. *Journal of the American Medical Association, 280*, 1569–1575.

Eisenberg, J.M., Kitz, D.S., & Webber, R.A. (1983). Development of attitudes about sharing decision-making: A comparison of medical and surgical residents. *Journal of Health and Social Behavior, 24*, 85–90.

Eiser, C. (1990). *Chronic childhood disease: An introduction to psychological theory and research*. Cambridge: Cambridge University Press.

Eisler, I., Dare, C., Russell, G.F., Szmukler, G., le Grange, D., & Dodge, E. (1997). Family and individual therapy in anorexia nervosa. A 5-year follow-up. *Archives of General Psychiatry, 54*, 1025–1030.

Ellingson, L.A., & Yarber, W.L. (1997). Breast self-examination, the health belief model and sexual orientation in women. *Journal of Sex Education and Therapy, 22*, 29–24.

Elliot, J., & White, H. (1990). Patients are patients [letter]. *New Zealand Medical Journal, 103*, 593.

Elliott, A.J., Russo, J., Bergam, K., Claypoole, K., Uldall, K.K., & Roy-Byrne, P.P. (1999). *Journal of Clinical Psychiatry, 60*, 226–231.

Ellis, A. (1962). *Reason and emotion in psychotherapy*. New York: Lyle Stuart.

Ellis, A. (1975). *How to live with a "neurotic"*. (rev. ed.). New York: Crown.

Ellis, A. (1994). The sport of avoiding sports and exercise: A rational emotive behavior therapy perspective. *The Sport Psychologist, 8*, 248–261.

Ellis, A. and Harper, B.A. (1975). *A new quide to rational living*. North Hollywood, California: Wilshire.

Ellison, L.F., Mao, Y., & Gibbons. (1995). Projected smoking-attributable mortality in Canada, 1991–2000. *Chronic Diseases in Canada, 16*, 84–89.

Ellison, L.F., Morrison, H.I., de Groh, M., &

Villeneuve, P.J. (1999). Health consequences of smoking among Canadian smokers: An update. *Chronic Diseases in Canada, 20*, 36–39.

Emanuel, E.J., & Emanuel, L.L. (1992). Four models of the physician-patient relationship. *Journal of the American Medical Association, 267*, 2221–2226.

Emergy, Hauck, E.R., Blumethal, J.A. (1992). Exercise adherence or maintenance among older adults: 1-year follow-up study. *Psychology and Aging, 7*, 466–470.

Emmons, K.M., Wechsler, H., Dowdall, G., & Abraham, M. (1998). Predictors of smoking among U.S. college students. *American Journal of Public Health, 88*, 104–107.

Emmott, S. (1991, June). Cognitive group therapy for coping with HIV infection. Paper presented to the VII International Conference on AIDS, Florence, Italy.

Engebretson, T.O., Clark, M.M., Niaura, R.S., Phillips, T., Albrecht, A., & Tilkemeier, P. (1999). Quality of life and anxiety in a phase II cardiac rehabilitation program. *Medical Science in Sports Exercise, 31*, 216–223.

Engel, G.L. (1977). The need for a new medical model: A challenge for biomedicine. *Science, 196*, 129–136.

Engel, J.M., Jensen, M.P., Schwartz, L., White, O.R. (1999, October). Outcome of biofeedback-assisted relaxation for pain in persons with cerebral palsy. Poster session presented at the annual meeting of the American Pain Society, Fort Lauderdale, FL.

Ennett, S.T., & Bauman, K.E. (1993). Peer group structure and adolescent cigarette smoking: A social network analysis. *Journal of Health and Social Behavior, 34*, 226–236.

Epp, J. (1986). Achieving health for all: A framework for health promotion. Canadian *Journal of Public Health, 77*, 393–430.

Epstein, L.H., & Cluss, P.A. (1982). A behavioral medicine perspective on adherence to long-term medical regimens. *Journal of consulting and Clinical Psychology, 50*, 950–971.

Erickson, M.H. (1967). An introduction to the study and application of hypnosis for pain control. In J. Lassner (Ed.), *Hypnosis and pscyhosomatic medicine* (p. 83). New York: Springer.

Erickson, M.H. (1967). An introduction to the study and application of hypnosis for pain control. In J. Lassner (Ed.), *Hypnosis and pscyhosomatic medicine* (p. 83). New York: Springer.

Esterling, B.A., Antoni, M.H., Kumar, M., & Schneiderman, N. (1993). Defensiveness, trait anxiety, and Eptstein-Barr virus capsid antigen antibody titers in healthy college students. *Health Psychology, 12*, 291–298.

Esterling, B.A., Kiecolt-Glaser, J.K., Bodnar, J.C., & Glaser, R. (1994). Chronic stress, social support, and persistent alterations in the natural killer cell response to cytokines in older adults. *Health Psychology, 13*, 291–298.

Etnier, J.L., Salazar, W., Landers, D.M., Petruzzello, S.J., Han, M., & Nowell, P. (1997). The influence of physical fitness and exercise upon cognitive functioning: A meta-analysis. *Journal of Sport and Exercise Psychology, 19*, 249–277.

Evans, D.L., Staab, J.P., Petitto, J.M., Morrison, M.F., Szuba,M.P., Ward, H.E., Wingate, B., Luber, M.P., & O'Reardon, J.P. (1999). Depression in medical settings: Biopsychological interventions and treatment considerations. *Journal of Clinical Psychiatry, 60 (Suppl 4)*, 40–55.

Evans, P.D, Bristow, M., Hucklebridge, F., Clow, A., & Walters, N. (1993). The relationship between secretory immuninity, mood and life-events. *British Journal of Clinical Psychology, 32*, 227–236.

Evans, P.D., Doyle, A., Hucklebridge, F., & Clow, A. (1997). Positive but not negative life-events predict vulnerability to upper respiratory illness. *British Journal of Health Psychology, 2*, 339–348.

Evans, R., Barer, M., & Marmot, T. (1994). *Why are some people healthy and others not?* New York: Aldine de Gruyter.

Evans, R.L., & Connis, R.T. (1995). Comparison of brief group therapy for depressed cancer patients receiving radiation treatment. *Public Health Reports, 110*, 306–311.

Evans, R.L., & Hendricks, R.D. (1993). Evaluating hospital discharge planning: A randomized clinical trial. *Medical Care, 31*, 358–370.

Everson, S.A., Goldberg, D.E., Kaplan, G.A., et al. (1996). Hopelessness and risk of mortality and incidence of myocardial infarction and cancer. *Psychosomatic Medicine, 58*, 113–121.

Eysenck, H.J. (1996). Personality and cancer. In C.L. Cooper (Ed.), *Stress, medicine and coping* (pp. 193–215). Boca Raton, FL: CRC Press.

Eysenck, H.J., Nias, D., & Cox. D.N. (1982). Sport and personality. *Advances in Behavioral Research and Therapy, 4*, 1–56.

Facione, N.C. (1993). Delay versus help seeking for breast cancer symptoms: A critical review of the literature on patient and provider delay. *Social Science and Medicine, 36*, 1521–1534.

Facione, N.C. (1999). Breast cancer screening in relation to access to health services. *Oncology Nursing Forum, 26*, 689–696.

Facione, N.C., & Giancarlo, C.A. (1998). Narratives of breast symptom discovery and cancer diagnosis: Psychologic risk for advanced cancer at diagnosis. *Cancer Nursing, 21*, 430–440.

Facione, N.C., & Giancarlo, C.A., & Ingram, C. (1999). Women's decisions to seek help for breast symptoms occur in a complex social context. *Western Journal of Medicine, 171*, 164.

Faden, R.R., Becker, C., Lewis, C., Freeman, J., Faden, A.I. (1981). Disclosure of information of patients in medical care. *Medical Care, 19*, 718–733.

Farrell, G.A. (1999). Aggression in clinical settings: Nurses' views—a follow-up study. *Journal of Advanced Nursing, 29*, 532–541.

Fawzy, F.I., & Fawzy, N.W. (1998). Group therapy in cancer settings. *Journal of Psychosomatic Research, 45*, 191–200.

Feifel, H. (1977). *New meanings of death*. New York: McGraw-Hill.

Felton, G.M., Parsons, M., & Bartoces, M.G. (1997). Demographic factors: Interaction effects on health promoting behavior and health related factors. *Public Health Nursing, 14*, 361–367.

Felton, J.S. (1998). Burnout as a clinical entity—its importance in health care workers. *Occupational Medicine, 48*, 237–250.

Feltz, D.L. (1988). Self-confidence and sports performance. In K.B. Pandolf (Ed.), *Exercise and sport sciences reviews* (pp. 423–457). New York: MacMillan.

Feltz, D.L., & Landers, D.M. (1983). The effects of mental practice on motor skill learning and performance: A meta-analysis. *Journal of Sport Psychology, 5*, 25–57.

Feltz, D.L., Bandura, A., & Lirgg, C.D. (1989). Perceived collective self-efficacy in hockey. In D. Kendzierski (chair) Self-Perceptions in Sport and Physical Activity: Self-Efficacy and Self-Image. Symposium conducted at a meeting of the American Psychological Association, New Orleans.

Fernandez, C.V., Stutzer, C.A., Macwilliam, L., & Fryer, C. (1998). Alternative and complementary therapy use in pediatric oncology patients in British Columbia: prevalence and reasons for use and nonuse. *Journal Of Clinical Oncology, 16*, 1279–1286.

Ferraro, d.P. (1980). Acute effects of marijuana on human memory and cognition. In R.C. Peterson (Ed.), *Marijuana research findings*. National Institute on Drug Abuse. Washington, DC: U.S. Government Printing Office.

Festinger, L. (1954). A theory of social comparison processes. *Human Relations, 7*, 117–140.

Finkelstein, P. (1986). Studies in the anatomy laboratory: A portrait of individual and collective defense. In R.H. Coombs, D.S. May, and G.W. Small (Eds.), *Inside doctoring: Stages and outcomes in the professional development of physicians* (pp. 22–42). New York: Praeger.

Finley, A., Chambers, C.T., McGrath, P.J., & Walsh, T. (1999, October). Further validation of the Parents' Postoperative Pain Measure. Poster session presented at the annual meeting of the American Pain Society, Fort Lauderdale, FL.

Finsen, V., Persen, L., Lovlien, M., Veslegaard, E., et al. (1988). Transcutaneous electrical nerve stimulation after major amputation. *British Journal of Bone and Joint Surgery, 70(B)*, 109–112.

Fischman, J. (1984). The mystery of Alzheimer's. *Psychology Today, 18(1)*, 27.

Fishbein, M., & Ajzen, I. (1975). Belief, attitude, intention, and behavior: An introduction to theory and research. Reading, MA: Addison-Wesley.

Fisher, J.D., & Fisher, W.A. (1992). Changing AIDs risk behavior. *Psychological Bulletin, 111*, 455–474.

Fisher, J.D., & Fisher, W.A. (1998). Theoretical approaches to individual level change in HIV risk behavior. In J. Peterson & R. Diclemente (Eds.), *HIV prevention handbook*. New York: Plenum.

Fisher, W.A., Dervaitis, K., Bryan, A., Silcox, J., & Kohn, H. (unpublished manuscript). Women's health status: Sexual health, reproductive health, sexual coercion, and partner abuse indicators in a Canadian obstetrics and gynaecology outpatient population.

Fitch, M.I., Gray, R.E., Greenberg, M., Labrecque, M., & Douglas, M.S. (1999). Nurses' perspectives on unconventional therapies. *Cancer Nursing, 22*, 238–245.

Flaherty, J.A., & Richman, J.A. (1993). Substance use and addiction among medical students, residents, and physicians. *Psychiatric Clinics of North America, 16*,

189–197.

Flakus, B.J. (1998). Stress relief for critical care nurses. *Nursing Management, 29*, 48D, 48H–48J.

Fletcher, A.B. (1988). Pain in the neonate. *The New England Journal of Medicine, 317*, 1347–1348.

Flor, H., Fydrich, T., & Turk, D.C. (1992). Efficacy of multidisciplinary pain treatment centers: A meta-analytic reveiw. *Pain, 49*, 221–230.

Flor, H., Kerns, R.D., & Turk, D.C. (1987). The role of spouse reinforcement, perceived pain, and activity levels of chronic pain patients. *Journal of Psychosomatic Research, 31*, 251–259.

Folkins, C.H., & Syme, W.E. (1981) Physical fitness training and mental health. *American Psychologist*, 373–389.

Folkman, S., & Lazarus, R.S. (1985). If it changes it must be a process: Study of emotion and coping during three stages of a college examination. *Journal of Personality and Social Psychology, 48*, 150–170.

Folkman, S., Lazarus, R.S., Dunkel-Schetter, C., DeLongis, A., & Gruen, R.J. (1986). Dynamics of a stressful encounter: Cognitive appraisal, coping and encounter outcomes. *Journal of Personality and Social Psychology, 50*, 992–1003.

Follick, M.J., Ahern, D. K, Attanasio, V., & Riley, J.F. (1985). Chronic pain programs: Current aims, strategies, and needs. *Annals of Behavioral Medicine, 7(3)*, 17–20.

Follick, M.J., Ahern, D.K., & Aberger, E.W. (1985). Development of an audiovisual taxonomy of pain behavior: Reliability and discriminant validity. *Health Psychology, 4*, 555–568.

Fordyce, W.E. (1976). *Behavioral methods for chronic pain and illness*. St. Louis: C.V. Mosby.

Fordyce, W.E. (1978). Learning processes in pain. In R.A. Sternbach (Ed.), *The psychology of pain*. New York: Raven Press.

Fordyce, W.E. (1995). *Back pain in the workplace*. Seattle: IASP Press.

Fordyce, W.E. (1996). Response to Thompson/Merskey/Teasell. *Pain, 65*, 112–114.

Forester, B., Kornfeld, D.S., Fleiss, J.L., & Thompson S. (1993). Group psychotherapy during radiotherapy: Effects on emotional and physical distress. *American Journal of Psychiatry, 150*, 1700–1706.

Fox, E.J., & Melzack, R. (1976). Transcutaneous electrical stimulation and acupuncture: Comparison of treatment for low-back pain. *Pain, 2*, 141–148.

Franco-Bronson, K. (1996). The management of treatment-resistant depression in the medically ill. *Psychiatric Clinics of North America, 19*, 329–350.

Frankel, R., & Beckman, H. (1989). Evaluating the patient's primary problem(s). In M. Stewart and D. Roter (Eds.), *Communicating with medical patients* (pp. 86–98). Newbury Park, Calif: Sage Publications.

Frankish, C.J., Milligan, C. D., & Reid, C. (1998). A review of relationships between active living and determinants of health. *Social Science and Medicine, 47*, 287–301.

Frasure-Smith, N., Lesperance, F., & Talajic, M. (1993). Depression following mycardial infarction: Impact on 6-month survival. *Journal of the American Medical Association, 270*, 1860–1861.

Frasure-Smith, N., Lesperance, F., & Talajic, M. (1995). Depression and 18-month prognosis after myocardial infarction. *Circulation, 91*, 999–1005.

Frasure-Smith, N., Lesperance, F., Juneau, M., Talajic, M., & Bourassa, M.G. (1999). Gender, depression, and one-year prognosis after myocardial infarction. *Psychosomatic Medicine, 61*, 26–37.

Freidson, E. (1961). *Patients' views of medical practice*. New York: Russell Sage Foundation.

French, J.R.P., Jr., & Raven, B. (1959). The bases of social power. In D. Cartwright (Ed.), *Studies in social power* (pp. 150–167). Ann Arbor: University of Michigan, Institute for Social Research.

Friedman, L.A., & Kimball, A.W. (1986). Coronary heart disease mortality and alcohol consumption in Framingham. *American Journal of Epidemiology, 124*, 481–489.

Friedman, M., & Rosenman, R.H. (1959). Association of specific overt behavior pattern with blood and cardiovascular findings—blood cholesterol level, blood clotting time, incidence of arcus senilis, and clinical coronary artery disease. *Journal of the American Medical Association, 162*, 1286–1296.

Friedman, M., & Rosenman, R.H. (1974). *Type A behavior and your heart*. New York: Knopf.

Frisoni, G.B., Fedi, V., Geroldi, C., Trabucchi, M. (1999). Cognition and perception of physical symptoms in the community-dwelling elderly. *Behavioral Medicine, 25*,

5–12.

Fuchs, C.S., Stampfer, M.J., Colditz, G.A., Giovannucci, E.L., et al. (1995). Alcohol consumption and mortality among women. *New England Journal of Medicine, 332*, 1245–1250.

Fulton, T.R. (1996). Nurses' adopption of patient-controlled analgesia approach. *Western Journal of Nursing Research, 18*, 383–396.

Futterman, A.D., Kemeny, M.E., Shapiro, D., & Fahey, J.L. (1994). Immunological and physiological changes associated with induced positive and negative mood. *Psychosomatic Medicine, 56*, 499–511.

Gallagher, E.J., Viscoli, C.M., & Horwitz, R.I. (1993). The relationship of treatment adherence to the risk of death after myocardial infarction in women. Journal of the *American Medical Association, 270*, 742–743.

Gallagher, E.M. & Scott, V.J. (1997). The STEPS Project: Participatory action research to reduce falls in public places among seniors and persons with disabilities. *Canadian Journal of Public Health, 88*, 129–133.

Gard, M.C.E., & Freeman, C.P. (1996). Dismantling of a myth: Review of eating disorders and socioeconomic status. International *Journal of Eating Disorders, 20*, 1–12.

Garner, D.M., & Garfinkel, P.E. (1980). Social-cultural factors in the development of anorexia nervosa. *Psychological Medicine, 10*, 647–656.

Garro, L.C. (1998). On the rationality of decision-making studies: Part 1: Decision models of treatment choice. *Medical Anthropology Quarterly, 12*, 319–340.

Gatrell, A.C., & Bailey, T.c. (1996). Interactive spatial data analysis in medical geography. *Social Science and Medicine, 42*, 843–855.

Gaudette, L.A., Richardson, A., & Huang, S. (1998). Which workers smoke? *Health Reports, 10(3)*, 35–45.

Gauvin, L. (1990). An experiential perspective on the motivational features of exercise and lifestyle. *Canadian Journal of Sport Sciences, 15*, 51–58.

Gauvin, L. and Spence, J.C. (1995). Psychological research on exercise and fitness: Current research trends and future challenges. *The Sport Psychologist, 9*, 434–448.

Gaziano, J.M., Buring, J.E., Breslow, J.L., Goldhaber, S.Z., et al. (1993). Moderate alcohol intake, increased levels of high-density lipoprotein and its subfractions, and decreased risk of myocardial infarction. *New England Journal of Medicine, 329*, 1829–1834.

Geist, R., Heinmaa, M., Katzman, D., & Stephens, D. (1999). A comparison of male and female adolescents referred to an eating disorder program. *Canadian Journal of Psychiatry, 44*, 374–378.

Gentry, W.D. (1979). Preadmission behavior. In W.D. Gentry & R.B. Williams (Eds.), *Psychological aspects of myocardial infarction and coronary care* (2nd ed., pp. 67–77). St. Louis: C.V. Mosby.

George, T.R. (1994). Self-confidence and baseball performance: A causal examination. *Journal of Sport and Exercise Psychology*, 16, 3181–399.

Geyer, S. (1991). Life events prior to manifestation of breast cancer: A limited prospective study covering eight years before diagnosis. *Journal of Psychosomatic Research, 35*, 335–363.

Ghosh, S., & Sallam, S. (1994). Patient satisfaction and postoperative demands on hospital and community services after day surgery. *British Journal of Surgery, 81*, 1635–1638.

Gibbons, B. (1990). Giving information to relatives. *Nursing Practice, 3(3)*, 19–23.

Gil, K.M., Keefe, F.J., Crisson, J.E., & Van Dalfsen, P.J. (1987). Social support and pain behavior. *Pain, 29*, 209–217.

Gilbar, O. (1989). Who refuses chemotherapy: A profile. *Psychological Reports, 64*, 1291–1297.

Gilmour, H., & Gentleman, J.F. (1999). Mortality in metropolitan areas. *Health Reports, 11(1)*, 9–19.

Gittelsohn, J., Silla, B., & Sanneh, K.M.L. (1991). Ethnographic study of acute respiratory infections in The Gambia. Department of International Health, Johns Hopkins School of Hygiene and Public health, Baltimore, MD, unpublished report.

Glaser, B.G., & Strauss, A. (1967). T*he discovery of grounded theory*. Chicago: Aldine Press.

Glaser, R., Kiecolt-Glaser, J.K., Bonneau, R., Malarkey, W., & Hughes, J. (1992). Stress-induced modulation of the immune response to recombinant hepatitis B vaccine. *Psychosomatic Medicine, 54*, 22–29.

Glaser, R., Kiecolt-Glaser, J.K., Speicher, C.E., & Holliday, J.E. (1985). Stress, loneliness, and changes in herpesvirus latency. *Journal of Behavioral Medicine, 8*, 249–260.

Glaser, R., Pearson, G.R., Bonneau, R.H., Esterling, B.A., et al. (1993). Stress and memory T-cell response to the Epstein-Barr virus in healthy medical students. *Health Psychology, 12*, 435–442.

Godin, G., Maticka-Tyndale, E, Adrien, A., Manson-Singer, S., et al. (1996). Cross-cultural testing of three social cognitive theories: An application to condom use. *Journal of Applied Social Psychology, 26*, 1556–1586.

Goffman, E. (1961). *Asylums*. Garden City, NY: Doubleday.

Gold, P.W., Gwirtsman, H., Avgerinos, P.C., Nieman, L.K., et al. (1986). Abnormal hypothalamic-pituitary-adrenal function in anorexia nervosa: Pathophysiologic mechanisms in under-weight and weight-corrected patients. *New England Journal of Medicine, 314,* 1335–1342.

Goldner, E.M., & Birmingham, C.L. (1994). Anorexia nervosa: Methods of treatment. In L. Alexander-Mott & D.B. Lumsden (Eds.), *Understanding eating disorders: Anorexia nervosa, bulimia nervosa, and obesity* (pp. 135–157). Washington, DC: Taylor & Francis.

Goodheart, C.D., & Lansing, M.H. (1997). *Treating people with chronic disease: A psychological guide.* Washington, DC: American Psychological Association.

Goodkin, K., Blaney, N.T., Feaster, D., Fletcher, M., Baum, M.K., Mantero-Atienza, E., Klimas, N.G., Millon, C., Szapocznic, J., & Eisdorfer, C. (1992). Active coping style is associated with natural killer cell cytotoxicity in asymptomatic HIV-1 seropositive homosexual men. *Journal of Psychosomatic Research, 36*, 535–650.

Goodman, G., & Dooley, D. (1976). A framework for help-intended communication. Psychotherapy: *Theory, Research and Practice, 13,* 106–117.

Goodwin, J.S., Hunt, W.C., Key, C.R., & Samet, J.M. (1987). The effect of marital status on stage, treatment, and survival of cancer patients. *Journal of the American Medical Association, 258*, 3125–3130.

Gotham, A.M., Brown, R.G., Marsden, C.D. (1986). Depression in Parkinson's disease: a quantitiative and qualitiative analysis. *Journal of Neorlogy, Neurosurgery and Psychiatry, 49*, 381–389.

Gough, J.G. (1967). Nonintellectual factors in the selection and evaluation of medical students. *Journal of Medical Education, 42*, 642–650.

Gould, D. Weiss, M., & Weinberg, R. (1981). The effects of model similarity and model task on self-efficacy and muscular endurance. *Journal of Sport Psychology, 3*, 17–29.

Gould, D., & Damarjian, N. (1996). Imagery training for peak performance. In J.L. Van Raaalte and B.W. Brewer (Eds.), *Exploring sport and exercise psychology* (pp. 25–50). Washington, D.C.: American Psychological Association.

Graham, N.M.H., Douglas, R.M., & Ryan, P. (1986). Stress and acute respiratory infection. *American Journal of Epidemiology, 124*, 389–401.

Grams, G.D., Herbert, C., Heffernan, C., Calam, B., Wilson, M.A., Grzybowski, S., & Brown, D. (1996). Haida perspectives on living with non-insulin-dependent diabetes. *Canadian Medical Association Journal, 155*, 1563–1568.

Gray, R.E., Fitch, M., Davis, C., & Phillips, C. (1997). Interviews with men with prostate cancer about their self-help group experiences. *Journal of Palliative Care, 13,* 15–21.

Green, E.E., Green, A.M., & Walters, E.D. (1972). Biofeedback for mind-body self-regulation: Healing and creativity. *Fields...Within Fields, 5*, n131–144.

Green, L., & Kreuter, M. (1991). *Health promotion planning: An educational and environmental approach.* Mountain View, CA: Mayfield Publishing.

Greenberg, J. (1978). The Americanization of Roseto. *Science News, 113*, 378–382.

Greenberg, J.S., & Pargman, D. (1989). *Physical fitness: A wellness approach*. Englewood Cliffs, New Jersey.

Greenfield, S. Kaplan, S.H., Ware, J.E., Jr., Yano, E.M., & Frank, H.J.L. (1988). Patient's participation in medical care: Effects on blood sugar control and quality of life in diabetes. *Journal of General Internal Medicine, 3*, 448–457.

Greenglass, E.R., & Burke, R.J. (1997). Hospital restructuring, anger and hostility in nurses. Paper presented at the Fifth European Congress of Psychology, July, 1997, Dublin, Ireland.

Greenglass, E.R., & Burke, R.J. (1999). Hospital restructuring and work-family conflict in nurses. Paper presented at the Fourth Interdisciplinary conference on occupational stress and health. Work, Stress and Health '99: Organization of Work in a Global Economy, March, 1999, Baltimore, Maryland.

Greenwald, A.G. (1968). Cognitive learning, cognitive response to persuasion, and attitude change. In Greenwald, A.G., Brock, T.C., & OstroM, T.M. (Eds.), *Psychological foundations of attitudes* (pp. 147–170). San Diego, CA: Academic Press.

Greenwood, J. (1998). Meeting the needs of patients' relatives. *Professional Nurse, 14*, 156–158.

Greer, S. (1991). Psychological response to cancer and survival. *Psychosomatic Medicine, 21*, 43–49.

Greer, S., & Moorey, S. (1997). Adjuvant psychological therapy for cancer patients. *Palliative Medicine, 11*, 240–244.

Gregoire, I., Kalogeropoulos, D., & Corcos, J. (1997). The effectiveness of a professionally led support group for men with prostate cancer. *Urological Nursing, 17*, 58–66.

Greist, J.H. (1984). Exercise in the treatment of depression. Coping with mental stress: The potential and limits of exercise intervention. Washington, DC: National Institute of Mental Health.

Griffin, M.J., Brennan, L., & McShane, A.J. (1998). Preoperative education and outcome of patient controlled analgesia. *Canadian Journal of Anaesthiology, 45*, 943–948.

Grinspoon, L., & Bakalar, J.B. (1995). Marijuana as medicine: A plea for reconsideration. *Journal of the American Medical Association, 273*, 1875–1876.

Gross, E.B. (1998). Gender differences in physician strss: Why the discrepant findings? *Women and Health, 26(3)*, 1–14.

Grossarth-Maticek, R., Eysenck, H.J., & Boyle, G.J. (1994). An empirical study of the diathesis-stress theory of disease. *International Journal of Stress Management, 1*, 3–18.

Grossarth-Maticek, R., Eysenck, H.J., & Vetter, H. (1988). Personality type, smoking habit, and their interaction on predictors of cancer and coronary heart disease. *Personality and Individual Differences, 9*, 479–495.

Grunau, R V.E. & Craig, K.D. (1987). Pain expression in neonates: Facial action and cry. *Pain, 28*, 395–410.

Gureje, O., Von Korff, M., Simon, G.E., & Gater, R. (1996). Persistent pain and well-being: A world Health Organization study in primary care. *Journal of the American Medical Association, 280*, 147–151.

Health Organization study in primary care. *Journal of the American Medical Association, 280*, 147–151.

Haan, N. (1993). The assessment of coping, defense, and stress. In L. Goldberger & S. Breznitz (Eds.) *Handbook of stress: Theoretical and clinical aspects* (2nd ed., pp 258–273). New York: Free Press.

Hadjistavropoulos, H.D., Craig, K.D., Grunau, R.E., & Johnston, C.C. (1994). Judging pain in newborns: Facial and cry determinants. *Journal of Pediatric Psychology, 19*, 485–491.

Hadjistavropoulos, H.D., Craig, K.D., Grunau, R.E., & Whitfield, M.F. (1997). Judging pain in infants: Behavioural, contextual, and developmental determinants. *Pain, 73*, 319–324.

Hadjistavropoulos, T. (1999). Chronic pain on trial: The influence of litigation and compensation on chronic pain syndromes. In A.R. Block, E.G. Kremer, & E. Fernandez (Eds.), *Handbook of pain syndromes* (pp. 59–76). Mahwah, NJ: Erlbaum.

Hadlow, J., & Pitts, M. (1991). The understanding of common terms by doctors, nurses and patients. *Social Science and Medicine, 32*, 193–196.

Hale, J.L., & Dillard, J.P. (1995). Fear appeals in health promotion campaigns: Too much, too little, or just right? In Maibach, E., & Parrott, R.L. (Eds.), *Designing health messages: Approaches from communication theory and public health practice*. Thousand Oaks, CA: Sage.

Halfens, R.G. (1995). Effect of hospital stay on health locus-of-control beliefs. Western *Journal of Nursing Research, 17*, 156–167.

Hall, R.A., Rappaport, M., Hopkins, H.K., & Griffin, R. (1973). Tobacco and evoked potential. *Science, 180*, 212–214.

Hall, S., & Smith, A. (1996). Investigation of the effects and aftereffects of naturally occurring upper respiratory tract illness on mood and performance. *Physiology and Behavior, 59*, 569–577.

Hamm, R.M., & Smith, S.L. (1998). The accuracy of patients' judgments of disease probability and test sensitivity and specificity. *Journal of Family Practice, 47*, 44–52.

Haney, C., Banks, C., & Zimbardo, P. (1973). Interpersonal dynamics in a simulated prison. *International Journal of Criminology and Penology, 1*, 69–97.

Hansen, R.G. (1986). The joy of stress. Fairway, Kansas: Andrews, McMeel and Parker.

Hansen, W.B., Graham, J.W., Sobel, J.L., Shelton, D.R., Flay, B.R., & Johnson, C.A. (1987). The consistency of peer and parent influences on tobacco, alcohol, and marijuana use among young adolescents. *Journal of Behavioral Medicine, 10*, 559–579.

Hardy, L., Jones, G., Gould, D. (1996). *Understanding psychological preparation for sport: Theory and practice of elite performers*. Chichester, England: John Wiley and Sons.

Hare, B.D., & Milano, R.A. (1985). Chronic pain: Perspectives on physical assessment and treatment. *Annals of Behavioral Medicine, 7(3)*, 6–10.

Harper, D.C. (1999). Presidential address: Social psychology of difference: Stigma, spread, and stereotypes in childhood. *Rehabilitation Psychology, 44*, 131–144.

Harris, J.C. (1995). *Developmental neuropsychiatry: Volume II Assessment, diagnosis and treatment of development disorders.* New York: Oxford University Press.

Harris, L.M., Robinson, J., & Menzies, R.G. (1999). Evidence for fear of restriction and fear of suffocation as components of claustrophobia. *Behaviour Research and Therapy, 37*, 155–159.

Harrison, A. (1999). All change? *British Medical Journal, 319*, 793.

Harrison, D., & Chick, J. (1994). Trends in alcoholism among make doctors in Scotland. *Addiction, 89,* 1613–1617.

Hart, I., & Poole, G.D. (1995). Individualism and collectivism and considerations in cross-cultural health research. *Journal of Social Psychology, 135*, 97–99.

Hasegawa, M., Hattori, S., Ishizaki, K., Suzuki, S., & Goto, F. (1996). The McGill Pain Questionnaire, Japanese version, reconsidered: Confirming the reliability and validity. *Pain Research and Management, 1(4)*, 233–237.

Haskell, W.L., Alderman, E.L., Fair, J.M., et al. (1994). Effects of intensive multiple risk factor reduction on coronary atherosclerosis and clinical cardiac events in men and women with coronary artery disease: The Stanford Coronary Risk Intervention Project (SCRIPT). *Circulation, 89*, 975–990.

Haug, M.R., & Lavin, B. (1981). Practitioner or patient—Who's in charge? *Journal of Health and Social Behavior, 22*, 212–229.

Haug, M.R., Musil, C.M., Warner, C.D., & Morris, D.L. (1997). Elderly persons' interpretation of a bodily change as an illness symptom. *Journal of Aging Research, 9*, 529–552.

Haupt, E., Herrmann, R., Benecke-Timp, A., Vogel, H., Haupt, A., & Walter, C. (1996). The KID Study II: Socioeconomic baseline characteristics, psycho-social strain, standard of current medical care education of the Federal Insurance for Salaried Employees' Institution (BfA) diabetic patients in inpatient rehabilitation. Kissingen Diabetes Intervention Study. *Experimental Clinics in Endocrinology and Diabetes, 104,* 378–386.

Hayes, M.V. (1996a). Editorial. *Health & Place, 2*, iii-v.

Hayes, M.V. (1996c). Foreword. *Social Science and Medicine, 42*, 787.

Hayes, M.V. (1996c). Introduction. *Social Science and Medicine, 42*, 789–790.

Haynes, R.B. (1976). A critical review of the "determinants" of patient compliance with therapeutic regimens. In D.L. Sackett & R.B. Haynes (Eds.), *Compliance with therapeutic regimens*. Baltimore: Johns Hopkins University Press.

Haynes, R.B., McKibbon, K.A., & Kanani, R. (1996). Systematic review of randomized trials of interventions to assist patients to follow prescriptions for medications. *Lancet, 348*, 383–386.

Haynes, S.G., Feinleib, M., & Kannel, W.B. (1980). The relationship of psychosocial factors to coronary heart disease in the Framingham Study: I. Methods and risk factors. *American Journal of Epidemiology, 107*, 362–383.

Hays, K. (1999). *Working it out: Using exercise in psychotherapy*. Washington, D.C: American Psychological Association.

Health Canada (1999). *Toward a healthy future: Second report on the health of Canadians.* Ottawa: Health Canada Publications.

Health Canada. (1995). *Horizon three: Young Canadians' alcohol and other drug use: Increasing our understanding.* Hewitt, D., Vinje, G., & MacNeil, P. (Eds.). Catalogue no. H39–307/3–1996E.

Health Canada. (1996). *Aids in Canada: Annual report on AIDS in Canada*. Division of HIV/AIDS Surveillance.

Health Canada. (1997). *AIDS and Aboriginal People: National AIDS Strategy, Phase II.* National AIDS Clearinghouse, Ottawa, Canada.

Hearn, J., & Higginson, T.J. (1998). Do specialist palliative care teams improve outcomes for cancer patients? A systematic literature review. *Palliative Medicine, 12*, 317–332.

Helgeson, V.S. (1992). Moderators of the relation between perceived control and adjustment to chronic illness. *Journal of*

Personality and Social Psychology, 63, 656–666.

Helweg-Larsen, M., & Collins, B.E. (1997). A social psychological perspective on the role of knowledge about AIDS in AIDS prevention. *Current Directions in Psychological Science, 6*, 23–26.

Henbest, R.J., & Fehrsen, G.S. (1992). Patient-centredness: Is it applicable outside the west? Its measurement and effect on outcomes. *Family Practice, 9*, 311–317.

Hendler, N.H., & Kozikowski, J.G. (1993). Overlooked physical diagnoses in chronic pain patients involved in litigation. *Psychosomtics, 34*, 494–501.

Hendricks, L.E., & Hendricks, R.T. (1998). Greatest fears of type 1 and type 2 patients about having diabetes: Implications for diabetes educators. *Diabetes Education, 24*, 168–173.

Henningfield, J.E., Cohen, C., & Pickworth, W.B. (1993). Psychopharmacology of nicotine. In C.T. Orleans & J. Slade (Eds.), *Nicotine addiction: Principles and management*. New York: Oxford University Press.

Henry, J.P., & Stephens, P.M. (1979). An animal model of neuropsychological factors in hypertension. In Y. Yamori, W. Lovenberg, W. Freis (Eds.), *Prophylactic approaches to hypertensive diseases* (pp. 299–307). New York: Raven.

Henthorne, T.L., LaTour, M.S., & Nataraajan, R. (1993). Fear appeals in print advertising: An analysis of arousal and ad response. *Journal of Advertising, 22*, 59–69.

Herbert, T.B., & Cohen, S. (1993). Stress and immunity in humans: A meta-analytic review. *Psychosomatic Medicine, 55*, 364–379.

Herbert, T.B., Cohen, S., Marsland, A.L., Bachen, E.A., Rabin, B.S., et al. (1994). Cardiovascular reactivity and the course of immune response to an acute psychological stressor. *Psychosomatic Medicine, 56*, 337–344.

Herrmann, C.K., Brand-Driehorst, S., Kaminsky, B., Leibing, E., Staats, H., & Rüger, U. (1998). Diagnostic groups and depressed mood as predictors of 22-month mortality in medical inpatients. *Psychosomatic Medicine, 60*, 570–577.

Hewson-Bower, B., & Drummond, P.D. (1996). Secretory immunoglobulin A increases during relaxation in children with and without recurrent upper respiratory tract infections. *Journal of Developmental and Behavioral Pediatrics, 17*, 311–316.

Hickson, G.B., Clayton, E.W., Entmman, S.S., Miller, C.S., et al. (1994). Obstetricians' prior malpractice experience and patients' satisfaction with care. *Journal of the American Medical Association, 272*, 1583–1587.

Hickson, G.B., Clayton, E.W., Githens, P.B., & Sloan, F.A. (1992). Factors that prompted families to file medical malpractice claims following perinatal injuries. *Journal of the American Medical Association, 267*, 1359–1363.

Hilgard, E.R., & Hilgard, J.R. (1975). *Hypnosis in the relief of pain*. Los Altos, CA: Kaufman.

Hill, A.J., Boudreau, F., Amyot, E., Dery, D., & Godin, G. (1997). Predicting the stages of smoking acquisition according to the theory of planned behavior. *Journal of Adolescent Health, 21*, 107–115.

Hill, C.E. Continuities and differences in the old and the new applied medical anthropology. In Hill, C.E. (Ed.), *Training manual in applied medical anthropology*. (pp. 14–22). Washington, D.C.: American Anthropological Association.

Hillhouse, J.J., Adler, C.M., Drinnon, J. & Turrisi, R. (1997). Applications of Ajzen's theory of planned behavior to predict sunbathing, tanning salon use, and sunscreen use intentions and behaviors. *Journal of Behavioral Medicine, 20*, 365–378.

Hinds, P.S., Sanders, C.B., Srivastava, D.K., Hickey, S., Jayawardene, D., Milligan, M., Olson, M.S., Puckett, P., Quargnenti, A., Randall, E.A., & Tye, V. (1998). Testing the stress-response sequence model in paediatric oncology nursing. *Journal of Advanced Nursing, 28*, 1146–1157.

Hirai, T. (1974). *The Psychophysiology of Zen*. Tokyo: Igaku Shoin Ltd.

Hislop, T.G., Waxler, N.E., Coldman, A.J., Elwood, J.M., & Kan, L. (1987). The prognostic significance of psychosocial factors in women with breast cancer. *Journal of Chronic Disease, 40*, 729–735.

Hobbs, N. & Perrin, J. (1985). *Issues in the care of children with chronic illness*. London: Jossey-Bass.

Hochstrasser, B., & Angst, J. (1996). The Zurich Study: XXII. Epidemiology of gastrointestinal complaints and comorbidity with anxiety and depression. *European Archives of Psychiatry and Clinical Neuroscience, 246*, 261–272.

Hoey, J. (1998). The arrogance of science and the pitfalls of hope. *Canadian Medical*

Association Journal, 159, 803–804.

Holland, C.K. (1993). An ethnographic study of nursing culture as an exploration for determining the existence of a system of ritual. *Journal of Advances in Nursing, 18*, 1461–1470.

Holland, J.C., Romano, S.J., Heiligenstein, J.H., Tepner, R.G., & Wilson, M.G. (1998). A controlled trial of fluoxetine and desipramine in depressed women with advanced cancer. *Psychooncology, 7*, 291–300.

Holmes, D.S. (1981). The use of biofeedback for treating patients with migraine headaches, Raynaud's disease, and hypertension: A critical evaluation. In C.K. Prokop & L.A. Bradley (Eds.), *Medical psychology: Contributions to behavioral medicine* (pp. 423–441). New York: Academic Press.

Holtgrewe, H.L. (1990). American Urological Association Survey of Transurethral Prostatectomy and the impact of changing medicare reimbursement. *Urologic Clinics of North America, 17*, 587–593.

Homo-Delarche, F., Fitzpatrick, F., Christeff, N., Nunez, E.A., Bach, J.F., & Dardenne, M. (1991). Sex steroids, glucocorticoids, stress and autoimmunity. *Journal of Steroid Biochemistry and Molecular Biology, 40*, 619–637.

Hope, A., Kelleher, C.C., & O'Connor, M. (1998). Lifestyle practices and the health promotion environment of hospital nurses. *Journal of Advanced Nursing, 28*, 438–447.

Hopkins, E.J., Pye, A.M., Solomon, M., & Solomon, S. (1967). A study of patient choice of doctor in an urban area. Journal of the Royal College of the General *Practitioners, 6*, 282.

Hornberger, J., Thom, D., & MacCurdy, T. (1997). Effects of a self-administered previsit questionnaire to enhance awareness of patients' concerns in primary care. *Journal of General Internal Medicine, 12*, 597–606.

Horwitz, R.I., Viscoli, C.M., Berkman, L., Donaldson, R.M., et al. (1990). Treatment adherence and risk of death after myocardial infarction. *Lancet, 336*, 5420–545.

Hoskins, C.N., Baker, S., Sherman, D., & Bohlander, J. (1996). Social support and patterns of adjustment to breast cancer. *Scholarly Inquiry For Nursing Practice, 10*, 99–123.

House, J.S. (1981). *Work stress and social support. Reading*, MA: Addison-Wesley.

House, J.S., Landis, K.R., & Umberson, D. (1988). *Social relationships and health. Science, 241*, 540–545.

Hovland, C.I., Janis, I.L., & Kelley, H.H. (1953). *Communication and persuasion: Psychological studies of opinion change*. New Haven, CT: Yale University Press.

Howard, G., Wagenknecht, L.E., Burk, G.L., Diez-Roux, A., et al. (1998). Cigarette smoking and progression of atherosclerosis: The Atherosclerosis Risk in Communities (ARIC) Study. *Journal of the American Medical Society, 279*, 119–124.

Howard, V.A. & Thurber. (1998). The interpretation of infant pain: Physiological and behavioral indicators. *Pediatric Nursing, 13(3)*, 164–174.

Howie, J.G., Porter, A.M., Heaney, D.J., & Hopton, J.L. (1991). Long to short consultation ratio: A proxy measure of quality of care for general practice. *British Journal of General Practice, 41(343)*, 48–54.

Hull, J.G. (1981). A self-awareness model of the causes and effects of alcohol consumption. *Journal of Abnormal Psychology, 90*, 586–560.

Hull, J.G. (1987). Self-awareness model. In H.T. Blane & K.E. Leonard (Eds.) *Psychological theories of drinking and alcoholism* (pp. 272–304). New York: Guilford Press.

Hull, J.G., & Bond, C.F. (1986). Social and behavioral consequences of alcohol consumption and expectancy: A meta-analysis. *Psychological Bulletin, 99*, 347–360.

Hunt, L.M., & Mattingly, C. (1998). Diverse rationalities and multiple realities in illness and healing. *Medical Anthropology Quarterly, 12*, 267–272.

Hunter, M. & Philips, C. (1981). The experience of headache: An assessment of the qualities of tension headache pain. *Pain, 10*, 209–219.

Hurley, A.D., Tomasulo, D.J. & Pfadt, A.G. (1998). Individual and group psychotherapy approaches for persons with mental retardation and developmental disabilities. *Journal of Developmental and Physical Disabilities, 10*, 365–386.

Ikard, F.F., & Tomkins, S. (1973). The experience of affect as a determinant of smoking behavior: A series of validity studies. *Journal of Abnormal Psychology, 81*, 172–181.

Ilacqua, G.E. (1994). Migraine headaches: Coping efficacy of guided imagery training. *Headache, 34*, 99–102.

Imrie, D.D. (1994). "Client" versus "patient"

[letter]. *Canadian Medical Association Journal, 150*, 123.

Irwin, M., Daniels, M., Smith, T.L., Bloom, E., & Weiner, H. (1987). Impaired natural killer cell activity during bereavement. *Brain, Behavior, and Immunity, 1*, 98–104.

Iserson, K.V. (1999). Hypnosis for pediatric fracture reduction. *Journal of Emergency Medicine, 17(1)*, 53–56.

Iverson, G. (1998). Mild head trauma: Epidemic in nature. *Recovery, 9*, 4–7.

Iwai, K. (1996). 1: The self-image of muscular dystrophy inpatients and the psychological effects of their disease. *Japanese Journal of Special Education, 33(5)*, 1–6.

Jackson and Csikszentmihalyi. (1999). *Flow in Sports*. Champaign, Illinois: Human Kinetics.

Jackson, W. (1999). *Methods: Doing social research, 2nd ed.* Scarborough, Ontario: Prentice Hall Allyn and Bacon.

Jacobson, A.M., & Weinger, K. (1998). Treating depression in diabetic patients: Is there an alternative to medications? *Annals of Internal Medicine, 129*, 656–657.

Jacobson, E. (1938). *Progressive relaxation: A physiological and clinical investigation of muscle states and their significance in psychology and medical practice (2nd ed.).* Chicago: University of Chicago Press.

Jacobson, L.D., Wilkinson, C., & Owen, P.A. (1994). Is the potential of teenage consultations being missed? A study of consultation times in primary care. *Family Practice, 11*, 296–299.

Jacobson, P.D., Bovbjerg, D.H., Schwartz, M.D., Hudis, C.A., Gilewski, T.A., & Norton, L. (1995). Conditioned emotional distress in women receiving chemotherapy for breast cancer. *Journal of Consulting and Clinical Psychology, 63*, 108–114.

JAMA. (1998). NIH Consensus Conference. Acupuncture. *Journal of the American Medical Association, 280(17)*, 1518–1524.

Jamison, K.R., Wellish, D.K., & Pasnau, R.O. (1978). Psychosocial aspects of mastectomy. I. The women's perspective. *American Journal of Psychiatry, 136*, 432–436.

Jamsa, K., & Jamsa, T. (1998). Technology in neonatal intensive care—a study on parents' experiences. *Technology and Health Care, 6*, 225–230.

Janis, I.L. (1983). Improving adherence to medical recommendations: Prescriptive hypotheses derived from recent research in social psychology. In A. Baum, S.E. Taylore, J. Singer (Eds.) *Handbook of psychology and health* (Vol. 4, pp. 113–148). Hillsdale, NJ: Erlbaum.

Jarvik, M.E. (1973). Further observations on nicotine as the reinforcing agent in smoking. In W.L. Dunn, Jr. (Ed.), *Smoking behavior: Motives and incentives* (pp. 33–50). Washington, DC: Winston.

Jasnoski, M.L., Holmes, D.S., Soloman, S., & Aguiar, C. (1981). Exercise, changes in aerobic capacity and changes in self-perception: An experimental investigation. *Journal of Research in Personality, 15,* 460–466.

Jasnowski, M.L., Holmes, D.S., & Banks, D.L. (1988). Changes in personality associated with changes in aerobic and anaerobic fitness in women and men. *Journal of Psychosomatic Research, 32*, 273–276.

Jed, E. (1999). Reflections on the NICU. A mother's perspective. *American Journal of Nursing, 99(3)*, 22.

Jellinek, E.M. (1960). *The disease concept of alcoholism*. New Haven, CT: College and University Press.

Jemmott, J.B. III, & Maglore, K. (1988). Academic stress, social support, and secretory Immunoglobulin A. *Journal of Personality and Social Psychology, 55*, 803–810.

Jemmott, JB III, Borysenko, M., Chapman, R., et al., (1983). Academic stress, power motivation, and decrease in secretion rate of salivary secretory Immunoglobulin A. *Lancet*, 1400–1402.

Jenkins, C., Carmody, T.J., & Rush, A.J. (1998). Depression in radiation oncology patients: A preliminary evaluation. *Journal of Affective Disorders, 50*, 17–21.

Jenkins, C.D. (1996). Where there's hope, there's life. Psychosomatic Medicine, 58, 122–124.

Jenner, B. It was too easy. Sport, 63. 67–78.

Jensen, M.P., & McFarland, C.A. (1993). Increasing the reliability and validity of pain intensity measurement in chronic pain patients. *Pain, 55*, 195–203.

Jensen, M.P., Turner, J.A., Romano, J.M., & Strom, S.E. (1995). The Chronic Pain Coping Inventory: Development and preliminary validation. *Pain, 60,* 203–216.

Jensen, T.S., Krebs, B., Nielsen, J. & Rasmussen, P. (1985). Immediate and long-term phantom limb pain in amputees; incidence, clinical characteristics and relationship to preamputation limb pain. *Pain, 21,* 267–278.

Johnson, B.G. (1984). Biofeedback, transcutaneous electrical nerve stimulation, acupuncture, and hypnosis. In G.K. Riggs & E.P. Gall (Eds.), *Rheumatic diseases: Rehabilitation and management*. Boston: Butterworth.

Johnson, C.G., Levenkron, J.C., Suchman, A.L., & Manchester, R. (1988). Does physician uncertainty affect patient satisfaction? *Journal of General Internal Medicine, 3*, 144–149.

Johnson, J.L. (1991). Learning to live again: The process of adjustment following a heart attack. In J.M. Morse & J.L. Johnson (Eds.), *The illness experience: Dimensions of suffering* (pp. 13–87). Newbury Park: Sage.

Johnson, M., & Vögele, C. (1993). Benefits of psychological preparation for surgery: A meta-analysis. *Annals of Behavioral Medicine, 15*, 245–256.

Johnson, S.B. (1985). The family and the child with chronic illness. In D.C. Turk & R.D. Kerns (Eds.), *Health, illness, and families: A life-span perspective* (pp. 220–254). New York: Wiley.

Jolly, A.M., Orr, P.H., Hammond, G., & Young, T.K. (1995). Risk factors for infection in women undergoing testing for Chlamydia trachomatis and Neisseria gonorrhoeae in Manitoba, Canada. *Sexually Transmitted Diseases, 22*, 289–295.

Jonasson, G., Carlsen, K.H., Sodal, A., Jonasson, C., & Mowinckel, P. (1999). Patient compliance in a clinical trial with inhaled budesonide in children with mild asthma. *European Respiratory Journal, 14*, 150–154.

Jones, K.S., & Rollman, G.B. (1999, October). Gender-related differences in response to experimentally-induced pain. Poster session presented at the annual meeting of the American Pain Society, Fort Lauderdale, FL.

Jones, S. (1996). Demographic distributions of literacy in Canada. In *Reading the future: A portrait of literacy in Canada.* Ottawa: Ministry of Industry.

Jorenby, D.E., Leischow, S.J., Nides, M.A., Rennard, S.I., et al. (1999). A controlled trial of sustained-release bupropion, a nicotine patch, or both for smoking cessation. *New England Journal of Medicine, 340*, 685–691.

Joyce, C.R.B., Zutshi, D.W., Hrubes, V., & Mason, R.M. (1975). Comparison of fixed interval and visual analogue scales for rating chronic pain. *European Journal of Clinical Pharmacology, 8*, 415–420.

Kabat-Zinn, J. (1993). Mindfulness meditation: Health benefits of an ancient Buddhist practice. In D. Goleman & J. Gurin (eds.), *Mind/body medicine: How to use your mind for better health* (pp. 259–275). Yonkers, NY: Consumer Reports Books.

Kaegi, E. (1998a). Unconventional therapies for cancer: 2. Green tea. Task Force on Alternative Therapies of the Canadian Breast Cancer Research Initiative. *Canadian Medical Association Journal, 158*, 1033–1035.

Kaegi, E. (1998b). Unconventional therapies for cancer: 3. Iscador. Task Force on Alternative Therapies of the Canadian Breast Cancer Research Initiative. *Canadian Medical Association Journal, 158*, 1157–1159.

Kaegi, E. (1998c). Unconventional therapies for cancer: 5. Vitamins A, C and E. Task Force on Alternative Therapies of the Canadian Breast Cancer Research Initiative. *Canadian Medical Association Journal, 158*, 1483–1488.

Kaegi, E. (1998d). Unconventional therapies for cancer: 6. 714-X Task Force on Alternative Therapies of the Canadian Breast Cancer Research Initiative. *Canadian Medical Association Journal, 158*, 1621–1624.

Kaegi, E. (1998e). A patient's guide to choosing unconventional therapies. *Canadian Medical Association Journal, 158*, 1161–1165.

Kahn, H.A. (1963). The relationship of reported coronary heart disease mortality to physical activity of work. *American Journal of Public Health, 53*, 1058–1067.

Kahneman, D. & Miller, D.T. (1986). Norm theory: Comparing reality to its alternatives. *Psychological Review, 80*, 136–153.

Kahneman, D., & Tversky, A. (1973). On the psychology of prediction, P*sychological Review, 80*, 237–251.

Kaler, S.R., Levy, D.A., & Schall, M. (1989). Sterotypes of professional roles. IMAGE: *Journal of Nursing Scholarship, 21(2)*, 85–89.

Kalisch, P.A., & Kalisch, B.J. (1987). *The changing image of the nurse*. Menlo Park, CA: Addison-Wesley.

Kanner, R. (1986). Pain management. *Journal of the American Medical Association, 256,* 2110–2114.

Kaplan, R.M. (1990). Behavior as the central outcome in health care. *American Psychologist, 45*, 1211–1220.

Kaplan, R.M., Sallis, J.F. and Patterson, T.L. (1993). *Health and human behavior.* New York: McGraw-Hill.

Kaplan, S.H., Gandek, B., Greenfield, S., Rogers, W. & Ware, J.E. (1995). Patient and visit characteristics related to physicians' participatory decision-making style: Results from the Medical Outcomes Study. *Medical Care, 33*, 1176–1187.

Kaps, E.C. (1994). The role of the support group, "Us Too". *Cancer, 74*, 2188–2189.

Karasek, R. (1979). Job demands, job decision latitude, and mental strain: Implications for job design. *Administrative Science Quarterly, 24*, 285–310.

Karoly, P. (1985). The assessment of pain: Concepts and procedures. In P. Karoly (Ed.), *Measurement strategies in health psychology*. New York: Wiley.

Karoly, P., & Ruehlman, L.S. (1996). Motivational implications of pain: Chronicity, psychological distress, and work global construal in a national sample of adults. *Health Psychology, 15*, 383–390.

Kasamatsu, A., & Hirai, T. (1966). An electroencephalographic study on the zen meditation (Zazen). Folia psychiatrica et neurological *Japonica, 20*, 315–336.

Kasamatsu, A., & Hirai, T. (1963). Science of Zazen. *Psychologia, 6,* 86–91.

Kashani, J., & Hakami, N. (1982). Depression in children and adolescents with malignancy. *Canadian Journal of Psychiatry, 27*, 474–477.

Kasl, S.V. (1975). Issues in patient adherence to health care regimens. *Journal of Human Stress, 1(3)*, 5–17.

Katz, J., Wowk, A., Culp, D., & Wakeling, H. (1999). A randomized, controlled study of the pain- and tension-reducing effects of 15 minute workplace massage treatments versus seated rest for nurses in a large teaching hospital. *Pain Research and Management, 4(2)*, 81–88.

Katz, R.C., Meyers, K., & Walls, J. (1995). Cancer awareness and self-examination practices in young men and women. *Journal of Behavioral Medicine, 18*, 377–384.

Katz, R.C., Wilson, L., & Frazer, N. (1994). Anxiety and its determinants in patients undergoing magnetic resonance imaging. *Journal of Behavior Therapy and Experimental Psychiatry, 25*, 131–134.

Kaufman, D.M., & Mann, K.V. (1998). Comparing achievement on the medical Council of Canada Qualifying Examination Part I of students in conventional and problem-based learning curricula. *Academic Medicine, 73*, 1211–1213.

Kavussanu, M. and McAuley, E. (1996). Exercise and optimism: Are highly active individuals more optimistic? *Journal of Sport and Exercise Psychology, 18*, 264–280.

Kawachi, I., Colditz, G.A., Stampfer, M.J., Willett, W.C., et al. (1993). Smoking cessation and decreased risk of stroke in women. *Journal of the American Medical Association, 269*, 232–236.

Keefe, F.J., & Block, A.R. (1982). Development of an observation method for assessing pain behavior in chronic low back pain patients. *Behavior Therapy, 13*, 363–375.

Kelly, B., Raphael, B., Judd, F., Perdices, M., Kernutt, G., Burnett, P., Dunne, M., & Burrows, G. (1998). Posttraumatic stress disorder in response to HIV infection. *General Hospital Psychiatry, 20,* 345–352.

Kelly, J.A. (1998). Group psychotherapy for persons with HIV and AIDS-related illnesses. *International Journal of Group Psychotherapy, 48*, 143–162.

Kemeny, M.E. (1994). Stressful events, psychological responses, and progression of HIV infection. In R. Glaser & J. Kiecolt-Glaser (Eds.), *Handbook of human stress and immunity* (pp. 245–266). New York: Academic Press.

Kendall, C., & Hailey, B.J. (1993). The relative effectiveness of three reminder letters on making and keeping mammogram appointments. *Behavioral Medicine, 19*, 29–34.

Kendler, K.S., Kessler, R.C., Heath, A.C., Neale, M.C., & Eaves, L.J. (1991). Coping: A genetic epidemiological investigation. *Psychological Medicine, 21*, 337–346.

Kent, H. (1997). Ignore growing patient interest in alternative medicine at your peril, MDs warned. *Canadian Medical Association Journal, 157*, 1427–1428.

Kerepcic, I., Jakovljevic, M., Ljubicic, D., Novy-Radonic, E., & Jurin, M. (1995). Psychoneuroimmunology of schizophrenia and depression. *Psychiatria Danubina, 7*, 105–112.

Kerns, R.D., Turk, D.C., & Rudy, T.E. (1985). The West Haven-Yale Multidimensional Pain Inventory. *Pain, 23*, 345–356.

Kerssens, J.J., Bensing, J.M., & Andela, M.G. (1997). Patient preference for genders of health professionals. *Social Science and Medicine, 44,* 1531–1540.

Kessler, M., Kronstorfer, R., & Traue, H.C. (1996). Depressive symptoms and disability in acute and chronic back pain patients. *International Journal of Behavioral Medicine, 3*, 91–104,

Kiecolt-Glaser, J.K., & Glaser, R. (1995). Psychoneuroimmunology and health consequences: Data and shared mechanisms. *Psychosomatic Medicine, 57*, 269–274.

Kiecolt-Glaser, J.K., Cacioppo, J.T., Malarkey, W.B., & Glaser, R. (1992). Acute psychological stressors and short-term immune changes: What, why, for whom, and to what extent? *Psychosomatic Medicine, 54*, 680–685.

Kiecolt-Glaser, J.K., Dura, J.R., Speicher, C.E., Trask, O.J., & Glaser, R.G. (1991). Spousal cargivers of dementia victims: Longitudinal changes in immunity and health. *Psychosomatic Medicine, 53*, 345–362.

Kiecolt-Glaser, J.K., Fisher, J.D., Ogrocki, P., Stout, J.C., Speicher, C.E., Glaser, R. (1987a). Marital quality, marital disruption, and immune function. *Psychosomatic Medicine, 49*, 13–34.

Kiecolt-Glaser, J.K., Garner, W., Speicher, C., Penn, G.M., Holliday, J., & Glaser, R. (1984). Psychosocial modifiers of immunocompetence in medical students. *Psychosomatic Medicine, 46*, 7–14.

Kiecolt-Glaser, J.K., Glaser, R., Cacioppo, J.T., & Malarkey, W.B. (1998). Marital stress: Immunologic, neuroendocrine, and autonomic correlates. *Annals of the New York Academy of Sciences, 840*, 656–663.

Kiecolt-Glaser, J.K., Glaser, R., Shuttleworth, E.C. Dyers, C.S., Ogroki, P., & Speicher, C.E. (1987b). Chronic stress and immunity in family caregivers of Alzheimer's disease victims. *Psychosomatic Medicine, 49*, 523–535.

Kiecolt-Glaser, J.K., Kennedy, S., Malkoff, S., Fisher, L., Speicher, C.E., & Glaser, R. (1988). Marital discord and immunity in males. *Psychosomatic Medicine, 50*, 213–229.

Kilborn, L.C., & Labbe, E.E. (1990). Magnetic resonance imaging scanning procedures: Development of phobic response during scan and at one-month follow-up. *Journal of Behavioral Medicine, 13*, 391–401.

Kindelan, K., & Kent, G. (1987). Concordance between patients' information preferences and general practitioners' perceptions. *Psychology and Health, 1*, 399–409.

King, A.J.C., Boyce, W.F., & King, M.A. (1999). Trends in the health of Canadian youth. Health Behaviors in School-Aged Children, a World Health Organization Cross-National Study. Canada: Health Canada.

King, K.M., & Teo, K.K. (1998). Cardiac rehabilitation referral and attendance: Not one and the same. *Rehabilitation Nursing, 23*, 246–251.

Kingston, G. (1999). Concussion leaves a gap in Long's memory. *Vancouver Sun*, October 18.

Kinsey, A.C., Pomeroy, W.B., & Martin, C.C. (1948). *Sexual behavior in the human male.* Philadelphia: Saunders.

Kinsey, A.C., Pomeroy, W.B., Martin, C.C., & Gebhard, P.H. (1953). *Sexual behavior in the human female*. Philadelphia: Saunders.

Kircaldy, B.D, & Shephard, R.J. (1990). Therapeutic implications of exercise. *International Journal of Sport Psychology, 21*, 165–184.

Kirkley, B.G., Schneider, J.A., Agras, W.J., Bachman, J.A. (1985). Comparison of two group treatments for bulimia. *Journal of Consulting and Clinical Psychology, 53*, 43–48.

Kirschenbaum, D. (1998). Using sport psychology interventions to improve health psychology outcomes. *The Health Psychologist, 20*, 16–23.

Kirschenbaum, D.S. (1997). *Mind matters: 7 Steps to smarter sport performance*. Carmel, Indiana: Cooper Publishing Group.

Kirschenbaum, K.S. (1997). Prevention of sedentary lifestyles: Rationale and methods. In W.P. Morgan (Ed.) *Physical activity and mental health* (pp.33–48). Washington, DC: Taylor and Francis.

Kitamura, A., Hiroyasu, I., Sankai, T., Naito, Y., et al. (1998). Alcohol intake and premature coronary heart disease in urban Japanese men. *American Journal of Epidemiology, 147*, 59–65.

Kivlahan, D.R., Marlatt, G.A., Fromme, K., Coppel, D.B., & Williams, E. (1990). Secondary prevention with college drinkers: Evaluation of an alcohol skills training program. *Journal of Consulting and Clinical Psychology, 58*, 805–810.

Kleinke, C.L., & Spangler, A.S. (1988). Psychometric analysis of the audiovisual taxonomy for assessing pain behavior in chronic back-pain patients. *Journal of Behavioral Medicine, 11*, 83–94.

Kleinman, A. (1980). *Patients and healers in the context of culture*. Berkeley, CA: University of California Press.

Klepp, K.I., Kelder, S.H., & Perry, C.L. (1995). Alcohol and marijuana use among adolescents: Long-term outcomes of the Class of 1989 Study. *Annals of Behavioral Medicine, 17*, 19–24U : D.

Klonoff, E.A., & Landrine, H. (1994). Culture and gender diversity in commonsense beliefs about the causes of six illnesses. *Journal of Behavioral Medicine, 17*, 407–418.

Knapp, P.H., levy, E.M., Giorgi, R.G., Black, P.H., Fox, B.H., & Heeren, T.C. (1992). Short-term immunological effects of induced emotion. *Psychosomatic Medicine, 54*, 133–148.

Knoerl, D.V., Faut-Callahan, M., Paice, J., & Shoot, S. (1999). Preoperative PCA teaching program to manage postoperative pain. *Medsurgical Nursing, 8*, 25–33,36.

Kohen, D., Burgess, A.P., Catalán, J., & Lant, A. (1998). The role of anxiety and depression in quality of life and symptom reporting in people with diabetes mellitus. *Quality of Life Research, 7*, 197–204.

Koltyn, K.F. & Vaughn, A.C. (1999, October) Pain responses in men and women exposed to three different noxious stimuli. Poster session presented at the annual meeting of the American Pain Society, Fort Lauderdale, FL.

Komproe, I.H., Rijken, M., Ros, W.J.G., Winnubst, J.A.M., & Harm't H. (1997). Available support and received support: Different effects under stressful circumstances. *Journal of Social and Personal Relationships, 14*, 59–77.

Kook, A.I., Mizruchin, A., Odnopozov, N., Gershon, H., et al. (1995). Depression and immunity. The biochemical interrelationship between the central nervous system and the immune system. *Biological Psychiatry, 37*, 817–819.

Korsch, B.M., Gozzi, E.K., & Francis, V. (1968). Gaps in doctor-patient communication. *Pediatrics, 42*, 855–871.

Kozlowski, L.T. (1979). Psychosocial influences on cigarette smoking. In Smoking and health: A report of the surgeon general. DHEW Publ. No. 79–40066. Washington, DC: GPA.

Kozlowski, L.T., Herman, C.P. (1984). The interaction of psychosocial and biological determinants of tobacco use: More on the boundary model. *Journal of Applied Social Psychology, 14*.

Krakowski, A.J. (1982). Stress and the practice of medicine: the myth and reality. *Journal of Psychosomatic Medicine, 26*, 91–98.

Krakowski, A.J. (1983). Stress and the practice of medicine: III. Physicians compared with lawyers. 7th World Congress of the International College of Psychosomatic medicine: Psychosomatic research and practice (1983, Hamburg, Germany).

Krakowski, A.J. (1985). Medicine and physicians: Rewards and burdens. *Psychiatria Fennica, 16*, 73–83.

Kramer, M. (1974). *Reality shock—Why nurses leave nursing.* St. Louis, MO: CV Mosby.

Krantz, D.S., & Deckel, A.W. (1983). Coping with cornary heart disease and stroke. In T.G. Burish & L.A. Bradley (Eds.), *Coping with chronic disease: Research and applications* (pp. 85–112). New York: Academic Press.

Krantz, D.S., Baum, A., & Wideman, M.V. (1980). Assessment for preferences for self-treatment and information in health care. *Journal of Personality and Social Psychology, 39*, 977–990.

Krantz, D.S., Grunberg, N.E., & Baum, A. (1985). Health psychology. *Annual Review of Psychology, 36*, 349–383.

Krause, J.S., Stanwyck, C.A., & Maides, J. (1998). Locus of control and life adjustment: Relationship among people with spinal cord injury. *Rehabilitation Counseling Bulletin, 4*, 162–172.

Krebs, B., Jensen, T.S., Kroner, K., Nielsen, J., & Jorgenssen, H.S. (1984). *Phantom limb phenomena in amputees 7 years after limb amputation. Pain (Suppl.), 2*, S85.

Krebs, L.U., Myers, J., Decker, G., Kinzler, J., Asfahani, P., & Jackson, J. (1996). The oncology nursing image: Lifting the mist. *Oncology Nursing Forum, 23*, 1297–1304.

Kreitler, H., & Kreitler, S. (1976). *Cognitive orientation and behavior.* Springer: New York.

Kremer, E., & Atkinson, S.H. (1981). Pain measurement: Construct validity of the affective dimension of the McGill pain questionnaire with chronic benign pain patients. *Pain, 11*, 93–100.

Kroner-Herwig, B., Jakle, C., Frettloh, J., Peters, K., et al. (1996). Predicting subjective disability in chronic pain patients. International *Journal of Behavioral Medicine, 3*, 30–41.

Krüger, S. McVey, G., & Kennedy, S.H. (1998). The changing profile of anorexia nervosa at the Toronto Programme for eating disorders. *Journal of Psychosomatic Research, 45*, 533–547.

Kübler-Ross, E. (1969). *On death and dying.* London: Macmillan.

Kuhl, J.P., Janal, M.N., Fletcher, D., Guastadisegni, P.E., & Clark, C. (1999, October). Cold pressor microchronography distinguishes pain-tolerant from pain-sensitive individuals, but not women from men.

Poster session presented at the annual meeting of the American Pain Society, Fort Lauderdale, FL.

Kulik, J.A., & Mahler, H.I.M. (1989). Social support and recovery from surgery. *Health Psychology, 8*, 221–238.

Kurtz, M.E., Kurtz, J.C., Given, C.W., & Given, B. (1995). Relationship of caregiver reactions and depression to cancer patients' symptoms, functional states and depression: A longitudinal view. *Social Science and Medicine, 40*, 837–846.

Kuttner, L. (1997). Mind body methods of pain management. Child and Adolescent *Psychiatric Clinics of North America, 6*, 783–796.

Kuuppelomäki, M., & Lauri, S. (1998). Cancer patients' reported experiences of suffering. *Cancer Nursing, 21*, 364–369.

La Greca, A.M., & Stone, W.L. (1985). Behavioral pediatrics. In N. Schneiderman & J.T. Tapp (Eds.), *Behavioral medicine: The biopsychosocial approach*. Hillsdale, NJ: Erlbaum.

La Via, M.F., Munno, I., Lydiard, R.B., Workman, E.W., Hubbard, J.R., Michel, Y., & Paulling, E. (1996). The influence of stress intrusion on immunodepression in generalized anxiety disorder patients and controls. *Psychosomatic Medicine, 58*, 138–142.

Labonte, R. (1987). Community health promotion strategies. *Health Promotion, 16*, 5–10, 32.

Labonte, R. (1990). Health promotion: From concepts to strategies. In Eikenberg, G. (Ed.), *The seeds of health: Promoting wellness in the '90s*. (pp. 129–146). Ottawa: Canadian College of Health Service Executives.

Laboratory Centre for Disease Control (LCDC) (1998). Diabetes.

Laboratory Centre for Disease Control, Bureau of HIV/AIDS and STD, Health Canada (May, 1997), Ottawa.

Laboratory Centre for Disease Control, Division of HIV/AIDS Surveillance, Bureau of HIV/AIDS and STD, Health Canada (May, 1997). *Epi update: HIV/AIDS epidemiology among Aboriginal people in Canada*. Ottawa: Health Canada. Ottawa.

Lack, D.Z. (1982). Women and pain: Another feminist issue. *Women Ther., 1*, 55–64.

Lacroix, J.M., Martin, B., Avendano, M., & Goldstein, R. (1991). Symptom schemata in chronic respiratory patients. *Health Psychology, 10*, 268–273.

Ladwig, K.H., Röll, G., Breithardt, G., & Borggrefe, M. (1999). Extracardiac contributions to chest pain perception in patients 6 months after acute myocardial infarction. *American Heart Journal, 137*, 528–534.

Ladwig, K.H., Schoefinius, A., Dammaun, G., Danner, R., Gurtler, R., & Herrmann, R. (1999). Long-acting psychotraumatic properties of a cardiac arrest experience. *American Journal of Psychiatry, 156*, 912–919.

Laforge, R.G., Greene, G.W., & Prochaska, J.O. (1994). Psychosocial factors influencing low fruit and vegetable consumption. *Journal of Behavioral Medicine, 17*, 361–374.

Laforge, R.G., Willey, C., Prochasska, J.O., & Levesque, D.A. (1995, March). Naturalistic evidence for a synergistic effect of nicotine patch with a stage matched smoking cessation intervention. Paper presented at the meeting of the Society of Behavioral Medicine, San Diego.

Laitinen, J. (1976). Acupuncture and transcutaneous electric stimulation in the treatment of chronic sacrolumbalgia and ischialgia. *American Journal of Chinese Medicine, 4*, 169–175.

Lalonde, M. (1974). *New perspectives on the health of Canadians.* Ottawa: Information Canada.

Lam, T.H., He, Y., Li, L.S., Li, L.S., et al. (1997). Mortality attributable to cigarette smoking in China. *Journal of the American Medical Association, 278*, 1505–1508.

Lambert, S.A. (1996). The effects of hypnosis/guided imagery on the postoperative course of children. *Journal of Developmental and Behavioral Pediatrics, 17*, 307–310.

Lamping, D.L., Abrahamowicz, M., Gilmore, N., Edgar, L., Grover, S.A., Tsoukas, C., Falutz, J., Lalonde, R., Hamel, M., & Darsigny, R. (1993, June). A randomized controlled trial to evaluate a psychosocial intervention to improve quality of life in HIV infection. Paper presented to the IX International Conference on AIDS, Berlin, Germany.

Landers, D.M., & Peruzzello, S.J. (1994). Physical activity, fitness, and anxiety. In C. Bouchard, R.J. Shephard, & T. Stephens (Eds.), *Physical activity, fitness, and health: International proceedings and consensus statement* (pp. 868–882). Champaign, Illinois: Human Kinetics.

LaPerriere, A., Fletcher, M.A., Antoni, M.H., et al. (1991). Aerobic exercise training in an

AIDS risk group. International *Journal of Sports Medicine, 12*, S53-S57.

Larocque, D. (1996). Absenteeism. *Canadian Nurse, 92(9)*, 42–46.

Larson, P.J., & Ferketich, S.L. (1993). Patients' satisfaction with nurses' caring during hospitalization. *Western Journal of Nursing Research, 15*, 690–707.

Larson, R., & Sutker, S. (1966). Value differences and value consensus by socioeconomic levels. *Social Forces, 44*, 563–569.

Larsson, U.S., Johanson, M., & Svardsudd, K. (1994). Sensitive patient-doctor communications relating to the breasts and prostate. *Journal of Cancer Education, 9*, 19–25.

Lau, R.R., Hartman, K.A., & Ware, J.E. Jr. (1986). Health as a value: Methodological and theoretical considerations. *Health Psychology, 5*, 25–43.

Lautenbacher, S., & Rollman, G.B. (1993). Sex differences in responsiveness to painful and non-painful stimuli are dependent upon the stimulation method. *Pain, 53*, 255–264.

Lauver, D. (1994). Care-seeking behavior with breast cancer symptoms in Caucasian and African-American women. *Research in Nursing Health, 17*, 421–431.

Lauver, D., Coyle, M., & Panchmatia, B. (1995). Women's reasons for and barriers to seeking care for breast cancer symptoms. *Women's Health Issues, 5*, 27–35.

Lauver, D., Nabholz, S., Scott, K., & Tak, Y. (1997). Testing theoretical explanations of mammography use. *Nursing Research, 46*, 32–39.

Lavie, CJ., Milani, R.V., Cassidy, M.M., & Gilliland, Y.E. (1999). Effects of cardiac rehabilitation and exercise training programs in women with depression, *American Journal of Cardiology, 83*, 1480–1483.

Lazarus, R.S., & Folkman, S. (1984). *Stress, appraisal, and coping*. New York: Springer.

Leathart, A. (1994). Communication and socialisation (1): An exploratory study and explanation for nurse-patient communication in ITU. *Intensive and Critical Care Nursing, 10*, 93–104.

Lee, I-M., Paffenberger, R.S., & Hsieh, C-C. (1992). Physical activity and risk of prostatic cancer among college alumni. *American Journal of Epidemiology, 146*, 413–417.

Lee, J., Parsons, G.F., & Gentleman, J.F. (1998). Falling short of the Pap test guidelines. *Health Reports, 10(1)*, 9–19.

Lee, P., Helewa, A., Smythe, H.A., Bombardier, C., & Goldsmith, C.H. (1985). Epidemiology of musculoskeletal disorders (complaints) and related disability in Canada. *Journal of Rheumatology, 12*, 1169–1173.

Leiter, M., Harvie, P., & Frizzel, C. (1998). The correspondence of patient satisfaction and nurse burnout. *Social Science and Medicine, 47*, 1611–1617.

LeRoy, P.L., & Filasky, R. (1990). Thermography. In J.J. Bonica (Ed.), *The management of pain* (2nd ed., pp. 610–621). Malvern, PA: Lea & Febiger.

Lespérance, F., Frasure-Smith, N., & Talijic, M. (1996). Major depression before and after myocardial infarction: Its nature and consequences. *Psychosomatic Medicine, 58*, 99–110.

Lester, N., Lefebvre, J.C., & Keefe, F.J. (1994). Pain in young adults: 1. Relationship to gender and family pain history. *Clinical Journal of Pain, 19*, 282–289.

Leszcz, M., & Goodwin, P.J. (1998). The rationale and foundations of group psychotherapy for women with metastatic breast cancer. *International Journal of Group Psychotherapy, 48*, 245–273.

LeUnes, A.D. and Nation, J.R. (1989). *Sport psychology: An introduction*. Chicago, Illinois: Nelson-Hall.

Leventhal, E.A., Hansell, S., Diefenbach, M., Leventhal, H., & Glass, D.C. (1996). Negative affect and self-report of physical symptoms: Two longitudinal studies of older adults. *Health Psychology, 15*, 193–199.

Leventhal, H. (1970). Findings and theory in the study of fear communications. In Berkowitz L., (Ed.), *Advances in experimental social psychology, 5* (pp. 119–186). San Diego, CA: Academic Press.

Leventhal, H., & Cleary, P.D. (1980). The smoking problem: A review of the research and theory in behavioral risk modification. *Psychological Bulletin, 88*, 370–405.

Leventhal, H., Prochaska T.R., & Hirschman, R.S. (1985). Public attitudes toward cancer pain. *Cancer, 56*, 2337–2339.

Levin, J.S., & Puchalski, C.M. (1997). Religion and spirituality in medicine: Research and education. JAMA. *Journal of the American Medical Association, 278*, 792–793.

Levinson, W. (1994). Physician-patient communication. A key to malpractice prevention. *Journal of the American Medical Association, 272*, 1619–1620.

Levinson, W. Roter, D.L., Mullooly, J.P., Dull, V.T., & Frankel, R.M. (1997). Physician-patient communication. The relationship with malpractice claims among primary care physicians and surgeons. *Journal of the American Medical Association, 277*, 553–559.

Levy, A.R., Bensiomon, D.R., Mayo, N.E., & Leighton, H.G. (1998). Inclement weather and the risk of hip fracture. *Epidemiology, 9*, 172–177.

Levy, S.M., Herberman, R.B., Whiteside, T., Sanzo, K., Lee, J., & Kirkwood, J. (1990). Perceived social support and tumor estrogen/progesterone receptor status as predictors of natural killer cell activity in breast cancer patients. *Psychosomatic Medicine, 52*, 73–85.

Ley, P. (1977). Psychological studies of doctor-patient communication. In Rachman, S., (Ed.) *Contributions to medical psychology, 1.* Oxford: Pergamon.

Ley, P. (1982). Satisfaction, compliance, and communication. *British Journal of Clinical Psychology, 21*, 241–254.

Linden, W. (1994). Autogenic training: A narrative and quantitative review of clinical outcome. *Biofeedback and Self-Regulation, 19*, 227–264.

Linden, W., & Chambers, L. (1994). Clinical effectiveness of non-drug treatment for hypertension: A meta-analysis. *Annals of Behavioral medicine, 16,* 35–45.

Linden, W., Chambers, L., Maurice J., & Lenz, J.W. (1993). Sex differences in social support, self-deception, hostility, and ambulatory cardiovascular activity. *Health Psychology, 12*, 376–380.

Linden, W., Stossel, C., & Maurice, J. (1996). Psychosocial interventions for patients with coronary artery disease: A meta-analysis. *Archives of Internal Medicine, 156,* 745–752.

Lindsay, E., Cameron, R., Walker, R., & Ferster, D. (1996). Planning and implementing the commit protocol in Brantford. Health and Canadian Society, 2, 237–267.

Linn, B.S., Linn, M.W., & Jensen, J. (1981). Anxiety and immune responsiveness. *Psychological Reports, 49*, 969–970.

Linn, S., Carroll, M., Johnson, C., Fulwood, R., Kalsbeek, W., & Briefel, R. (1993). High-density lipoprotein cholesterol and alcohol consumption in US White and Black adults: Data from NHANES II. *American Journal of Public Health, 83*, 811–816.

Liossi, C. & Hatira, P. (1999). Clinical hypnosis versus cognitive vehavioral training for pain management with pediatric cancer patients undergoing bone marrow aspirations. *International Journal of Clinical Experimental Hypnosis*,

Lipkus, I.M., Barefoot, J.C., Williams, R.B., & Siegler, I.C. (1994). Personality measures as predictors of smoking initiation and cessation in the UNC Alumni Heart Study. *Health Psychology, 13*, 149–155.

Litt, M.D., Nye, C., & Shafer, D. (1995). Preparation for oral surgery: Evaluating elements of coping. *Journal of Behavioral Medicine, 18*, 435–459.

Lloyd, E.C., Mathews, K.A., Wing, R.R., & Orchard, T.I. (1992). Psychosocial factors and complications of IDDM. The Pittsburgh Epidemiology of Diabetes Complications Study VIII. *Diabetes Care, 15,* 166–172.

Locke, E.A., & Latham, G.P. (1985). The application of goal setting to sports. *Journal of Sports Psychology, 7*, 205–222.

Locke, E.A., & Latham, G.P. (1990) *A theory of goal-setting and task performance.* Englewood Cliffs, New Jersey: Prentice-Hall.

Locke, E.A., (1968). Toward a theory of task motivation and incentives. Organizational Behaviour and Human *Performance, 3,* 157–189.

Loeser, J.D. (1996). The IASP report on back pain in the work place. *Pain Research and Management, 1*, 180.

Lollis, C.M., Johnson, E.H., & Antoni, M.H. (1997). The efficacy of the health belief model for predicting condom usage and risky sexual practices in university students. *AIDS Education and Prevention, 9,* 551–563.

Lorber, J. (1975). Good patients and problem patients: Conformity and deviance in a general hospital. *Journal of Health and Social Behavior, 16,* 213–225.

Lox, C.L., McAuley, E., & Tucker, R.S. (1995). Exercise as an intervention for enhancing subjective well-being in an HIV-1 population. *Journal of Sport and Exercise Psychology, 17,* 345–362.

Luce, G. and Peper, E. (1971). Mind over body, mind over mind. *New York Times Magazine*, September.

Ludwick,-Rosenthal, R., & Neufeld, R.W.J. (1988). Stress management during noxious medical procedures: An evaluative review of outcome studies. *Psychological Bulletin, 104*, 326–342.

Lukins, R., Davan, I.G.P., & Drummond, P.D. (1997). A cognitive behavioural approach to preventing anxiety during magnetic resonance imaging. *Journal of Behavior Therapy and Experimental Psychiatry, 28*, 97–104.

Lurie, J.D., & Sox, H.C. (1999). Principles of medical decision making. *Spine, 24*, 493–498.

Lurie, N., Rank, B., Parenti, C., Woolley, T., & Snoke, W. (1989). How do house officers spend their nights? A time study of internal medicine staff on call. *New England Journal of Medicine, 320* 1673–1677.

Lurie, N., Slater, J., McGovern, P., Ekstrum, J., Quam, L., & Margolis, K. (1993). Preventive care for women: Does the sex of the physician matter? *New England Journal of Medicine, 329*, 478–482.

Luschen, G., Cockerham, W., & Kunz, G. (1996). The sociocultural context of sport and health problems of causal relations and structural interdependence. *Sociology of Sport Journal, 13*, 197–213.

Lustman, P.J., Freedland, K.E., Griffith, L.S., & Clouse, R.E. (1998). Predicting response to cognitive behavior therapy of depression in type 2 diabetes. *General Hospital Psychiatry, 20*, 302–306.

Lustman, P.J., Griffith, L.S., Freedland, K.E., & Clouse, R.E. (1998). Cognitive behavior therapy for depression in type 2 diabetes mellitus. A randomized, controlled trial. *Annals of Internal Medicine, 129*, 613–621.

Lutsky, I., Hopwood, M., Abram, S.E., Cerletty, J.M., Hoffman, R.G., & Kampine, J.P. (1994). Use of psychoactive substances in three medical specialties: Anaesthesia, medicine and surgery. *Canadian Journal of Anaesthesiology, 41*, 561–567.

Lutsky, I., Hopwood, M., Abram, S.E., Jacobson, G.R., Haddox, J.D., & Kampine, J.P. (1993). Psychoactive substances use among American anesthesiologists: A 30-year retrospective study. *Canadian Journal of Anaesthesiology, 40*, 915–921.

Lyketsos, C.G., Hoover, D.R., Guccione, M., Dew, M.A., Wesch, J.E., Bing, E.G., & Treisman, G.J. 91996). Changes in depressive symptoms as AIDS develops. *American Journal of Psychiatry, 153*, 1430–1437.

Lyketsos, C.G., Hoover, D.R., Guccione, M., et al., (1993). Depressive symptoms as predictors of medical outcomes in HIV infection. *Journal of the American Medical Association, 270*, 2563–2567.

Lykken, D.T. (1987). Psychophysiology. In R.J. Corsini (Ed.), *Concise encyclopedia of psychology*. New York: Wiley.

Lynch, G.P. (1988). Athletic injuries and the practicing sport psychologist: Practical guidelines for assisting athletes. *The Sport Psychologist, 2*, 161–167.

Macciocchi, S.N., Barth, J.T., Alves, W.A., Rimel, R.W., & Jane, J.J. (1996). Neuropsychological functioning and and recovery after mild head injury in collegiate athletes. *Neurosurgery, 39*, 510–514.

MacDonald, N.E., Wells, G.A., Fisher, W.A., Warren, W.K., et al. (1990). High-risk STD/HIV behavior among college students. *Journal of the American Medical Association, 263*, 3155–3159.

MacDonald, T.K., MacDonald, N.E., Zanna, M.P., & Fong, G.T. (2000). Alcohol, sexual arousal, and intentions to use condoms: applying alcohol myopia to risky sexual behavior. Manuscript submitted for publication.

MacDonald, T.K., Zanna, M.P., & Fong, G.T. (1996). Why common sense goes out the window: Effects of alcohol on intentions to use condoms. *Personality and Social Psychology Bulletin, 22*, 763–775.

MacDonald, T.K., Zanna, M.P., & Fong, G.T. (1998). Alcohol and intentions to engage in risky behaviors: Experimental evidence for a causal relationship. In J.G. Adair, D. Belanger, & K. Dion (Eds.), *Advances in Psychological Science: Vol. 1. Social, personal, and cultural aspects* (pp. 407–428). East Sussex, UK: Psychology Press.

MacDonald, T.K.,, Zanna, M.P., & Fong, G.T. (1995). Decision making in altered states: Effects of alcohol on attitudes toward drinking and driving. *Journal of Personality and Social Psychology, 68*, 973–985.

Maclure, M. (1993). Demonstration of deductive meta-analysis: Ethanol intake and risk of myocardial infarction. *Epidemiology Review, 15*, 328–351.

Magni, G., Rossi, M.R., Rigatti-Luchini, S., & Merskey, H. (1992). Chronic abdominal pain and depression. Epidemiologic findings in the United States. Hispanic Health and Nutrition Examination Survey. *Pain, 49*, 549–559.

Maguire, P. & Rutter, D. (1976). History-taking for medical students. 1. Deficiencies in performance. Lancet, 2, 556–558.

Mahler, H.I.M., & Kulik, J.A. (1991). Health care involvement preferences and social-emotional recovery of male coronary-artery-bypass patients. *Health Psychology, 10*, 399–408.

Mahoney, M. (1996). Foreward. In J.L. Van Raalte and B.W. Brewer (Eds.), *Exploring sport and exercise psychology*. Washington,

D.C.: American Psychological Association.

Mahoney, M.J., & Avener, M. (1977). Psychology of the elite athlete: An exploratory study. *Cognitive Therapy and Research, 1*, 135–141.

Mahoney, M.J., Gabriel, T.J., & Perkins, T.S. (1987). Psychological skills and exceptional athletic performance. *The Sport Psychologist, 1*, 181–199.

Maier, S.F., Watkins, L.R., Fleshner, M. (1994). Psychoneuroimmunology: The interface between behavior, brain, and immunity. *American Psychologist, 49*, 1004–1017.

Main, C.J., & Spanswick, C.C. (1995). "Functional overlay", and illness behaviour in chronic pain: Distress or malingering? Conceptual difficulties in medicolegal assessment of personal injury claims. *Journal of Psychosomatic Research, 39*, 737–753.

Malcarne, V.L., Compas, B.E., Epping-Jordan, J.E., & Howell, D.C. (1995). Cognitive factors in adjustment to cancer: Attributions of self-blame and perceptions of control. *Journal of Behavioral Medicine, 18*, 401–417.

Manga, P. (1993). Socio-economic inequalities. In Stephens, T., & Fowler, G.D. (Eds.), Canada's Health Promotion Survey, 1990 Technical Report. Ottawa: Ministry of Supply and Services (Catalogue No. H39–263/2–1990E).

Mann, T., Nolen-Hoeksema, S., Huang, K., Burgard, D., et al. (1997). Are two interventions worse than none? Joint primary and secondary prevention of eating disorders in college females. *Health Psychology, 16*, 215–225.

Manne, S.L., Jacobsen, P.B., Gorfinkle, K., Gerstein, F., & Redd, W.H. (1993). Treatment adherence difficulties among children with cancer: The role of parenting style. *Journal of Pediatric Psychology, 18*, 47–62.

Manuck, S.B., Cohen, S., Rabin, B.S., Muldoon, M.F., & Bachen, E.A. (1991). Individual differences in cellular immune response to stress. *Psychological Science, 2*, 111–115.

Marcoux, B.C., & Shope, J.T. (1997). Application of the theory of planned behavior to adolescent use and misuse of alcohol. *Health Education Research, 12*, 323–331.

Marlatt, G.A., & Gordon, J.R. (1980). Determinants of relapse: Implications for the maintenance of behavior change. In P.O. Davidson and S.M. Davidson (Eds.), *Behavioral medicine: Changing health lifestyles.* (pp. 410–452). New York: Brunner/Mazel.

Marrero, D.G., Guare, J.C., Vandagriff, J.L., & Fineberg, N.S. (1997). Fear of hypoglycemia in the parents of children and adolescents with diabetes: Maladaptive or health response? *Diabetes Education, 23*, 281–286.

Marsh, H.W., Hey, J., Johnson, S., & Perry, C. (1997). Elite Athlete Self Description Questionnaire: Hierarchical confirmatory factor analysis of responses by two distinct groups of elite athletes. *International Journal of Sport Psychology, 3*, 237–252.

Marsh, H.W., Richards, G.E. Johnson, S., Roche, L., & Tremayne, P. (1994). Physical Self-Description Questionnaire: Psychometric properties and a multitrait-multimethod analysis of relations to existing instruments. *Journal of Sport and Exercise Psychology, 16*, 270–305.

Marshall, J.R. & Funch, d.P. (1986). Gender and illness behavior among colorectal cancer patients. *Women's Health, 11*, 67–82.

Marshall, S.P., Smith, M.S., & Weinberger, E. (1995). Perceived anxiety of pediatric patients to magnetic resonance. *Clinical Pediatrics, 34*, 59–60.

Marsland, A.L., Manuck, S.B., Fazzari, T.V., Steward, C.J., & Rabin, B.S. (1995). Stability of individual differences in cellular immune responses to acute psychological stress. *Psychosomatic Medicine, 57*, 295–298.

Martelli, M.F., Auerbach, S.M., Alexander, J., & Mercuri, L.G. (1987). Stress management in the health care setting: Matching interventions with patient coping styles. *Journal of Consulting and Clinical Psychology, 56*, 856–872.

Martin, D.P., Diehr, P., Conrad, D.A., Davis, J.H., Leickly, R., & Perrin, E.B. (1998). Randomized trial of a patient-centered hospital unit. Patient Education and *Counseling, 34*, 125–133.

Martinsen, E.W. (1990). Benefits of exercise for the treatment of depression. *Sports Medicine, 9*, 380–389.

Martinsen, E.W. (1993). Therapeutic implications of exercise for clinically anxious and depressed patients. *International Journal of Sport Psychology, 24*, 185–199.

Martinsen, E.W. (1994). Physical activity and depression: Clinical experience. *Actua Psychiatrca Scandinavica, 377*, 23–27.

Martinson, E.W., & Morgan, W.P. (1997). Antidepressant effects of physical activity. In W.P. Morgan (Ed.), *Physical activity and mental status* (pp.93–106). Washington, DC:

Taylor and Francis.

Marvel, M.K. (1993). Involvement with the psychosocial concerns of patients. *Archives of Family Medicine, 2,* 629–633.

Marvel, M.K., Epstein, R.M., Flowers, K., & Beckman, H.B. (1999). Soliciting the patient's agenda: Have we improved? *Journal of the American Medical Association, 281,* 283–287.

Maslach, C. (1979). The burn-out syndrome and patient care. In C. Garfield (Ed.), *The emotional realities of life-threatening illness* (pp. 111–120). St. Louis, MO: CV Mosby.

Masur, F.T., III. (1981). Adherence to health care regimens. In C.K. Prokop & L.A. Bradley (Eds.), *Medical psychology: Contributions to behavioral medicine.* New York: Academic Press.

Matarazzo, J.D. (1980). Behavioral health and behavioral medicine. American *Psychologist, 35,* 807–817.

Matarazzo, J.D., Weiss, S.M., Herd, J.A., Miller, N.E., Weiss, S., (Eds.) (1984). *Behavioral Health: A handbook of health enhancement and disease prevention.* New York: Wiley.

Matrunola, P. (1996). Is there a relationship between job satisfaction and absenteeism? *Journal of Advanced Nursing, 23,* 827–834.

Mattila-Lindy, S., Hemminki, E., Malin, M., Makkonen, K., Topo, P., Maentyranta, T., & Kangas, I. (1998). Physicians' gender and clinical opinions of reproductive health matters. *Women and Health, 26(3),* 15–26.

Mauer, M.H., Burnett, K.F., Ouellette, E.A., Ironson, G.H., & Dandes, H.M. (1999). Medical hypnosis and orthopedic hand: pain perception, postoperative recovery, and therapeutic comfort. *International Journal of Clinical and Experimental Hypnosis, 47(2),* 144–161.

Maunsell, E., Jacques, B., & Deschenes, L. (1995). Social support and survival among women with breast cancer. *Cancer, 76,* 631–637.

Mayled, A. (1998). Medical admissions units: The role of the nurse practitioner. *Nursing Standard, 12,* 44–47.

Mayne, T.J., & Ambrose, T.K. (1999). Research review on anger in psychotherapy. *Journal of Clinical psychology, 55,* 353–363.

Mazullo, J.M., Lasagna, L., Griner, P.F. (1974). Variations in interpretation of prescription instructions. *Journal of the American Medical Association, 227,* 929–931.

McAuley, E. (1991). Efficacy, attributional and affective responses to exercise participation. *Journal of Sport and Exercise Psychology, 13,* 382–393.

McAuley, E. and Corneya, K.S. (1992). Self-efficacy relationships with affective and exertion responses to exercise. *Journal of Applied Social Psychology, 22,* 312–326.

McAuley, Schaffer, & Rudolph. (1995). Affective responses to acute exercise in elderly impaired males: The moderating effects of self-efficacy and age. *International Journal of Aging and Human Development, 41,* 13–35.

McAuliffe, W.E., Rohman, M., Santangelo, S., Feldman, B., Magnuson, E., Sobol, A., & Weissman, J. (1986). Psychoactive drug use among practicing physicians and medical students. *New England Journal of Medicine, 315,* 805–810.

McCain, G.C., & Morwessel, N.J. (1995). Pediatric nurses' knowledge and practice related to infant pain. *Issues in Comprehensive Pediatric Nursing, 18,* 277–286.

McCaul, K.D., Schroeder, D.M., & Reid, P.A. (1996). Breast cancer worry and screening. Some prospective data. *Health Psychology, 15,* 430–433.

McClelland, D.C., Ross, G., & Patel, V. (1985). The effect of an academic examination on salivary norepinephrine and immunoglobulin levels. *Journal of Human Stress,* 52–59.

McCracken, L.M., Zayfert, C., & Gross, R.T. (1993). The pain anxiety symptoms scale (PASS): A multi-modal measure of pain specific anxiety symptoms. *Behaviour Research and Therapy, 31,* 647–652.

McCreary Centre Society (1993). Adolescent Health Survey: Province of British Columbia. Richmond, BC: New Leaf Computer.

McCreary Centre Society (1999). *Healthy Connections: Listening to BC Youth.* Burnaby, BC: The McCreary Centre Society.

McDade, T. (1996). Prostates and profits: The social construction of benign prostatic hyperplasia in American men. *Medical Anthropology, 17,* 1–22.

McDaniel, J.S. (1996). Stressful life events and psychoneuroimmunology. In T.W. Miller (Ed.), *Theory and assessment of stressful life events,* pp. 3–36. Madison, CT: International Universities Press.

McDonald, D.D. (1994). Gender and ethnic stereotyping and narcotic analgesic administration. Res. *Nurs. Health, 17,* 45–49.

McFarland, C., & Buehler, R. (1997). Negative affective states and the motivated retrieval of positive life events: The role of affect acknowledgement. *Journal of Personality and Social Psychology, 73*, 200–214.

McFarland, C., & Buehler, R. (1998). The impact of negative affect on autobiographical memory: The role of self-focused attention to moods. *Journal of Personality and Social Psychology, 75*, 1424–1440.

McFarland, K.F., & Rhoades, D.R. (1998). Gender-related values and medical specialty choice. *Academic Psychiatry, 22*, 236–239.

McGehee, D.S., Heath, M.J.S., Gelber, S., Devay, P., & Role, L.W. (1995). Nicotine enhancement of fast excitatory transmission in CNS by presynaptic receptors. *Science, 269*, 1692–1696.

McGinnis, J.M., Shopland, D., & Brown, C. (1987). Tobacco and health: Trends in smoking and smokeless tobacco consumption in the United States. In L. Breslow, J.E. Fielding, & L.B. Lave (Eds.). *Annual review of public health (Vol. 8)*. Palo Alto, CA: Annual Reviews.

McGrath, P.A. (1987). An assessment of children's pain: A review of behavioral, physiological and direct scaling techniques. *Pain, 31*, 147–176.

McGuire, W.J. (1985). Attitudes and attitude change. In G. Lindzey, & E. Aronson, (Eds.), *Handbook of social psychology (3rd ed.), Vol. 2*, pp. 233–346. New York: Random House.

McIsaac, H.K., Thordarson, D.S., Shafran, R., Rachman, S., & Poole, G. (1998). Claustrophobia and the magnetic imaging procedure. *Journal of Behavioral Medicine, 31*, 255–268.

McKinlay, J.B. (1975). Who is really ignorant—physician or patient? *Journal of Health and Social Behavior, 16*, 3–11.

McKinlay, J.B., Burns, R.B., Feldman, H.A., Freund, K.M., Irish, J.T., Kasten, L.E., Moskowitz, M.A., Potter, D.A., & Woodman, K. (1998). Physician variability and uncertainty in the management of breast cancer. Results from a factorial experiment. *Medical Care, 36*, 385–396.

McKinnon, W., Weisse, C.S., Reynolds, C.P., Bowles, C.A., & Baum, A. (1989). Chronic stress, leukocyte subpopulations, and humoral response to latent viruses. *Health Psychology, 8*, 389–402.

McLennon, B., & Gauthier, (1998). Presentation to The Standing Committee on Finance Roundtable on Research. October, 1999, Ottawa.

McMurran, M. (1994). *The psychology of addiction*. London: Taylor & Francis.

McQuaid, E.L., & Nassau, J.H. (1999). Empirically supported treatments of disease-related symptoms in pediatric psychology: asthma, diabetes, and cancer. *Journal of Pediatric Psychology, 24*, 333–334.

Meichenbaum, D. (1975). Enhancing creativity by modifying what subjects say to themselves. *American Educational Research Journal, 12*, 129–145.

Meichenbaum, D. (1977). *Cognitive-behavior modification: An integrative approach*. New York: Plenum Press.

Melamed, B.G., & Siegal, L, J. (1975). Reduction of anxiety in children facing surgery by modeling. *Journal of Consulting and Clinical Psychology, 43*, 511–521.

Melendez, J.C., & McCrank, E. (1993). Anxiety-related reactions associated with magnetic resonance imaging examinations. *Journal of the American Medical Association, 270*, 745–747.

Melzack, R. (1973). *The puzzle of pain*. New York: Basic Books.

Melzack, R. (1975). The McGill Pain Questionnaire: Major properties and scoring methods. *Pain, 1*, 277–299.

Melzack, R. (1987). The short-form McGill Pain Questionnaire. *Pain, 30*, 191–197.

Melzack, R. (1989). Folk medicine and the sensory modulation of pain. In P.D. Wall & R. Melzack (Eds.), *Textbook of pain (2nd ed.)*. Edinburgh: Churchill Livingstone.

Melzack, R. (1991). The gate control theory 25 years later: new perspectives on phantom limb pain. In M.R. Bond, J.E. Charloton, & C.J. Woolf (Eds.), *Proceedings of the VIth World Congress on Pain* (pp. 9–21). Amsterdam: Elsevier Science Publishers.

Melzack, R. (1992). Phantom limbs. *Scientific American, 266*, 120–126.

Melzack, R. (1993). Pain: Past, present and future. *Canadian Journal of Experimental Psychology, 47(4)*, 615–629.

Melzack, R. (1998). Pain and stress: Clues toward understanding chronic pain. In M. Sabourin, F. Craik, and M. Robert (Eds.), *Advances in psychological science: Vol. 2. Biological and Cognitive Aspects.* Hove: Psychology Press Limited.

Melzack, R., & Loeser, J.D. (1978). Phantom body pain in paraplegics: evidence for a central 'pattern generating mechanism' for pain. *Pain, 4*, 195–210.

Melzack, R., & Wall, P.D. (1965). Pain mechanisms: A new theory. *Science, 150,* 971–979.

Melzack, R., & Wall, P.D. (1996). *The Challenge of Pain. (updated 2nd ed.).* New York: Basic Books.

Melzack, R., Israel, R., Laxroix, R., & Schultz, G. (1997). Phantom limbs in people with congenital limb deficiency or amputation in early childhood. *Brain, 120*, 1603–1620.

Mendes-de-Leon, C.F., Powell, L.H., & Kaplan, B.H. (1991). Change in coronary-prone behaviors in the Recurrent Coronary Prevention Project. *Psychosomatic medicine, 53*, 407–419.

Merskey, H. (1970). On the development of pain. *Headache, 10*, 116–123.

Merskey, H. (1986). Psychiatry and pain. In R.A. Sternbach (Ed.), *The psychology of pain (2nd ed.)*. New York: Raven Press.

Merskey, H. (1996a). Back pain, psychology and money. *Pain Research and Management, 1*, 13.

Merskey, H. (1996b). Re: Back pain in the work place. *Pain, 65*, 111–112.

Messing, K. (1998). Hospital trash: Cleaners speak of their role in disease prevention. *Medical Anthropology Quarterly, 12*, 168–187.

Meyerowitz, B.E., Heinrich, R.L., & Schag, C.C. (1983). A competency-based approach to coping with cancer. In T.G. Burish & L.A. Bradley (Eds.), *Coping with chronic disease: Research and applications* (pp. 137–158). New York: Academic Press.

Michalko, S.L., McAuley, E., & Bane, S. (1996). Self-efficacy and affective responses to acute exercise in middle-aged adults. *Journal of Social Behavior and Personality, 11*, 375–385.

Miles, F., & Meehan, J.W. (1995). Visual discrimination of pigmented skin lesions. *Health Psychology, 14*, 171–177.

Millar, M.G. (1997). The effects of emotion on breast self-examination: Another look at the Health Belief Model. *Social Behavior and Personality, 25*, 223–232.

Millar, W.J., & Hill, G.B. (1994). Hip fractures: Mortality, morbidity and sugical treatment. *Health Reports, 6,* 323–337.

Miller, A.L. (1993, March). The U.S. smoking-material fire problem through 1990: The role of lighted tobacco products in fire. Paper presented at the meeting of the National Fire Protection Association, Quincy, MA.

Miller, D.L., & Stark, L.J. (1994). Contingency contracting for improving adherence in pediatric populations. Journal of the *American Medical Association, 271*, 81–83.

Miller, N.E. (1969). Learning of visceral and glandular responses. *Science, 163*, 434–445.

Miller, N.E. (1983). Behavioral medicine: Symbiosis between laboratory and clinic. *Annual Review of Psychology, 34*, 1–31.

Miller, N.E., & DiCara, L.V., (1967). Instrumental learning of heart rate changes in curarized rats: Shaping, and specificity to discriminate stimulus. *Journal of Comparative and Physiological Psychology, 63*, 1–6.

Miller, S.M. (1980). When is a little information a dangerous thing? Coping with stressful life-events by monitoring vs. blunting. In Levine, S., & Ursin, H. (Eds.), *Coping and health*. New York: Plenum Press.

Miller, S.M., & Mangan, C.E. (1983). Interacting effects of information and coping style in adapting to gynecologic stress: Should the doctor tell all? *Journal of Personality and Social Psychology, 45*, 223–236.

Miller, T.D., Balady, G.J., & Fletcher, G.F. (1997). Exercise and its role in the prevention and rehabilitation of cardiovascular disease. *Annals of Behavioral Medicine, 19*, 220–229.

Miller, W.R., & Hester, R.K. (1980). Treating the problem drinker: Modern approaches. In W.R. Miller (Ed.), *The addictive behaviors* (pp. 11–141). Oxford, England: Pergamon Press.

Millstein, S.G. (1996). Utility of the theories of reasoned action and planned behavior for predicting physician behavior: A prospective analysis. *Health Psychology, 15*, 398–402.

Minor, M.A., & Sanford, M.K. (1993). Physical interventions in the management of pain in arthritis. *Arthritis Care and Research, 6*, 197–206.

Misovich, S.J., Fisher, J.D., & Fisher, W.A. (1996). The perceived AIDS-preventive utility of knowing one's partner well: A public health dictum and individuals' risky sexual behaviour. *The Canadian Journal of Human Sexuality, 5*, 83–90.

Misovich, S.J., Fisher, J.D., & Fisher, W.A. (1997). Close relationships and elevated HIV risk behavior: Evidence and possible underlying psychological processes. *Review of General Psychology, 1*, 72–107.

Mitchell, J.E., & de Zwaan, M. (1993). Pharmacological treatments of binge eating. In C.G. Fairburn & G.T. Wilson (Eds.), *Binge eating: Nature, assessment, and treat-*

ment (pp. 250–269). New York: Guilford Press.

Mittelmark, M.B., Murray, D.M., Luepker, R.V., Pechacek, T.F., et al. (1987). Predicting experimentation with cigarettes: The Childhood Antecedents of Smoking Study (CASS). *American Journal of Public Health, 77*, 206–208.

Monane, M. Bohn, R.L., Gurwitz, J.H., Glynn, R.J., Levin, R., & Avorn, J. (1996). Compliance with antihypertensive therapy among elderly Medicaid enrollees: The rates of age, gender, and race. *American Journal of Public Health, 86*, 1805–1808.

Moore, K.L., & Persaud, T.V.N. (1993). *Before we are born. (4th ed.)*. Philadelphia: W.B. Saunders.

Moore, S.M., Barling, N.R., & Hood, B. (1998). Predicting testicular and breast self-examination behaviour: A test of the theory of reasoned action. *Behaviour Change, 15*, 41–49.

Mor, V., Masterson-Allen, S., Goldberg, R., Guadagnoli, E., & Wool, M.S. (1990). Prediagnostic symptom recognition and help seeking among cancer patients. *Journal of Community Health, 15,* 253–266.

Morgan, S.B. Bieberich, A.A., Walker, M., & Schwerdtfeger, H. (1998). Children's willingness to share activities with a physically handicapped peer: Am I more willing than my classmates? *Journal of Pediatric Psychology, 23*, 367–375.

Morgan, W.P. (Ed.). (1997). *Physical activity in mental health*. Washington, D.C.: Taylor and Francis.

Morgan, W.P., & Ellickson, K.A. (1989). Health, anxiety and physical exercise. In D. Hackfort & Spielberger, C. (Eds.) *Anxiety in sports: An international perspective.* New York: Hemisphere Publishing.

Morley, J.E. (1998). The elderly Type 2 diabetic patient: Special considerations. *Diabetes Medicine, 15 (Suppl 4)*, S41-S46.

Morris, E. (1999). Reflections on the NICU. A nurse's perspective. *American Journal of Nursing, 99(3)*, 23.

Morrison, D.M., Gillmore, M., & Baker, S.A. (1995). Determinants of condom use among high-risk heterosexual adults: A test of the theory of reasoned action. *Journal of Applied Social Psychology, 25*, 651–676.

Moyer, A. (1997). Psychosocial outcomes of breast-conserving surgery versus mastectomy: A meta-analytic review. *Health Psychology, 16*, 284–298.

Mpofu, E., & Houston, E. (1998). Assessment of value change in persons with acquired physical disabilities: Current and prospective applications for rehabilitation counselors. *Canadian Journal of Rehabilitation, 12*, 53–61

Mulvihill, C.K. (1996). AIDS education for college students: Review and proposal for a research-based curriculum. *AIDS Education and Prevention, 8*, 11–25.

Munro, L., Rodwell, J., & Harding, L. (1998). Assessing occupational stress in psychiatric nurses using the full job strain model: The value of social support to nurses. *International Journal of Nursing Studies, 35*, 339–345.

Murphy, H., Dickens, C., Creed, F., & Bernstein, R. (1999). Depression, illness perception and coping in rheumatoid arthritis. *Journal of Psychosomatic Research, 46,* 155–164.

Murphy, K.J., & Brunberg, J.A. (1997). Adult claustrophobia, anxiety and sedation in MRI. *Magnetic Resonance Imaging, 15*, 51–54.

Murphy, L.R. (1996). Stress management in work settings: A critical review of the health effects. *American Journal of Health Promotion, 11*, 112–135.

Murry, M. (1980). *Seeking the master*. London: Neville Spearman.

Muscroft, J., & Hicks, C. (1998). A comparison of psychiatric nurses' and general nurses' reported stress and counselling needs: A case study approach. *Journal of Advanced Nursing, 27*, 1317–1325.

Mushlin, A.I., Kouides, R.W., & Shapiro, D.E. (1998). Estimating the accuracy of screening mammography: A meta-analysis. *American Journal of Preventative Medicine, 14,* 143–153.

Musselman, D.L., Evans, D.L., & Nemeroff, C.B. (1998). The relationship of depression to cardiovascular disease. *Archives of General Psychiatry, 55*, 580–592.

Muustedt, K., Muller, H., Blauth-Eckmeyer, E., Stenger, K., Zygmunt, M., & Vahrson, H. (1999). Role of dexamethoasone dosage in combination with 5-HT3 antagonists for prophylaxis of acute chemotherapy-induced nausea and vomiting. *British Journal of Cancer, 79*, 637–639.

Nair, B.R. (1998). Patient, client or customer? *Medical Journal of Australia, 169*, 593.

Nam, R.K., Fleshner, N., Rakovitch, E., Klotz, L., Trachtenberg, J., Choo, R., Morton, G., & Danjoux, C. (1999). Prevalence and patterns of the use of complementary therapies among prostate cancer patients: An epidemiological analysis. *Journal of Urology, 161*, 1521–1524.

Naranjo, C. (1971). *On the Psychology of Meditation*. New York: The Viking Press.

National Advisory Council on Aging (1994). NACA aging vignettes. Ottawa: NACA.

National Advisory Council on Aging (1996). NACA aging vignettes. Ottawa: NACA.

National Advisory Council on Aging (1997). NACA aging vignettes. Ottawa: NACA.

National Cancer Institute of Canada, Canadian Cancer Statistics 1998, Toronto, 1998.

National Highway Traffic Safety Administration. (1993–1996). Fatality analysis reporting system, 1992–1995. Washington, DC: U.S. Department of Transportation.

National Institute on Alcohol Abuse and Alcoholism (NIAAA). (1988). Alcohol and aging. *Alcohol Alert, 2*, 1–4.

Negri, E., La Vecchia, C., D'Avanzo, B., Nobili, A., et al. (1994). Acute myocardial infarction: Association with time since stopping smoking in Italy. *Journal of Epidemiology and Community Health, 48*, 129–133.

Neittaanmäki, L., & Luhtala, R. (1993). More women enter medicine: Young doctors' family origin and career choice. *Medical Education 27*, 440–445.

Neittaanmäki, L., Gross, E.B., Virjo, I, Hyppölä, H., Kumpusalo, E. (1999). Personal values of male and female doctors: Gender aspects. *Social Science and Medicine, 48*, 559–568.

Nerenz, D.R., & Leventhal, H. (1983). Self-regulation theory in chronic illness. In T.G. Burish & L.A. Bradley (Eds.), *Coping with chronic disease: Research and applications* (pp. 13–87). New York: Academic Press.

Neumarker, K.J. (1997). Mortality and sudden death in anorexia nervosa. *International Journal of Eating Disorders, 21*, 202–212.

Newport, D.J., & Nemeroff, C.B. (1998). Assessment and treatment of depression in the cancer patient. *Journal of Psychosomatic Research, 45*, 215–237.

Newsom, J.T., Knapp, J.E., & Schulz, R. (1996). Longitudinal analysis of specific domains of internal control and depressive symptoms in patients with recurrent cancer. *Health Psychology, 15*, 323–331.

Nezu, A.M.,Nezu, C.M., Fridman, S.H., Faddis, S., & Houts, P.S. (1998). *Helping cancer patients cope: A problem-solving approach*. Washington, D.C.: American Psychological Association.

Ng, B., Dimsdale, J.E., Shragg, G.P., & Deutsch, R. (1996). Ethnic differences in analgesic consumption for post-operative pain. *Psychosomatic Medicine, 58*, 125–129.

Ng, E., Wilkins, R., Pole, J., & Adams, O.B. (1997). How far to the nearest physician? *Health Reports, 8(4)*, 19–31.

Ng, K., & von Gunten, C.F. (1998). Symptoms and attitudes of 100 consecutive patients admitted to an acute hospice/palliative care unit. *Journal of Pain and Symptom Management, 16*, 307–316.

Nichols, A. (1987). Women's preference for sex of doctor: A postal survey. *Journal of the Royal College of the General Practitioners, 37*, 540.

Nideffer, R.M. (1985). *Athlete's guide to mental training*. Champaign, Illinois: Human Kinetics.

Nideffer, R.M., & Sharpe, R.C. (1978). *Attention control training: How to get control of your mind through total concentration*. New York: Wideview Books.

Nigl, A.J. (1984). *Biofeedback and behavioral strategies in pain treatment*. New York: Medical and Scientific Bookds.

North, T.C., McCullagh, P., & Tran, Z.V. (1990). Effects of exercise on depression. *Exercise and Sport Science Reviews, 18*, 379–415.

Norton, G.R., Norton, P.J., Asmundson, G.J.G., Thompson, L.A., & Larsen, M.A. (in press). Neurotic butterflies in my stomach: The role of anxiety, anxiety sensitivity and depression in functional gastrointestinal disorders. *Journal of Psychosomatic Research*.

O'Connor, P.G., & Spickard, A. Jr. (1997). Physician impairment by substance abuse. *Medical Clinics of North America, 81*, 1037–1052.

O'Leary, A., Shoor, S., Lorig, K., & Holman, H.R. (1988). A cognitive-behavioral treatment for rheumatoid arthritis. *Health Psychology, 7*, 527–544.

O'Brien, M.K. (1997). Compliance among health professionals. In A. Baum, S. Newman, J., Weinman, R., West, & C. McManus (Eds.), *Cambridge handbook of psychology, health and medicine* (pp. 278–281). Cambridge, United Kingdom: Cambridge University Press.

O'Neill, M., Rootman, I., & Pederson, A. (1994). Beyond Lalonde: Two decades of Canadian health. In Pederson, A., O'Neill, M., & Rootman, I. (Eds.), *Health promotion in Canada: Provincial, national and international perspectives.* (pp. 374–386). Toronto, ON: Saunders.

Ockene, J.K., Kuller, L.H., Svendsen, K.H., & Meilahn, E. (1990). The relationship of smoking cessation to coronary heart disease and lung cancer in the Multiple Risk Factor Intervention Trial (MRFIT). *American Journal of Public Health, 80,* 954–958.

Odenheimer, G.L., (1993). Dementia and the older driver. *Clinical Geriatric Medicine, 9,* 349–364.

Öhlund, C., Lundström, I., Areskoug, B., Eek, C., et al. (1994). Pain behavior in industrial subacute low back pain: Part 1. Reliability: concurrent and predictive validity of pain behavior assessments. *Pain, 58,* 201–209.

Ohnhaus, E.E., & Adler, R. (1975). Methodological problems in the measurement of pain: A comparison between the verbal ratings scale and the visual analogue scale. *Pain, 1,* 379–384.

Olivotto, I.A., Kan, L., & Coldman, A.J. (1998). False positive rate of screening mammography. *New England Journal of Medicine, 339,* 560.

Olson, J.M., & Zanna, M. (1987). Understanding and promoting exercise: A social psychological perspective. *Canadian Journal of Public Health, 78,* S1-S7.

Onions, C.T. (Ed.). (1986). *Shorter Oxford English dictionary on historical principles (3rd ed.).* Oxford: Oxford University Press.

Orlick, T., & Partington, J. (1988). Mental links to excellence. *The Sport Psychologist, 2,* 105–130.

Orne, M.T. (1962). On the social psychology of the psychological experiment: With particular reference to demand characteristics and their implications. *American Psychologist, 17,* 776–783.

Orne, M.T. (1989). On the construct of hypnosis: How its definition affects research and its clinical application. In G.D. Burrows & L. Dennerstein (Eds.), *Handbook of hypnosis and psychosomatic medicine.* Amsterdam: Elsevier.

Orne, M.T., & Dinges, D.F. (1989). Hypnosis. In P.D. Wall & R. Melzack (Eds.), *Textbook of pain (2nd ed.).* Edinburgh: Churchill Livingstone.

Osowiecki, D., & Compas, B.E. (1998). Psychological adjustment to cancer: Control beliefs and coping in adult cancer patients. *Cognitive Therapy and Research, 22,* 483–499.

Osterhouse, R.A., & Brock, T.C. (1970). Distraction increases yielding to propaganda by inhibiting counterarguing. *Journal of Personality and Social Psychology, 15,* 344–358.

Ostrea, E.M., Romero, A., & Yee, H. (1993). Adaptation of the meconium drug test for mass screening. *Journal of Pediatrics, 122,* 152–154.

Ostrow, A.C. (Ed.). (1996). *Directory of psychological tests in the sport and exercise sciences (2nd ed.).* Morgantown, West Virginia: Fitness Information Technology.

Otto, M.W., & Dougher, M.J. (1985). Sex differences and personality factors in responsivity to pain. Percept. *Mot Skills, 61,* 383–390.

Owen, H., & Plummer, J. (1997). Patient-controlled analgesia: Current concepts in acute pain management. *CNS Drugs, 8,* 203–218.

Paffenberger, R.S., Wing, A.L., & Hyde, R.T. (1978). Physical activity as an index of heart attack risk in college alumni. *American Journal of Epidemiology, 108,* 161–175.

Paice, J.A., Toy, C., & Shott, S. (1998). Parriers to cancer patin relief: Fear of tolerance and addiction. *Journal of Pain Symptom Management, 16,* 1–9.

Pallavicini-Gonzalez, J., Venegas-Ramirez, L., & Espinoza, M.A. (1995). The experience of intensive care patients of J.J. Aguirre Hospital: 1989–1992. *Revista de Psiquiatria Clinica, 32(1–2),* 25–36.

Parasuraman, R., & Nestor, P. (1993). Attention and driving: Assessment in elderly individuals with dementia. *Clinical Geriatric Medicine, 9,* 377–387.

Parboosingh, E.J., Anderson, G., Clark, E.A., et al. (1996). Cervical cancer screening: Are the 1989 recommendations still valid? *Canadian Medical Association Journal, 154,* 1867–1869.

Pargman, D. (1998). *Understanding sport behavior.* Upper Saddle River, New Jersey: Prentice –Hall.

Park, D.C., Hertzog, C., Leventhal, H., Morrell, R.W., et al. (1999). Medication adherence in rheumatoid arthritis patients: Older is wiser. *Journal of the American Geriatric Society, 47(2),* 172–183.

Parker, D.R., McPhillips, J.V., Derby, C.A., Gans, K.M., et al. (1996). High-density-lipoprotein cholesterol and types of alcoholic beverages consumed among men and women. *American Journal of Public Health, 86,* 1022–1027.

Parker, P.A., & Kulik, J.A. (1995). Burnout, self- and supervisor-related job performance, and absenteeism among nurses. *Journal of Behavioral Medicine, 18,* 581–599.

Parrish, J.M. (1986). Parent compliance with medical and behavioral recommendations. In N.A. Krasnegor, J.D. Arasteh, & M.F. Cataldo (Eds.), *Child health behavior: A behavioral pediatrics perspective*. New York: Wiley.

Parsons, T. (1951). *The social system*. Glencoe, IL: Free Press.

Paskett, E.D., & Rimer, B.K. (1995). Psychosocial effects of abnormal Pap tests and mammograms: A review. *Journal of Women's Health, 4*, 73–82.

Pate, R.R., Pratt, M., Blair, S.N., Haskell, W.L., et al. (1995). Physical activity and public health: A recommendation from the Centers for Disease Control and Prevention and the American College of Sports Medicine. *Journal of the American Medical Association, 273*, 402–407.

Patton, G.C., Selzer, R., Coffey, C., Carlin, J.B., & Wolfe, R. (1999). Onset of adolescent eating disorders: Population based cohort study over 3 years. *British Medical Journal, 318*, 765–768.

Payne, D.K., Hoffman, R.G., Theodoulou, M., Dosik, M., & Massie, M.J. (1999). Screening for anxiety and depression in women with breast cancer: Psychiatric and medical oncology gear up for managed care. *Psychosomatics, 40*, 64–69.

Payne, S.A., Dean, S.J., & Kalus, C. (1998). A comparative study of death anxiety in hospice and emergency nurses. *Journal of Advanced Nursing, 28*, 700–706.

Pearlin, L.I. (1993). The social contexts of stress. In L. Goldberger and S. Breznitz (Eds.) *Handbook of stress: Theoretical and clinical aspects* (2nd ed., pp. 303–315). New York: Free Press.

Peck, C.L., & King, N.J. (1985). Compliance and the doctor-patient relationship. *Drugs, 30*, 78–84.

Pederson, L.L. (1982). Compliance with physician advice to quit smoking: A review of the literature. *Preventive Medicine, 11*, 71–84.

Pelto, P.J., & Pelto, G.H. (1997). Studying knowledge, culture, and behavior in applied medical anthropology. *Medical Anthropology Quarterly, 11*, 147–163.

Pennebaker, J.W. (1983). Accuracy of symptom perception. In A. Baum, S.E. Taylor, & J. Singer (Eds.), *Handbook of psychology and health (Vol. 4)*. Hillsdale, NJ: Erlbaum.

Pennebaker, J.W. (1994). Psychological bases of symptom reporting: Perceptual and emotional aspects of chemical sensitivity. *Toxicology and Industrial Health, 10*, 497–511.

Penninx, B.W., Guralnik, J.M., Mendes de Leon, C.F., Pahor, M., Visser, M., Corti, M.C., & Wallace, R.B. (1998). Cardiovascular events and mortality in newly and chronically depressed persons > 70 years of age. *American Journal of Cardiology, 81*, 988–94.

Pereles, L., & Russell, M.L. (1996). Needs for CME in geriatrics. Part 2: Physician priorities and perceptions of community representatives. *Canadian Family Medicine, 42,* 632–640.

Perkins, D.O., Stern, R.A., Golden, R.N., et al., (1994). Mood disorders in HIV infection: Prevalence and risk factors in a nonepicenter of the AIDS epidemic. *American Journal of Psychiatry, 151*, 233–236.

Perna, R.B., Durgin, D.L., & Geller, S.E. (1999, October). Patient ratings of modalities in multidisciplinary pain management. Poster session presented at the annual meeting of the American Pain Society, Fort Lauderdale, FL.

Perretta, P., Akiskal, H.S., Nisita, C., Lorenzetti, C., Zaccagnini, E., Della-Santa, M., & Cassano, G.B. (1998). The high prevalence of bipolar II and associated cyclothymic and hyperthymic temperaments in HIV patients. *Journal of Affective Disorders, 50,* 215–224.

Persky, V.W., Kempthorne,Rawson, J., & Shekelle, R.B. (1987). Personality and risk of cancer: 20-year follow-up of the Western Electric Study. *Psychosomatic Medicine, 49*, 435–449.

Peterkin, A.D. (1998). *Staying human during residency training*. Toronto, ON: University of Toronto Press.

Peterson, L., & Schick, B. (1993). Empirically derived injury prevention rules. Special section: Behavioral pediatrics. *Journal of Applied Behavior Analysis, 26*, 451–460.

Petruzzello, S.J., Landers, D.M., Hatfield, B.D. Kubitz, K.A., & Salazar, W. (1991). A meta-analysis on the anxiety reducing effects of acute and chronic exercise. *Sports Medicine, 11*, 301–310.

Petty, R.E., & Cacioppo, J.T. (1981). *Attitudes and persuasion: Classic and contemporary approaches*. Dubuque, IA: Brown.

Phares, F. (1957). Expectancy changes in skill and chance situations. *Journal of Abnormal and Social Psychology, 54*, 339–342.

Philips, S.P. (1997). Problem-based learning in

medicine: New curriculum, old stereotypes. *Social Science and Medicine, 45*, 497–499.

Phillips, K.D., & Morrow, J.H. (1998). Nursing management of anxiety in HIV infection. *Issues in Mental Health Nursing, 19*, 375–397.

Phillips, S. (1996). Sexual harassment of female physicians by patients. What is to be done? *Canadian Family Physician, 42*, 73–76.

Pickett, W., Hartling, L., & Brison, R.J. (1997). A population-based study of hospitalized injuries in Kingston, Ontario, identified via the Canadian Hospitals Injury Reporting and Prevention Program. *Chronic Diseases in Canada, 18*, 61–69.

Pierce, J.P., Choi, W.S., Gilpin, E.A., Farkas, A.J., & Berry, C.C. (1998). Tobacco industry promotion of cigarettes and adolescent smoking. *Journal of the American Medical Association, 279*, 511–515.

Pinder, R. (1990). *The management of chronic disease: patient and doctor perspectives on Parkinson's disease*. London: MacMillan Press.

Piotrowski, C. (1998). Assessment of pain: A survey of practicing clinicians. *Perceptual and Motor Skills, 86*, 181–182.

Pisano, E.D., Earp, J., & Gallant, T.L. (1998). Screening mammography behavior after a false positive mammogram. *Cancer Detection and Prevention, 22*, 161–167.

Pisano, E.D., Earp, J., Schell, M., Vokaty, K., & Denham, A. (1998). Screening behavior of women after a false-positive mammogram. *Radiology, 208*, 245–249.

Pistrang, N., Barker, C., & Rutter, C. (1997). Social support as conversation: Analysing breast cancer patients' interactions with their partners. *Social Science and Medicine, 45*, 773–782.

Plotnik, R. (1989). *Introduction to psychology, 2nd edition*, New York: McGraw-Hill.

Polleri, A. (1992). Pain and sex steroids. In F. Sicuteri (Ed.), *Advances in pain research and therapy: Vol. 20.* (pp. 253–259). New York: Raven.

Pomerleau, O.F. (1979). Behavioral factors in the establishment, maintenance, and cessation of smoking. In *Smoking and health: A report of the Surgeon General*, pp. 16–31. Washington, D.C.: GPO.

Pomerleau, O.F., & Pomerleau, C.S. (1989). A biobehavioral perspective on smoking. In T. Ney & A. Gale (Eds.), *Smoking and human behavior*. New York: Wiley.

Pomerleau, O.F., Collins, A.C., Shiffman, S., & Pomerleau, C.S. (1993). Why some people smoke and others do not: New perspectives. *Journal of Consulting and Clinical Psychology, 61*, 723–731.

Pomeroy, W.B. (1972). *Dr. Kinsey and the institute for sex research*. New York: Harper & Row.

Poole, G. D., & Kallhood, L. (1996). Technologists' perceptions of patient stress and technologists' helping strategies: Survey results. *Radiaction*, April, pp. 19–20.

Poole, G.D., & Craig, K.D. (1992). Judgments of genuine, suppressed, and faked facial expressions of pain. *Journal of Personality and Social Psychology, 63*, 797–805.

Poole, G.D., & Ting, K. (1995). Cultural differences between Euro-Canadian and Indo-Canadian maternity patients. *Journal of Social Psychology, 135*, 631–644.

Poole, G.D., Poon, C., Achille, M., White, K., Franz, N., Jittler, S., Watt, K., Cox, D.N., Doll, R. Social Support for Prostate Cancer Patients: The Effect of Support Groups (submitted for publication).

Porteous, A. & Tyndall, J. (1994). Yes, I want to walk to the OR. *Canadian Operating Room Nursing Journal, 12*, 15–25.

Posse, M., & Haellstrom, T. (1998). Alexithymia, personality characteristics, and somatization tendency in different physical diseases. *European Journal of Psychiatry, 12*, 215–224.

Pound, P., Bury, M, Gompertz, P., & Ebrahim, S. (1995). Stroke patients' views on their admission to hospital. *British Medical Journal, 311*, 18–22.

Pratt, J.P., Overfield, T., & Hilton, H.G. (1994). Health behaviours of nurses and general population women. *Health Values, 18(5)*, 41–46.

Pratt, L.A., Ford, D.E., Crum, R.M. et al., (1996). Depression, psychotropic medication, and risk of myocardial infarction: Prospective data from the Baltimore ECA follow-up. *Circulation, 94*, 3123–3129.

Prescott, L.M., Harley, J.P., & Klein, D.A. (1999). *Microbiology, 4th ed.* Boston: WCB/McGraw-Hill.

Prochaska, J.O., & DiClemente, C.C. (1983). Stages and processes of self-change of smoking: Toward an integrative model of change. *Journal of Consulting and Clinical Psychology, 51*, 390–395.

Prochaska, J.O., & DiClemente, C.C. (1986). Toward a comprehensive model of change. In Miller, W.R., Heather, N. et al., (Eds.) *Treating addictive behaviors: Processes of change. Applied clinical psychology*. (pp. 3–27). New York: Plenum Press.

Prochaska, J.O., & Velicer, 1997). The transtheoretical model of health behavior change. *American Journal of Health Promotion, 12*, 38–48.

Prokop, C.K., Bradley, L.A., Burish, T.G., Anderson, K.O., & Fox, J.E. (1991). *Health psychology: Clinical methods and research*. New York: MacMillan.

Pryse-Phillips, W., Findlay, H., Tugwell, P., Edmeads, J., et al. (1992). A Canadian population survey on the clinical, epidemiological and societal impact of migraine and tension-type headache. *Canadian Journal of Neurol Sci, 19*, 333–339.

Ptacek, J.T., Fries, E.A., Eberhardt, T.L., & Ptacek, J.J. (1999). Breaking bad news to patients: Physicians; perceptions of the process. *Support and Care for Cancer, 7(3)*, 113–120.

Quirk, M., & Wapner, S. (1995). Environmental psychology and health. *Environment and Behavior, 27*, 90–99.

Rachman, S., & Taylor, S. (1993). Analysis of claustrophobia. *Journal of Anxiety Disorders, 7*, 1–11.

Radojevic, V., Nicassio, P.M., & Weisman, M.H. (1992). Behavioral intervention with and without family support for rheumatoid arthritis. *Behavior Therapy, 23*, 13–30.

Raglan, J.S., & Morgan, W.P. (1987). Influence of exercise and "distraction therapy" on state anxiety and blood pressure. *Medicine and Science in Sport and Exercise, 19*, 456–463.

Rains, J.C., Penzien, D.B., & Jamison, R.N. (1992). A structured approach to the management of chronic pain. In L. VandeCreek, S. Knapp, & T.L. Jackson (Eds.), I*nnovations in clinical practice: A source book. Vol. 11* (pp. 521–539). Sarasota, FL: Professional Resource Press.

Ramachandran, V.S. (1993). Behavioral and magnetoencephalographic correlates of plasticity in the adult human brain. *Proceedings of the National Academy of Science USA, 90*, 10413–10420.

Ramirez, A.J., T.K., Craig, Watson, J.P., Fentiman, I.S., North, W.R., & Rubens, R.D. (1989). Stress and relapse of breast cancer. *British Medical Journal, 298*, 291–293.

Ramirez, A.J., Westcombe, A.M., Burgess, C.C., Sutton, S., Littlejohns, P. & Richards, M.A. (1999). Factors predicting delayed presentation of symptomatic breast cancer: A systematic review. *The Lancet, 353*, 1127–1131.

Raphael, B., & Emmerson B. (1991). Are patients clients or people? *Medical Journal of Australia, 154*, 183–184.

Rapp, R. (1993). Accounting for amniocentisis. In S. Lindenbaum, & M. Lock (Eds.), Knowledge, power & practice: *The anthropology of medicine and everyday life* (pp. 55–76). Berkeley, CA: University of California Press.

Raps, C.S., Peterson, C., Jonas, M., & Seligman, M.E.P. (1982). Patient behavior in hospitals: Helplessness, reactance, or both? *Journal of Personality and Social Psychology, 42*, 1036–1041.

Raven, B.H. (1974). The comparative analysis of power and influence. In J.T. Tedeschi (Ed.), *Perspectives on social power*. Chicago: Aldine.

Raven, B.H., Freeman, H.E., & Haley, R.W. (1982). Social science perspectives in hospital infection control. In A.W. Johnson, O. Grusky, & B. Raven (Eds.), *Contemporary health services: Social science perspectives* (pp. 139–176). Boston, MA: Auburn House.

Reading, A.E. (1989). Testing pain mechanisms in persons in pain. In P.D. Wall & R. Melzack (Eds.), *Textbook of pain (2nd ed.)*. Edinburgh: Churchill Livingstone.

Reading, J. (1997). The tobacco report. First Nations and Inuit Regional Health Survey. Ottawa, ON: Health Canada.

Rehm, J.T., Bondy, S.J., Sempos, C.T., & Vuong, C.V. (1997). Alcohol consumption and coronary heart disease morbidity and mortality. *American Journal of Epidemiology, 146*, 495–501.

Reiss, D., Steinglass, P. & Howe, G. (1993). The family's organization around the illness. In R.E. Cole & D. Reiss (Eds.), *How do families cope with chronic illness* (pp. 173–213). Hillsdale, New Jersey: Lawrence Erlbaum.

Rejeski, W.J., Hardy, C.H., & Shaw, J. (1991). Psychometric confounds of assessing state anxiety in conjunction with acute bouts of vigorous exercise. *Journal of Sport and Exercise Psychology, 13*, 65–74.

Report on the health of Canadians. Prepared by the Federal, Provincial, and Territorial Advisory Committee on Population Health for the meeting of Ministers of Health, Toronto, Canada, September 10–11, 1996.

Resnick, B. (1996). Motivation in geriatric rehabilitation. IMAGE: *Journal of Nursing Scholarship, 28*, 41–45.

Reverby, S.M. (1993). Other tales of the nursing-feminism connection. *Nursing and*

Health Care, 14, 296–301.

Reynolds, D.V. (1969). Surgery in the rat during electrical anesthesia induced by focal brain stimulation. *Science, 164*, 444–445.

Reynolds, P., & Kaplan, G.A. (1990). Social connections and risk for cancer: Prospective evidence from the Alameda County Study. *Behavioral Medicine, 16*, 101–110.

Rice, P.R. *Stress and health (3rd ed.)*. Pacific Grove, California: Brooks/Cole.

Richards, J.S., Nepomuceno, C., Riles, M., & Suer, Z. (1982). Assessing pain behavior: The UAB Pain Behavior Scale. *Pain, 14*, 393–398.

Richards, M.A., Westcombe, A.M., Love, S.B., Littlejohns, P., & Ramirez, A.J. (1999). Influence of delay on survival in patients with breast cancer: A systematic review. *The Lancet, 353*, 1119–1126.

Richards, T. (1990). Chasms in communication. *British Medical Journal, 301*, 1407–1408.

Richardsen, A.M., & Burke, R.J. (1991). Occupational stress and job satisfaction among Canadian physicians. *Work and Stress, 5*, 301–313.

Richardson, J.L., Zarnegar, Z., Bisno, B, et al. (1990). Psychosocial status at initiation of cancer treatment and survival. *Journal of Psychosomatic Research, 34*, 189–201.

Rieger, E., Touyz, S.W., & Wain, G.V. (1998). *Journal of Psychosomatic Research, 45*, 201–214.

Riley, J.L. III., Robinson, M.E., Wise, E.A., Myers, C.D., & Fillingim, R.B. (1998). Sex differences in the perception of noxious experimental stimuli: A meta-analysis. *Pain, 74*, 181–187.

Rithotz, M.D., & Jacobson, A.M. (1998). Living with hypoglycemia. *Journal of General Internal Medicine, 13*, 799–804.

Roberts, C.M., & Smith, P.R. (1999). Attitudes and behaviour of children toward peers with disabilities. *International Journal of Disability, Development and Education, 46*, 35–50.

Robins, L.N. (1995). Editorial: the natural history of substance use as a guide to setting drug policy. *American Journal of Public Health, 85*, 12–13.

Robinson, D. (1973, July 15). Ten noted doctors answer ten tough questions. Parade.

Robinson, M.E., Riley, J.L., Myers, C.D., Papas, R.K., et al. (1999, October). Gender role expectations of pain: Do they explain the sex differences? Poster session presented at the annual meeting of the American Pain Society, Fort Lauderdale, FL.

Rodin, J. & Janis, I.L. (1982). In H.S. Friedman & M.R. DiMatteo (Eds.), *Interpersonal Issues in Health Care* (pp. 33–49). New York: Academic Press.

Rodin, J., & Salovey, P. (1989). Health psychology. *Annual Review of Psychology, 40*, 533–579.

Rodrigue, J.R., & Hoffman, R.G. (1994). Caregivers of adults with cancer: multidimensional correlates of psychological distress. *Journal of Clinical Psychology in Medical Settings, 1*, 231–244.

Roland, M.O., Bartholomew, J., Courtney, M.J.F., Morris, R.W., & Morrell, D.C. (1986). The "five minute" consultation: Effect of time constraint on verbal communication. *British Medical Journal, 292*, 874–876.

Rose, J.S., Chassin, L., Presson, C.C., & Sherman, S.J. (1996). Prospective predictors of quit attempts and smoking cessation in young adults. *Health Psychology, 15*, 261–268.

Rosen, D.M., Lam, A.M., Carlton, M.A., Cario, G.M., & McGride, L. (1998). Analgesia following major gynecological laparoscopic surgery—PCA versus intermittent intramuscular injection. *Journal of the Society of Laparoendoscopic Surgery, 2(1)*, 25–29.

Rosen, D.S., & Neumark-Sztainer, D. (1997). Review of options for primary prevention of eating disturbances among adolescents. *Journal of Adolescent Health, 23(6)*, 354–363.

Rosenberger, P.H., Bornstein, R.a., nasrallay, R.H., et al., (1993). Psychopathology in human immunodeficiency virus infection: Lifetime and current assessment. *Comprehensive Psychiatry, 34*, 150–158.

Rosenstock, I.M. (1974). Historical origins of the health belief model. Health Education *Monographs, 2*, 328–335.

Rosenstock, I.M., Strecher, V.J., & Becker, M.H. (1994). The Health Belief Model and HIV risk behavior change. In R.J. DiClemente & J.L. Peterson (Eds.), *Preventing AIDS: Theories and methods of behavioral interventions* (pp. 5–25). New York: Plenum.

Roseveare, C., Seavell, C., Patel, P., Criswell, J., Kimble, J., Jones, C., & Shepherd, H. (1998). Patient-controlled sedation and analgesia, using propofol and alfentanil, during colonoscopy: A prospective randomized controlled trail. *Endoscopy, 30*, 768–773.

Ross, C.E., & Duff, R.S. (1982). The effects of client characteristics, type of practice and experiences with care. *Journal of Health and Social Behavior, 23*, 119–131.

Ross, D. (1998). Rethinking child poverty. *Canadian Council on Social Development, 22*, 9–11.

Rosser, W.W. (1996). Approach to diagnosis by primary care clinicians and specialists: Is there a difference? *Journal of Family Practice, 42*, 139–144.

Roter, D.L., & Hall, J.A. (1998). Why physician gender matters in shaping the physician-patient relationship. *Journal of Women's Health, 7*, 1093–1097.

Roter, D.L., Hall, J.A., Merisca, R., Nordstrom, B., et al. (1998). Effectiveness of interventions to improve patient compliance: A meta-analysis. *Medical Care, 36*, 1138–1161.

Roter, D.L., Stewart, M., Putnam, S.M., Lipkin, M., Jr., et al. (1997). Communication patterns of primary care physicians. *Journal of the American Medical Association, 277*, 350–356.

Rotter, J. (1996). Generalized expectancies for internal versus external control of reinforcement. *Psychological Monographs, 80*, (Whole issue).

Rouse, B.A. (Ed.). (1998). Substance abuse and mental health statistics source book. Rockville, MD: Department of Health and Human Services: Substance Abuse and Mental Health Services Administration.

Roux, S., Markle, L., & Diamond, A. (1998). False positive rate for screening mammography. *New England Journal of Medicine, 339*, 561.

Rowbotham, M.C., & Lowenstien, D.H. (1990). Neurolgic ocnsequences of cocaine use. In W.P. Creger, C.H. Coggins, & E.W. Hancock (Eds.), *Annual review of medicine (Vol. 41)*. Palo Alto, CA: Annual Reviews.

Rowley, B.B., Baldwin, D.C., & McGuire, M.B. (1991). Selected characteristics of graduate medical education in the United States. *Journal of the American Medical Association, 266*, 933–943.

Rozanski, A., Blumenthal, J.A., & Kaplan, J. (1999). Impact of psychological factors on the pathogenesis of cardiovascular disease and implications for therapy. *Circulation, 99*, 2192–2217.

Rudolph, D.L., & Butki, B.D. (1998). Self-efficacy and affective responses to short bouts of exercise. *Journal of Applied Sport Psychology, 10*, 268–280.

Rudolph, K.D., Dennig, M.D., & Weisz, J. R. (1995). Determinants and consequences of children's coping in the medical setting: Conceptualization, review and critique. *Psychological Bulletin, 118*, 328–357.

Ruedy, J., Kaufman, D.M., & MacLeod, H. (1999). Alternative and complementary medicine in Canadian medical schools: A survey. *Canadian Medical Association Journal, 160*, 816–817.

Rushall, B.S., (1984). The content of competition thinking. In W.F. Straub and J.M. Williams (Eds.), *Cognitive Sport Psychology*. Lansing, Michigan: Sport Science Associates.

Russell, N.K., & Roter, D.L. (1993). Health promotion counseling of chronic-disease patients during primary care visits. *American Journal of Public Health, 83*, 979–982.

Russell, S. (1999). An exploratory study of patients' perceptions, memories and experiences in an intensive care unit. *Journal of Advanced Nursing, 29*, 783–791.

Rutledge, T., & Linden, W. (in press). Psychological risk factors moderate pharmacological treatment effects among ischemic heart disease patients. *Psychosomatic Medicine*.

Rutter, D.R., Quine, L., & Chesham, D.J. (1995). Predicting safe riding behaviour and accidents: Demography, beliefs, and behaviour in motorcycling safety. *Psychology and Health, 10*, 369–386.

Saarinen-Rahiika, H., & Binkley, J.M. (1998). Problem-based learning in physical therapy: A review of the literature and overview of the McMaster University experience. *Physical Therapy, 78*, 195–207.

Sabir, S., Godwin, M., & Birtwhistle, R. (1997). Men and women residents' experiences with women's health care in a family medicine center. *Academic Medicine, 72*, 293–295.

Sacco, R.L., Elkind, M., Boden-Albala, B.I., Feng, L., et al. (1999). The protective effect of moderate alcohol consumption on ischemic stroke. *Journal of the American Medical Association, 281*, 53–60.

Sachs, B.C. (1992). Coping with cancer. *Stress medicine, 8*, 167–170.

Safer, M.A., Tharps, Q.J., Jackson, T.C., & Leventhal, H. (1979). Determinants of three stages of delay in seeking care at a medical care clinic. *Medical Care, 17*, 11–29.

Sainsbury, R., Johnston, C., & Haward, B. (1999). Effect on survival of delays in referral of patients with breast-cancer symptoms: A retrospective analysis. *The Lancet, 353*, 1132–1135.

Saldana, L. & Peterson, L. (1997). Preventing injury in children: The need for parental involvement. In T.S. Watson & F.M. Gresham (Eds.), *Handbook of child behavior therapy* (pp. 221–238). New York: Plenum Press.

Salmenperae, L., Suominen T., & Lauri, S. (1998). Oncology nurses' attitudes towards alternative medicine. *Psycho-oncology, 7*, 453–459.

Salovey, P., O'Leary, A., Stretton, M.S., Fishkin, S.A., & Drake, C.A. (1991). Influence of mood on judgments about health and illness. In J.P. Firgas (Ed.), *Emotion and social judgments* (pp. 241–262).

Samora, J., Saunders, L., & Larson, R.F. (1961). Medical vocabulary knowledge among hospital patients. *Journal of Health and Social Behavior, 2*, 83–89.

Sampson, W. (1999). Alternative Medicine: How to spot the flaws in published research. Presentation to Simon Fraser University, Burnaby, B.C., November 16, 1999.

Sanderson, B.K., Raczynski, J.M., Cornell, C.E., Hardin, M., & Taylor, H.A., Jr. (1998). *American Journal of Epidemiology, 149*, 489.

Sarafino, E.P. (1998). *Health psychology: Biopsychosocial interactions*. New York: John Wiley and Sons.

Savage, S.A., & Clarke, V.A. (1996). Factors associated with screening mammography and breast self-examination intentions. *Health Education Research, 11*, 409–421.

Schachter, S. (1981). Recidivism and self-cure of smoking and obesity. *American Psychologist, 31*, 436–444.

Schacter, S. (1982). Recidivism and self-cure of smoking and obesity. *American Psychologist, 37*, 436–444.

Scheifer, S.J., Keller, S.E., Camerino, M., Thornton, J.C., & Stein, M. (1983). Suppression of lymphocyte stimulation following bereavement. *Journal of the American Medical Association, 250*, 374–377.

Scheifer, S.J., Keller, S.E., Meyerson, A.T., Raskin, M.J., Davis, K.L., & Stein, M. (1984). Lymphocyte function in major depressive disorder. *Archives of General Psychiatry, 41*, 484–486.

Schleifer, S.J., Macari-Hinson, M.M., Coyle, D.A., Slater, W.R., Kahn, M., Gorlin, R., et al., (1989). The nature and course of depression following myocardial infarction. *Archives of Internal Medicine, 149*, 1785–1789.

Schmale, A.H., Jr., & Engel, G.L. (1967). The giving up-given up complex illustrated on film. *Archives of General Psychiatry, 17*, 135–145.

Schroder, I.M. (1971). Conceptual complexity and personality organization. In Schroder, H.M. & Suedfeld, P. (Eds.), *Personality theory and information processing* (pp. 240–273). New York: Ronald Press.

Schubert, D., Burns, Paras, W., & Sioson, E. (1992). Increase of medical hospital length of stay by depression in stroke and amputation patients: A pilot study. *Psychotherapy and Psychosomatics, 57*, 61–66.

Schuckit, M.A. (1996). Recent developments in the pharmacotherapy of alcohol dependence. *Journal of Consulting and Clinical Psychology, 64*, 669–676.

Schulz, R., Bookwalla, J., Knapp, J.E., Scheier, & Williamson, G.M. (1996). Pessimism, age, and cancer mortality. *Psychology and Aging, 11*, 304–309.

Schutz, J., & Luthe, W. (1959). *Autogenic training: A psychophysiological approach to psychotherapy.* New York: Grune and Stratton.

Schwam, K. (1998). The phenomenon of compassion fatigue in perioperative nursing. *AORN Journal, 68*, 642–645, 647–648.

Schwartz, G.E., & Weiss, S.M. (1978). Behavioral medicine revisited: An amended definition. *Journal of Behavioral Medicine, 1*, 249–251.

Scott, C.G., & Ambroson, D.L. (1994). The rocky road to change: Implications for substance abuse programs on college campuses. *Journal of American College Health, 42*, 291–296.

Scott, V.J., & Gallagher, E.M. (1999). Mortality and morbidity related to injuries from falls in British Columbia. *Canadian Journal of Public Health, 90*, 343–347.

Segall, A., & Roberts, L.W. (1980). A comparative analysis of physician estimates and levels of medical knowledge among patients. *Sociology of Health and Illness, 2(3)*, 317–334.

Seligman, M.E.P. (1975). *Helplessness*. San Francisco: Freeman.

Sellick, S.M., & Zaza, C. (1998). Critical review of 5 nonpharmacologic strategies for managing cancer pain. *Cancer Prevention and Control, 2(1)*, 7–14.

Sellwood, W., & Tarrier, N. (1994). Demographic factors associated with extreme non-compliance in schizophrenia. *Social Psychiatry and Psychiatric Epidemiology, 29*, 172–177.

Selye, H. (1974). *Stress without distress*. Philadelphia: Lippincott.

Selye, H. (1976). *Stress in health and disease*. Woburn, MA: Butterworth.

Selye, H. (1956). *The stress of life*. New York: McGraw-Hill.

Selye, H. (1993). History of the stress concept. In L. Goldenberger and S. Breznitz (Eds.), *Handbook of stress: Theoretical and clinical aspects* (pp. 7–17). New York: Free Press.

Sexton, M.M. (1979). Behavioral epidemiology. In O.F. Pomerleau & J.P. Brady (Eds.), *Behavioral medicine: Theory and practice* (pp. 3–22). Baltimore MD: Williams & Wilkins.

Seymour, G.J., Savage, N.W., & Walsh, L.J. (1995). *Immunology: An introduction for the health sciences*. Roseville, NSW: McGraw-Hill Australia.

Sgoutas-Emch, S.A., Cacioppo, J.T., Uchino, B.N., Malarkey, W., Pearl, D., Kiecolt-Glaser, J.K., & Glaser, R. (1994). The effects of an acute psychological stressor on cardiovascular, endocrine, and cellular immune response: A prospective study of individuals high and low in heart reactivity. *Psychophysiology, 31*, 264–271.

Shapiro, S. (1977). Evidence on screening for breast cancer from randomised trial. *Cancer, 39*, 2772–2782.

Shekelle, R.B., Raynor, W.J., Ostfeld, A.M., Garron, D.C., Bieliauskas, L.A., Liu, S.C., Maliza, C., & Paul, O. (1981). Psychological depression and 17-year risk of death from cancer. Psychosomatic *Medicine, 43*, 117–125.

Sheps, D.S., Sheffield, D., & Carney, R.M. (1999). Does depression predict more symptoms or more disease? *American Heart Journal, 137*, 386–387.

Sher, K.J., & Levenson, R.W. (1982). Risk for alcoholism and individual differences in the stress-response-dampening effect of alcohol. *Journal of Abnormal Psychology, 91*, 350–367.

Sheridan, M. (1992). *Pain in America*. Tuscaloosa: University of Alabama Press.

Shields-Poe, D., & Pinelli, J. (1997). Variables associated with parental stress in neonatal intensive care units. *Neonatal Network, 16*, 29–37

Shiffman, S., Paty, J.A., Gnys, M., Kassel, J.D., & Elash, C. (1995). Nicotine withdrawal in chippers and regular smokers: Subjective and cognitive effects. *Health Psychology, 14*, 301–309.

Shifren, K., Bauserman, R., & Carter, D.B. (1993). Gender role orientation and physical health: A study among young adults. *Sex Roles, 29*, 421–432.

Shlain, L. (1979). Cancer is not a four-letter word. In C.A. Garfield, (Ed.), *Stress and survival: The emotional realities of life-threatening illness*. St. Louis: C.V. Mosby.

Shopland, D.R., & Burns, D.M. (1993). Medical and public health implications of tobacco addiction. In C.T. Orleans & J. Slade (Eds.) *Nicotine addiction: Principles and management*. New York: Oxford University Press.

Shuler, M.E., & Nair, P. (1999). Brief report: Frequency of maternal cocaine use during pregnancy and infant neurobehavioural outcome. *Journal of Pediatric Psychology, 24*, 511–514.

Sidney, S., Beck, J.E., Tekawa, I.S., Quesenberry, C.P., & Friedman, G.D. (1997). Marijuana use and mortality. *American Journal of Public Health, 87*, 585–590.

Silverman, J., Kurtz, S. & Draper, J. (1998). *Skills for communicating with patients*. Radcliffe Medical Press: Abingdon, Oxon, UK.

Simkins, L. (1982). Biofeedback: Clinically valid or oversold? *Psychological Record, 32*, 3–17.

Simpson, M., Buckman, R., Stewart, M., Maguire, P., et al. (1991). Doctor-patient communication: The Toronto consensus statement. *British Medical Journal, 303*, 1385–1367.

Sinclair, S. (1997). *Making doctors: An institutional apprenticeship*. Oxford: Berg.

Sist, T.C., Florio, G.A., Miner, M.F., Lema, M.J., & Zevon, M.A. (1998). The relationship between depression and pain language in cancer and chronic non-cancer pain patients. *Journal of Pain and Symptom Management, 15*, 350–358.

Sluijs, E.M., Kerssens, J.J., van der Zee, J., & Myers, L.B. (1998). Adherence to physiotherapy. In L.B. Meyers, Midence, K., et al., (Eds.), *Adherence to treatment in medical conditions*. Amsterdam: Harwood Academic.

Smart, G. (1997). Helping children relax during magnetic resonance imaging. American

Journal of Maternity and Child Nursing, 22, 236–241.

Smith, J.C. (1993). *Understanding stress and coping*. New York: MacMillan.

Smith, L., & Bassett, C. (1996). Introducing change to the post-anaesthetic care unit. *Nursing Standard, 11(9)*, 36–38.

Smith, R.E. (1980). Development of an integrated coping response through cognitive-affective stress management training. In I.G. Sarason and C.D. Spielberger (Eds.), *Stress and anxiety (Vol.7)*. Washington, D.C.: Hemisphere Publishing Corporation.

Smith, R.E. (1999). Generalization effects in coping skills training. *Journal of Sport and Exercise Psychology, 21*, 189–204.

Sobel, L.C., Sobel, M.B., Toneatto, T., & Leo, G.I. (1993). What triggers the resolution of alcohol problems without treatment? *Alcoholism: Clinical and Experimental Research, 17*, 217–224.

Sohara, N., Takagi, H., Abe, T., Hashimoto, Y., Kojiina, A., Takahashi, H., Nagamine, T., & Mori, M. (1999). *Supportive Care in Cancer, 7(2)*, 84–88.

Solomon, G.F., & Moos, R.H. (1964). Emotions, immunity and disease: A speculative theoretical integration. *Archives of General Psychiatry, 11*, 657–674.

Sonstroem, R.J. (1997). Physical activity and self-esteem. In W.P. Morgan (Ed.), *Physical activity and mental health* (pp. 127–143). Washington, DC: Taylor and Francis.

Spencer, J., Young, M.E., Rintala, D., & Bates, S. (1995). Socialization to the culture of a rehabilitation hospital: an ethnographic study. *Journal of Occupational Therapy, 49*, 53–62.

Spiegel, D. & Bloom, J.R. (1983). Group therapy and hypnosis reduce metastatic breast carcinoma pain. *Psychosomatic Medicine, 45*, 333–339.

Spiegel, D., Bloom, J.R., Kraemer, H.C., & Gottheil, E. (1989). Psychological support for cancer patients. *Lancet, 2*, 1447.

Spiegel, D., Sephton, S.E., Terr, A.I., & Stites, D.P. (1998). Effects of psychosocial treatment in prolonging cancer survival may be mediated by neuroimmune pathways. *Annals of the New York Academy of Sciences, 840*, 674–683.

Stacy, A.W., Sussman, S., Dent, C.W., Burton, D., & Flay, B.R. (1992). Moderators of peer social influence in adolescent smoking. *Personality and Social Psychology Bulletin, 18*, 163–172.

Stainer, U.M., Grond, S., & Maier, C. (1999). Responders and non-responders to post-operative pain treatment: The loading dose predicts analgesic needs. *European Journal of Anaesthesiology, 16,* 103–110.

Stanton, W.R., Mahalski, P.A., McGee, R., & Silva, P.A. (1993). Reasons for smoking or not smoking in early adolescence. *Addictive Behaviors, 18*, 321–329.

Starfield, B., Wray, C., Hess, K., Gross, R., et al. (1981). The influence of patient-practitioner agreement on outcome of care. *American Journal of Public Health, 71*, 127–131.

Statistics Canada (1999). *Toward a Healthy Future: Second Report on the Health of Canadians*. Ottawa, Ontario.

Steele, C.M., & Josephs, R.A. (1990). Alcohol myopia: Its prized and dangerous effects. *American Psychologist, 45*, 921–933.

Steffens, D.C., O'Connor, C.M., Jiang, W.J., Pieper, C.F., et al. (1999). The effect of major depression on functional status in patients with coronary artery disease. *Journal of the American Geriatric Society, 47*, 319–322.

Stegen, K., Neujens, A., Crombez, G., Hermans, D., et al. Negative affect, respiratory reactivity, and somatic complaints in a CO2 enriched air inhalation paradigm. *Biological Psychology, 49*, 109–122.

Steginga, S., Occhipinti, S., Wilson, K., & Dunn, J. (1998). Domains of distress: The experience of breast cancer in Australia. *Oncology Nursing Forum, 25*, 1063–1070.

Stein, P.N., & Motta, R.W. (1992). Effects of aerobic and nonaerobic exercise on depression and self-concept. *Perceptual Motor Skills, 74*, 79–89.

Steinhausen, H.C., Winkler, C., & Meier, M. (1997). Eating disorders in adolescence in a Swiss epidemiological study. *International Journal of Eating Disorders, 22*, 247–251.

Stenstroem, U., Wikby, A., Andersson, P., & Ryden, O. (1998). Relationship between locus of control beliefs and metabolic control in insulin-dependent diabetes mellitus. *British Journal of Health Psychology, 3*, 15–25.

Sternbach, R.A. (1968). *Pain: A psychophysiological analysis*. New York: Academic Press.

Sternbach, R.A. (1974). *Pain patients: Traits and treatment*. Academic Press, New York.

Sternbach, R.A. (1986). Clinical aspects of pain. In R.A. Sternbach (Ed.), *The psychology of pain (2nd ed.)*. New York: Raven Press.

Sternbach, R.A. (1989). Acute versus chronic pain. In P.D. Wall & R. Melzack (Eds.), *Textbook of pain (2nd ed.)*. Edinburgh: Churchill Livingstone.

Stewart, M. A, Brown, J. B, Levenstein, J.H. , McCracken, E., & McWhinney, I.R. (1986). The patient-centered clinical method: Changes in residents' performance over two months of training. *Family Practice, 3*, 164–167.

Stewart, M.A., Brown, J.B., Weston, W.W., McWhinney, I.R., et al. (1999). *Patient-centred medicine: Transforming the clinical method*. Thousand Oaks: Sage.

Stewart, M.A., McWhinney, I.R., & Buck, C.W. (1979). The doctor-patient relationship and its effect upon outcome. *Journal of the Royal College of General Practice, 29*, 77–82.

Stice, E. (1994). Relation of media exposure to eating disorder symptomology: An examination of mediating mechanisms. *Journal of Abnormal Psychology, 103*, 836–840.

Stoller, E.P. (1984). Self-assessments of health by the elderly: The impact of informal assistance. *Journal of Health and Social Behavior, 25*, 260–270.

Stone, A.A., Cox, D.S., Valdimarsdottir, H., Jandorf, L., & Neale, J.M. (1987). Evidence that secretory IgA antibody is associated with daily mood. *Journal of Personality and Social Psychology, 52*, 988–993.

Stone, A.A., Neale, J.M., Cox, D.S., Napoli, A., Valdimarsdottir, H., & Kennedy-Moore, E. (1994). Daily events are associated with a secretory immune response to an oral antigen in men. *Health Psychology, 13*, 440–446.

Story, M., French, S.A., Resnick, M.D., et al. (1995). Ethnic/racial and socioeconomic differences in dieting behaviors and body image perceptions in adolescents. International *Journal of Eating Disorders, 18*, 173–179.

Strauss, G.J. (1996). Psychological factors in intensive management of insulin dependent diabetes mellitus. *Nursing Clinics of North America, 31*, 737–745.

Strauss, R. (1957). The nature and status of medical sociology, *American Sociological Review, 22*, 200–204.

Strecher, V.J., Champion, V.L., & Rosenstock, I.M. (1997). The health belief model and health behavior. In Gochman, D.S. et al. (Eds.). *Handbook of health behaviour research 1: Personal and social determinants* (pp. 71–91). New York: Plenum Press.

Streltzer, J. (1997). Pain. In W-S. Tseng, & J. Streltzer (Eds.), *Culture and psychopathology: A guide to clinical assessment* (pp. 87–100). New York: Brunner/Mazel.

Struckman-Johnson, C., Struckman-Johnson, D., Gilliland, R.C., & Ausman, A. (1994). Effective persuasive appeals in AIDS PSAs and condom commercials on intentions to use condoms. *Journal of Applied Social Psychology, 24*, 2223–2244.

Stuber, M.L. (1995). Stress responses to pediatric cancer: A family phenomenon. *Family Systems Medicine, 13*, 163–172.

Stuijs, E.M., Kerssens, J.J., van der Zee, J., Myers, L.B. (1998). Adherence to physiotherapy. In L.B. Myers, K. Midence et al. (Eds.), *Adherence to treatment in medical conditions* (pp. 363–382). Amsterdam: Harwood Academic Publishers.

Suinn, R. (1972). Behavioral rehearsal training for ski racers. *Behavior Therapy, 3*, 519.

Sullivan, P. (1990). Women close in on 50% share of places in Canada's medical schools. *Canadian Medical Association Journal, 143*, 781–783.

Sunshine, A., & Olson, N.Z. (1989). Non-narcotic analgesics. In P.D. Wall & R. Melzack (Eds.), *Textbook of pain (2nd ed.)*. Edinburgh: Churchill Livingstone.

Susser, M., & Susser, E. (1996). Choosing a future for epidemiology: I. Eras and paradigms. *American Journal of Public Health, 86*, 668–673.

Sutton, S., Saidi, G., Bickler, G., & Hunter, J. (1995). Does routine screening for breast cancer raise anxiety? Results from a three wave prospective study in England. *Journal of Epidemiology and Community Health, 49*, 413–418.

Sutton, S.R., & Eiser, J.R. (1984). The effect of fear-arousing communications on cigarette smoking: An expectancy-value approach. *Journal of Behavioral Medicine, 7*, 13–34.

Svarstad, B.L. (1974). The doctor-patient encounter: an observational study of communication and outcome. Doctoral dissertation, University of Wisconsin, Madison.

Swain, L., Catlin, G., & Beaudet, M.P. 91999). The National Population Health Survey—its longitudinal nature. *Health Reports, 10(4)*, 69–82.

Szasz, T.S., & Hollender, M.H. (1956). A contribution to the philosophy of medicine. The basic models of the doctor-patient relationship. *Archives of Internal Medicine, 97*, 585–592.

Tabar, L., Fagerberg, G., Duffy, S., & Day, N.

(1989). The Swedish two-country trial of mammographic screening for breast cancer: Recent results and calculations of benefit. *Journal of Epidemiology and Community Health, 43*, 107–114.

Taggart, H.M., & Connor, S.E. (1995). The relation of exercise habits to health beliefs and knowledge about osteoporosis. *Journal of American College Health, 44*, 127–130.

Tagliacozzo, D.L., & Mauksch, H.O. (1972). The patient's view of the patient's role. In E.G. Jaco (Ed.), *Patients, physicians, and illness* (2nd ed., pp. 172–185).

Takeda, W., & Wessel, J. (1994). Acupuncture for the treatment of pain in osteoarthritic knees. *Arthritis Care and Research, 7*, 118–122.

Tannock, I.F., & Warr, D.G. (1998). Unconventional therapies for cancer: A refuge from the rules of evidence? *Canadian Medical Association Journal, 159*, 801–802.

Tate, A.K., & Petruzzello, S.J. (1995). Varying the intensity of acute exercise: Implications for changes in affect. *Journal of Sports Medicine and Physical Fitness, 35*, 1–8.

Tatemichi, T.K., Sacktor, N., and Mayeus, R. (1994). Dementia associated with cerebrovascular disease, other degenerative diseases, and metabolic disorders. In R.D. Terry, R. Katzman and K.L. Blick (Eds.), *Alzheimer's Disease* (pp. 167–178). New York: Raven Press.

Taylor, J. (1994). On exercise and sport avoidance: A reply to Dr. Albert Ellis. *The Sport Psychologist, 8*, 262–271.

Taylor, J. (1996). Intensity regulation and athletic performance. In J.L. Van Raalte and B.W. Brewer (Eds.), *Exploring sport and exercise psychology* (pp. 75–106). Washington, D.C.: American Psychological Association.

Taylor, J., & Taylor, S. (1997). *Psychological approaches to sports injury rehabilitation*. Gaithersburg, MD: Aspen Publishers.

Taylor, N., Hall, G.M., & Salmon, P. (1996). Is patient-controlled analgesia controlled by the patient? *Social Science and Medicine, 43*, 1137–1143.

Taylor, S., White, B., & Muncer, S. (1999). Nurses' cognitive structural models of work-based stress. *Journal of Advanced Nursing, 29*, 974–983.

Taylor, S.E. (1979). Hospital patient behavior: Reactance, helplessness, or control? *Journal of Social Issues, 35*, 156–184.

Taylor, S.M., Goldsmith, C.H., & Best, J.A. (1996). The community intervention trial for smoking cessation (COMMIT). *Health and Canadian Society, 2,* 179–195.

Taylor, S.M., Ross, N.A., Cummings, K.M., Glasgow, R.E., et al. (1998). Community intervention trial for smoking cessation (COMMIT): Changes in community attitudes toward cigarette smoking. *Health Education Research, 13*, 109–122.

Taylor, V.M., Anderson, G.M., McNeney, B., Diehr, P., Lavis, J.N., Deyo, R.A., Bombardier, K C. Malter, A., & Axcell, T. (1998). Hospitalizations for back and neck problems: a comparison between the Province of Ontario and Washington State. *Health Services Research, 33*, 929–945.

Tell, G.S., Polak, J.F., Ward, B.J., Kittner, S.J., et al., (1994). Relation of smoking with carotid artery wall thickness and stenosis in older adults.: The Cardiovascular Health Study. *Circulation, 90*, 2905–2908.

Teno, J.M., & Coppola, K.M. (1999). For every numerator, you need a denominator: A simple statement but key to measuring the quality of care of the "dying" *Journal of Pain and Symptom Management, 17*, 109–113.

Thackwray, D.E., Smith, M.C., Bodfish, J.W., & Meyers, A.W. (1993). A comparison of behavioral and cognitive-behavioral intervention for bulimia nervosa. *Journal of Consulting and Clinical Psychology, 61*, 639–645.

Theorell, T., Blomkvist, V., Jonsson, H., Schulman, S., Berntorp, E., & Stigendel, L. (1995). Social support and the development of immune function in human immunodeficiency virus infection. *Psychosomatic Medicine, 57*, 32–36.

Thomas, K.B. (1987). General practice consultations: Is there any point in being positive? *British Medical Journal, 294*, 1200–1202.

Thomas, P.D., Goodwin, J.M., & Goodwin, J.S. (1985). Effects of social support on stress-related changes in cholesterol level, urine acid level, and immune function in an elderly sample. *American Journal of Psychiatry, 142*, 735–737.

Thomas, R.E. (1997). Problem-based learning: measurable outcomes. *Medical Education, 31*, 320–329.

Thomas, W., White, C.M., Mah, J., Geisser, M.S., et al. (1995). Longitudinal compliance with annual screening for fecal occult blood. *American Journal of Epidemiology, 142*, 176–182.

Thomason, T.E., McCune, J.S., Bernard, S.A., Winer, E.P., Tremont, S., & Lindley C.M.

(1998). Cancer pain survey: Patient-centered issues in control. *Journal of Pain Symptom Management, 15*, 275–284.

Thompson, C.L., & Pledger, L.M. (1993). Doctor-patient communication: Is patient knowledge of medical terminology improving? *Health communication, 5*, 89–97

Thompson, D.S., & Shear, M.K. (1998). Psychiatric disorders and gynecological oncology: A review of the literature. *General Hospital Psychiatry, 20*, 241–247.

Thompson, J.K. (1986, April). Larger than life. *Psychology Today*, pp. 38–44.

Thompson, R.A., & Sherman, R.T. (1993). *Helping athletes with eating disorders*. Champaign, IL: Human Kinetics Publishers.

Thun, M.J., Day-Lally, C.A., Calle, E.E., Flanders, W.D., & Heath, C.W., Jr. (1995). Excess mortality among cigarette smokers: Changes in a 20-year interval. *American Journal of Public Health, 85*, 1223–1230.

Tierney, A.J., Taylor, J., Closs, S.J. (1992). Knowledge, expectations and experiences of patients receiving chemotherapy for breast cancer. *Scandinavian Journal of Caring Sciences, 6(2)*, 75–80.

Timko, C. (1987). Seeking medical care for a breast cancer symptom: Determinants of intentions to engage in prompt or delay behavior. *Health Psychology, 6*, 305–328.

Tims, F.M., Fletcher, B.W., & Hubbard, R.L. (1991). Treatment outcomes for drug abuse clients. In R.W. Pickens, C.G. Leukefeld, & C.R. Schuster (Eds.), *Improving drug abuse treatment*. Rockville, MD: National Institute on Drug Abuse.

Tinsley, J.A. (1998). Reverse gender bias—a caution to women faculty. *Academic Medicine, 73*, 1130–1131.

Tomasi, T.B., Jr. (1971). *The immune system of secretions*. Englewood Cliffs, NJ: Prentice-Hall.

Tomkins, S.S. (1966). Psychological model for smoking behavior. *American Journal of Public Health, 56 (Suppl. 12)*, 17–20.

Tomkins, S.S. (1968). A modified model of smoking behavior. In E.F. Borgatta & R.R. Evans (Eds.), *Smoking, health and behavior* (pp. 165–188). Chicago: Aldine.

Tomporowski, P.D., & Ellis, N.R. (1986). Effects of exercise on cognitive process: A review. *Psychological Bulletin, 99*, 338–346.

Toynbee, P. (1977). *Patients*. New York: Harcourt Brace.

Triandis, H.C., Bontempo, R., Villareal, M.J., Asai, M., & Lucca, N. (1998). Individualism and collectivism: Cross-cultural perspectives on self-ingroup relationships. *Journal of Personality and Social Psychology, 54*, 323–338.

Trotter, R.T., II. (1991). Ethnographic research methods for applied medical anthropology. In Hill, C.E. (Ed.), *Training manual in applied medical anthropology* (pp. 180–212). Washington, D.C.: American Anthropological Association.

Tsoh, J.Y., McClure, J.B., Skaar, K.L., Wetter, D.W., et al. (1997). Smoking cessation 2: Components of effective intervention. *Behavioral Medicine, 23*, 15–27.

Tuokko, H., Tallman, K., Beattie, B.L., Cooper, P., & Weir, J. An examination of driving records in a dementia clinic. *Journal of Gerontology, 50*, S173-S181.

Turk, D.C. (1997). The role of demographic and psychosocial factos in transition from acute to chronic pain. In T.S. Jensen, J.A. Turner, & Z. Wiesenfeld-Hallin (Eds.), *Proceedings of the 8th World Congress on Pain: Progress in pain research and management* (pp. 185–213). Seattle: International Association for the Study of Pain Press.

Turk, D.C., & Meichenbaum, D. (1991). Adherence to self-care regimens: the patient's perspective. In R.H. Rozensky, J.J. Sweet, & S.M. Tovian (Eds.), *Handbook of clinical psychology.I. Medical settings* (pp. 249–266). New York: Plenum.

Turk, D.C., & Okifuji, A. (1996). Perception of traumatic onset, compensation status, and physical findings: Impact on pain severity, emotional distress, and disability in chronic pain patients. *Journal of Behavioral Medicine, 19*, 435–454.

Turk, D.C., & Stacey, B.R. (in press). Multidisciplinary pain centers in the treatment of chronic back pain. In J.W. Frymoyer, T.B. Ducker, N.M. Hadler, J.P., Kostuik, J.N. Weinstein, & T.S. Whitcloud (Eds.), *The adult spine: Principles and practice (2nd ed.)*. New York: Raven Press.

Turk, D.C., Kerns, R.D., & Rosenberg, R. (1992). Effects of marital interaction on chronic pain and disability: Examining the downside of social support. *Rehabilitation Psychology, 37*, 259–274.

Turk, D.C., Litt, M.D., Salovey, P., & Walker, J. (1985). Seeking urgent pediatric treatment: Factors contributing to frequency, delay, and appropriateness. *Health Psychology, 4*, 43–59.

Turk, D.C., Meichenbaum, D., & Genest, M.

(1983). *Pain and behavioral medicine: A cognitive-behavioral perspective*. New York: Guilford Press

Turk, D.C., Wack, J.T., & Kerns, R.D. (1985). An empirical examination of the "pain-behavior" construct. *Journal of Behavioral Medicine, 8*, 119–130.

Turk, D.C., Zacki, H.S., & Rudy, T.E. (1993). Effects of intraoral appliance and biofeedback/stress management alone and in combination in treating pain and depression in TMD patients. *Journal of Prosthetic Dentistry, 70*, 158–164.

Turk, M. (1993). High anxiety. *The New Physician*, September, pp. 16–22.

Turncock, C. (1991). Communicating with patients in the ICU. *Nursing Standard, 5(15)*, 38–40.

Turner Cobb, J.M., & Steptoe, A. (1996). Psychosocial stress and susceptibility to upper respiratory tract illness in an adult population sample. *Psychosomatic Medicine, 58*, 404–412.

Turner Cobb, J.M., & Steptoe, A. (1998). Psychosocial influences on upper respiratory infectious illness in children. *Journal of Psychosomatic Research, 45*, 319–330.

Turner, L., Linden, W., van der Wal, R., & Schamberger, W. (1995). Stress management for patients with heart disease: A pilot study. *Heart and Lung, 24,* 145–153.

Twycross, R.G. & McQuay, H.J. (1989). Opioids. In P.D. Wall & R. Melzack (Eds.), *Textbook of pain (2nd ed.)*. Edinburgh: Churchill Livingstone.

Tyc, V.L., Fairclough, D., Fletcher, B., Leigh, L., et al. (1995). Children's distress during magnetic resonance imaging procedures. *Children's Health Care, 24*, 5–19.

U.S. Department of Health and Human Services (USDHHS). (1998). Preliminary results from the 1997 National Household Survey on Drug Abuse (DHHS Publication No. SMA 98–3251). Washington, DC: U.S. Government Printing Office.

Uchino, B.N., Cacioppo, J.T., & Kiecolt-Glaser, J.K. (1996). The relationship between social support and physiological processes: A review with emphasis on underlying mechanisms and implications for health. *Psychological Bulletin, 119*, 448–531.

Unruh, A.M. (1996). Gender variations in clinical pain experience. *Pain, 65*, 123–167.

Unruh, A.M., Ritchie, J., & Merskey, H. (1999). Does gender affect appraisal of pain and pain coping strategies? *Clinical Journal of Pain, 15(1)*, 31–40.

Vaillant, G.E., Sobowale, N.C., & McArthur, C. (1972). Some psychologic vulnerabilities of physicians. *New England Journal of Medicine, 287*, 372–375.

Vallerand, A.H. (1995). Gender differences in pain. *Image J Nurs Sch , 27(3)*, 235–237.

Van Elderen, T., Maes, S., Rouneau, C., & Seegers, G. (1998). Perceived gender differences in physician consulting behaviour during internal examination. *Family Practice, 15*, 147–152.

Van Wel, F., & Knobbout, J. (1998). Adolescents and fear appeals. *International Journal of Adolescence and Youth, 7*, 121–135.

VanIneveld, C.H., Cook, D.J., Kane, S.L., & King, D. (1996). Discrimination and abuse in internal medicine residency. *The Internal Medicine Program Directors of Canada. Journal of General Internal Medicine, 11*, 401–405.

Varni, J.W., & Thompson, K.L. (1986). Biobehavioral assessment and management of pediatric pain. In N.A. Krasnegor, J.D. Arasteh, & M.F. Cataldo (Eds.), *Child health behavior: A behavioral pediatrics perspective*. New York: Wiley.

Varni, J.W., Thompson, K.L., & Hanson, V. (1987). The Varni/Thompson Pediatric Pain Questionnaire I: Chronic musculoskeletal pain in juvenile rheumatic arthritis. *Pain, 28*, 27–38.

Vealey, R. (1988). Future directions in psychological skills training. *The Sports Psychologist, 2*, 318–336.

Verbrugge, L.M. (1985). Triggers of symptoms and health care. *Social Science and Medicine, 20*, 855–876.

Verdes, D.M.M. (1999). First Nations gender differences in the frequency of health care use: A health belief model perspective. Unpublished Master's Thesis, The University of Northern British Columbia.

Verhoef, M.J., Hagen, N., Pelletier, G., & Forsyth, P. (1999). Alternative therapy use in neurologic diseases: Use in brain tumor patients. *Neurology, 52*, 617–622.

Viemeroe, V., & Krause, C. (1998). Quality of life in individuals with physical disabilities. *Psychotherapy and Psychosomatics, 67*, 317–322.

Villareal, M.C., Brown, C.M., & Lawson, K.A. (1998). Differences in morphine consumption administered by PCA and traditional IV methods in a pediatric population. *Journal of Pharmaceutical Care in Pain and Symptom Control, 6*, 75–94.

Vincent, C. Young, M., & Phillips, A. (1994). Why do people sue doctors? A study of patients and relatives taking legal action. *Lancet, 343*, 1609–1613.

Vincent, M.O. (1983). Some sequelae of stress in physicians. *Psychiatric Journal of the University of Ottawa, 8(3)*, 120–124.

von Baeyer, C.L., Baskerville, S., & McGrath, P.J. (1998). Everyday pain in three- to five-year-old children in day care. *Pain Research and Management, 3(2)*, 111–116.

von Baeyer, C.L., Johnson, M.E., & McMillan, M.J. (1984). Consequences of nonverbal expression of pain: Patient distress and observer concern. *Social Science and Medicine, 19*, 1319–1324.

Von Koch, L., Wottrich, A. W., & Holmqvist, L.W. (1998). Rehabilitation in the home versus the hospital: The importance of context. *Disability and Rehabilitation: An International Multidisciplinary Journal, 20*, 367–372.

Vuckovic, N. (1999). Fast relief: Buying time with medications. *Medical Anthropology Quarterly, 13*, 51–68.

Waite, B.T., Gansneder, B., & Rotella, R.J. (1990). A sport-specific measure of self-acceptance. *Journal of Sport and Exercise Psychology, 12*, 264–279.

Waitzkin, H. (1984). Doctor-patient communication: Clinical implications of social scientific research. *Journal of the American Medical Association, 252*, 2441–2446.

Waitzkin, H. (1985). Information giving in medical care. *Journal of Health and Social Behavior, 26*, 81–101.

Walerstein, S.J., & Rosner, F. (1989). House staff stress. *New York State Journal of Medicine, 89*, 454–457.

Wall, P.D. (1984). Introduction. In P.D. Wall & R. Melzack (Eds.), *Textbook of pain* (2nd ed., pp. 1–16). Edinburgh: Churchill Livingstone.

Walsh, J.D., Blanchard, E.B., Kremer, J.M., & Blancard, C.G. (1999). The psychosocial effects of rheumatoid arthritis on the patient and the well partner. *Behaviour Research and Therapy, 37*, 259–271.

Walsh, N.E., & Dimitru, D. (1988). The influence of compensation on recovery from low back pain. *Occupational Medicine: State of the Art Reviews, 3*, 109–120.

Walston, K.A., Wallston, B.S., & DeVellis, R. (1978). Development of the Multidimensional Health Locus of Control (MHLC) scale. *Health Education Monographs, 6*, 161–170.

Walters, E.E., & Kendler, K.S. (1995). Anorexia nervosa and anorexic-like syndromes in a population-based female twin sample. *American Journal of Psychiatry, 152*, 64–71.

Wannamethee, G., Sharper, A.G., & MacFarlane, P.W. (1993). Heart rate, physical activity, and mortality rate from cancer and other noncardiovascular diseases. *American Journal of Epidemiology, 137*, 735–748.

Ward, K.G. (1999). A TEAM approach to NICU care. *RN, 62(2)*, 47–49.

Wardle, J., & Pope, R. (1992). The psychological costs of screening for cancer. *Journal of Psychosomatic Research, 36*, 609–624.

Warrick, P.D., Irish, J.C., Morningstar, M., Gilbert, R., Brown, D., & Gullane, P. (1999). Use of alternative medicine among patients with head and neck cancer. *Archives of Otolaryngolical Head and Neck Surgery, 125*, 573–579.

Watkins, L.L., & Grossman, P. (1999). Association of depressive symptoms with reduced baroreflex cardiac control in coronary artery disease. *American Heart Journal, 137*, 453–457.

Watson, J. (1988). New dimensions in human caring theory. *Nursing Science Quarterly, 4*, 175–181.

Waxler-Morrison, N., Hislop, T.G., Mears, B., & Kan, L. (1991). Effects of social relationships on survival for women with breast cancer: A prospective study. *Social Science and Medicine, 33*, 177–183.

Weinberg, R.S. (1996). Goal setting in sport and exercise: Research to practice. In J.L. Van Raalte and B.W. Brewer (Eds.), *Exploring sport and exercise psychology* (pp. 3–24). Washington, D.C.: American Psychological Association.

Weintraub, M. (1976). Intelligent noncompliance and capricious compliance. In L. Lasagna (Ed.), *Patient compliance*. Mt. Kisco, NY: Futura.

Weiss, M.R., Wiese, D.M., & Klint, K.A. (1989). Head over heels with success: The relationship between self-efficacy and performance in competitive youth gymnastics. *Journal of Sport and Exercise Psychology, 11*, 444–451.

Weiss, S.R., McFarland, B.H., Burkhart, G.A., & Ho, P.T. (1998). Cancer recurrences and secondary primary cancers after use of antihistamines or antidepressants. *Clinical Pharmacology Therapy, 63*, 594–599.

Weisse, C.S., Sanders, K., Syat, B.I., & Sorum, P.C. (1999, October). When treating pain, male and female doctors are impacted differently by patient gender and race. Poster session presented at the annual meeting of the American Pain Society, Fort Lauderdale, FL.

Weller, A., & Hener, T. (1993). Invasiveness of medical procedures and state anxiety in women. *Behavioral Medicine, 19*, 60–65.

Weller, S.C. (1983). New data on intracultural variability: The hot-cold concept of medicine and illness. *Human Organization, 42*, 341–351.

Wells, D. (1997). A critical ethnography of the process of discharge decision-making for elderly patients. *Canadian Journal on Aging, 16*, 682–699.

Wenger, M., Bagchi, B., & Anand, B. (1961). Experiments in India on "voluntary" control of the heart and pulse. *Circulation, 24*, 1319–1325.

West C. (1993). Reconceptualizing gender in physician-patient relationships. *Social Science and Medicine, 36*, 57–66.

Whelan, T.A., & Kirby, R.J. (1998). Advantages for children and their families of psychological preparation for hospitalisation and surgery. *Journal of Family Studies, 4*, 35–51.

While, A.E., & Wilcox, V.K. (1994). Paediatric day surgery: day-case unit admission compared with general paediatric ward admission. *Journal of Advances in Nursing, 19*, 52–57.

White, S.A., & Duda, J.L. (1991, October). The interdependence between goal perspectives, psychological skill, and cognitive interference among elite skiers. Paper presented at the annual meeting of the Association for the Advancement of Applied Sport Psychology, Savannah, Georgia.

Whitehead, W.E., Busch, C.M., Heller, B.R., & Costa, P.T. (1986). Social learning influences on menstrual symptoms and illness behavior. *Health Psychology, 5*, 13–23.

Whitemore, A.S., Perlin, S.A., & DiCiccio, Y. (1995). Chronic obstructive pulmonary disease in lifetime nonsmokers: Results from NHANES. *American Journal of Public Health, 85*, 702–706.

Wickersham, B.A. (1984). The exercise program. In G.K. Riggs & E.P. Gall (Eds.), *Rheumatic diseases: Rehabilitation and management*. Boston: Butterworth.

Wiegmann, S.M., & Berven, N.L. (1998). Health locus-of-control beliefs and improvement in physical functioning in a work-hardening, return-to-work program. *Rehabilitation Psychology, 43*, 83–100.

Wilcox, S., & Storandt, M. (1996). Relations among age, exercise, and psychological variables in a community sample of women. *Health Psychology, 15*, 110–113.

Wilkins, K. (1995). Causes of death: How the sexes differ. *Health Reports, 7(2)*, 33–43.

Wilkins, K., & Beaudet, M.P. (1998). Work stress and health. *Health Reports, 10(3)*, 47–62.

Wilkins, K., & Park, E. (1997). Characteristics of hospital users. *Health Reports, 9(3)*, 27–36.

Wilkins, R. (1993). The use of postal codes and addresses in the analysis of health data. *Health Reports, 5(2)*, 157–177.

Williams, J.M., & Leffingwell, T.R. (1996). Cognitive strategies in sport and exercise psychology. In J.L. Van Raalte and B.W. Brewer (Eds.), *Exploring sport and exercise psychology* (pp. 51–74). Washington, D.C.: American Psychological Association.

Williams, P.A., Dominick-Pierre, K., Vayda, E., Stevenson, M., & Burke, M. (1990). Women in medicine: Practice patterns and attitudes. *Canadian Medical Association Journal, 143*, 194–201.

Williams, S., Weinman, J., Dale, J., & Newman, S. (1995). Patient expectations: What do primary care patients want from the GP and how far does meeting expectations affect patient satisfaction? *Family Practice, 12(2)*, 193–201.

Wilson, J.T. (1973). Compliance with instruction in the evaluation of therapeutic efficacy. *Clinical Pediatrics, 12*, 333.

Wing, P.C. (1997). Patient or client? If in doubt, ask. *Canadian Medical Association Journal, 157(3)*, 287–289.

Winters, R. (1985). Behavioral approaches to pain. In N. Schneiderman & J.T. Tapp (Eds.), *Behavioral medicine: The biopsychosocial approach.* Hillsdale, NJ: Erlbaum.

Wise, E.A., Papas, R.K., Campbell, L.C., Riley, J.L. III, & Robinson, M.E. (1999, October). A quantitative review of cultural differences in experimental pain. Poster session presented at the annual meeting of the American Pain Society, Fort Lauderdale, FL.

Witte, K. (1992). Putting fear back into fear appeals: The extended parallel process model. *Communication Monographs, 59*, 329–349.

Witte, K. (1994). Fear control and danger control: A test of the extended parallel process model (EPPM). *Communication Monographs, 61*, 113–134.

Wolf, S. (1997). Visceral responses to the social environment. *Acta Physiologica Scandinavica, 640*, 140–143.

Wolf, S.L., Nacht, M., & Kelly, J.L. (1982). EMG feedback training during dynamic movement for low back pain patients. *Behavior Therapy, 13*, 395–406.

Wolf, Z.R. (1993). Nursing rituals: doing ethnography. *NLN Publications,* August, 269–310.

Wolpe, J. (1958). *Psychotherapy by reciprocal inhibition*. Stanford, California: Stanford University Press.

Wonderlich, S.A., Brewerton, T.D., Jocic, Z., Dansky, B.S., & Abbott, D.W. (1997). Relationships of childhood sexual abuse and eating disorders. J*ournal of the American Academy of Child and Adolescent Psychiatry, 36*, 11.

Wong, H.C. (1999). Educating medical students about alternative therapies. *Canadian Medical Association Journal, 161*, 128–129.

Woods, J.H. (1966). T*he yoga-system of Patanjali*. Delhi, India: Motilal Banarsidass.

Woodward, N.J., & Wallston, B.S. (1987). Age and health care beliefs: Self-efficacy as a mediator of low desire for control. *Psychology and Aging, 2*, 3–8.

World Health Organization. (1986). Ottawa Charter for Health Promotion, Ottawa, Canada. Canadian Public Health Association.

World Health Organization. (1998). *Malaria, Fact Sheet No. 94.*

Wright, L. (1988). The Type A behavior pattern and coronary heart disease. *American Psychologist, 43*, 2–14.

Yalom, I.D., & Vinogradov, S. (1988). Bereavement groups: Techniques and themes. *International Journal of Group Psychotherapy, 38*, 419–446.

Yogananda, P. (1969). *Autobiography of a yogi*. Bombay, India: Jaico Publishing House.

Young, J.C. (1981). *Medical choice in a Mexican village*. New Brunswick. NJ: Rutgers University Press.

Zador, P.L., & Ciccone, M.A. (1993). Automobile driver fatalities in frontal impacts: Air bags compared with manual belts. *American Journal of Public Health, 83,* 661–666.

Zajonc, R.B. (1968). Attitudinal effects of mere exposure. *Journal of Personality and Social Psychology Monograph Supplements, 9,* 1–27.

Zalewski, C., Keller, B., Bowers, C., Miske, P. et al. (1994). Depressive symptomatology and post-stroke rehabilitation outcome. *Clinical Gerontologist, 14*, 62–67.

Zanna, M., Cameron, R., Goldsmith, C.H., Poland, B., et al. (1996). Critique of the COMMIT study based on the Brantford experience. *Health and Canadian Society, 2,* 319–336.

Zatzick, d.F., & Dimsdale, J.E. (1990). Cultural variations in response to painful stimuli. *Psychosomatic Medicine, 52*, 544–557.

Zborowski, M. (1958). Cultural components in response to pain. *Journal of Social Issues, 8,* 16–30.

Zifferblatt, S.M. (1975). Increasing patient compliance through applied analysis of behavior. *Preventive Medicine, 4*, 173–182.

Zimbardo, P.G. (1970). The human choice: Individuation, reason, and order versus deindividuation, impulse, and chaos. In W.J. Arnold & D. Levine (Eds.), *Nebraska symposium on motivation, 1969*. Lincoln, NE: University of Nebraska Press.

Zucker, T.P., Flesche, C.W., Germing, U., Schroeter, S., Willers, R., Wolf, H.H., & Hevil, A. (1998). Patient-controlled versus staff-controlled analgesia with pethidine after allogeneic bone marrow transplantation. *Pain, 75*, 305–312.

Zussman, R. (1993). Life in the hospital: A review. *Milbank Quarterly, 71*, 167–185.

Zyzanski, S.J., Strange, K.C., Langa, D., & Flocke, S.A. (1998). Trade-offs in high-volume primary care practice. *Journal of Family Practice, 46*, 397–402.

Index

N

O

P

Q

R

S